Anspaugh Chapter Objectives and Outcomes

https://wps.pearsoned.com/bc_anspaugh_health_10/216/55399/14182252.cw/index.html

Chapter 1: The Need for Health Education

Valued Outcomes:

- Define health, health education, and health promotion.
- List and describe the components that make up wellness.
- Identify why health education is a necessary component in the nation's schools.
- Discuss the significance of the Youth Risk Behavior Surveillance System.
- Identify the components of a comprehensive school education.
- Discuss the components of a coordinated school health education program.
- Discuss the implications of the School Health Policies and Program Study (SHPPS).

1. Provide a detailed explanation about the relevance and need for health education in school curricula today. Include several reasons why health education is important to school children and how the Youth Risk Behavior Surveillance System can assist in the development of a Coordinated School Health Program

Chapter 2: The Role of the Teacher in Coordinated School Health Programs

Valued Outcomes:

- Discuss the academic and personal qualifications of an effective health educator.
- Describe how a teacher of health has an opportunity to be a significant model in students' lives.
- Explain the unique challenges health educators face.
- Explain the barriers that make health instruction more difficult to teach than other subjects.
- Discuss the minimum competencies needed by a health educator.
- Describe the legal liability associated with teaching.
- Discuss how the educator can work with other members of the school staff to enhance the wellness of each student.

Discuss at least three barriers to effective health teaching and offer at least one solution for overcoming the barriers.

Chapter 3: Planning for Health Instruction

Valued Outcomes:

- Identify the potential content areas of health education.
- Describe scope and sequence of health education.
- Discuss the HECAT assessment tool.
- Identify the National Health Education Standards.
- Discuss why the National Health Education Standards are important.
- Describe various curriculum approaches to teaching health education.
- Develop an effective lesson plan.
- Write effective performance objectives.

Describe the components of a well-developed health curriculum and list several ways the Michigan Model includes these components.

Chapter 4: Strategies for Implementing Health Instruction

Valued Outcomes:

- List the factors that affect selection of teaching strategies.
- Discuss the elements of an effective decision-making model.
- Describe reasons why teaching refusal skills is important.
- Discuss styles of learning.
- Select learning strategies that appeal to the various styles of learning.
- Describe how to effectively use various strategies for teaching.
- Discuss ways to use technology in the classroom.

Explain how you would select learning strategies for a diverse class of 35 fifth graders for the topic of alcohol and drugs. List at least three factors which would determine your selections. Provide detailed examples of strategies.

Chapter 5: Measurement and Evaluation of Health Education

Valued Outcomes:

- Explain the difference between measurement and evaluation.
- List the skills needed to be competent in measuring and evaluating student progress.
- Discuss the steps necessary for developing a teacher-designed test.
- Describe how to write effective test items.
- Identify alternative methods of assessing student progress.
- Explain various grading strategies.
- Discuss the use of rubrics in grading.
- Discuss the use of benchmarks, standards, and performance indicators in assessment of learning.
- Explain how to assess students from a variety of cultures.
- Discuss how to assess students with different learning styles.

Discuss the benefits of effective evaluation in health education. List at least three benefits in your discussion.

Chapter 6: Mental Health and Stress Reduction

Valued Outcomes:

- Define mental health.
- Identify the characteristics of emotionally healthy students.
- Describe how psychosocial factors contribute to mental health.
- Describe the importance of self-esteem in fostering mental health.
- Discuss strategies for enhancing self-esteem of students.
- Discuss the characteristics of students with learning disabilities.
- Discuss the indicators of psychiatric problems in students.
- Identify the potential problems associated with latchkey children or children from separated/divorced families.
- Identify the means of dealing with students who have experienced the death of a pet, friend, grandparent, parent, or sibling.
- Define the terms stress and stressor.
- List the detrimental health effects of prolonged stress.

- Identify strategies for dealing with stress.
- Discuss the role of the family in maintaining and influencing the emotional health of students.
- Discuss the effects of bullying on students.

What can you do, as a teacher, to identify and address mental health problems in your classroom? Discuss the benefits of effective evaluation in health education. List at least three benefits in your discussion.

Chapter 7: Strategies for Teaching Mental Health and Stress Reduction

Valued Outcomes:

- Realize every person is unique and special with many good qualities.
- Understand that all people share basic human needs for physical safety, love, security, emotional support, and acceptance from others.
- Discuss how personality development is affected by one's self-concept and acceptance from others.
- Develop strategies that illustrate the expression of emotions in mentally and emotionally healthy ways.
- Discuss why open and honest communication is an essential part of good mental health.
- Develop and utilize strategies to identify stressors and effectively deal with stressful situations.
- Help students learn personal responsibility in their conduct and interactions with others.

Chapter 8: Body Systems

Valued Outcomes:

- Describe the function and structure of skin, hair, and nails.
- Explain the different roles of the brain.
- Discuss the function of selected components (structures) of the nervous system.
- Describe the functions of selected glands and hormones associated with the endocrine system.
- Discuss the role of each component of the respiratory system in the breathing process.
- Trace a drop of blood through the circulatory and pulmonary systems.
- Describe the major function of red blood cells.
- Explain the function of white blood corpuscles in fighting off infection.
- Describe how food travels through the body.
- Describe the function of the skeletal system.
- Describe how liquid and solid wastes are filtered in the body.
- Differentiate between voluntary and involuntary muscles.

Relate the three criteria for indelible learning to the anatomy of the brain.

Chapter 9: Personal Health

Valued Outcomes:

- Discuss the proper care of the skin, nails, and hair.
- Define *posture*, and explain its importance to personal health.
- Describe the function of the five major senses, and discuss their possible impairments and care.
- List the behavioral indications of vision and hearing problems.
- Describe how to maintain good dental health.

- Define *fitness*, and name its five components.
- Discuss the importance and appropriate amounts of physical activity, relaxation, and sleep for children.
- Discuss the *Healthy People 2020* objectives that are related to fitness and physical activity.

Discuss three aspects of personal appearance that are considered important for the health of elementary school children.

Chapter 10: Strategies for Teaching Body Systems and Personal Health

Valued Outcomes: Body Systems

- Daily care and maintenance of the human body and an understanding of how its systems operate serve as the foundation for personal health and well-being.
- The integumentary system is the first line of defense for the body and functions to help maintain body temperature.
- The nervous system receives, interprets, and sends messages that help direct and guide all other body systems.
- The endocrine system helps maintain balance among all body systems through the secretion of hormones.
- The reproductive system is activated in puberty and creates and perpetuates human life.
- The respiratory system provides the pathway and mechanics for oxygen to enter the body, and the carbon dioxide to leave it.
- The circulatory system, through the heart's pumping of blood, delivers oxygen and other essential chemicals to the body.
- The digestive and excretory systems break down food so that it can be used for all body processes. Substances that cannot be used are eliminated from the body as waste products.
- The skeletal/muscular system provides the body and its parts with shape, support, protection, and movement.

Valued Outcomes: Personal Health

- Adequate dental care and regular visits to health care professionals are important in maintaining personal health.
- Consistent, routinely scheduled, prescribed exercise programs promote personal health and well-being.
- Relaxation and sleep allow bodily processes and functions to renew their energy sources.

Chapter 11: Sexuality Education

Valued Outcomes:

- Identify the goals of a sexuality education program.
- Discuss the social aspects of sexuality and family living.
- Discuss marriage, parenthood, and divorce.
- Trace the psychological development of sexuality.
- Describe the anatomy and physiology of the male and female reproductive systems.
- Explain the problems of family abuse and violence.

List the four goals that should be included in a school-based sexuality education program. Name three topics that should be included under each goal.

Chapter 12: Strategies for Teaching Sexuality Education

Valued Outcomes:

After completing this chapter, you should be able to:

- Provide learning opportunities for a variety of topics related to sexuality education.
- Discuss the different types of families.
- Help students identify why each member of a family is important and what roles each member has.
- Present the interpersonal skills necessary for strengthening individual and family relationships.
- Help students identify why a positive self-image is necessary.
- Help students identify why the understanding of self is a foundation for successful transition to adulthood.
- Discuss children's rights; no one should be mistreated, taken advantage of, or abused by another person.
- Discuss the physical, social, and emotional growth of the male/female.
- Discuss procreation.
- Discuss menstruation and the process that healthy females experience.
- Help students develop wholesome attitudes toward sexuality.
- Help students understand how sexual values and decisions are often individual decisions.

Chapter 13: Substance Use and Abuse

Valued Outcomes:

After completing this chapter, you should be able to:

- Define *substance use*, *misuse*, and *abuse*.
- Identify reasons that people abuse substances.
- Describe the various effects of different drugs on the body.
- Describe how tobacco advertising influences youth to use tobacco products.
- List recommendations for schools to reduce alcohol, tobacco, and other drug abuse problems among their students.
- Give examples of the signs and symptoms of substance use and abuse.
- Describe the most effective drug abuse education and prevention programs.

Young people misuse or abuse drugs for a variety of reasons. Identify five reasons for substance abuse among young people as stated in your text. Support each reason with a clear and specific explanation relevant to young people and their experiences.

Chapter 14: Strategies for Teaching about Substance Use and Abuse

Valued Outcomes:

After completing this chapter, you should be able to convey the following to your students:

- Dealing effectively with personal problems is important in preventing substance abuse.
- Poor self-image increases the potential for substance abuse.
- Drugs should be taken only when a doctor prescribes them and only in the amount prescribed.
- People use and abuse drugs for physical, emotional, and social reasons.

- Certain drugs can be legally purchased only with a doctor's prescription.
- Some drugs, called over-the-counter drugs, can be purchased without a doctor's prescription.
- Smoking is dangerous to health.
- Tobacco smoke can be harmful to those who do not smoke, as well as to smokers themselves.
- Alcohol is a drug.
- Misuse of alcohol can cause physical, emotional, and social problems.
- Alcoholism is a disease.
- Alcoholism can lead to many health problems.
- Barbiturates can cause both physical and psychological dependency.
- Cocaine and crack are very dangerous drugs and should not be used under any circumstances.
- Amphetamines, like barbiturates, can be dangerous if abused.
- Illegal drugs, including narcotics and hallucinogens, can have unpredictable and serious health consequences.

Chapter 15: Infectious and Noninfectious Conditions

Valued Outcomes:

After completion of this chapter, you should be able to:

- Describe the disease agents for infectious and noninfectious conditions.
- Describe the typical stages through which a disease progresses.
- Describe how the body is protected from disease.
- Discuss the major childhood communicable diseases.
- Discuss the human immunodeficiency virus.
- Discuss cardiovascular disease and several types of cancer.
- Identify the risk factors associated with the major noninfectious diseases.
- Discuss the recent trends in the diagnosis and treatment of diseases.

List the six body defenses and provide at least two means by which each defense protects against disease causing agents.

Chapter 16: Strategies for Teaching Infectious and Noninfectious Conditions

Valued Outcomes:

After completing this chapter, you should be able to convey the following to your students:

- Discuss the diseases that are the leading causes of deaths.
- Explain how pathogens cause disease.
- Describe how the immune system protects against disease.
- Identify how the heart works.
- Discuss how noninfectious diseases often develop over time and are affected by lifestyle.

Chapter 17: Nutrition

Valued Outcomes:

After completing this chapter, you should be able to:

- Discuss the *Healthy People 2010* objectives for nutrition.

- Describe children's eating patterns.
- Explain the economic, personal, and lifestyle factors that determine our food choices.
- Discuss the *Dietary Guidelines for Americans, 2010*.
- Discuss categories of nutrients.
- Understand and use the Nutrition Facts panel.
- Discuss vitamins and minerals.
- Compare food selections from fast food restaurants.
- Discuss USDA's MyPlate and ChooseMyPlate.gov.
- Describe nutritional problems, such as undernutrition, anorexia nervosa, and bulimia.
- Explain the factors that have led to an increase in childhood obesity.
- Read and understand a food label.
- Discuss food quackery.

Identify specific antioxidants, and explain how antioxidants reduce the risk of chronic disease.

Chapter 18: Strategies for Teaching Nutrition

Valued Outcomes:

After completing this chapter, you should be able to convey the following to your students:

- There is a close relationship between dietary practices and overall health.
- Food serves several functions in meeting body needs.
- Food fads and fallacies can affect an individual's food behavior.
- There are healthy and unhealthy ways of losing weight.
- The essential nutrients in food are carbohydrates, lipids, proteins, water, minerals, and vitamins.
- Eating a variety of carefully selected foods is the best way to ensure that the body receives the proper amounts of the nutrients it needs.
- MyPlate, with ChooseMyPlate.gov, can serve as an aid in planning balanced meals.
- The lack of certain nutrients can lead to certain diseases.
- Being underweight or overweight can lead to physical and emotional problems.
- Maintaining a proper weight is an individual responsibility, but others can help if there is a weight problem.
- A person who does not have a weight problem can be malnourished.
- Many people in the world do not have enough to eat.
- Food labels can provide useful nutritional information.

Chapter 19: Injuries: Accident and Violence Prevention

Valued Outcomes:

- Discuss the difference between intentional and unintentional injuries.
- Discuss the major human and environmental causes of accidents.
- Describe the characteristics of an accident-prone person.
- Discuss young people's attitudes toward violence.
- List the ways for a child to protect himself or herself against violence.
- List the ways for a child to protect himself or herself against adult and stranger abuse.
- Describe why risk taking is a necessary evil.
- Discuss the major parts of a school safety program.
- Contrast a positive approach to safety education with a negative approach.
- Discuss the growing violence problem in U.S. society.

It has been shown that certain people are more prone to accidents than others are. Identify and discuss eight characteristics of the "accident prone" individual and suggest an intervention to reduce his or her risk.

Chapter 20: Strategies for Teaching Injuries: Accident and Violence Prevention

Valued Outcomes:

- Each person is to a large degree responsible for his or her own personal safety.
- Peers exert a tremendous influence over safety practices.
- Obedience to safety rules enhances the quality of life.
- Risk taking is a part of living, but unnecessary risk taking greatly increases the risk of harm to oneself and to others.
- The degree of risk in any particular activity can often be determined by analytical thinking.
- Rules and procedures for safe behavior help prevent accidents in the home, school, and community.
- Hazardous conditions should be corrected whenever possible.
- There are many people and community agencies that can help when accidents occur.
- Elementary school children have more fatal accidents than any other age group.
- More than half of all accidents involving children happen at school.
- Playground rules are important for safe activities.
- Elementary students need to practice safe behavior in traffic.
- Home and school fire escape routes should be practiced frequently.
- Acting without thinking often results in an accident.
- Basic first-aid skills are important for everyone.
- Improper first aid can do more harm than good.
- Safety is not just a matter of luck. Safe behavior must be learned.

Chapter 21: Consumer Health

Valued Outcomes:

- Analyze the role of advertising in consumer purchases.
- List various advertising approaches.
- Discuss how quackery affects health care.
- State criteria for selecting a health care professional.
- State criteria for selecting a health care facility.
- List the rights of the consumer.
- Discuss private and governmental agencies that help protect the consumer.

Many people use the Internet to obtain health information, products, and services. Explain why consumers need to be cautious when using the Internet for these purposes, and discuss how one can determine whether web-based health information is credible and trustworthy.

Chapter 22: Strategies for Teaching Consumer Health

Valued Outcomes:

- Discuss why it is important to obtain accurate information concerning health care information.
- Describe why not all products and services are worthwhile or necessary.

- List ways that advertising seeks to persuade or induce use of a product.
- Describe why many advertising claims are inflated or misleading.
- Discuss why all labels on health care products should be read carefully.
- List ways in which quackery in health care products can be identified.
- Understand that many health care products are not useful and are even dangerous.
- Discuss why medical treatment should be obtained only from qualified professionals.
- List the governmental and private agencies that work to protect the consumer.
- Realize that making wise consumer decisions concerning health care products and services is a personal responsibility.

Chapter 23: Aging, Dying, and Death

Valued Outcomes:

- Discuss aging as a normal part of the life cycle.
- Describe how ageism affects the elderly in our society.
- Describe the current demographic aspects of the elderly in the United States.
- Explain the factors that can help delay or retard the physiological changes that occur in aging.
- List the reasons why elderly people have problems with nutrition.
- Describe Alzheimer's disease.
- Suggest intergenerational contact programs for school-age students and the elderly.
- Discuss the factors that will lead to better quality lives for the elderly in the future.
- Discuss the fears of a dying person.
- Describe the relationship of personal beliefs in facing dying and death.
- List ways in which family members cope with and help in times of a relative's death.
- Describe healthy ways to grieve.
- Discuss the purposes of funerals, hospice care, and living wills.
- Describe the warning signs for suicide in children.
- Describe effective methods of teaching death education.

Why is death education an important topic to teach in school? Include at least three reasons. Describe how educators might effectively approach the topic of death in their classroom.

Chapter 24: Strategies for Teaching about Aging, Dying, and Death

Valued Outcomes: Aging

- Aging is a natural part of the life cycle.
- Exercise and proper diet can slow down the aging process to some degree.
- Most elderly people are healthy and alert.
- People use their retirement years for different activities from those done in preretirement times.
- Elderly people make positive contributions to society.
- Nutritional needs change as one ages.
- The elderly in the United States are often discriminated against.
- Many social agencies provide services for the elderly.

Valued Outcomes: Dying and Death

- Death is a natural end to the life cycle.
- Our society generally avoids the topics of death and dying in discussion and conscious thought.
- Dying people and the family of a dying person have special needs.
- Grief and bereavement naturally follow the death of a close friend or relative.

- Funeral and burial rituals have significant meaning in our society.
- There are ways to help a friend who is contemplating suicide to reconsider the action.
- Organ donation can be considered an "ultimate gift of life."

Chapter 25: Environmental Health

Valued Outcomes:

- Discuss the responsibility of people in caring for the environment.
- Describe an ecosystem.
- Discuss the impact of pollution on all aspects of the ecosystem.
- Understand the connection between overpopulation and environmental pollution.
- Explain the impact of air pollution on the environment.
- State the conditions that lead to water pollution.
- Discuss what individuals can do to remedy the different types of environment pollution.
- List the sources of indoor pollution.
- Discuss the Environmental Protection Agency's Superfund attempt to control and clean up solid waste.
- Discuss how to live a greener lifestyle.

What strategies and life skills would you emphasize to elementary students to teach them how they and their families can protect the environment?

Chapter 26: Strategies for Teaching Environmental Health

Valued Outcomes:

- Understand that high levels of wellness can only be sustained if the environment is conducive to well-being.
- Describe how all the animals, plants, and natural resources in any habitat form a self-sustaining ecosystem.
- Discuss how all parts of an ecosystem are interdependent.
- Discuss how ecosystems are linked to each other and form a global network called an ecosphere and how a change in one ecosystem has the potential to affect other ecosystems.
- Understand how human activities have the greatest impact on ecosystems.
- Describe the major sources of pollution.
- Discuss how overpopulation has resulted in environmental problems.
- Understand how conservation of natural resources, preservation of ecosystems, and protection of the environment from pollution are essential for preserving the ecosphere.
- Discuss why the preservation of the ecosphere must stem from individual and community action

Teaching Today's Health

Tenth Edition

David J. Anspaugh   Ed.D, CHES, AAHE fellow
Professor Emeritus, University of Memphis

Gene Ezell   Ed.D, CHES, AAHE fellow
Professor, University of Tennessee at Chattanooga

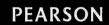

BOSTON   COLUMBUS   INDIANAPOLIS   NEW YORK   SAN FRANCISCO   UPPER SADDLE RIVER
AMSTERDAM   CAPE TOWN   DUBAI   LONDON   MADRID   MILAN   MUNICH   PARIS   MONTRÉAL   TORONTO
DELHI   MEXICO CITY   SÃO PAULO   SYDNEY   HONG KONG   SEOUL   SINGAPORE   TAIPEI   TOKYO

Executive Editor: Sandra Lindelof

Project Editor: Emily Portwood

Editorial Assistant: Briana Verdugo

Development Manager: Barbara Yien

Managing Editor: Deborah Cogan

Associate Production Project Manager: Megan Power

Production Management and Composition,
  and Interior Design: Integra

Cover Designer: Jana Anderson

Photo Researchers: Jessica Bruah and Tim Herzog

Image Rights and Permissions Manager: Donna Kalal

Manufacturing Buyer: Stacey Weinberger

Executive Marketing Manager: Neena Bali

Text Printer: LSC Communications Harrisonburg

Cover Printer: LSC Communications Harrisonburg

Cover Photo Credit: Claudia Rehm/Glow Images

Credits and acknowledgments borrowed from other sources and reproduced, with permission, in this textbook appear on the appropriate page within the text or on page 539.

Library of Congress Cataloging-in-Publication Data

Anspaugh, David J.

  Teaching today's health / David J. Anspaugh, Gene Ezell.—10th ed.

   p. cm.

   ISBN-13: 978-0-321-79391-1

   ISBN-10: 0-321-79391-9

 1. Health education (Elementary)—United States.   I. Ezell, Gene.   II. Title.

   LB1588.U6A83 2013

   372.37—dc23   2011031679

7   18

PEARSON

www.pearsonhighered.com

ISBN 10:   0-321-79391-9

ISBN 13: 978-0-321-79391-1

This book is dedicated to Susan and Connor, and to the students who have touched my life throughout the years.—DJA

This book is dedicated to my wife, Cynthi, and Megan, Alex, and Sam, all of whom complete me.—GE

Brief Contents

Contents

Preface

As the tenth edition of *Teaching Today's Health* comes to fruition, the goal has remained the same: to produce a product that will serve pre-professional teachers by helping them envision the possibilities for influencing students' lives through teaching quality health education. The opportunity to provide quality health education has never been greater than today. With the National Health Education Standards and the Coordinated School Health Model, the benchmarks, model, and philosophy are all in place for achieving great things in health education. There has never been a greater need for comprehensive quality health education. Our nation is facing a crisis in childhood obesity, type 2 diabetes, poor nutrition, poor cardiovascular fitness, and mental and emotional health concerns. Unfortunately many of the problems society and our youth have faced for decades are still present. Smoking, drug use, sexually transmitted infections, and problem pregnancies are still significant issues.

We as teachers must ensure that elementary and middle school students are better served, are provided correct health education information, and are ensured personalizing opportunities to assess their own value system. Ultimately, we want students to develop positive, healthy lifestyles. If students do not understand the value of health information, they will have no incentive to adopt a healthy lifestyle. To ensure this outcome, teachers must give students opportunities for critical thinking and provide an environment that fosters positive self-esteem, a sense of self-efficacy, and an internal locus of control. Finally, teachers should be role models for positive health behavior and making effective health decisions.

Like previous editions, the tenth edition of *Teaching Today's Health* presents the background, content, and strategies necessary for optimal teaching of health education in elementary and middle schools. Health education relies upon the National Health Education Standards and state-level and community-level health education standards and must originate from a solid cognitive knowledge base. From this cognitive base, teachers can provide multiple opportunities for students to personalize information. It is through the personalizing of basic information that children begin to make decisions that will ultimately result in positive health habits. Ingrained in these concepts is the continuing development of critical thinking skills.

Teachers continually deal with controversy and are bombarded by new information in many areas. Clearly, it is difficult to remain on the cutting edge of health information. Recognizing this need, we have attempted to include here the material needed for a solid foundation in teaching elementary and middle school health. Obviously, it still requires that teachers continue to update their knowledge and seek information related to health. The desire is that the content found in the tenth edition will serve as the starting point for effective teaching of health education.

New to the Tenth Edition

This edition has been updated with the latest available data for the health information covered in the theory-based chapters. Significant updates include the following:

- Chapter 3 (Planning for Health Instruction) includes the most recent version of the full National Health Education Standards and the coverage of the Michigan Model for Health has been significantly expanded and updated, now including full scope and sequence charts for grades K-12.

- The coverage of bullying in Chapter 6 (Mental Health and Stress Reduction) has been significantly updated and now incorporates coverage of cyber bullying.

- New sections in Chapter 8 (Body Systems) will help students make connections among the functions of the body systems, further exploring how each system is necessary and contributes to the overall healthy functioning of the body.

- Chapter 13 (Substance Use and Abuse) has been revised to offer a new overview of the most commonly abused drugs and their properties, and new subsections have been added to facilitate easier movement through the chapter.
- A new overview of infectious diseases and an updated schedule for recommended childhood immunizations is available in Chapter 15 (Infectious and Noninfectious Conditions).
- Coverage of nutrition information has been revised and expanded in Chapters 17 and 18, including updates based on *Healthy People 2020*, the *Dietary Guidelines for Americans, 2010*, and the MyPlate initiative.
- Chapter 23 (Aging, Dying, and Death) has been revised to reflect new statistics and research studies, as well as current advice on healthy aging, dementia, and caring for the elderly.
- Activities presented in the strategies chapters have been thoroughly examined and updated to reflect current instructional methods and resources (such as the new MyPlate initiative), and reorganized to fall under the seven teaching methods detailed in the new "Appendix A: Index of Teaching Strategies" (pages 465–476).
- New Creativity in the Classroom suggestions have been added to select theory chapters; these suggestions can help teachers engage student interest in fun and surprising ways.
- A new "Glossary" (including definitions for all the **bold** terms in the book) has been added to this edition.
- New and updated worksheets, to accompany new strategy activities or to supplement existing strategies, are provided at the end of the book. The puzzle worksheets (crosswords, word searches) are now available only on the companion website, www.pearsonhighered .com/anspaugh.

Organization

As with previous editions, the tenth edition of *Teaching Today's Health* is organized to present a strong foundation of health education theory along with an abundance of strategies to help teachers develop the skills required to become competent health teachers. Chapters 1 through 5 discuss the necessity for health education, the National Health Education Standards, the role of the teacher, planning effective health education, strategies for teaching, and implementing effective evaluation. All these topics are covered within the framework of the contemporary theory of wellness and optimal well-being.

Chapters 6 through 26 consist of specific content areas followed by strategies for making the content come alive for students. The strategies include values clarification activities, dramatizations, decision stories, experiments and demonstrations, puzzles, games, and bulletin board suggestions. Strategy activities have been correlated to related National Health Education Standards, and many of these activities can be adapted to meet additional standards. Additionally, many of the strategy activities that call for worksheets or game boards are accompanied by worksheets, which are located at the back of the textbook and have been designed to be ready to use in the classroom. Each strategy chapter has two examples of fully detailed lesson plans for classroom use.

Each theory-based chapter concludes with a bulleted chapter summary, as well as questions for students to consider (discussion questions and/or critical thinking questions). Additional review strategies, study aids, worksheets, and resources can be found on the *Teaching Today's Health* website at www.pearsonhighered.com/anspaugh.

Resources for Instructors and Students

▪ Companion Website

The tenth edition is accompanied by a companion website, www.pearsonhighered.com/anspaugh, which is full of dynamic resources that can make health education more effective. The website includes quizzes for each theory-based chapter. Website activities, websites of interest, and worksheets for puzzle-based activities (crosswords, word searches) are posted online for increased convenience. Information about first aid training is also available on the website. The website now includes the glossary and flash cards.

▪ Instructor's Manual and Test Bank

The *Instructor's Manual and Test Bank* includes valued outcomes, lecture outlines, multiple-choice questions, and essay questions for each theory chapter of the text. The "Strategies" chapter content includes valued outcomes and activities. Finally, the supplement includes transparency masters. This material can be downloaded from the "Instructor's Resource Center," accessible from www.pearsonhighered.com/educator.

▪ PowerPoint® Presentations

These updated PowerPoint® presentations can be used to support instruction. The files can be downloaded from the "Instructor's Resource Center," accessible from www.pearsonhighered.com/educator.

Acknowledgments

It is our sincere desire that a great many elementary and middle school children will benefit from the information gathered in this text. A sincere word of heartfelt thanks to

Emily Portwood, our Project Editor for this edition; we thank her for her great suggestions and gentle guidance on this project. Thanks are also due to Megan Power, our production supervisor, for expertly guiding the book through the production process, and to the talented team at Integra for their painstaking work on the composition of this edition.

Finally, we appreciate the worthwhile comments and suggestions of our reviewers: Cynthia Butler, Florida Atlantic University-Davie; Beth McNeill, Texas A&M University; Marianne Fahlman, Wayne State University; Peggy McGuire, Eastern Kentucky University; Katie Crosslin, Texas Women's University; Tammy Washington, USC-Aiken at USC-Salkehatchie; Monica Webb, University of Florida; Matt Lucas, Longwood University; and Bill Thompson, Belmont University.

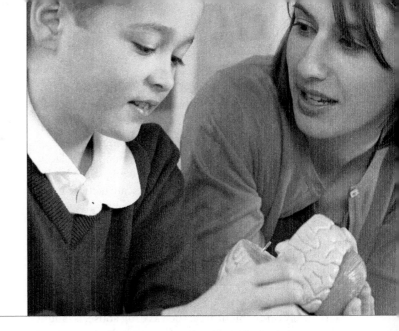

1 The Need for Health Education

The health of young people is strongly linked to their academic success, and the academic success of youth is strongly linked with their health. Thus, helping students stay healthy is a fundamental part of the mission of schools.

—*Centers for Disease Control and Prevention (2011)*

Valued Outcomes

After completion of this chapter, you should be able to:

- State definitions of health, health education, and health promotion.
- List and describe the components that make up wellness.
- Identify why health education is a necessary component in the nation's schools.
- Discuss the significance of the Youth Risk Behavior Surveillance System.
- Identify the components of a comprehensive school education.
- Discuss the components of a coordinated school health education program.
- Discuss the implications of the School Health Policies and Program Study (SHPPS).

Reflections

The raising of a child requires much love, care, and concern from many different sources, including the home, community, community agencies, and school. As you read this chapter, think of how and in what manner these components of our society can provide positive support and guidance for children and their families. How can the family become part of the coordinated school program? How can other agencies provide input and services? What is the role of the school health team?

The Evolution of Health Education

Formal health education first took the form of instruction in anatomy and physiology. Health was taught purely as a science, and emphasis was placed on retention of facts. When the "facts-alone" model did not work, some health educators began to use "preaching" or "scare tactics" to try to persuade students to include positive health behaviors in their lives. These approaches not only caused students to have a negative attitude toward health behaviors, but also diminished the credibility of the teachers from the students' perspective. Following these approaches, some health educators used a crisis-oriented approach; that is, if a problem arises, then address it. The problem with this approach is that typically one content area, such as drug abuse, is taught in a vacuum, and other aspects of a comprehensive school health program are not taught in context. As health education evolved, health teachers became more concerned with students' attitudes and behaviors. Today, the emphasis is on improving resiliency skills in students. It is interesting to note that, since the 1970s, early-age death rates have declined at a significant rate. This decline reflects a decrease in deaths due to cardiovascular disease and coincides with the declining use of tobacco, the reduction in dietary intake of fats and cholesterol, and increased exercise among adults. Society is in a period in which lifestyle, more than medicine, can lead to decreases in death rates.

Americans are currently in the middle of a health promotion movement. Data from governmental sources indicate that over the past three decades, childhood obesity in the United States has tripled, with one in three children being overweight or obese. The statistics for African Americans and Hispanics are even higher, with nearly 40 percent of children in these demographic areas overweight or obese. Statistics such as these have caused professionals and laypeople to focus their attention on more health promotion programs for our nation's youth (U.S. Department of Health and Human Services 2011).

For teachers, the charge today is to motivate students to improve their own health status through positive self-direction. Health education offers students an opportunity for personal growth and enhancement that is not duplicated anywhere else in the school curriculum.

What Is Health?

Health topics are everywhere. On television, radio, the Internet, and in popular magazines, Americans are continually bombarded with health-related information. For years, the World Health Organization's (WHO) 1947 definition of health—"a state of complete physical, mental and social well-being and not merely the absence of disease or infirmity" (WHO 2006)—was the accepted definition. A newer definition formulated by the Joint Committee on Health Education Terminology (Gold 2002) points to the essence of the concept. The committee stated that **health**

"is an integrated method of functioning which is oriented toward maximizing the potential of which the individual is capable. It requires that the individual maintain a continuum of balance and purposeful direction with the environment where he (*sic*) is functioning." This concept goes beyond simply not being ill or sick. It implies, as Hoyman suggested in 1975, that health has several dimensions, each having its own continuum.

Health is also referred to as **wellness**. Figure 1.1 shows a conceptualization of these components.

1. **Spiritual**—includes such aspects as meaning and purpose in life; self-awareness; and connectedness with self, others, and a larger reality. The spiritual component may involve, for example, imagery, meditation, and group support activities.
2. **Social**—the ability to interact successfully with people and one's personal environment. This component involves the ability to develop and maintain intimacy with others and to have respect and tolerance for those with different opinions and beliefs.
3. **Physical**—the ability to carry out daily tasks, develop cardiovascular and muscular fitness, maintain adequate nutrition and proper weight, avoid abusing drugs and alcohol, and avoid tobacco products.
4. **Environmental**—maintaining safe water, food, and air: having a safe emotional and physical environment in which we can live and carry out our daily activities.
5. **Emotional**—the ability to control stress and to express emotions appropriately and comfortably. This involves the ability to recognize and accept feelings and not to be defeated by setbacks and failures.
6. **Intellectual**—the ability to learn and use information effectively for personal, family, and career development. It means striving for continued growth and learning to deal with new challenges effectively.

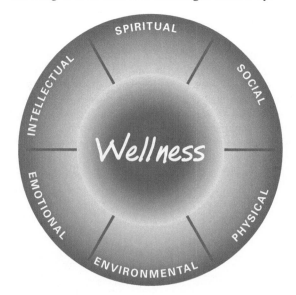

Figure 1.1
The Components of Wellness

The first assumption of the wellness approach to living is that an individual achieves good health by balancing each of these dimensions. A second assumption is that each individual is ultimately responsible for her or his well-being. That is, we—not the government, physicians, nurses, or some other institution—must accept personal responsibility for our health. Each person must foster attitudes that will improve the quality of life and expand the human potential. To accomplish this, teachers must empower their students to see themselves as being *in control* of improving their quality of life. Such students have an **internal locus of control**. (This trait contrasts with **external locus of control**, in which an individual believes that he or she cannot control many of the factors that contribute to a higher level of wellness.)

Another vital concept in a wellness lifestyle is self-efficacy. Self-efficacy is the belief in one's ability to accomplish a specific task or behavior. Self-efficacy is something each student can give himself or herself, if the teacher can provide the support and encouragement necessary to acquire a personal sense of competence.

The sooner students begin the lifelong process of becoming healthy, the more likely they will be successful. Teachers must recognize that children bring to schools many values and behaviors. These values represent both the beneficial and negative aspects of a student's living practices. At the same time, teachers should be aware of the powerful influence they exert on the lives of their students. Nowhere in the entire educational spectrum can a teacher make such an impression as at the elementary level. Consequently, the teacher who exemplifies a lifestyle conducive to high-level wellness—who exhibits a style of living that is physically, socially, and psychologically healthy—enhances the probability that his or her students will attempt to incorporate those beneficial aspects in their own lives.

What Is Health Education and Health Promotion?

As with the term *health*, **health education** has taken on new meanings over the years. Although there are many ways of defining *health education*, the Joint Committee on Health Education Terminology stated that the health education process is the "continuum of learning which enables people, as individual members of social structures, to voluntarily make decisions, modify, and change social conditions in ways which are health enhancing" (1991, 103).

The Society for Public Health Education (SOPHE) states that health education is: "any combination of learning experiences that promote voluntary actions and informed decisions conducive to health." SOPHE further states that health education is "concerned with the health behavior of individuals and with the living and working conditions that influence their health" (NCSOPHE 2006).

The term **health promotion** is sometimes used incorrectly in reference to health education. *Health promotion* is defined by Michael O'Donnell, editor of the *American Journal of Public Health*, as "any combination of health education, and related organizational, political, and economic intervention designed to facilitate behavioral and environmental changes conducive to health" (National Center for Health Fitness 2006). Health promotion is therefore broader in scope than health education, and health education is an intricate part of health promotion. Health education is one of several different formats that can be used to influence health and quality of life.

From the elementary teacher's perspective, health education is the process of developing and providing planned learning experiences in such a way as to supply information, change attitudes, and influence behavior. In other words, health education is helping children develop the concept of wellness (discussed in the previous section). This process should result in children developing a sense of individual responsibility for their health, leading to health enhancement or high-level wellness. As part of this process, a child should develop assertiveness, decision-making skills, self-esteem, self-confidence, and a sense that he or she can achieve success not only in health-related matters, but also in life in general.

The teacher accomplishes all this through creating and facilitating learning experiences that develop the child's decision-making ability. With good decision-making skills, the child will make better choices about the personal, family, peer, and societal factors that influence quality of life. An effective school health program must have a direct influence on children's lives and behavior.

Health education is a lifelong process. As people develop awareness of the many components of health and incorporate them into their own lives, they

- assume responsibility for their own health and health care and actively participate with a medical professional in the decision-making process.

- respect the benefits of medical technology but are not so in awe of medical equipment and tests that they fail to question medical professionals on their use of the technology.

- try new behaviors and modify others.

- are skeptical of health fads and trends.

- ask questions, seek evidence, and evaluate information regarding health matters.

- strive for self-reliance in personal health matters.

- voluntarily adopt practices consistent with a healthy lifestyle.

Accomplishing Health Education

With the school day already crowded, many elementary teachers wonder how to find time to teach health education. But time must be found. Our nation's children are an invaluable resource. Health education can help ensure that this generation is fit physically, psychologically, and socially to assume the difficult tasks of adulthood. Still, the problem remains: When and how should health education be taught in the classroom? How can it be accomplished?

Health education that is relevant and motivating for the student requires careful planning. The quality of health instruction is reflected in the amount of planning and organization the teacher carries out. There are many approaches to teaching health (several of which will be discussed in Chapter 4). However, the responsibility rests with each teacher to create and facilitate direct instruction in health and to infuse other health-related topics whenever the opportunity arises.

As previously stated, time must be allotted for direct health instruction during the school day. There is no substitute for this. However, if the time that can be allotted is minimal, health instruction can be incorporated or integrated into other parts of the curriculum. There are some advantages to integrating a part of health instruction into other subject areas, including opportunities for a significant amount of creativity in learning and teaching. Many of the activities presented in the Strategies chapters in this book can be integrated into other subject areas in this way. Look for this icon ◯ which highlights activities that can be readily integrated into math, science, reading, writing, physical education, social studies, or art. However, the greatest need is for health to receive its just place in the elementary school day.

In health education, topics must be appropriate to the developmental level of the child. Health must be taught every semester at every grade level from kindergarten throughout the high school experience. The planned curriculum must be sequential and address the physical, emotional, mental, and social dimensions of the child's health at a particular grade level. Only in this way can it become a meaningful part of each child's learning experience. Meaningful health education influences a child's decision-making skills. To do this, health instruction must blend information giving with attitudinal experiences. In short, a child will be better able to make personal decisions concerning health behavior if the teacher has provided cognitive and affective opportunities for growth. Part of this process is providing children with a decision-making model with ample opportunities to practice decision making.

Presenting factual information alone—the cognitive aspect of health education—is not enough. Knowledge of facts *alone* does not lead to changes in behavior, as evidenced by the failure of many cognitive health education programs in the past. Knowledge must become personalized if it is to have an effect. This personalization is the affective aspect of health education. Strategies for accomplishing this personalization component will be presented throughout this text. To accomplish its objectives, health education must be:

- **Sequential**—instruction should be provided throughout the educational experience, grades K through 12. The curriculum at each level should be based on what has been learned in previous years and serve as the basis for curricula in future years.

- **Planned**—instruction should be based on goals, outcome-related objectives, and evaluation criteria. It should be taught within the total curriculum framework; teaching within other subjects, such as science, should not serve as a substitute.

- **Comprehensive**—instruction should include all the identified health content areas. More important than the individual subjects, however, is an understanding of how all subjects interrelate with the components of high-level wellness and quality of life.

- **Taught by qualified health teachers**—individuals who have a concern for the total wellness of their students and who have been trained in the content as well as the strategies of health education. Effective health teaching requires more than the accumulation of knowledge. It requires that students have opportunities to personalize and incorporate positive health habits into their daily lives.

The need for health education continues to grow each year. It is important to remember that in the last twenty years, topics such as childhood obesity, drug abuse, smoking, heart disease prevention, teenage pregnancy, adolescent suicide, stress control, incest, child abuse, human immunodeficiency virus (HIV), and cardiopulmonary resuscitation (CPR) have been added to an already long list of topics that includes nutrition, disease, mental health, sexuality, personal health, environmental health, first aid, and consumerism.

It would seem that the task of creating health education programs is overwhelming. How does the school help children acquire knowledge, develop awareness and skills, provide personalizing experiences, and reinforce healthful behaviors? Equally important, how does the school interact with the community and the family to maximize the potential for assuming healthful behaviors?

Conceptually, the family, community, and school all play important roles in children's learning, and each segment must seek to cooperate with the others to provide opportunities to learn, practice, and reinforce healthful lifestyles. It is imperative that schools recognize the importance of working within the community and with the family in attaining the healthy development of each child. This process is discussed more completely in the section dealing with the coordinated school health program later in this chapter.

Why Health Education?

Perhaps the best argument for teaching health education is that health behaviors are the most important determinant of health status. Health-related behaviors are both learned and changeable, so there is no better time to start formal health education than in the elementary school years, when the child is more flexible and more apt to accept positive health behaviors. In addition, this approach can help students avoid the health problems that result from smoking, poor nutrition, overweight, lack of exercise, stress, abuse of drugs and alcohol, and unsafe personal behavior.

Unfortunately, health education still suffers from a lack of priority in the school curriculum and a lack of adequately trained teachers. If we wish to help prevent many of the conditions that are now the leading causes of death (Table 1.1), then we must emphasize prevention in our educational efforts.

The Centers for Disease Control and Prevention (CDC) has indicated that during childhood and adolescence, behaviors are established that later contribute significantly to heart disease, cancer, and injuries. Such behaviors include the use of tobacco products, unhealthy eating habits, inactivity, use of alcohol and drugs, and unprotected sex.

The consequences of unprotected sex are manifest in HIV infections, sexually transmitted infections (STIs), and unintended pregnancies (CDC 2011).

Not every area of concern in a comprehensive health education program has been covered here, but it is hoped that the pressing need for health education has been established. The scope of health education is a broad one. Personal, family, and community problems must be effectively addressed if we are to live personally and socially satisfying lives. The time to begin effective health education is in the elementary school.

Today parents, administrators, and students no longer perceive health education as a peripheral or secondary activity. Parent and teacher organizations, such as the Michigan PTSA, are encouraging local schools to implement coordinated health programs (Michigan PTSA 2004). The window of opportunity is there for providing comprehensive health education. As teachers, parents, and as a society, we must begin to effectively deal with the challenges facing children and youth today. The Health Highlight boxes in this chapter illustrate some facts and statistics that help emphasize the continuing need for health education.

More tragic is the loss in human potential. Today, the diseases that are killing Americans are chronic diseases

Table 1.1	Leading Causes of Death by Age in 2009[1]		
	Age Groups		
Rank	**1–4**	**5–14**	**15–24**
1	Accidents (4,448)	Accidents (1,667)	Accidents (12,351)
2	Congenital Anomalies (485)	Malignant Neoplasms (893)	Homicide (4,820)
3	Homicide (385)	Congenital Anomalies (350)	Suicide (4,341)
4	Malignant Neoplasms (349)	Homicide (319)	Malignant Neoplasms (1,659)
5	Heart Diseases (154)	Suicide (266)	Heart Diseases (1,010)
6	Influenza & Pneumonia (132)	Influenza & Pneumonia (230)	Congenital Anomalies (451)
7	Septicemia (70)	Heart Diseases (200)	Influenza & Pneumonia (410)
8	Chronic Lower Respiratory Diseases (60)	Chronic Lower Respiratory Diseases (116)	Pregnancy, Childbirth, Puerperium (202)
9	Perinatal Period Conditions (58)	Other Neoplasms (84)	Cerebrovascular Diseases (198)
10	Neoplasms (51)	Cerebrovascular Diseases (69)	Chronic Lower Respiratory Diseases (182)

[1] Actual number of deaths (preliminary estimates) are shown in parentheses.
Source: National Vital Statistics System, National Center for Health Statistics, CDC.

What Is a Comprehensive School Health Education Curriculum?

The Division of Adolescent and School Health has provided details of a comprehensive school health education (CSHE). The following list describes key elements of CSHE, which itself is part of an overall coordinated school health program:

1. A documented, planned, and sequential program of health instruction for students in kindergarten through grade 12
2. A curriculum that addresses and integrates education about a range of categorical health problems and issues at developmentally appropriate ages
3. Activities that help young people develop the skills they need to avoid tobacco use; dietary patterns that contribute to disease; sedentary lifestyle; sexual behaviors that result in HIV infection, other STIs, and unintended pregnancy; alcohol and other drug use; and behaviors that result in unintentional and intentional injuries
4. Instruction provided for a prescribed amount of time at each grade level
5. Management and coordination by an education professional trained to implement the program
6. Instruction from teachers who are trained to teach the subject
7. Involvement of parents, health professionals, and other concerned community members
8. Periodic evaluation, updating, and improvement

Source: CDC April 27, 2011

---

such as cancer, heart disease, and AIDS. Many of these deaths could be prevented by helping people alter their lifestyles through improved eating habits, regular exercise, eliminating smoking, and practicing safer sex. The incidence of these diseases will be decreased not through additional medical care or greater medical expenditures, but through educating people to live healthful lives and, thereby, prevent disease. As a nation, our resources must be invested in helping people take control of their lives.

National Initiatives for Comprehensive School Health

Several national initiatives have created support for a comprehensive school health education program. A most important document is *Healthy People 2020* (Office of Disease Prevention and Health Promotion 2010). This document focuses on improving the quality of life for all citizens of the United States. Many of the objectives either relate directly to, or have implications for, coordinated school health education.

Other initiatives have helped to emphasize the importance of coordinated school health programs. They include The National Education Goals for 2000 and the federally enacted Safe and Drug-Free Schools and Communities Act (SDFSCA) of 1994. Two of the eight goals set forth by the National Education Goals emphasized health education (National Education Goals Panel 2002). Goal 1 states, "All children [in America] will start school ready to learn." A component of this goal states that every child would receive nutrition, physical activity experiences, and health care to enable them to arrive at school with healthy minds and bodies. Goal 7 states, "Every school in the United States will be free of drugs, violence, and the unauthorized presence of firearms and alcohol and will offer a disciplined environment conducive to learning." The objectives for this goal include implementing a firm and fair policy on possession, use, and distribution of drugs and alcohol; having parent, business, government, and community organizations work together to provide a learning environment free of violence, drugs, crime, and the presence of weapons; schools should provide a healthy environment and safe haven for all; all local educational agencies should develop a sequential comprehensive K through 12 drug and alcohol program; community-based teams should be organized to provide support for students and teachers; and every school should work to eliminate sexual harassment (Joint Committee on Health Education Standards 1995).

The Youth Risk Behavior Surveillance System

The Youth Risk Behavior Surveillance System (YRBSS) provides information on the health behaviors practiced by young people. It is another source of information that helps educators determine the health practices and status of American youth. The YRBSS also serves to illustrate the necessity for a coordinated school health program. This system was developed by the CDC along with cooperation and collaboration with federal, state, and private-sector partners. It includes a national survey as well as surveys conducted by state and local education

HEALTH HIGHLIGHT | *Healthy People 2020*: Some Objectives with Implications for Health Education

Adolescent Health

- Increase the proportion of adolescents who have had a wellness checkup in the past twelve months
- Decrease school absenteeism among adolescents due to illness or injury
- Increase the proportion of middle and high schools that prohibit harassment based on a student's sexual orientation or gender identity

Health Education

- Increase the proportion of elementary, middle, and senior high schools that require school health education
- Increase the proportion of schools that require cumulative instruction in health education that meet the U.S. National Health Education Standards for elementary, middle, and senior high schools
- Increase the proportion of required health education classes or courses with a teacher who has had professional development related to teaching personal and social skills for behavior change within the past two years

Immunization and Infectious Diseases

- Reduce, eliminate, or maintain elimination of cases of vaccine-preventable diseases
- Increase the proportion of children aged 19 to 35 months who receive the recommended doses of DTaP, polio, MMR, Hib, hepatitis B, varicella and PCV vaccines
- Maintain vaccination coverage levels for children in kindergarten
- Increase the percentage of children and adults who are vaccinated annually against seasonal influenza

Injury and Violence Prevention

- Increase the proportion of public and private schools that require students to wear appropriate protective gear when engaged in school-sponsored physical activities
- Reduce bullying among adolescents
- Reduce weapon carrying by adolescents on school property
- Reduce child maltreatment deaths
- Reduce abusive sexual contact other than rape or attempted rape
- Reduce children's exposure to violence

Mental Health

- Reduce suicide attempts by adolescents
- Reduce the proportion of adolescents who engage in disordered eating behaviors in an attempt to control their weight
- Increase the proportion of children with mental health problems who receive treatment

Nutrition and Weight Status

- Increase the proportion of schools that offer nutritious foods and beverages outside of school meals
- Reduce the proportion of children and adolescents who are considered obese
- Increase the contribution of fruits to the diets of the population aged 2 years and older
- Increase the variety and contribution of vegetables to the diets of the population aged 2 years and older
- Reduce consumption of calories from solid fats and added sugars in the population aged 2 years and older

Physical Activity

- Increase the proportion of adolescents who meet current federal physical activity guidelines for aerobic physical activity and for muscle-strengthening activity
- Increase the proportion of the nation's public and private schools that require daily physical education for all students

Sleep Health

- Increase the proportion of students in grades 9 through 12 who get sufficient sleep

Substance Abuse

- Increase the proportion of adolescents never using substances
- Increase the proportion of adolescents who perceive great risk associated with substance abuse
- Reduce the proportion of persons engaging in binge drinking of alcoholic beverages
- Reduce steroid use among adolescents

Tobacco Use

- Reduce the initiation of tobacco use among children, adolescents, and young adults
- Reduce the proportion of nonsmokers exposed to secondhand smoke
- Increase tobacco-free environments in schools, including all school facilities, property, vehicles, and school events
- Reduce the proportion of adolescents and young adults grades 6 through 12 who are exposed to tobacco advertising and promotion
- Reduce the illegal sales rate to minors through enforcement of laws prohibiting the sale of tobacco products to minors

Source: U.S. Department of Health and Human Services, *Healthy People 2020* (2010). Full report available at www.healthypeople.gov.

---

agencies. The CDC conducts national surveys every two years to produce data representative of students in grades 9 through 12 in both public and private schools in the fifty states and the District of Columbia. In 2009 nearly 16,410 students in forty-two states took the survey (CDC 2011). Summary results certainly indicate the need for beginning a coordinated school health education in the elementary school. Tables 1.2, 1.3, and 1.4 provide information on risk behaviors that improved, worsened, or either did not change or demonstrated inconsistent patterns of change. The data represent the years in which the YRBSS was given.

Table 1.2	Trends in Unintentional Injuries for Students in Grades 9–12 (1991–2009)					
1991	**1995**	**1999**	**2003**	**2007**	**2009**	**Changes from 1991–2009[1]**
Rarely or never wore a seat belt (when riding in a car driven by someone else)						
25.9%	21.7%	16.4%	18.2%	11.1%	9.7%	Decreased
Rarely or never wore a bicycle helmet (among students who had ridden a bicycle during the twelve months before the survey)						
96.2%	92.8%	85.3%	85.9%	85.1%	84.7%	Decreased, 1991–2001 No change, 2001–2009
Rode with a driver who had been drinking alcohol one or more times (in a car or other vehicle during the thirty days before the survey)						
39.9%	38.8%	33.1%	30.2%	29.1%	28.3%	Decreased
Drove when drinking alcohol one or more times (in a car or other vehicle during the thirty days before the survey)						
16.7%	15.4%	13.1%	12.1%	10.5%	9.7%	No change, 1991–1997 Decreased, 1997–2009

[1] Based on trend analyses using a logistic regression model controlling for sex, race/ethnicity, and grade.

Source: U.S. Department of Health and Human Services, National Youth Risk Behavior Survey (YRBS) 2010. Available at www.cdc.gov/healthyyouth.

The Coordinated School Health Program

A total school health program is needed if the school is to function as an effective institution for promoting high-level wellness. As shown in Figure 1.2, a coordinated

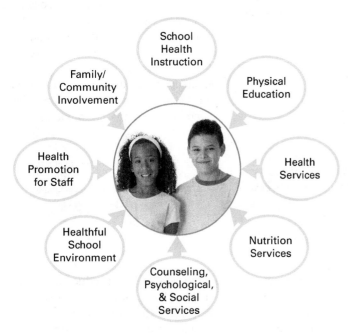

Figure 1.2
The Coordinated School Health Program

school health program includes eight components. The following are working descriptions of the eight components of a coordinated school health program.

1. **Healthful school environment**—The healthful school environment includes both the physical and the emotional environment of the classroom. The physical environment includes the actual physical environment in and around the school building, and the physical conditions, such as temperature, noise, and lighting, in the school and classroom. The psychological (or emotional) environment includes the relationships between the students and teachers as well as the relationships between the students themselves.

2. **School health instruction**—Health instruction is most effective when it is planned and sequential and taught by qualified, trained teachers each year in a K through 12 curriculum. School health instruction should include the physical, mental, emotional, spiritual, and social dimensions of health. The curriculum should include interactive learning experiences that are designed to motivate and help students maintain and improve their health, prevent disease, and reduce health-related risk behaviors. Well-rounded school health instruction includes teaching about knowledge, attitudes, skills, and practices. The comprehensive health education curriculum includes a variety of topics, such as personal health, family health, community health, consumer

Table 1.3 Trends in Sexual Behaviors for Students in Grades 9–12 (1991–2009)

	1991	1995	1999	2003	2007	2009	Changes from 1991–2009[1]
Ever had sexual intercourse							
	54.1%	53.1%	49.9%	46.7%	47.8%	46.0%	Decreased
Had sexual intercourse with four or more persons (during their life)							
	18.7%	17.8%	16.2%	14.4%	14.9%	13.8%	Decreased
Had sexual intercourse with at least one person (during the three months before the survey)							
	37.5%	37.9%	36.3%	34.3%	35.0%	34.2%	Decreased
Used a condom during last sexual intercourse (among students who were currently sexually active)							
	46.2%	54.4%	58.0%	63.0%	61.5%	61.1%	Increased, 1991–2003 No change, 2003–2009
Used birth control pills or Depo-Provera before last sexual intercourse to prevent pregnancy (among students who were currently sexually active)							
	NA[2]	NA	19.5%	20.7%	18.8%	22.9%	No change
Drank alcohol or used drugs before last sexual intercourse (among students who were currently sexually active)							
	21.6%	24.8%	24.8%	25.4%	22.5%	21.6%	Increased, 1991–2001 Decreased, 2001–2009
Were ever taught in school about AIDS or HIV infection							
	83.3%	86.3%	90.6%	87.9%	89.5%	87.0%	Increased, 1991–1997 Decreased, 1997–2009

[1] Based on trend analyses using a logistic regression model controlling for sex, race/ethnicity, and grade.

[2] Not available.

Source: U.S. Department of Health and Human Services, National Youth Risk Behavior Survey (YRBS). 2010. Available at www.cdc.gov/healthyyouth

---

health, environmental health, sexuality education, mental and emotional health, injury prevention and safety, nutrition, prevention and control of disease, and substance use and abuse. See Health Highlight, "What Is a Comprehensive School Health Education Curriculum?" (page 6).

3. **School health services**—Many educators mistakenly think that school health services should be left to the school nurse and support staff; however, the classroom teacher can play a major role in this area of the comprehensive school health program. School health services include those that help students, faculty, and staff to appraise, protect, and promote health. These services are designed to ensure access, referral, or both to primary health care services. For example, staff might provide vision screening for the students, and the teacher and staff can work together

to inform the parents of any vision need and help the parents find the appropriate medical service for the child. The teacher and staff should be able to direct the parents to health care services, whether the student's family can afford privately funded health care, whether they need financially assisted health care, or whether they require free health care. School health services are intended also to prevent and control communicable disease and other health problems in and around the school. The classroom and school environment is conducive to the spread of communicable diseases. The teachers and staff should ensure that the instruction and facilities are such that the students are provided as much protection as possible from such diseases. Other school health services include the following: providing emergency care for illness or injury; promoting and

Table 1.4 Trends in Tobacco, Alcohol, and Illegal Drug Use on School Property for Students in Grades 9–12 (1991–2009)

1991	1995	1999	2003	2007	2009	Changes from 1991–2009[1]
Smoked cigarettes on school property on at least one day (during the thirty days before the survey)						
NA[2]	16.0%	14.0%	8.0%	5.7%	5.1%	No change, 1993–1995 Decreased, 1995–2009
Used chewing tobacco, snuff, or dip on school property on at least one day (during the thirty days before the survey)						
NA	6.3%	4.2%	5.9%	4.9%	5.5%	No change
Had at least one drink of alcohol on school property on at least one day (during the thirty days before the survey)						
NA	6.3%	4.9%	5.2%	4.1%	4.5%	Decreased
Used marijuana on school property one or more times (during the thirty days before the survey)						
NA	8.8%	7.2%	5.8%	4.5%	4.6%	Increased, 1993–1995 Decreased, 1995–2009
Offered, sold, or given an illegal drug by someone on school property (during the twelve months before the survey)						
NA	32.1%	30.2%	28.7%	22.3%	22.7%	Increased, 1993–1995 Decreased, 1995–2009

[1] Based on trend analyses using a logistic regression model controlling for sex, race/ethnicity, and grade.

[2] Not available.

Source: U.S. Department of Health and Human Services, National Youth Risk Behavior Survey (YRBS) 2010. Available at www.cdc.gov/healthyyouth.

providing optimum sanitary conditions for a safe school facility and school environment; and providing educational and counseling opportunities for promoting and maintaining individual, family, and community health. Qualified professionals such as physicians, nurses, dentists, health educators, classroom teachers, and other allied health personnel provide these services.

4. **Physical education**—Like health instruction, physical education should be a planned, sequential K through 12 curriculum. Instruction in physical education should provide cognitive content and learning experiences in a variety of activity areas, such as basic movement skills; physical fitness; rhythm and dance; games; team, dual, and individual sports; tumbling and gymnastics; and aquatics. With the current emphasis on preventing obesity in children, quality physical education should promote through a variety of planned physical activities each student's optimum physical, mental, emotional, and social development, and should promote activities and sports that all students enjoy and can pursue throughout their lives. As with school health

instruction, physical education should be taught by qualified, trained teachers.

5. **Nutrition and food services**—Though these services are mainly provided by a qualified school cafeteria staff, the classroom teacher can enhance this aspect of the comprehensive school health program though nutrition-related instruction and activities. The students should be provided access to a variety of nutritious and appealing meals that accommodate the health and nutrition needs of all students and that reflect the U.S. Dietary Guidelines for Americans and other criteria to achieve nutritional integrity. The school nutrition services can utilize nutrition-related community services to augment the instruction and services provided by the school.

6. **School-based counseling (psychological and social services)**—These services should be designed to improve students' mental, emotional, and social health. Though the majority of schools may not have their own qualified professionals such as school counselors, social workers, or school psychologists on staff, schools can partner with the community to provide these services. These

services include individual and group assessments, interventions, and referrals. Organizational assessment and consultation skills of counselors and psychologists contribute not only to the health of students but also to the health of the school environment.

7. **Schoolsite health promotion for staff—** Opportunities in this area include those intended for school staff to improve their health status through activities such as health assessments, health education, and health-related fitness activities. For example, competitions can be held between classrooms or between teachers, in which competitors accumulate so many points a day for exercising or for eating the appropriate number of vegetables each day. Also, workout sessions for faculty, staff, and students can be held before and/or after school to further augment the school's physical education program. These opportunities encourage school staff to pursue a healthy lifestyle that contributes to their improved health status, improved morale, and a greater personal commitment to the school's overall coordinated health program. When students see the teachers and staff of their school involved in such activities, students are more likely to view these professionals as positive health models and therefore involve themselves in such activities. Health promotion activities have improved productivity, decreased absenteeism, and reduced health insurance costs.

8. **School, family, community health promotion partnerships**—Simply stated, when school officials, parents, and community organizations partner together to deliver a cohesive and accurate health message, the students are more likely to perceive that the message is important and credible. School health advisory councils, coalitions, and broadly based constituencies working together for school health can greatly enhance school health program efforts. To respond more effectively to students' health-related needs, schools need to actively solicit parent involvement and engage community resources and services (U.S. Department of Health and Human Services, CDC 2005).

The Status of Health Education

The School Health Policies and Programs Study (SHPPS) is a national survey conducted periodically to assess school health programming and policies at the classroom, school, and district state levels. All fifty states were surveyed. The SHPPS survey was designed to answer four questions: (1) What were the characteristics of school health program components at the state, district, school, and classroom levels and across elementary, middle, and high school? (2) Were there persons responsible for coordinating and delivering each health program component, and what were the qualifications or educational backgrounds of this group? (3) What was the collaboration among staff from each component of the school health program and outside agencies/education? (4) What key policies and practices have changed over time?

The portion of the survey that investigated health education looked at fourteen health topics. Nationwide, 88.2 percent of states (forty-four states) had adopted a policy requiring that elementary schools teach at least one of fourteen health topics. Almost 63 percent (thirty-one states) had a policy requiring that elementary schools teach at least seven of the fourteen topics. Only about 6 percent (three states) required that all fourteen be taught (SHPPS 2006).

At the state level, only about 6 percent required the use of a particular course of study or curriculum. Only 15.7 percent of the states recommended one particular curriculum. The curricula generally contained expectations of what the student should know and be able to do at the end of a grade or multiple grades for the various subject areas. Most of these curricular plans contained detailed directions, strategies, and materials to foster learning and the teaching of content. The states were more likely to provide plans on how to evaluate and assess students' performance. Both the states and districts provided a variety of materials for elementary health education (SHPPS 2006).

The professional preparation of individuals teaching health at the elementary school level required undergraduate or graduate training in health education in 34 percent of the states surveyed nationwide. School districts required such training in 33.7 percent of schools nationwide. The policy of requiring training in health education applied only to newly hired personnel. Nationwide, 94 percent of all states offered some type of certification, licensure, or endorsement to teach health. At the elementary level, slightly more than 26 percent of all states had a policy stating that newly hired staff must be certified, licensed, or endorsed. At the middle school level, slightly more than 72 percent of states required newly hired staff to be certified licensed, or endorsed in health education (SHPPS 2006).

Nationwide, at the time of the survey, only 22 percent of states had adopted a policy stating that each school district should have someone to supervise or coordinate school health education. Nationwide, almost 43 percent of districts had adopted a policy to have someone supervise the health education at the school district level. Continuing education was required by almost 62 percent of states, and 39 percent of districts had such a policy. Staff development was defined to include workshops, conferences, continuing education, graduate courses, or any other kind of in-service experience on health topics or teaching strategies. During the two years preceding the survey, 94 percent of all states had provided funding for staff development. At the district level, almost 95 percent had provided funding for staff development.

At the state level, collaboration among health education staff was quite extensive. During the year prior to the survey, state-level health education staff had worked with nutrition and food service staff in 94 percent of the states, with physical education staff in 82 percent of the states, and with health service staff in 75 percent of the states. In nearly half of the states, state-level health education staff had worked with state health departments (98 percent), with the state-level school health committee council (94 percent), colleges/universities (92 percent), organizations such as the American Heart Association or American Cancer Society (90 percent), the American Alliance for Health, Physical Education, Recreation, and Dance (86 percent), state-level nurses' associations (82 percent), and state mental health or social services (74 percent) (SHPPS 2006).

The last part of the survey attempted to discover changes that had occurred between the first survey in 2000 and the follow-up survey in 2006. The percentage of states that had adopted a policy requiring districts or schools to follow national or state health education standards increased from 60.8 to 74.5 percent. The number of districts requiring schools to follow national, state, or district health education standards also increased, from 68.8 to 79.3 percent. Interestingly, the percentage of states and districts requiring schools to teach topics related to human sexuality, violence prevention, and injury prevention increased at the elementary and middle school levels. The percentage of states providing scope and sequence of instruction for elementary schools decreased from 62 to 51 percent. The percentage of states providing one or more recommended health education curricula decreased for elementary schools from 56 to 39.2 percent and in middle schools from 56 to 39 percent. The percentage of states requiring certification, licensure, or endorsement to teach health education increased from 48 to 62 percent. Accompanying this increased demand for some form of certification for teaching health was increased funding for staff development, which rose from 39.6 percent in 2000 to 61.7 percent in 2006. Finally, the evaluation of health education curricula at the district level increased from 53.2 percent in 2000 to to 66.6 percent in 2006 (Kann et al. 2007).

Obviously the effort to provide quality comprehensive health education is making strides. There is still much work to do, but administrators, educators, and parents are beginning to see the validity of health education. Health educators have an opportunity to become proactive rather than reactive in meeting the needs of students. There is a window of opportunity to better prepare our students emotionally, mentally, and physically. The charge is for the teachers to view health education and the coordinated health model as the framework for helping our students to become better citizens, healthier individuals, and more productive members of society.

Family Structure and the Well-Being of Children

Population and Family Characteristics

According to the Federal Interagency Forum on Child and Family Statistics, children ages 0 to 17 comprised 24 percent of the population in the United States in 2009, which is well below the peak of 36 percent at the end of the baby boom in 1964 (2011). By 2050, children are projected to comprise 23 percent of the total population in the United States. Additionally, American children continue to be more diverse ethnically. In 2009, 55 percent of U.S. children were white, non-Hispanic; 15 percent were black; and 4 percent were Asian. The fastest-growing ethnic group is Hispanic, which increased from 9 percent to slightly more than 22.5 percent of U.S. children between 1980 and 2009.

As the population of children has changed over time, so too has family structure changed. Fewer children today live with two married parents. The percentage of American children living with two married parents decreased from 77 percent in 1980 to 67 percent in 2009. This later percentage has been fairly stable since 1994. Data indicate that children who live with their married, biological parents are healthier (86 percent in excellent or very good health) than children who live with a married stepparent (80 percent in excellent or very good health), children who lived with a single parent (76 percent in excellent or very good health), and children who lived with neither parent (67 percent in excellent or very good health).

Birth rates for unmarried teenagers have dropped considerably since 1994. Children who live with their married, biological parents are less likely to become unmarried mothers. Pooled data from 1996 and 2009 show that 2 percent of all females ages 15 to 17 who lived with their married biological parents became unmarried mothers by age 17 to 19, compared with 9 percent of those who lived with a single parent and 27 percent of those who did not live with either parent (Federal Interagency Forum on Child and Family Statistics 2011).

Economic Security

Among the concerns of school-aged children and their families are poverty, parental employment, housing, and the availability of health insurance. In 2010, 19 percent of children ages 0 to 17 lived in poverty. In contrast, 22 percent of children lived in poverty in 1993. In 2009, 77 percent of children ages 0 to 17 had at least one parent who was employed full time. However, about 36 percent of children ages 0 to 17 experienced housing problems such as crowding or physically inadequate buildings. A majority of children (89 percent) had health insurance coverage in 2004. However, although government insurance coverage has continued its upward trend since 1999, the proportion of children covered by private health insurance has dropped since 2000. In 2009, about 10 percent of children had no regular source of health care (Federal Interagency Forum on Child and Family Statistics 2009).

Health and Mortality

Overweight and obesity are continual health concerns for American families. More and more of America's children ages 6 to 18 are overweight, rising from 6 percent in 1976 to 19 percent in 2007–2008.

Many children suffer from asthma and other respiratory disorders. Between 1980 and 1995, the percentage of children who had asthma more than doubled. In 2008, nine percent of children had asthma.

Exposure to lead remains a persistent concern. The percentage of children who have been exposed to lead has decreased significantly, but some children are still affected by lead. In 1999–2002, fewer than 2 percent of children aged 1 to 5 years had blood lead levels greater than 10 micrograms per deciliter (µg/dL). The median concentration of lead in the blood of children aged 1 to 5 years dropped from 14 µg/dL in 1976–1980 to about 2 µg/dL in 2001–2002.

Depression is a significant concern that can adversely affect the well-being of students. In 2008, 8 percent of adolescents aged 12–17 years had at least one major depressive disorder (MDE). The rate for the occurrences was lowest for ages 12–13 (5 percent), with ages 14–15 next (8 percent), and the highest rates for those ages 16–17 (11 percent). Females had nearly three times the rate of depression (12 percent) than males (4 percent). Only 40 percent of adolescent females and 38 percent of adolescent males received treatment for their depression.

For the first time in decades, the infant mortality rate decreased in 2007 to 6.75 per 1,000 live births. Infant mortality dropped from 6.89 in 2000 to 6.75 in 2007. (Both rates are per 1,000 live births.) Low birth weight is the primary causative factor for infant mortality. Children born to married mothers are less likely to experience low birth weight. For example, in 2002, 7 percent of infants born to married mothers were of low birth weight, compared with 10 percent to unmarried mothers. In the same year, the mortality rate for infants born to married mothers was 5 per 1,000 live births, compared with 10 per 1,000 live births for infants born to unmarried mothers.

Another positive health change is the decline in deaths from firearm injuries among adolescents between 1994 and 2007. The largest decrease in deaths from firearm injuries was among black and Hispanic males (Federal Interagency Forum on Child and Family Statistics 2011).

Drug Usage

In general, tobacco, alcohol, and drug use has declined between 1999 and 2009. According to information ascertained from the Youth Risk Behavior Survey (YRBS) for students grades 9–12 in 2009, 46.3 percent of students had tried cigarette smoking; this represented a decrease from 70.1 percent in 1999. In 2009, 8.9 percent of students had used smokeless tobacco on at least one day during the thirty days before the survey. In the case of alcohol usage, 72.5 percent of students had at least one alcoholic drink at some point in their lives, and 24 percent had five or more drinks in a row on at least one day during the thirty days prior to the survey. Other drug related behaviors reported in the YRBS indicated that at some point in their life 36.8 percent of adolescents had used marijuana, 2.8 percent had used some form of cocaine, 11.7 percent had sniffed glue or other inhaled substances, 4.1 percent had used methamphetamines, and 3.3 percent used steroids (pills or shots) without a doctor's prescription. All of the percentages represented the same or decreased usage of the various substances (YRBSS 2009).

Politics and Health Education

The No Child Left Behind Act of 2001 (NCLB) was a controversial United States federal law. The law seeks to improve the performance of the primary and secondary schools by increasing the standards of accountability for states, school districts, and individual schools. The law was based on the belief that high expectations and setting of goals will result in success for all students. The Act required "highly qualified" teachers to teach in the schools. A highly qualified teacher was one who has fulfilled state certification and licensing requirements, obtained at least a bachelor's degree, and demonstrated subject matter expertise. Additionally, the Act required all public schools to assess annually for math and reading skills in grades 3 to 8 and at least once during high school. Also, by the end of the 2007–2008 school year, testing in science was to be conducted once during grades 3 to 8 and once in grades 10 to 11.

Although the Act may have increased accountability for the schools and increased federal funding for education, it totally ignored health and physical education as significant contributors not only to enhancing the lives of students but also to improving standardized test scores. In an attempt to provide what President Barack Obama has called a "world class education," and to overcome some of the criticisms expressed concerning the No

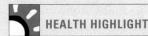

- **74,494,000 children** live in the United States
- **Every 8* seconds** a high school student drops out
- **Every 34 seconds** a baby is born into poverty
- **Every minute** a baby is born to a teen mother
- **Every 4 minutes** a child is arrested for a drug offense

- **Every 8 minutes** a child is arrested for a violent crime
- **Every 45 minutes** a child/teen dies from an accident
- **Every 3 hours** a child/teen is killed by a firearm
- **Every 5 hours** a child/teen commits suicide
- **Every 5 hours** a child is killed by abuse or neglect

- **36.4 percent** of two-year olds are not fully immunized
- **70 percent** of 8th graders in public school are not reading at their grade level

* Based on calculation per school day (180 days of seven hours each)

Source: Children's Defense Fund, State of America's Children® 2011. Available at www.childrensdefense.org/soac. Used by permission.

Child Left Behind legislation, the Reauthorization of the Elementary and Secondary Education Act (ESEA) was passed in 2011. The priorities of the ESEA are centered around four areas: (1) Improving teacher and principal effectiveness to ensure that every classroom has a great teacher and every school has a great leader; (2) providing information to families to help them evaluate and improve their children's schools, and to educators to help them improve their students' learning; (3) Implementing college- and career-ready standards and developing improved assessments aligned with those standards; and (4) Improving student learning and achievement in America's lowest-performing schools by providing intensive support and effective interventions (ESEA 2011).

These four priorities seem to advance the rationale the Coordinated School Health Model advocates. Although not directly stated, a component of the ECSA supports the concept of providing safe schools for students to learn in and to enhance the health of students through classroom and community support while providing greater opportunities to engage families in their children's education. Although the Coordinated School Health Model seems to provide a very viable model for these goals to be attained, policymakers must recognize that what they are advocating for is what health education seeks to provide and clearly state that health education has a significant role in promoting the goals for quality education.

Health improvement and school improvement are interrelated and critical to each other. Some people will always put forth the argument that the basics of reading, science, and math are the path to success. However, if health education is not proactively addressed, the schools will have to deal with health-related problems when they become a crisis (Health Is Academic 2004). To help our children realize their true potential, we must first make sure they are truly prepared to meet the challenges not only of achievement testing but also of preparation for life. The political

establishment must do what is right for our students and emphasize the need for health education as an essential part of students' total education.

School-Based Health Centers—The School Nurse

School-based health centers (SBHCs) began in the 1970s as a result of the increasing number of students who needed better access to health care directed to their individual needs. SBHCs operate in school and complete health evaluations, diagnoses, and treatment of a variety of health needs. Most SBHCs provide preventive care, health assessments, treatment of acute illness, screenings, immunizations, and counseling. The number of SBHCs has grown dramatically in the past twenty years. There are now over 1,400 SBHCs in forty-five states. SBHCs are commonly sponsored by community health organizations, including hospitals, local health departments, community health centers, academic medical centers, and nonprofit organizations (National Assembly on School-based Health Care 2005).

Even if SBHCs are not available on a broad scale, schools should have access to a school nurse. Unfortunately, many school districts have been forced to cut back or underdevelop the role of the school nurse by assigning one nurse responsibility for several schools. This does not allow nurses sufficient time in a given school to completely develop the school health service. Even worse, in some communities school health services are performed by parents, school secretaries, or some other inadequately trained person.

The services provided by school nurses are extremely important to children's welfare. Most frequently, nurses provide direct care to sick or injured children. Important functions are gathering information through assessment of the children, recordkeeping, and routine assessments. These assessments should help provide for appropriate follow-up care and some type of interpretation to the parent.

Nurses are excellent resources. They should be included on any health education curriculum planning committee and should be involved in planning the education of special populations. Nurses have become increasingly involved in planning the educational programs of handicapped children. Nurses can assist these children in becoming self-sufficient in the classroom and help alleviate the fears and concerns of the teachers. Finally, the nurse should ensure that emergency procedures for injuries, accidents, and sickness are developed because of legal concerns that surround giving aid in any of these situations. The nurse can help ensure proper care by helping to develop guidelines and workshops for teachers, aides, and office personnel in emergency procedures.

Chapter In Review

Summary

- *Health* is defined as an integrated method of functioning that is oriented toward maximizing personal potential.
- *Wellness* implies that individuals engage in attitudes and behaviors that enhance quality of life and maximize personal potential.
- Wellness consists of six components: spiritual, social, emotional, intellectual, physical, and environmental.
- To achieve wellness, students must feel they can control their lives (locus of control) and believe in their ability to accomplish a specific task or behavior (self-efficacy).
- Self-esteem, self-confidence, and a sense that one can achieve success are key to optimal learning.
- Health promotion is the aggregate of all purposeful activities designed to improve personal and public health through a combination of strategies, including health education, health protection measures, health enhancement, and health maintenance.
- Health education is the process of developing and providing planned experiences to supply information, change attitudes, and influence behavior.
- To accomplish its goals, health education must be sequential, planned, comprehensive, and taught by qualified teachers.
- Quality health education includes providing a decision-making model that helps students make informed, appropriate decisions concerning their health.
- Factual information does not ensure behavioral change.
- Students must be given opportunities to personalize the information they learn so that they can formulate attitudes as precursors to behavior.
- Significant categories of risk behaviors: behaviors that may result in unintentional and intentional injuries; tobacco use; alcohol and other drug use; sexual behaviors that result in HIV infections, other STIs, and unintended pregnancy; unhealthy dietary behaviors; and inadequate physical activity.
- A comprehensive school health education program has a planned, sequential K through 12 program; addresses a range of categorical health problems and issues; helps students develop skills to avoid negative behaviors; provides for a prescribed amount of time at each grade level; is managed and coordinated by a trained professional; contains instruction from teachers who are trained to teach health; involves parents and health professionals; and includes periodic evaluation, updating, and improvement.

- Several national initiatives have created support for a coordinated school health program.
- The YRBSS is an excellent source of information that helps identify the need for a comprehensive school health education curriculum and coordinated health program.
- Problems that indicate the need for comprehensive health education include child and adolescent accident rates, transmission of HIV and other STIs, smoking, lack of activity, poor nutrition, alcohol and drug use, problem pregnancies, suicides, and chronic diseases.
- An effective coordinated school health program has eight components: healthful school environment; school health instruction; school health services; physical education; nutrition and food services; school-based counseling (psychological and social services); schoolsite health promotion; and school, family, and community health promotion partnerships.
- The School Health Policies and Programs Study (SHPPS) is a national survey conducted by the Centers for Disease Control and Prevention. The study assesses the characteristics of school health at the state and district levels and across elementary, middle, and high school classrooms.
- SHPPS found that there is more emphasis on health education, more emphasis on the training of teachers, greater collaboration among state and school health education staffs and outside agencies, and more policies that enhance the quality of health education requirements.
- Consideration of the well-being of children within the family structure includes an examination of economic security, general health (physical, mental, emotional), and risk education.
- Federal and state policies and politics have a significant impact on health education programs.
- A school-based health center can be an important component of an effective school health program.

Discussion Questions

1. Discuss the various definitions of health and the implications of the definitions.
2. Define the term *wellness*; discuss the implications of the different components of wellness.

3. What is the difference between health promotion and health education?

4. How would you justify the need for health education in the elementary school?

5. What are some of the initiatives that support the need for health education?

6. Why is prevention the best approach to affecting the quality of life?

7. Why is self-responsibility so important to develop when teaching health?

8. Discuss why the YRBSS is an important tool for all classroom teachers as well as health educators.

9. What are the various components of a coordinated school health program, and why are they important?

10. How can the classroom teacher aid in the development of a healthy school environment?

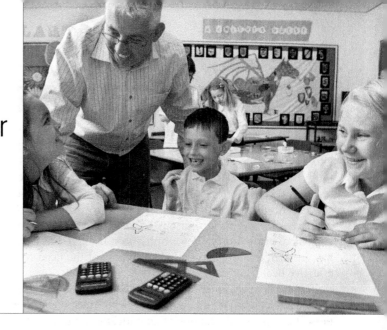

2 The Role of the Teacher in Coordinated School Health Programs

Valued Outcomes

After completion of this chapter, you should be able to:

- Discuss the academic and personal qualifications of an effective health educator.

- Describe how a teacher of health has an opportunity to be a significant model in students' lives.

- Explain the unique challenges health educators face.

- Explain the barriers that make health instruction more difficult to teach than other subjects.

- Discuss the minimum competencies needed by a health educator.

- Describe the legal liability associated with teaching.

- Discuss how the educator can work with other members of the school staff to enhance the wellness of each student.

Reflections

Because of their important status as role models for children and their responsibilities *in loco parentis* (in the place of parents), teachers are expected to live up to higher social standards and expectations than people in other occupations. As you read through this chapter, reflect on your personal qualities relative to the material being discussed. Are there areas in which you could improve? Is it fair to ask teachers to measure up to some of the qualities expected by parents and other people? Are the legal and ethical responsibilities of teaching fair? How will you ensure that your classroom is free of bias and discrimination?

Health educators spend much of their time working with people and must be comfortable working with both individuals and groups. They need to be good communicators and comfortable speaking in public as they may need to teach classes or give presentations. Health educators often work with diverse populations, so they must be sensitive to cultural differences and open to working with people of varied backgrounds. Health educators often create new programs or materials, so they should be creative and skilled writers.

—*United States Department of Labor, Bureau of Labor Statistics (2011)*

The Challenge of Health Education

Health education professionals and professional organizations have been working for more than twenty years to improve the preparation and competency of health educators. Health education has become a focal point during the last few years as our nation has worked toward reaching specific health goals (such as the *Healthy People 2020* objectives for the nation, discussed in Chapter 1) for the citizens of our country. The emphasis on health education has, in turn, led to an increased awareness of the need for effective health educators.

To be effective, an educator must concentrate not only on academic preparation, but also on personal qualifications. Personal qualifications of an educator are important because of the significance of and emphasis on the teacher's behavior and attitudes.

Teaching health is unlike teaching any other topic in the curriculum. For example, in other classes the teacher may get immediate feedback from the students regarding the learning of a concept. However, in health education the teacher may never know whether a student actually applies a health concept in his or her life because the opportunity to apply that concept may not surface until several years later. Furthermore, the methodology used in health education is unlike other subject areas in that it demands an open, accepting environment in the classroom during instruction.

A philosophy that should govern every teacher is the following: "Every teacher is a health teacher"; that is, every teacher in the school is a health teacher, regardless of what discipline he or she is actually teaching. This implies that, regardless of the subject matter you happen to be teaching, you are making an impact on your students through your behavior. Health education may be the only subject matter in which the teacher must embody the content. You can teach as much by what you do as what you say in the health classroom; you as a teacher are on display before your students, and you have the opportunity to portray a positive health image through your behavior. For example, if the students observe you eating a good diet in the lunchroom, they will see that the healthy diet aspect of health is important to you. Therefore, they are more likely to adopt the same value.

Another challenge facing today's classroom teacher is that most schools are becoming increasingly diverse. Teachers want their students to be able to learn in an environment that is free from bias and discrimination, but the reality is that we live in a world in which racism and other forms of bias continue to affect us. To better address diversity and encourage a successful learning environment, the Institute for Educational Leadership (2011) recommends focusing on these areas:

- Cultural factors must be incorporated into school curricula, including historical and present treatment of racial and ethnically diverse groups. Educators must also reflect cultural sensitivity in their interactions with students, parents, colleagues, and community members.

- School policies and practices should be reviewed for discriminatory language and action taken to eliminate such language and policies.

- Develop political action committees and support legislators who actively support the diverse population in our state and nation.

- Formulate programs and activities to ensure that all school personnel are culturally sensitive through culturally specific inservice training; assessment and modification of inservice training; and inclusion of cultural sensitivity as part of teacher administrator performance evaluations.

- Use available valid research on cultural sensitivity and apply it effectively in schools.

Elementary school children are very impressionable, and you can teach skills and influence behavior positively through your own behavior and attitudes. You have an excellent opportunity to become a good health role model by practicing safe and healthy habits.

You must emphasize to students that they cannot become healthy passively. Involving them in active learning opportunities, in which they are allowed to clarify their values and taught how to make wise decisions, will personalize their health education. Your students will then be better able to make their own responsible choices for healthful behavior.

■ Barriers to Successful Health Teaching

Most schools and school districts face challenges when trying to implement and teach programs such as a new health education program. Health educators will face the emphasis on standardized test scores, the narrowing of the school's focus on curriculum, and limited budgets for resources to teach health education (Wechsler, Howell, et al. 2004).

For example, elementary education majors in most colleges receive very little instruction in health content and in methodology that specifically relates to health instruction. Because the elementary teacher must teach many subjects, most college programs emphasize methods and materials instead of specific subject areas. This puts the elementary teacher at a distinct disadvantage because teaching health requires a different methodology from other subjects. Teaching content alone is not sufficient in health education.

Students may be able to pass a paper-and-pencil test on health knowledge, but this does not ensure that they will put that knowledge into practice. This phenomenon, known as cognitive dissonance, concerns the discrepancy between personal health knowledge and general health behavior. Consider: it is common knowledge that wearing safety belts in cars provides significant protection, yet a number of Americans do not wear them regularly.

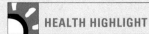

HEALTH HIGHLIGHT | **State Teaching Standards and Qualifications**

Each state department of education has its own standards and qualifications for teachers. Many states delineate specific abilities that health educators should possess in order to be able to teach health education effectively; one of these states is California. The *Subject Matter Abilities Applicable to the Content Domains in Health Science* for the California Department of Education are included here as a sample of state health education standards. You should of course pay close attention to the standards that are given in the state in which you intend to teach.

1. Candidates apply knowledge of behavioral and scientific principles to the content area of health science/health education and apply health-related skills across multiple health topics. They demonstrate problem-solving and critical-thinking skills that develop confidence in the decision making process and promote healthy behaviors.

2. Candidates recognize differences in individual growth and development and variation in culture and family life. They assess individual and community needs for health education by interpreting health related data about social and cultural environments. They differentiate between health education practices that are grounded on sound scientific research and those that are not research based. They identify opportunities for collaboration among health educators in all settings, including school and community health professions. They apply laws, regulations, and policies affecting school health education.

3. Candidates use their analytical skills to identify behaviors that enhance and/or compromise personal health and well-being and recognize the short-term and long-term effects of the lifestyle choices and habits of individuals. They apply a variety of risk assessment skills and prevention strategies to health related issues. They evaluate sources of health-related information and differentiate between reliable and unreliable sources.

4. Candidates demonstrate effective communication and advocacy skills as they relate to personal, family, and community health and health education needs. They understand the role of communication in interpersonal relationships and identify strategies that encourage appropriate expression. They emphasize the importance of the communication process, including listening, assertiveness, and refusal skills.

Source: California Commission on Teacher Credentialing (revised) 2010. *Health Science Teacher Preparation in California: Standards of Quality and Effectiveness for Subject Matter Programs: A Handbook for Teacher Educators and Program Reviewers.* (Available at www.ctc.ca.gov/educator-prep/standards/SSMP-Handbook-Health.pdf.)

Therefore, health instruction requires an active involvement of the student in the learning process; you must give the student opportunities to experience situations (even though they may be simulated) in which they focus their values and make decisions regarding health behavior. Again, this teaching process is no guarantee that every student will make a healthy decision in each case, but it will help the student learn the concept being taught as well as apply the concept to his or her lifestyle.

Health instruction further demands the inclusion of teaching methodologies that enable the student to consider a healthy behavior valuable enough to incorporate into his or her lifestyle. To overcome these specific barriers to health education, take as many courses as you can that emphasize health content and health instruction. (For a more detailed discussion of value-based instruction, see Chapter 4.)

Effective health instruction, ironically, is hindered by the tremendous wealth of health information currently available. Health education is by its nature interdisciplinary in that it borrows not only from educational theory but also from many social sciences, such as psychology and sociology, as well as from physical science, biology, and even religion. It is difficult enough for a health education specialist to stay current in health, much less the elementary teacher, who must master several other subject areas.

Health information is changing constantly—the results of new studies related to health information appear virtually every day. The teacher has an obligation to follow these new developments. One way to do so is to attend educational seminars and workshops.

Further, some health information is conflicting; two studies on the same health topic might reach different conclusions. Some physicians consider megadoses of vitamin C to be the answer to preventing colds; other physicians disagree. Such disagreements between authorities cause a dilemma for the conscientious teacher who wishes to present *all* the information. Also, the conflicting information can be confusing for the student who is trying to make a wise, informed decision.

Another problem surfaces when teachers must deal with information that is inconclusive. For example, much information about nutrition appears contradictory. Normally, teachers think that to command the respect of students, they need to know everything, but this is impossible in situations where even the authorities have not discovered all the answers.

Another barrier to effective health instruction is that so many issues in health education are controversial. Teachers who handle controversial issues risk offending students and/or parents. Even some subjects that would not appear controversial, such as nutrition, might offer opportunities to offend some groups. If you teach that servings of meat are recommended for a balanced diet, you may risk offending vegetarians. Further, controversial topics tend to polarize students. The more controversial the topic, the more emotional the students become about the issue. When this occurs, there is a greater likelihood of dissension and ill feeling among the students. Such dissension can disrupt the optimal teaching/learning environment that is necessary in health instruction.

Many times, as an instructor, you will be battling against students' negative image of health and health education. Health educators are sometimes viewed as "warriors against pleasure," meaning that students think of health educators as those who tell them to quit doing what they like to do, such as eating desserts, and to do what they don't like to do, such as exercising. This may translate into negative feelings that the teacher must overcome, especially when the student perceives that the teacher's ideas conflict with those of parents or the peer group. Also, some students come into the health education classroom with preconceived notions, habits, and misconceptions about health information. This misinformation might have come from the home, media, older siblings, or peers. Teachers should be very knowledgeable of their students' backgrounds and subcultural perspectives. This understanding is critical in understanding a student's behavior and knowing what will motivate a student.

This makes the job of the educator doubly difficult because she or he not only must provide the correct information, but also may be spending much of the time in the classroom dispelling many myths that the students bring with them.

Finally, some administrators place a low priority on health education by allowing other activities to substitute for health instruction or by not placing health education in the curriculum at all. One way to overcome this problem is to help other teachers integrate health education with the other main subjects in the curriculum. There are many ways to integrate health into content and activities at the elementary level. Figuring one's heart rate can be integrated into mathematics. For language arts, the students can read a story about a health topic. The students can do many experiments in health class that are related to science. Many of the activities presented in the Strategies chapters in this book can be integrated into other subject areas in this way. Look for this icon ◯, which highlights activities that can be readily integrated into math, science, language arts, social studies, or art.

Professional Preparation

Continuing education and training for teachers is critical for professional development and the implementation of effective school health education. Health education professional development should focus on strategies that actively engage students and help them master important health information and skills (Brener, McManus, et al. 2009). In an effort to strengthen the professional preparation of health educators, health education was formally joined with the National Council for Accreditation of Teacher Education (NCATE) in 1986. The purpose for this alliance was to establish an accreditation process for teacher training programs. It involved (1) assessment of the competencies for health educators, (2) the inclusion of the recognized content areas of comprehensive school health instruction, and (3) key professional issues relative to health education in a school setting. These three components are included in the criteria for accreditation standards for health education. These standards provide university health education teacher training programs with guidance in planning, implementing, and evaluating their professional preparation programs. Further, the National Transition Task Force on Accreditation in Health Education, sponsored by the Society for Public Health Education and the American Association for Health Education, has developed a unified accreditation process for professional preparation in health education (National Transition Task Force on Accreditation in Health Education 2004). Additionally, one of the priorities of ESEA is to improve teacher effectiveness. This professional preparation should include all teachers, including teachers of health education.

School health education has been criticized as being ineffective. This is largely the result of poor teacher preparation. Ideally, a preschool or elementary school health teacher should be a specialist, but this is not feasible when so many subjects must be taught. Therefore, elementary school teachers are forced to teach subjects such as health with less professional preparation than their secondary school colleagues. Many states still allow teachers who have dual certification in health and physical education to teach health at the secondary level and allow those who have a general elementary certification to teach health at the elementary level.

There are several reasons for recommending that a teacher of health be a certified specialist. Health is different from other subjects in that the content comes from a variety of sources and is not limited to one distinct discipline (as discussed previously). Also, the behavioral outcomes desired of the student in a health class differ remarkably from those of other subjects. Because these outcomes are not easily measured, a health teacher should have specific training in making empirical observations that indicate whether the desired outcomes are being acquired.

Even when a teacher is dually prepared—say, in health and physical education—the health portion is typically slighted in favor of the physical education portion. The reduced amount of higher education coursework in this dual major hinders effective teacher preparation.

Coursework dealing with the personal health of the individual is also desirable. In taking this course, prospective teachers learn more about their own personal health behavior. Further, coursework in first aid and emergency skills is very helpful.

The National Task Force on the Preparation and Practice of Health Educators, composed of professionals from several national organizations with an interest in health education, has been working since 1978 to develop a framework of minimum competencies that should be required of health educators. These competencies are included in the document *A Framework for the Development of Competency-Based Curricula for Entry-Level Health Educators* (later revised and retitled *A Competency-Based Curriculum Framework for the Professional Preparation of Entry-Level Health Educators*—National Task Force on the Preparation and Practice of Health Educators 1988) and are intended to guide certifying institutions in the professional preparation of students intending to teach health. This curriculum was developed with a generic health educator in mind, that is, an individual who might be teaching health in a variety of settings, including the school classroom. Eventually, NCATE accreditation of teacher credential programs in health will require the use of the guidelines specified in this framework.

As an outgrowth of the work of this task force, the National Commission for Health Education Credentialing (NCHEC) was formed to oversee the professional credentialing process for health educators. The elected volunteers that serve as the directors and commissioners of the NCHEC help develop and administer a national competency-based examination; develop standards for professional preparation; and promote professional development through continuing education for health education professionals (National Commission for Health Education Credentialing 2008).

Credentialing refers to the licensing of those who have met or exceeded established standards. Credentialing might come in the form of certification, registration, or licensure of individuals, or accreditation of organizations. The health education profession uses certification as the method of individual credentialing for the profession. Certification is the process by which a nongovernmental agency or association grants recognition to an individual who has met predetermined qualifications specified by the agency or association. Typical qualifications include the following:

- Graduation from an accredited or approved program
- Acceptable performance on a qualifying examination or series of examinations

It differs from state and local certifications and registries in that the requirements do not vary from one locale to another. National certification benefits practitioners and the public in that it

- Establishes a national standard.
- Attests to the individual's knowledge and skills.
- Assists employers in identifying qualified health education practitioners.
- Promotes a sense of pride and accomplishment.
- Promotes continued professional development. (National Commission for Health Education Credentialing 2011)

Certification is granted through a process of both meeting basic academic eligibility requirements and receiving a passing score on the certified health education specialist national examination. The certification exam itself consists of questions developed around responsibilities of health educators (National Commission for Health Education Credentialing 2002). Students can find detailed information about required responsibilities and competencies for health educators at www.nchec.org.

As discussed earlier, a teacher's preparation does not end upon receipt of a diploma and teaching certificate. You can continue to educate yourself by taking graduate courses in specific content areas or in advanced teaching methods; by joining local, state, regional, and national health education professional organizations; and by attending professional health conferences. Staying current also requires reading up-to-date textbooks, journals, and other health education publications. Finally, in-service workshops that deal with health-related topics are extremely valuable. To continue professional development beyond undergraduate training, many school health educators join one of the following professional associations:

- American Association for Health Education (AAHE), www.aahperd.org/aahe, under the umbrella of the American Alliance for Health, Physical Education, Recreation and Dance (AAHPERD). Its current emphasis includes health professionals in several types of work environments, such as K through 12 school, university, hospital, business and industry, and community.
- American School Health Association (ASHA), www.ashaweb.org. This professional organization emphasizes all areas of school health, including services and environment as well as education; membership includes health educators as well as school nurses, physicians, dentists, and dental hygienists.
- Society for Public Health Education (SOPHE), www.sophe.org. This professional association is made up of a diverse membership of health education professionals and students. Its primary focus is on public health education.

Becoming a Quality Health Teacher

There are many influences on a child, such as the media and peer pressure, that may be detrimental. Teachers should be positive role models, because educators are an important factor in students' health behavior development. Students desire positive role models who are honest, sincere, energetic, knowledgeable, and caring.

Stay Motivated. If you hope to motivate your students to work hard, your own efforts should reflect your commitment to hard work. Motivation for teachers includes finding ways to get students to do things they might not want to do on their own. Students need to

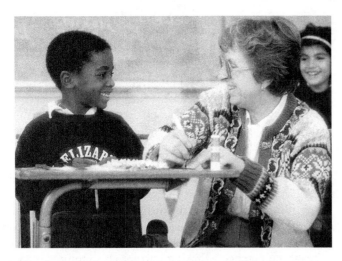

A teacher's task is to motivate students to want to learn.

do more than "know" health—get them to put into action what they know. Use motivating techniques to discover new ways to persuade youngsters to act in healthy ways. If students are motivated about the subject, we can teach them the skills they'll need to make healthy decisions and to act in healthy ways. No small part of our task as teachers is to motivate them beyond apathy. The problem lies in fostering the kind of attitude that includes sacrifice and discipline, both among the students and among ourselves.

There is probably no phase of teaching health that is more grossly misunderstood by teachers than the area of motivation. Teachers tend to be highly motivated individuals, and they sometimes have trouble understanding or dealing with students who do not share equally their enthusiasm and love for education or healthy behaviors.

You cannot motivate students who feel no sense of responsibility or commitment to you or your program. Your task, then, is obvious—motivate your students to want to learn and to want to be healthy. Students will more likely be motivated when they know you care enough about them to work as hard as you can to try to improve their skills.

Many young people are simply waiting for someone to guide them and care about them, and those are the students that we have to find and motivate to act in healthy ways. If we accept as true that none of them will accept the challenge of excelling, we're doing them a grave disservice—we're prejudging them toward the mediocrity we want them to avoid. Not all young people are selfish and apathetic; many have not had the opportunity to challenge themselves to a higher purpose.

One cannot overstate or overestimate the effect of motivation (or lack of motivation) on the level of intensity of a student's performance.

Be Organized. Students, especially young students, want and need the kind of guidance, leadership, and professionalism that is evidenced in teachers' efforts to organize their classes. Practice organization and attention to detail. Convey your concern for your program to your students in terms more vivid than you could ever express in words.

Good organization is a habit. Anyone can become more organized by making lists of tasks to accomplish and assigning priorities to those that are most important. Then, approximate the amount of time needed for each task, and try to work through the list in order of priority.

Be Consistent in Your Relations with Your Students. Being consistent doesn't mean that you have to treat all students alike. Students are not alike, and you should not treat them as though they were. Their motivations as well as their personalities vary widely. Some students thrive on praise and compliments, whereas others treat a compliment as a signal that it is all right to quit working in class. Be aware of the differences in your students, and learn what motivates them best.

Students have the right to fair and equitable treatment, attention, and discipline, regardless of skin color, ethnicity, sex, or physical abilities.

Avoid Forming Hasty (or Permanent) Negative Opinions of Students. When we pay attention to the teacher's lounge gossip about students who we are going to have in class, it's all too easy to form a hasty opinion. When we prejudge, the student never has a chance. Once we label a student, he or she tends to live up (or down) to that level of expectation.

Never Be Too Busy to Listen to Your Students. Communication is a two-way street. Students are expecting—or demanding through various forms of behavior—that teachers be concerned about them as human beings as well as students. When a student has a problem, the teacher should be willing to give the student a chance to talk it out. Sometimes all a youngster needs is an adult to give a pat on the back that says, "I care," and to listen when the youngster needs to talk. Genuine communication does not always require words; it grows out of a mutual sense of concern for others.

Show Care and Concern to Your Students. Teachers may view their teaching as just a job, but students need guidance and a sense of belonging that grows out of a teacher's personal and professional behavior toward his or her students. Many teachers prefer not to become involved in the personal lives of their students. Increasingly, however, teachers are being required to deal with problems in students' personal lives that affect their in-class performance.

Be a Success Yourself. To paraphrase Thomas Edison, success, like genius, is 1 percent inspiration and 99 percent perspiration. Successful people invest in themselves. They go to seminars, read a lot, and consult with others. They are natural and eager learners. This doesn't necessarily mean they go back to school, but they believe there is something to be learned from every encounter that they have with other people and their ideas. Successful people believe they're in control of their own lives (internal locus of control) and their fates. They know that effort means more than luck. Good luck comes from hard work. A surprising number of opportunities seem to open up for those people who work hardest at putting themselves on a successful path.

Successful people have self-confidence. They believe they can overcome obstacles.

Be Positive. A key ingredient of success is the ability to eliminate from your own environment things that tend to put you in a negative or unresourceful state, while installing positive ones in yourself and in others. Positive thinking and unswerving dedication to making a dream a reality will provide the incentive to carry on through whatever hard times and negativism on the part of others lie in your path. Change your vocabulary. Instead of "Why don't they do something about it?" make it "I know what I'm going to do." Expect, anticipate, and welcome change. Change is normal and inevitable. With every change there is the unfamiliar and the unexpected. Risk it!

Use positive self-talk on a daily basis. Think uplifting thoughts. This is especially true regarding your students.

Seek Role Models. Benefit from others—if you think about why you are the way you are, chances are it has a lot to do with trying to be like someone you admired. Teachers usually have a teacher in their past who inspired them to become teachers. Goad yourself to meet new challenges, set new goals, and then top your previous behavior so you can perhaps be a role model for others.

Set Goals. Another key to success is knowing what you want. People's abilities to fully tap their resources are directly affected by their goals. Before you can operate efficiently, you must develop specific goals. Outline your goals clearly. Concrete goals are easily understood by you and by your students. Goals don't have to be elaborate. Set goals and develop a plan to achieve those goals.

Work Hard. The road to success is never easy. To be a success, you have to work. This is not popular advice, but work and achievement are irrevocably linked.

Stay Mentally Fresh. No matter how well you are doing what you are doing, you can do it better by exposing yourself to interests and ideas outside your immediate, day-to-day activities. These ideas will spark your imagination and give you ideas you can use in your own work. Try using exercise to simultaneously stay mentally fresh and get physically healthy.

The Teacher as Part of the Health Team

Legal Responsibilities of the Teacher

Because we live in a litigious society, one major concern of today's teacher is liability. Negligence can be charged when children are under your care and supervision, such as in the classroom, on the playground, and entering or departing buses. You are considered *in loco parentis* when a child is under your supervision. Your primary responsibility is to act responsibly to prevent injury to students. You should be well aware of first-aid and emergency procedures to care for a student in your charge without aggravating an existing injury or illness.

You should follow your school system's procedure for filing a report for each accident. Each school should provide in-service preparation of faculty for preventing and handling accidents, and each school should have an active safety program. (Safety procedures and accident reports are discussed in Chapter 19.) Further, be sure to heed Title VII of the Civil Rights Act when interacting with students. The Act prohibits discriminating on the basis of race or color, religion, sex, and national origin (including membership in a Native American tribe). It also prohibits retaliating against a student who asserts his or her rights under the law. Also, the Americans with Disabilities Act (ADA) prohibits discriminating against people with disabilities. You can read the text of these laws at www.eeoc. gov/policy/laws.html.

The State of Minnesota has developed a good example of the legal responsibilities for teachers, including specific rules regarding teachers' responsibilities and standards of conduct. These include responsibilities related to non-discrimination, health and safety, dealing with confidential student information, delivering reasonable discipline, not taking advantage of professional relationships (with students, parents, or colleagues), and avoiding malicious statements about students or colleagues. (See the Minnesota Rules 2011, part 8700.7500, published by the Office of the Revisor of Statutes).

Working with Students

One of the teacher's responsibilities is to counsel students in health-related matters. Counseling should be straightforward and free of moral judgment, preaching, or scare tactics. In the role of counselor, you must have good listening skills and communication skills. Sometimes it is difficult to get to the heart of the problem; these skills will help you offer sound advice. Also, you need to show genuine sympathy toward a student's problem.

No matter how concerned you are about a student's problem, you must recognize the limitations of your ability to help. Do not try to diagnose or assign blame for a health problem. Either of these actions can lead to legal problems. If you perceive that a student is having problems, it is best to record your observations, without

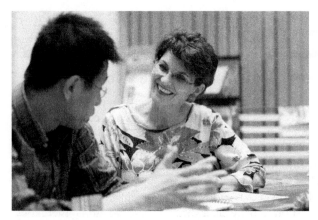

Health educators can keep other professionals informed of health matters.

personal opinions, and discuss them with an administrator. The student may require additional guidance beyond the initial crisis counseling you can supply. Make sure you are familiar with available services in the school or community so you can refer the student to the most appropriate one. Most teachers are not professionally trained in counseling, nor are they expected to replace those who are.

▪ Working with Parents

Always notify a student's parents when an illness or serious deviation from normal health occurs. Follow school policy when notifying parents. Some schools require teachers to contact parents through the administrative offices. A good policy is to ensure that a member of the school administration is present at any parent–teacher conference. The third party can clear up any confusion in communication and can serve as an arbitrator in case of misunderstanding. Share your observations without including personal opinions or diagnoses. Explain to the parents the significance of the issue of concern, and encourage them to obtain needed care for the child. If a parent asks for guidance in seeking care, refer the person to the proper agency or individual. Be sure to take an active role in following up on any case reported to parents.

Health educators can proactively involve parents in the health education of their children by sending information home in a newsletter and designing activities in which the parents help the children.

▪ Working with Other Teachers and the School Administration

A major responsibility of the health teacher is to keep other teachers and the administrators informed of health matters related to the community and students. This information will help other faculty members and the administration to understand the students and to recognize the continuing need for health education in the school.

You can represent the school on health-related committees of teacher–parent and community organizations. You can also help other faculty and administrators become aware of the environmental conditions in the school that might be unhealthy to the students, staff, and faculty. You should also attempt to become involved in textbook selection committees. Look for sound, up-to-date content, but beware of textbooks that propagate stereotypes.

A primary duty of the health educator is to plan the health education curriculum and make recommendations to the administration regarding the health education program within the school. You can help interpret and implement any state requirement for the health curriculum. Also, make suggestions concerning the health service program and health environment.

You also must work closely with the school administration when notifying parents about a child's health, referring parents to appropriate health resources, and following up on student cases. You should keep the administration informed about a child's progress in school after a child returns from an illness.

▪ Working with the School or Clinic Nurse

Because you daily observe each child in your class, you can help the school nurse understand the health behavior of students. You can also assist the nurse in various aspects of the screening program—by preliminary screening in the classroom, by preparing students for screening tests to reduce their anxiety, and by referring students who are in particular need of screening. Teachers and nurses can participate in in-service workshops for the other faculty members. Finally, teachers who are properly trained can complement the school's emergency care program by offering their services when needed.

▪ Working with Outside Agencies

One of your objectives should be to promote health education and awareness in the community. You can help volunteer organizations educate the community in health matters. Many of these agencies, such as the American Heart Association and American Dental Association, have health curricula and need help to implement their programs in the schools. Through this cooperation, you can learn about other health professionals in your community and acquaint yourself with the services these agencies offer to students. Determine which agencies will provide services for paying students and which agencies will provide services for students for a reduced or waived fee. You should also become involved with the local public health department and cooperate with department staff members in providing services to the students and community.

Finally, in this time of budget cuts and termination of health programs, you are strongly urged to become active in lobbying for health services and programs. Work with local teacher groups to educate legislators about health matters.

Chapter In Review

Summary

- The nation's emphasis on health education has, in turn, led to a need for effective educators.

- An effective educator must concentrate on academic preparation and personal qualifications.

- Teaching health is different from teaching other disciplines in the curriculum.

- Teachers must be aware that they are modeling health behavior to students through their own lifestyles.

- Educators who model good health behavior have a positive impact on their students.

- There are several barriers to successfully implementing health education.

- There are several unique challenges to teaching health education.

- Teachers can overcome these hindrances by keeping their knowledge of health current, learning how to present controversial information in the classroom, and helping administrators see how health education can be integrated with other required subjects.

- Teamwork with parents, the school nurse, the school physician, administrators, community organizations, and students is the key to a successful school health program.

- As part of the team, the teacher is aware of his or her legal responsibilities, observes each student for any deviation from normal health, reports to the proper authority within the schoolm, and is available to refer the student and parent to the appropriate community resource or to counsel the student and/or parent concerning the child's health.

Discussion Questions

1. Describe the challenges in the role of the health teacher.

2. How does health education differ from instruction in other subject areas?

3. Discuss the interdisciplinary nature of health as a barrier to implementing good health instruction.

4. Describe the role of the NCHEC in promoting the health education profession.

5. How can a teacher be a positive role model in health behavior to the students?

6. List the characteristics and actions that will help you become a quality educator.

7. Discuss the ways in which a teacher can work with other teachers to improve the coordinated school health program.

8. Why should an administrator be present at any parent–teacher conference?

9. Discuss how a teacher can involve parents in their child's health education.

Critical Thinking Questions

1. What do you consider to be the greatest challenge for today's health educator?

2. How would you propose to overcome the barriers to successful health teaching as described in this chapter?

3. What do you consider to be the primary benefits of becoming a certified health educator? What are the drawbacks?

4. Considering the list of personal qualities detailed in this chapter, how can you develop these in yourself?

5. Describe the process you would use in scheduling and implementing a teacher–parent–administrator meeting.

6. How will you ensure that you do not discriminate against any student?

Access more material online at www.pearsonhighered.com/anspaugh. At this companion website for *Teaching Today's Health*, you'll find chapter quizzes, web links, flashcards, a glossary, additional Worksheets, and more to help you succeed.

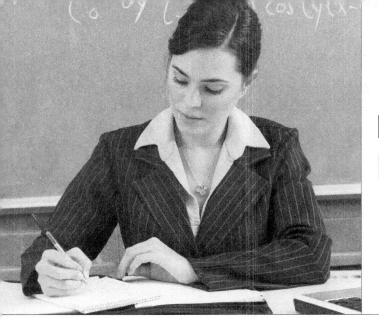

Planning for Health Instruction

3

When it comes to the education of our children... failure is not an option.

—*President George W. Bush (2001)*

Valued Outcomes

After completion of this chapter, you should be able to:

- Identify the potential content areas of health education.
- Describe scope and sequence for health education.
- Discuss the HECAT assessment tool.
- Identify the National Health Education Standards.
- Discuss why the National Health Education Standards are important.
- Describe various curriculum approaches to teaching health education.
- Develop an effective lesson plan.
- Write effective performance objectives.

Reflections

As you read this chapter, reflect on why it is necessary to begin to utilize the concepts of standards-based education and performance indicators in planning and teaching health education. What are the advantages and disadvantages of this approach? What might be the concerns of teachers in implementing such an approach? Can the National Health Education Standards really enhance the teaching of health? Why?

Traditional Content Areas in the Elementary School

Teaching health education, like teaching any subject, requires careful planning. Teachers must know what to teach, when to teach it, and how to teach it so that the content is internalized, or personalized, by the students. First-graders are vastly different from eighth-graders. Health instruction at each grade level must be tailored to the maturational, intellectual, and interest levels of the students.

Virtually every state department of education has a health education curriculum that can be used as a guide for planning. All teachers should read it carefully because it contains a recommended list of topics to present at each grade level. Teachers must recognize the complexity of life and attempt to incorporate the dimensions of wellness (physical, social, intellectual, emotional, environmental, and spiritual) into health instruction.

The general public often visualizes elementary health instruction merely in terms of rules for brushing teeth and riding bicycles safely. It is, of course, far more than that. Teaching health is a complicated process. For one thing, it takes time to effectively impact students' lives. To make an impact on the cognitive, affective, and psychomotor domains, forty to fifty hours of formal health instruction are necessary in each of the three domains. Various health education authorities cite from ten to twenty different content areas, depending on how the areas are grouped or separated. Most health educators agree on the following content areas for elementary health instruction:

- Mental and emotional health
- Personal health
- Nutrition
- Family health
- Prevention of substance use and abuse
- Injury prevention and safety
- Growth and development
- Consumer and community health
- Prevention and control of disease
- Environmental health

Unfortunately, many school districts are unable to provide instruction in all ten content areas, particularly at the elementary and middle school level. The problem seems to stem from a lack of time in the school day and a lack of knowledge for teaching the ten areas.

■ CDC Health Risk Behavior Content Areas

The Centers for Disease Control and Prevention (CDC) has provided direction in content areas by organizing the leading causes of illness and death in America into six health-risk behavior areas. It is generally thought that these health-risk behaviors contribute to most of the death, disability, and social problems found in the United States today. Many of the behaviors that contribute to these problems begin during childhood and early adolescence. The six areas are as follows (Dash 2005):

1. Tobacco use
2. Unhealthy dietary behaviors
3. Inadequate physical activity
4. Alcohol and other drug use
5. Sexual behaviors that may lead to HIV infection, other sexually transmitted diseases, and unintended pregnancies
6. Behaviors that contribute to unintentional injuries

It is easier to establish healthy behavior during childhood than it is to change unhealthy behaviors during adulthood. Whatever approach a state, school district, or individual may take, it is essential that schools accept the critical role of establishing lifelong healthy behavior patterns. Whatever curriculum philosophy is adopted, it is imperative that the education framework include opportunities to learn correct information, assess personal feelings concerning that information, and practice using the information in a healthy way. Table 3.1 provides a correlation of content areas and CDC youth risk behaviors to the National Health Education Standards, described in more detail later in this chapter.

The ultimate reason for all health education is to increase each student's **health literacy,** or "the capacity of the individual to obtain, interpret, and understand basic health information and services and the competence to use such information and services in ways which are health enhancing" (Association for the Advancement of Health Education 1995, 75). Content areas and topics also change in emphasis to reflect current knowledge and health concerns.

Developing Scope and Sequence

Once a state district or school identifies what content areas to cover, it must also determine how to order and organize that content. The **scope** outlines the breadth and arrangement of essential health topics and concepts across grade levels, and the **sequence** specifies logical progression of health knowledge, skills, and behaviors to address at each grade level from grades K through high school.

When done correctly, a scope and sequence chart should outline what students should know and do at the end of each grade level experience: Scope and sequence state what should be taught and when, while allowing this content to align with the National Health Education Standards, which are described throughout this chapter. See the Health Highlight box (page 29) for more information about effectively planning scope and sequence.

Table 3.1 Correlation of Content Areas and CDC Risk Behaviors to National Health Education Standards

National Health Education Standards	Corresponding Health Education Content Areas	Corresponding CDC Adolescent Risk Behaviors (Prevention)
Students will comprehend concepts related to health promotion and disease prevention to enhance health.	• Mental and emotional health • Personal health • Nutrition • Injury prevention and safety • Growth and development • Prevention and control of disease • Community health	• Tobacco use • Unhealthy dietary behaviors • Inadequate physical activity • Alcohol and other drug use • Sexual behaviors that may lead to sexually transmitted diseases and unintended pregnancies • Behaviors that contribute to unintentional injuries
Students will analyze the influence of family, peers, culture, media, technology, and other factors on health behaviors.	• Personal health • Family health • Consumer and community health • Environmental health	• Tobacco use • Alcohol and other drug use • Behaviors that contribute to unintentional injuries
Students will demonstrate the ability to access valid information and products and services to enhance health.	• Personal health • Consumer and community health	• Unhealthy dietary behaviors
Students will demonstrate the ability to use interpersonal communication skills to enhance health and avoid or reduce health risks.	• Personal health • Prevention of substance use and abuse • Injury prevention and safety	• Tobacco use • Alcohol and other drug use • Behaviors that contribute to unintentional injuries
Students will demonstrate the ability to use decision-making skills to enhance health.	• Personal health • Prevention of substance use and abuse • Injury prevention and safety	• Tobacco use • Alcohol and other drug use • Behaviors that contribute to unintentional injuries
Students will demonstrate the ability to use goal-setting skills to enhance health.	• Personal health • Prevention of substance use and abuse • Injury prevention and safety	• Tobacco use • Unhealthy dietary behaviors • Inadequate physical activity • Alcohol and other drug use
Students will demonstrate the ability to practice health-enhancing behaviors and avoid or reduce risks.	• Personal health • Nutrition • Prevention of substance use and abuse • Injury prevention and safety	• Tobacco use • Unhealthy dietary behaviors • Inadequate physical activity • Alcohol and other drug use • Sexual behaviors that may lead to sexually transmitted diseases and unintended pregnancies • Behaviors that contribute to unintentional injuries
Students will demonstrate the ability to advocate for personal, family, and community health.	• Personal health • Family health • Consumer and community health	• Unhealthy dietary behaviors • Inadequate physical activity • Behaviors that contribute to unintentional injuries

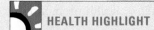

To help formulate scope and sequence health education curricula, the National Center for Chronic Disease Prevention and Health Promotion has developed the Health Education Curriculum Analysis Tool, or **HECAT** (CDC 2007). This assessment tool provides state, regional, and local health agencies with guidance, analysis, scoring, rubric, and resources for examining health education curricula. The HECAT articulates the National Health Education Standards. The information gathered can then be used to develop or modify health education scope and sequence. HECAT entails eight general steps:

1. Determine the necessary health education standard and additional benchmarks required at the local level.
2. Clarify health priorities by using local, community, and national health data on youth health-related behaviors, including health problems and risk-taking behaviors among school-aged youth.
3. Select key health topics, based on data, that should be addressed pre-K through grade 12.
4. For each topic, identify and prioritize expected behavioral outcomes for students that will meet the needs of the community and school district.
5. Determine the essential concepts and skills for each health topic that directly relate to the behavioral outcomes. The concepts and skills should specify what students should know and be able to do relevant to each of the key health topics and aligned with standards or benchmarks.
6. For each of the essential health education concepts and skills, decide specifically *what* should be taught and *when* it should be taught *across* the curriculum for all ages.
7. Determine the overall amount of instructional time. Allow sufficient time for students to master each concept and skill; to successfully develop the breadth and depth of knowledge of all health education concepts; and to be able to perform all health behavior skills.
8. Review and validate the scope and sequence.

The use of HECAT helps (1) ensure a complete, thorough review of the health education curriculum; (2) clarify what should be included in the health education curriculum; (3) ensure the curriculum is aligned with the National Health Education Standards; (4) identify instructional strategies for improving teaching; and (5) provide sound and defensible justification for curriculum decisions (CDC 2010). For more detailed information abut how to use the HECAT, visit the CDC's Division of Adolescent and School Health at www.cdc.gov/healthyyouth/HECAT.

The eight National Health Education Standards can be found in the pages that follow. These standards should serve as the foundation for curriculum development and instruction in health education. These standards are a framework for health educators in the United States. The goal is to create an instructional program that will enable students to experience comprehensive health education, which in turn will enable them to become/remain healthy and to achieve academic success (American Association for Health Education 2006).

Effective Health Education Curriculum

The Health Education Curriculum Analysis Tool (HECAT) provides an excellent framework for evaluating and formulating health curriculum. In developing health curriculum for today's students the Centers for Disease Control and Prevention (CDC) has determined criteria for effective health education. As outlined by the CDC, an extensive review of health curriculum research and evaluation found that today's curricula should reflect the teaching of functional information (essential concepts); shape personal values that support healthy behaviors; shape group norms that value a healthy lifestyle; and develop the health skills necessary to incorporate, practice, and maintain health-enhancing behaviors (CDC 2011). The HECAT says effective health education curriculum:

1. *Focuses on clear health goals and related behavioral outcomes.* Instructional strategies and learning experiences are directly related to the behavioral outcomes.
2. *Is research-based and theory driven.* Curricula go beyond the cognitive level and address health determinants such as social factors, attitudes, values, and skills shown to influence specific health-related behaviors.
3. *Addresses individual values and group norms that support health-enhancing behaviors.* Instructional strategies help students assess the level of risk taking among peers, correct misconceptions of peer norms, and reinforce health-enhancing beliefs.
4. *Focuses on increasing personal perceptions of risk and harmfulness of engaging in specific health risk behaviors and reinforcing protective factors.* Students are allowed opportunities to assess their vulnerability to health problems and to validate health-enhancing beliefs, intentions, and behaviors.
5. *Addresses social pressures and influences* (peer pressure, media influence, and social barriers).
6. *Builds personal competence, social competence, and self-efficacy by addressing skills* (development of communication, refusal, decision making, and self-management skills). Students should be guided through the skill as well as the relevance of the skill; presented with the steps to develop the skill; model the skill, practice and rehearse the skill in real life scenarios; and provide feedback and reinforcement.
7. *Provides functional health knowledge that is basic, accurate, and directly contributes to health-promoting decisions and behaviors.*
8. *Uses strategies designed to personalize information and engage students.* Use of student centered activities such as group discussion, problem solving, role playing, and cooperative learning.
9. *Provides age-appropriate and developmentally appropriate information, learning strategies, teaching methods, and materials.*
10. *Incorporates learning strategies, teaching methods, and materials that are culturally inclusive.*
11. *Provides adequate time for instruction and learning.*
12. Provides opportunities to reinforce skills and positive health behaviors.
13. *Provides opportunities to make positive connections with influential others;* links with students and other

influential people who reinforce health-promoting behaviors.
14. *Includes teacher information and plans for professional development and training that enhance effectiveness of instruction and student learning.* Teachers should be personally interested in promoting healthful activities, knowledgeable about the curriculum, and skilled in presenting instructional strategies that promote health enhancement.

What this criteria provides is a set of guidelines for developing a comprehensive curriculum plan for kindergarten through twelfth grade that will encompass pertinent health concerns and provide learning experiences throughout the school years. Student interests that grow and develop based on their ages and levels of intellectual, physical, and emotional maturity can also be considered in developing an appropriate curriculum. If these guidelines are followed a plan should develop to help promote responsible decisions and practices regarding personal, family, and community health. A comprehensive school curriculum should be either developed or purchased for every school district. There are numerous commercial programs that may be reviewed to determine if those materials meet the needs of a particular school or district. The CDC *Healthy Youth!* training manual can help in the curriculum evaluation process (apps.nccd. cdc.gov/SHI/default.aspx).

The Place of Values in the Curriculum

The affective domain can be defined as what one holds important or values in relationship to a given topic or component of our lives. Attitudes and values can be viewed as one's predisposition toward action. Thus, values (attitudes) give direction to life and help determine behavior. One of the ways educators can assess the effectiveness of teaching is through attempting to measure student values through tests, checklists, writing about issues, and group discussion. Members of our society share many of the same general values. However, each community, family, and individual has a more specific set of values. Values are closely linked with personal feelings and must be carefully considered when you plan health instruction. Failure to do so can result in the blocking of effective learning and in opposition from parents and community organizations. Values are learned through a variety of experiences and interactions with the environment. The family, peer group, school, church, and media all influence personal value formation. In other words, value formation is a continual process. Yet many parents become concerned when formal teaching about values takes place in the schools. There is concern that values contrary to the parents' values will be taught. Any recommendation or point of emphasis by a teacher can be construed as the imposition of values.

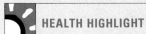 **HEALTH HIGHLIGHT** | **National Health Education Standards for Pre-K–12***

The following National Health Education Standards, including the rationales and performance indicators, were developed by the Joint Committee on National Health Standards, supported by the American Cancer Society. These standards are intended "to reinforce the positive growth of health education and to challenge schools and communities to continue efforts toward excellence in health education" (CDC 2011).

Health Education Standard 1

Students will comprehend concepts related to health promotion and disease prevention to enhance health.

Rationale

The acquisition of basic health concepts and functional health knowledge provides a foundation for promoting health-enhancing behaviors among youth. This standard includes essential concepts that are based on established health behavior theories and models. Concepts that focus on both health promotion and risk reduction are included in the performance indicators.

Performance Indicators

Pre-K–Grade 2	Grades 3–5	Grades 6–8	Grades 9–12
1.2.1 identify that healthy behaviors impact personal health.	**1.5.1** describe the relationship between healthy behaviors and personal health.	**1.8.1** analyze the relationship between healthy behaviors and personal health.	**1.12.1** predict how healthy behaviors can affect health status.
1.2.2 recognize that there are multiple dimensions of health.	**1.5.2** identify examples of emotional, intellectual, physical, and social health.	**1.8.2** describe the interrela-tion-ship of emotional, intel-lectual, physical, and social health in adolescence.	**1.12.2** describe the inter-relationships of emotional, intellectual, physical, and social health.
1.2.3 describe ways to prevent communicable diseases.	**1.5.3** describe ways in which a safe and healthy school and community environment can promote personal health.	**1.8.3** analyze how the environment affects personal health.	**1.12.3** analyze how environment and personal health are interrelated.
		1.8.4 describe how family history can affect personal health.	**1.12.4** analyze how genet-ics and family history can impact personal health.
1.2.4 list ways to prevent common childhood injuries.	**1.5.4** describe ways to prevent common childhood injuries and health problems.	**1.8.5** describe ways to reduce or prevent injuries and other adolescent health problems.	**1.12.5** propose ways to reduce or prevent injuries and health problems.
1.2.5 describe why it is important to seek health care.	**1.5.5** describe when it is important to seek health care.	**1.8.6** explain how appropriate health care can promote personal health.	**1.12.6** analyze the relationship between access to health care and health status.
		1.8.7 describe the benefits of and barriers to practicing healthy behaviors.	**1.12.7** compare and contrast the benefits of and barriers to practicing a variety of healthy behaviors.
		1.8.8 examine the likelihood of injury or illness if engaging in unhealthy behaviors.	**1.12.8** analyze personal susceptibility to injury, illness, or death if engaging in unhealthy behaviors.
		1.8.9 examine the potential seriousness of injury or illness if engaging in unhealthy behaviors.	**1.12.9** analyze the potential severity of injury or illness if engaging in unhealthy behaviors.

(continued)

HEALTH HIGHLIGHT | **National Health Education Standards for Pre-K–12 (*continued*)**

Health Education Standard 2

Students will analyze the influence of family, peers, culture, media, technology, and other factors on health behaviors.

Rationale

Health is impacted by a variety of positive and negative influences within society. This standard focuses on identifying and understanding the diverse internal and external factors that influence health practices and behaviors among youth including personal values, beliefs, and perceived norms.

Performance Indicators

Pre-K–Grade 2	Grades 3–5	Grades 6–8	Grades 9–12
2.2.1 identify how the family influences personal health practices and behaviors.	**2.5.1** describe how family influences personal health practices and behaviors.	**2.8.1** examine how the family influences the health of adolescents.	**2.12.1** analyze how family influences the health of individuals.
	2.5.2 identify the influence of culture on health practices and behaviors.	**2.8.2** describe the influence of culture on health beliefs, practices, and behaviors.	**2.12.2** analyze how culture supports and challenges health beliefs, practices, and behaviors.
	2.5.3 identify how peers can influence healthy and unhealthy behaviors.	**2.8.3** describe how peers can influence healthy and unhealthy behaviors.	**2.12.3** analyze how peers influence healthy and unhealthy behaviors.
2.2.2 identify what the school can do to support personal health practices and behaviors.	**2.5.4** describe how the school and community can support personal health practices and behaviors.	**2.8.4** analyze how the school and community can support personal health practices and behaviors.	**2.12.4** evaluate how the school and community can affect personal health practices and behaviors.
2.2.3 describe how the media can influence health behaviors.	**2.5.5** explain how media can influence thoughts, feelings, and health behaviors.	**2.8.5** analyze how messages from media influence health behaviors.	**2.12.5** evaluate the effect of media on personal and family health.
	2.5.6 describe ways technology can influence personal health.	**2.8.6** analyze the influence of technology on personal and family health.	**2.12.6** evaluate the impact of technology on personal, family, and community health.
		2.8.7 explain how the perceptions of norms influence healthy and unhealthy behaviors.	**2.12.7** analyze how the perceptions of norms influence healthy and unhealthy behaviors.
		2.8.8 explain the influence of personal values and beliefs on individual health practices and behaviors.	**2.12.8** analyze the influence of personal values and beliefs on individual health practices and behaviors.
		2.8.9 describe how some health risk behaviors can influence the likelihood of engaging in unhealthy behaviors.	**2.12.9** analyze how some health risk behaviors can influence the likelihood of engaging in unhealthy behaviors.
		2.8.10 explain how school and public health policies can influence health promotion and disease prevention.	**2.12.10** analyze how public health policies and government regulations can influence health promotion and disease prevention.

HEALTH HIGHLIGHT | **National Health Education Standards for Pre-K–12 (*continued*)**

Health Education Standard 3

Students will demonstrate the ability to access valid information and products and services to enhance health.

Rationale

Accessing valid health information and health-promoting products and services is critical in the prevention, early detection, and treatment of health problems. This standard focuses on how to identify and access valid health resources and how to reject unproven sources. Application of the skills of analysis, comparison, and evaluation of health resources empowers students to achieve health literacy.

Performance Indicators

Pre-K–Grade 2	Grades 3–5	Grades 6–8	Grades 9–12
3.2.1 identify trusted adults and professionals who can help promote health.	**3.5.1** identify characteristics of valid health information, products, and services.	**3.8.1** analyze the validity of health information, products, and services.	**3.12.1** evaluate the validity of health information, products, and services.
3.2.2 identify ways to locate school and community health helpers.	**3.5.2** locate resources from home, school, and community that provide valid health information.	**3.8.2** access valid health information from home, school, and community.	**3.12.2** use resources from home, school, and community that provide valid health information.
		3.8.3 determine the accessibility of products that enhance health.	**3.12.3** determine the accessibility of products and services that enhance health.
		3.8.4 describe situations that may require professional health services.	**3.12.4** determine when professional health services may be required.
		3.8.5 locate valid and reliable health products and services.	**3.12.5** access valid and reliable health products and services.

Reprinted, with permission, from the American Cancer Society. *National Health Education Standards: Achieving Excellence, Second Edition.* (Atlanta, GA: American Cancer Society, 2007), cancer.org/bookstore.

(continued)

Conversely, to take no stand at all can imply an anything-goes attitude.

Therefore, in planning health instruction, you must make clear how values will be a part of the teaching. Your job is not to impose your values; it is to help children develop their own values by making wise decisions about health-related matters. Children will form values with or without your assistance, but you can help them make positive decisions that will lead to high-level wellness by providing factual knowledge about health and by allowing children to clarify their own feelings.

Attitudes and behavior are intertwined. To achieve a balance between knowledge and attitudes toward health education, you will need to address student feelings. In other words, the study of health must be personalized if it is to have an impact. By providing opportunities for children to identify feelings and personalize health information, teachers can help children understand how information, attitudes, and behavior affect quality of life. In doing so, children become better equipped to deal with peer pressure, communicate more effectively, and develop sound decision-making skills.

Each person must weigh the importance or value of a decision against perceived rewards and costs involved. To brush one's teeth regularly, to smoke, to have regular physical examinations, and to experiment with drugs are all examples of decisions that affect health. Individuals make such decisions for themselves; consequently, teachers must make a planned effort to help children think through the possible consequences of health-related decisions.

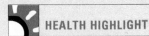 **HEALTH HIGHLIGHT** | **National Health Education Standards for Pre-K–12 (continued)**

Health Education Standard 4

Students will demonstrate the ability to use interpersonal communication skills to enhance health and avoid or reduce health risks.

Rationale

Effective communication enhances personal, family, and community health. This standard focuses on how responsible individuals use verbal and nonverbal skills to develop and maintain healthy personal relationships. The ability to organize and convey information and feelings is the basis for strengthening interpersonal interactions and reducing or avoiding conflict.

Performance Indicators

Pre-K–Grade 2	Grades 3–5	Grades 6–8	Grades 9–12
4.2.1 demonstrate healthy ways to express needs, wants, and feelings.	**4.5.1** demonstrate effective verbal and nonverbal communication skills to enhance health.	**4.8.1** apply effective verbal and nonverbal communication skills to enhance health.	**4.12.1** use skills for communicating effectively with family, peers, and others to enhance health.
4.2.2 demonstrate listening skills to enhance health.	**4.5.2** demonstrate refusal skills that avoid or reduce health risks.	**4.8.2** demonstrate refusal and negotiation skills to avoid or reduce health risks.	**4.12.2** demonstrate refusal, negotiation, and collaboration skills to enhance health and avoid or reduce health risks.
4.2.3 demonstrate ways to respond when in an unwanted, threatening, or dangerous situation.	**4.5.3** demonstrate nonviolent strategies to manage or resolve conflict.	**4.8.3** demonstrate effective conflict management or resolution strategies.	**4.12.3** demonstrate strategies to prevent, manage, or resolve interpersonal conflicts without harming self or others.
4.2.4 demonstrate ways to tell a trusted adult if threatened or harmed.	**4.5.4** demonstrate how to ask for assistance to enhance personal health.	**4.8.4** demonstrate how to ask for assistance to enhance the health of self and others.	**4.12.4** demonstrate how to ask for and offer assistance to enhance the health of self and others.

Curriculum Approaches

Many helpful resources are available to help teachers plan a course of health education for the classroom. As noted, these resources include the state health education guidelines, commercial health education textbook series, and materials from government and private health-related agencies. There are also numerous websites that offer content and strategy suggestions. The discussion that follows includes resources that might help you find useful health education materials. Some of the listed programs require the purchase of materials; other programs are provided free or at minimal cost. Most of the mentioned materials have websites that provide greater detail about the nature of the resource. The websites usually contain information on the training necessary to use the material, the philosophy of the curriculum approach, and the type(s) of information the curriculum provides. Most of the criteria in the essentials for effective health education can be found in the Michigan Model.

■ The Michigan Model—A State Model

Although there is no officially mandated national curriculum, several models have been suggested as possibilities. An excellent model that states have adopted is the Michigan Model for Health®. The original model was a result of a coalition of eight state agencies that included the Department of Education, Department of Public Health, Department of Social Services, Department of Mental Health, Department of State Police, Office of Substance Abuse Services, Office of Health and Medical Affairs, and

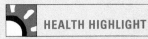

HEALTH HIGHLIGHT | **National Health Education Standards for Pre-K–12 (*continued*)**

Health Education Standard 5

Students will demonstrate the ability to use decision-making skills to enhance health.

Rationale

Decision-making skills are needed in order to identify, implement, and sustain health-enhancing behaviors. This standard includes the essential steps needed to make healthy decisions as prescribed in the performance indicators. When applied to health issues, the decision-making process enables individuals to collaborate with others to improve their quality of life.

Performance Indicators

Pre-K–Grade 2	Grades 3–5	Grades 6–8	Grades 9–12
		5.8.1 identify circumstances that can help or hinder healthy decision making.	**5.12.1** examine barriers that can hinder healthy decision making.
5.2.1 identify situations when a health-related decision is needed.	**5.5.1** identify health-related situations that might require a thoughtful decision.	**5.8.2** determine when health-related situations require the application of a thoughtful decision-making process.	**5.12.2** determine the value of applying a thoughtful decision-making process in health-related situations.
5.2.2 differentiate between situations when a health-related decision can be made individually or when assistance is needed.	**5.5.2** analyze when assistance is needed in making a health-related decision.	**5.8.3** distinguish when individual or collaborative decision making is appropriate.	**5.12.3** justify when individual or collaborative decision making is appropriate.
	5.5.3 list healthy options to health-related issues or problems.	**5.8.4** distinguish between healthy and unhealthy alternatives to health-related issues or problems.	**5.12.4** generate alternatives to health-related issues or problems.
	5.5.4 predict the potential outcomes of each option when making a health-related decision.	**5.8.5** predict the potential short-term impact of each alternative on self and others.	**5.12.5** predict the potential short- and long-term impact of each alternative on self and others.
	5.5.5 choose a healthy option when making a decision.	**5.8.6** choose healthy alternatives over unhealthy alternatives when making a decision.	**5.12.6** defend the healthy choice when making decisions.
	5.5.6 describe the outcomes of a health-related decision.	**5.8.7** analyze the outcomes of a health-related decision.	**5.12.7** evaluate the effectiveness of health-related decisions.

Reprinted, with permission, from the American Cancer Society. *National Health Education Standards: Achieving Excellence, Second Edition.* (Atlanta, GA: American Cancer Society, 2007), cancer.org/bookstore.

(continued)

the Office of Highway Safety Planning. The model, originally developed in 1985, has been revised several times, including the addition of new topics since the original materials were created.

Eighty percent of Michigan's public schools have implemented the model, and it is also being implemented in a large number of Michigan's private schools. Throughout the United States, other public and private school systems have also adopted the program. Over one million students have been reached through implementation of the Michigan Model.

The **Michigan Model for Health** is a comprehensive and sequential K–12 health education curriculum that provides students the knowledge and skills needed

| | HEALTH HIGHLIGHT | **National Health Education Standards for Pre-K–12 (*continued*)** |

Health Education Standard 6

Students will demonstrate the ability to use goal-setting skills to enhance health.

Rationale

Goal-setting skills are essential to help students identify, adopt, and maintain healthy behaviors. This standard includes the critical steps that are needed to achieve both short-term and long-term health goals. These skills make it possible for individuals to have aspirations and plans for the future.

Performance Indicators

Pre-K–Grade 2	Grades 3–5	Grades 6–8	Grades 9–12
		6.8.1 assess personal health practices.	**6.12.1** assess personal health practices and overall health status.
6.2.1 identify a short-term personal health goal and take action toward achieving the goal.	**6.5.1** set a personal health goal and track progress toward its achievement.	**6.8.2** develop a goal to adopt, maintain, or improve a personal health practice.	**6.12.2** develop a plan to attain a personal health goal that addresses strengths, needs, and risks.
6.2.2 identify who can help when assistance is needed to achieve a personal health goal.	**6.5.2** identify resources to assist in achieving a personal health goal.	**6.8.3** apply strategies and skills needed to attain a personal health goal.	**6.12.3** implement strategies and monitor progress in achieving a personal health goal.
		6.8.4 describe how personal health goals can vary with changing abilities, priorities, and responsibilities.	**6.12.4** formulate an effective long-term personal health plan.

Reprinted, with permission, from the American Cancer Society. *National Health Education Standards: Achieving Excellence, Second Edition.* (Atlanta, GA: American Cancer Society, 2007), cancer.org/bookstore.

to practice and maintain healthy behaviors and lifestyles. The curriculum provides age-appropriate lessons addressing the most serious health issues facing school-aged children, including social and emotional health; nutrition and physical activity; the use of alcohol, tobacco and other drugs; personal health and wellness; safety; and a new HIV component. The Model facilitates learning through a variety of interactive teaching and learning techniques with skill development through demonstration and guided practice.

The Michigan Model is based on the Adapted Health Belief Model and the merging of several behavior change theories. A key principle of the Adapted Health Belief Model is that a health education program is more likely to impact behavior change if it includes all of the following components: knowledge, skills, self-efficacy, and environmental support. The Michigan Model for Health is designed for implementation as a component of the core school curriculum, with each of the lessons lasting 30–45 minutes in length. The lessons may be integrated in various disciplines such as language arts, science, social studies, etc. (Michigan Model 2011). Tables 3.2 and 3.3 contain the scope and sequence of activities for grades K–6 and

grades 7–12. Visit the website www.pearsonhighered.com/anspaugh for a link to the Michigan Model for Health.

To help encourage family involvement, "Family Resource" sheets are included within the lessons of the Model. These resource sheets provide information concerning topics being studied as well as suggested activities the family can do to help enhance the classroom experience.

▪ Examples of Teaching Materials: Lessons, Information, and Websites

Agencies such as the American Cancer Society, American Heart Association, March of Dimes, American Red Cross, American Dental Association, and American Dairy Association provide free and inexpensive materials through their local affiliates. Some websites that contain information for teachers include the following:

- **Open Heart Surgery**—*www.cosi.org/files/Flash/openHeart/heart.html* Includes anatomy, prevention, disease, and surgery of the heart. Students can make mock diagnoses and give treatment or undertake virtual surgery.

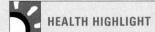

| HEALTH HIGHLIGHT | **National Health Education Standards for Pre-K–12 (*continued*)** |

Health Education Standard 7

Students will demonstrate the ability to practice health-enhancing behaviors and avoid or reduce risks.

Rationale

Research confirms that practicing health-enhancing behaviors can contribute to a positive quality of life. In addition, many diseases and injuries can be prevented by reducing harmful and risk-taking behaviors. This standard promotes accepting personal responsibility for health and encourages the practice of healthy behaviors.

Performance Indicators

Pre-K–Grade 2	Grades 3–5	Grades 6–8	Grades 9–12
	7.5.1 identify responsible personal health behaviors.	**7.8.1** explain the importance of assuming responsibility for personal health behaviors.	**7.12.1** analyze the role of individual responsibility in enhancing health.
7.2.1 demonstrate healthy practices and behaviors to maintain or improve personal health.	**7.5.2** demonstrate a variety of healthy practices and behaviors to maintain or improve personal health.	**7.8.2** demonstrate healthy practices and behaviors that will maintain or improve the health of self and others.	**7.12.2** demonstrate a variety of healthy practices and behaviors that will maintain or improve the health of self and others.
7.2.2 demonstrate behaviors that avoid or reduce health risks.	**7.5.3** demonstrate a variety of behaviors that avoid or reduce health risks.	**7.8.3** demonstrate behaviors to avoid or reduce health risks to self and others.	**7.12.3** demonstrate a variety of behaviors to avoid or reduce health risks to self and others.

Reprinted, with permission, from the American Cancer Society. *National Health Education Standards: Achieving Excellence, Second Edition.* (Atlanta, GA: American Cancer Society, 2007), cancer.org/bookstore.

(continued)

- **Infection Detection Prevention**—*www.amnh.org/nationalcenter/infection/* Online magazine from the American Museum of Natural History. The website is divided into sections on the various pathogens and contains an excellent explanation of how pathogens break through the immune system.
- **Kids Health**—*www.kidshealth.org* Explains to kids how the human body works, what makes them sick, and how to be safe. The website is divided into sections for adults, teens, and children and contains games and activities.
- **It's My Life (PBS Kids)**—*pbskids.org/itsmylife/* Organized by topics such as friends, family, school, and body. Printable activities include journal pages and discussion questions. The website includes lesson plans on bullies, staying home alone, smoking, eating disorders, and drug abuse.

▪ Teaching Units

A **teaching unit** is an organized method for developing lesson plans for a particular group of students and thus can be tailored to each classroom. The resource unit serves as a guide, whereas the teaching unit is the plan for student learning. Unlike the resource unit, which is prepared by a curriculum committee, the teaching unit is developed by the classroom teacher. It is specific; the resource unit is general. The teacher selects the specific concepts to be studied, as well as the objectives, content, learning strategies, evaluation methods, and references that will be used in class. Given a well-developed resource unit that identifies major concepts, creating a teaching unit is fairly easy. In addition to the resource unit, the state health education guidelines, the teacher's edition of the classroom textbook, and various materials from health-related agencies can all be used to develop the teaching unit. In preparing a teaching unit, a teacher can use a variety of formats, depending on individual preference.

▪ Lesson Planning—Selected Strategies

Once the teaching unit has been developed, the next step is to plan how to teach the unit. This is done by creating daily lesson plans that provide a logical progression of the unit from start to finish. Each lesson plan must be based on concepts taught in previous lessons so that learning builds on the established base. There are several components that must go into effective lesson planning. For example, the growth and development characteristics of the age group for which the lesson is being planned must be understood to enable the teacher to plan age-appropriate content and strategies for learning. To help

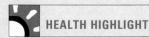

Health Education Standard 8

Students will demonstrate the ability to advocate for personal, family, and community health.

Rationale

Advocacy skills help students promote healthy norms and healthy behaviors. This standard helps students develop important skills to target their health-enhancing messages and to encourage others to adopt healthy behaviors.

Performance Indicators

Pre-K–Grade 2	Grades 3–5	Grades 6–8	Grades 9–12
8.2.1 make requests to promote personal health.	**8.5.1** express opinions and give accurate information about health issues.	**8.8.1** state a health-enhancing position on a topic and support it with accurate information.	**8.12.1** use accurate peer and societal norms to formulate a health-enhancing message.
8.2.2 encourage peers to make positive health choices.	**8.5.2** encourage others to make positive health choices.	**8.8.2** demonstrate how to influence and support others to make positive health choices.	**8.12.2** demonstrate how to influence and support others to make positive health choices.
		8.8.3 work cooperatively to advocate for healthy individuals, families, and schools.	**8.12.3** work cooperatively as an advocate for improving personal, family, and community health.
		8.8.4 identify ways in which health messages and communication techniques can be altered for different audiences.	**8.12.4** adapt health messages and communication techniques to a specific target audience.

Reprinted, with permission, from the American Cancer Society. *National Health Education Standards: Achieving Excellence, Second Edition.* (Atlanta, GA: American Cancer Society, 2007), cancer.org/bookstore.

with this process, Tables 3.2 and 3.5 should be reviewed prior to writing the lesson plan. How students learn (learning styles) will be discussed later (see Chapter 4), but in planning an effective lesson there should be a variety of activities and strategies that appeal to the various styles of learning found in the classroom.

The Teaching in Action box on page 39 shows a sample daily lesson plan for grade 3. A conceptual statement is presented as the Instructional Objective, and a performance indicator is outlined for that day. **Performance indicators** are the expectations of what the students will demonstrate if the intended instruction and learning have taken place. The content outline provides a summary of the main topics to be covered. The strategies are the heart of the lesson plan. They should be described in detail and listed in the order in which they are to be used.

As shown in the daily lesson plan example, each strategy should be followed by an evaluation activity ("Closure for Strategies"). Through this activity, the teacher will be able to judge to some extent how well the students have learned the concept presented. Because the strategy is a performance in nature, it can also be used to determine how well the objectives have been achieved.

Another lesson plan format works exceptionally well with the National Health Education Standards. The format for this lesson plan is shown in the Teaching in Action box on page 45. This format begins with the listing of the national health standard or standards that are addressed in the lesson, followed by a second section that lists the national health education performance indicator or indicators. The third section, valued outcomes, describes performance expectations for the students. The fourth section, description of strategies, lists content and learning experiences that provide for the assimilation of material and facilitate assessment of attitudes and positive health behaviors. The materials required to successfully teach the lesson are listed in the fifth section. Most noteworthy in this lesson format is the formative evaluation section. The benchmarks listed in this section are indicators of the depth of understanding and insight into the area studied. This last

---

TEACHING IN ACTION | **Sample Daily Lesson Plan**

<u>**Lesson Title:**</u> Mental Health—Getting to Know Me

<u>**Date:**</u> February 19, 2012   <u>**Time:**</u> 10:00 A.M.   <u>**Grade:**</u> Three   <u>**Teacher:**</u> Avery

<u>**Instructional Objective:**</u> Students will identify several emotions and state acceptable ways to express them.

<u>**Teacher Needs:**</u> Pictures of people expressing emotions, crayons, paper. Write role-playing situations.

Content (Progression)

Emotion—the way we feel
1. Anger
2. Love
3. Sadness
4. Fear
5. Excitement

Expressing Emotions
1. Facial expression
   A. Smile
   B. Frown
   C. Tears
   D. Eyes
2. Talking
   A. Soft voice
   B. Loud voice
   C. Excited voice
   D. Fast voice
   E. Slow voice
3. Body language
   A. Using arms
   B. Kissing
   C. Clapping

Strategies (Full Description)

1. Discuss what feelings are and list on the board. Show pictures of people displaying different emotions. Use several pictures that reflect certain emotions.
2. Discuss ways we express emotions. Ask students to give ways that are acceptable/unacceptable means of expressing feelings. Have students role-play these ways to express the various emotions.

Closure for Strategies

1. Give children crayons and have them draw a face of the emotion requested.
   Processing Questions
   A. How many of you have used one of the emotions drawn?
   B. What are some of the reasons we express an emotion?
2. Give the children a situation that illustrates an expression of a particular emotion. Have them role-play an acceptable way to express the emotion.
   Processing Questions
   A. What ways are best for expressing our emotions?
   B. What are some ways we should not express our emotions?
   C. Is it "OK" to get angry? Cry? Hit someone?

Teacher Evaluation
1. Keep the lesson as taught?   yes _____ no _____
2. What I need to improve _____
3. Next time make sure _____
4. Strengths of lesson _____

---

section provides for the essential elements or content to be emphasized in the lesson.

Dr. David Lohrmann of Indiana University uses a most interesting approach to lesson planning. Again, this format bases effective lesson planning on the National Health Education Standards. Twelve questions to be addressed before lesson planning are presented in Table 3.4. These questions are basic to any successful planning of a lesson and should be considered regardless of the format. The lesson planning format is easily understood once the

questions in Table 3.4 have been answered. What makes this planning approach so valuable is the incorporation of an assessment component in initial planning. Once the learning objectives have been established, the teacher must then select the types and number of assessments to use for the aligning of instruction and assessment. Drawn from Ferrara and McTighe (1992), there are five types of assessments (discussed further in Chapter 5). Lohrmann uses these five types of assessments in his lesson planning format. Another important function of

Table 3.2 Michigan Model for Health: Scope and Sequence for Grades K-6

	Kindergarten	Grade One	Grade Two	Grade Three
Social and Emotional Health	- Showing respect and caring - Making and keeping friends - Caring touch in positive relationships - Identifying and describing feelings - Managing strong feelings - Recognizing and expressing feelings - Giving and receiving compliments and appreciation - Being responsible at home and school - Identifying people who can help	- Skills for predicting potential feelings of others - Skills for finding out how others feel - Showing courtesy to others - Demonstrate giving and receiving compliments or appreciation - Ways family members and friends help each other - Listening skills for friendships - Decision-making and problem-solving skills	- Identifying and expressing feelings - Handling mixed feelings - Expressing feelings respectfully - Listening with respect - Everyone deserves respect - Showing respect - Managing strong feelings - Making good decisions: WIN - Practicing WIN	- Positive role models and friends - Making and keeping friends - Everyone has special talents - Respecting differences - Helping others by protecting them from bullies - Helping others and getting help - Expressing thanks and appreciation - Expressing annoyance respectfully
Nutrition and Physical Activity	- Variety in foods and snacks for good health - Drinking water for good health - Categorize foods and snacks into the five food groups - Importance of physical activity for good health - Examples of ways to be physically active	- Importance of eating a variety of foods from all five food groups - Benefits of eating healthy snacks - Benefits of drinking water - Benefits of physical activity - How sleep, rest, and physical activity maintain health	- Food groups - Combining foods and foods to limit - Benefits of physical activity	- Magic Numbers: 5 and 60 - Food advertising and impact on eating - Three types of physical activity - Developing a plan to be physically active - Advocate for healthy eating and daily activity
Safety	- Dangerous and destructive situations that need adult help - Pedestrian safety - Rule for dangerous objects and weapons - How and when to dial 911 - Avoiding inappropriate touch - Trusted adults who can help	- Wheeled recreation hazards, safety, and safety gear - Fire and burn hazards and how to prevent - Actions to take in a fire emergency - Situations that are dangerous, destructive, and disturbing and need adult help - Escaping dangerous situations - Define emergency and how to make emergency phone call - Avoiding inappropriate touch - Trusted adults who can help	- Wheeled recreation safety: bicycles, skateboards, skates - Water safety - Internet safety - Personal safety - Practicing personal safety skills	- Three keys to passenger safety: safety belts, booster seats, back seat - Safety belt smarts - Identifying and responding to unsafe situations - Street smarts: internet, personal, safety, weapons
Alcohol, Tobacco, and Other Drugs	- How to safely use over-the-counter and prescription medicines - Household products that can be dangerous - Rules for avoiding poisons - Trustworthy sources of information	- How to safely use over-the-counter and prescription medicines - Illicit drugs - Household products that can be dangerous - Rules for avoiding poisons - Trustworthy sources of information - Harmful chemicals in tobacco products - Dangers of secondhand smoke and ways to avoid or reduce exposure	- Caffeine - Staying away from nicotine and alcohol - Saying "No" to second-hand smoke	- Medicines and poisons - Negative effects of tobacco use - Tobacco and media - Alcohol and alcoholism - Positive influences - Refusal skills
Personal Health and Wellness	- Hand washing GERMS - Taking care of teeth - Encouraging peers to make positive choices for personal health	- Skills for stopping the spread of germs: covering sneezes and washing hands - Taking care of teeth		- Basic hygiene: Care of the Body - Hand washing GERMS - Planning for good hygiene
HIV				

Source: Michigan Model for Health, Scope and Sequence for Grades K-6. Used by permission of Educational Materials Center, Central Michigan University. 2011. Available at http://www.emc.cmich.edu/mm/

Grade Four	Grade Five	Grade Six
- Managing strong feelings, including I-messages - Positive self-talk - Effects of teasing and bullying and what to do to protect self and others - Decision-making and problem-solving skills - Non-violent conflict resolution skills	- Identifying feelings of different intensities in self and others - Managing strong feelings, including I-messages & positive self-talk - Effects of teasing and bullying & what to do to protect self and others - Assertive communication - Listening skills - Identifying situations that could lead to trouble - Decision-making and problem-solving skills - Importance of telling adults if self or others are in dangerous situations - Non-violent conflict resolution skills - Goal setting - Advocate for a healthy school environment	- Positive and negative risks of friendships - Listening skills - Appreciation - Assertive communication, including I-messages - Managing strong feelings - Angry feelings versus angry behavior - Criteria for getting help - Decision-making and problem-solving skills - Criteria for evaluating solutions - Non-violent conflict resolution skills - Stress management
- Food groups and their benefits - Daily amounts to eat from each food group and how to estimate amounts - "Fill Your Plate" visual - Influence of food & beverage advertising - Daily recommended amounts of physical activity and sleep - Personal assessment and goal setting to get adequate sleep, rest, and physical activity	- Six nutrients and their benefits - Using food labels to determine information about a food - Water as a preferred beverage - Use of Dietary Guidelines when choosing foods - "Fill Your Plate" visual - Analyze a favorite meal - Evaluate a peer's meal and make recommendations for improvement	- Prevention of foodborne illness - Benefits of healthy eating and physical activity - Dietary guidelines applied to individuals - Body image and healthy weight - Influences on eating, activity and sleep - Use of Dietary Guidelines to make a personal plan - Supporting others to eat healthy and be active
- Fire and burn hazards and how to prevent - Home fire escape plan - Home safety hazards and how to prevent injuries - Home alone safety strategies - Define emergency and how to make emergency phone call - How to prevent injury from dangerous objects, including weapons - Child sexual abuse and abduction prevention	- Safety hazards around water and ice and how to prevent injuries - Sun safety - Home alone safety strategies - How to make emergency phone call - Safety strategies when in public places, including when alone in public places - Child sexual abuse and abduction prevention	- Seatbelt safety and impact of car passenger behavior - Safety strategies when in public places, including escaping when weapons are present - School procedures for school crisis situations - Strategies to be safe when using the Internet - How to get adult help - Advocacy for others to practice safe behaviors - Child sexual abuse and abduction prevention
- Dangers of secondhand smoke and ways to avoid or reduce exposure - Reasons individuals choose to drink or not to drink - Decisions about alcohol and other drug use impact family and friends - Family and friends influence alcohol and other drug use decisions - Influence of advertising - Refusal skills	- Dangers of inhalant use and how to avoid exposure - Influence of family and peers on drug use - Rules for safety around dangerous or unknown products - Effects of smoking tobacco, secondhand smoke, & use of spit tobacco - Advocate for someone to avoid tobacco use or quit using - Analyze tobacco advertisements - Refusal skills - Effects of alcohol, especially on driving a vehicle - Impact of alcohol and tobacco use on friends and family - Ways to avoid riding with a driver who has been drinking and what to do if it can't be avoided	- Possible reasons people use or don't use drugs - Negative health effects of drug use - Analysis of drug use data - Persuasion skills for encouraging others to stay drug free - Influence of family, society and peers on drug use - Impact of drug use on goals - School rules and laws related to tobacco - Refusal skills - Valid resources for drug problems - Ways to avoid riding with a driver who has been drinking and what to do if it can't be avoided - Benefits of remaining drug free and making a drug-free commitment
	- Importance of and rationale for keeping the body clean - Hygiene concerns and solutions - Influence of media, including advertisements on products purchased and on body image - Analyze advertisements for information	- Skills for reducing the spread of germs
- Define HIV and AIDS - How HIV isn't transmitted - How HIV is transmitted: blood-to-blood contact and touching used needles or syringes - How to protect self and others - Importance of being compassionate when others are ill	- Define HIV and AIDS - How HIV isn't transmitted - How HIV is transmitted: sharing used needles or syringes, having sex with infected person, infected mother to child - How to protect self and others - Importance of being compassionate when others are ill	

Table 3.3 Michigan Model for Health: Scope and Sequence for Grades 7–12

	Tobacco Use	Drug and Alcohol Use	Dietary Behaviors That Contribute to Nutrition-Related Conditions Including Obesity	Physical Inactivity	Unintentional Injuries and Violence	Sexual Behaviors That Contribute to Unintended Pregnancy and STIs, Including HIV
Grades 7–8 (Middle School)	**The Power Is Yours to Be Tobacco Free** **Content** • Healthy ways to meet needs without tobacco use • Health, legal, social, and financial consequences of use **Skills** • Analyze influences to use tobacco • Use refusal skills to avoid tobacco use • Support those who abstain and those who are trying to quit • Identify risky situations that could lead to tobacco use • Solve problems • Avoid secondhand smoke • Access resources • Compose persuasive advice for peers on how to stay tobacco free	**Protect a Friend—Share Your Skills** **Content** • Influences that promote drug* use in young people • Rules and laws related to drugs • Health, social, and legal consequences of drug use • Resources for drug-related information and help **Skills** • Evaluate internal and external pressures to use drugs • Express opinions, thoughts, and feelings • Solve problems • Refuse to use drugs • Identify trouble • Promote drug-free messages to peers • Apply a personal commitment to living drug free • Access resources * "Drug" refers to alcohol, tobacco, and other drugs.	**A Winning Team: Healthy Eating and Physical Activity** **Content** • Health benefits of healthy eating, hydration, and being physically active • Federal guidelines for diet and physical activity • Factors in weight control • Identify moderate-intensity physical activities • Healthy body image, body type and healthy body weight • Nutrition information on food labels, health claims, and advertisements **Skills** • Analyze personal food intake • Assess personal barriers to healthy eating and getting physical activity and develop solutions • Access resources for weight management and unhealthy eating patterns • Analyze influences of sedentary activities on physical activity • Select foods with most nutritional value • Analyze nutrition information to identify healthier food options when eating out • Persuade peers to eat healthy and be physically active • Set goals to improve healthy eating and increase physical activity		**The Two "R's" for Stopping Assault and Preventing Violence** **Content** • Healthy and harmful relationships • Causes of conflict; how conflicts can escalate • Influences that promote and discourage violence • Characteristics and laws related to sexual harassment and abusive relationships • Resources to stop assault and prevent violence **Skills** • Resolve conflicts: – listen – express emotions and thoughts – show empathy – manage anger – respond appropriately to anger – solve problems and negotiate • De-escalate intimidation • Avoid and escape violence • Maintain personal safety • Deal with sexual harassment • Deal with abusive relationships • Help others • Advocate for nonviolence • Access resources	**Growing Up and Staying Healthy: Understanding HIV and Other STIs** **Content** • How STIs are and are not transmitted • Consequences of infection with HIV and other STIs • Health risks of various behaviors • Negative consequences of having sexual intercourse and ways to reduce risks* • Benefits of staying within behavioral limits and remaining abstinent **Skills** • Evaluate influences on decisions regarding sexual behavior. • Analyze behaviors and situations that may increase the risk for HIV and other STIs • Apply strategies to abstain from sex and/or reduce risk* • Locate and describe reliable sources of information and help, and when it is needed • Avoid and escape risky situations • Communicate respectfully and assertively • Refuse peer pressure verbally and nonverbally • Set goals to stay free of STIs, to stay within behavioral boundaries, and reduce the risk of having sex • Advocate for healthy behavioral choices among peers *This module offers two tracks: abstinence-only, abstinence-based, with condoms.
Grades 9–12 (High School)	**Teens Campaign Against Tobacco** **Content** • Factors that contribute to positive health behaviors • Health benefits of abstaining from use • Resources for information, help, and cessation • Financial, political, social, health, and legal issues related to tobacco • Messages that will encourage youth not to use or to quit **Skills** • Advocate for the prevention, reduction, or elimination of use among peers • Promote a tobacco-free environment • Abstain from use (refusal)	**Teens Voice Solutions** **Content** • Scope of adolescent drug* use • Physical, emotional, social, and economic consequences of drug use • Impact of environment on the problem of drug use • Legal issues related to drug use among adolescents **Skills** • Evaluate internal and external pressures to use drugs • Synthesize and communicate research findings on reducing drug use • Communicate assertively • Refuse to use drugs • Solve personal and social problems	**Help Yourself to Good Nutrition** **Content** • Health benefits of eating: – foods from the five food groups – recommended number and size of servings from each food group • Weight management principles and myths regarding weight loss • Influence of body image on eating patterns • Healthy and unhealthy eating patterns **Skills** • Plan – healthy weight loss or maintenance – nutritious meals within a budget – nutritious meals at fast food restaurants	**Stay Physically Active—For Life** **Content** • Six components of wellness • Contribution of physical activity to physical wellness • Recommended amount and types of physical activity for health benefits • Benefits of regular physical activity • Consequences of being inactive • Strategies to overcome barriers **Skills** • Analyze barriers to being active • Assess current level of activity	**Managing Conflicts and Preventing Violence** **Content** • Healthy and harmful relationships • Causes of conflict; how conflicts can escalate • Factors that contribute to and prevent violence • Consequences of violence • Characteristics and laws related to sexual harassment and abusive relationships • Resources to prevent and avoid violence • Individual's responsibility for safety of self and others **Skills** • Resolve conflicts: – listen – express emotions and thoughts – show empathy – manage anger – respond appropriately to anger – solve problems and negotiate • De-escalate intimidation	**Healthy and Responsible Relationships: HIV, Other STIs, and Pregnancy Prevention** **Content** • Characteristics of healthy relationships • Consequences of infection with STIs* • How STIs are and are not transmitted • Health risks of various behaviors • STI testing • Costs of pregnancy and teen parenting • Situations requiring professional health services **Skills** • Apply strategies to abstain from sex and/or reduce risk** • Access reliable sources of information and help • Avoid and escape risky situations • Communicate respectfully and assertively • Refuse pressure • Identify trouble • Analyze influences on sexual behaviors • Set goals to reach personal goals

Drug (alcohol, tobacco, and other drugs)

- Encourage others to abstain
- Encourage others to quit
- Support others who want to quit
- Access resources
- Propose and evaluate possible solutions for reducing drug use among adolescents
- Communicate a proposed solution to the problem of drug use to school and/or community representatives
- Access resources

* "Drug" refers to alcohol, tobacco, and other drugs.

Nutrition / Physical Activity

- Set personal physical activity goals
- Advocate for school and community support of physical activity
- for improved personal nutrition
- Analyze effects of nutrition on:
  - physical activity
  - athletic performance
  - pregnancy
  - fetal development
- Analyze nutrition information and resources
- Synthesize and communicate research findings on nutrition

Violence

- Avoid and escape violence
- Maintain personal safety
- Prevent violence
- Deal with sexual harassment
- Deal with abusive relationships
- Access resources

STIs

- Advocate for peers to prevent STIs and pregnancy

* "STIs" includes HIV
** This module offers three tracks: abstinence-only, abstinence-plus-condoms, or abstinence-plus-contraceptives.

Sun Safety

Take Control of Your Sun Exposure

Content
- Incidence and detection of skin cancer
- Harmful versus helpful sun exposure
- Consequences of sun exposure
- Safe alternatives to UV ray exposure for a tanned appearance
- Sunscreens, sunglasses, and fabrics that protect from UV rays

Skills
- that pose risks from the sun's UV rays
- Take protective steps when exposed to sun
- Make a plan to stay safe in the sun

Look Young and Stay Healthy–Your Choice

Content
- Consequences of UV exposure on health and appearance
- Incidence of skin cancer
- Risk factors for and recognition of skin cancer
- Safe alternatives to UV ray exposure for a tanned appearance
- Selection and use of sunscreens

Skills
- Access help for skin problems
- Use protective measures when exposed to sun
- Make a personal plan to stay safe in the sun
- Advocate for peers to avoid UV rays

High School

Gambling

All "Bets" Are Off!

Content
- Possible health, social, and legal consequences of gambling
- Different types of gamblers
- Laws related to gambling
- Influences that encourage or discourage gambling
- Resources for gambling information and help
- Assess personal risk

Skills
- Analyze influences and advertising related to gambling
- Abstain from gambling, using refusal skills
- Communicate concern for others
- Access resources
- Promote awareness of gambling risks

Don't Bet On It!

Content
- Possible health, social, and legal consequences of gambling
- Different types of gamblers
- Warning signs of problem and compulsive gamblers
- Phases compulsive gamblers experience
- Laws related to gambling
- Influences that encourage or discourage gambling
- Resources for gambling information and help
- Assess personal risk

Skills
- Analyze influences and advertising related to gambling
- Communicate concern for others
- Access resources
- Advocate for abstinence from gambling by youth

Service Learning

Building Character Through Service-Learning

Content
- Six essential character traits
- What service learning is and is not
- Needs assessment
- Project planning strategies

Skills
- Assess community needs
- Apply planning skills to develop a service-learning project
- Participate in teamwork with peers and community members
- Interview people and present ideas
- Reflect on personal experiences and Learning

Character Education

Choosing Who I Am – Choosing Who I Become

Content
- Six essential character traits
- Core democratic values and the common good
- Impact of character traits on individuals and society
- Warning signs of stress
- Resources for help with stress management

Skills
- Investigate the meanings of the character traits
- Analyze situations for character traits
- Advocate for behaviors that demonstrate character
- Use assertive communication skills
- Analyze situations that call for simple acts of caring and those requiring getting the help of a caring adult.
- Make a self-assessment of character traits and develop a personal plan

Managing Life in a Less-Than-Perfect World (Alternative Version)

Content
- Six essential character traits
- Ways to manage emotions
- Communication skills
- Warning signs of stress and resources for stress management
- Review of decision-making model
- Focus on personal skills

Skills
- Analyze how character traits are demonstrated in behavior
- Apply the character traits to situations
- Communicate effectively:
  - listen
  - speak assertively
- Develop an anger management plan
- Examine respect for people in authority
- Examine the importance of caring and citizenship
- Make a self-assessment regarding character traits, and develop a personal plan to demonstrate positive character

Building Character in Ourselves and Our School

Content
- Six essential character traits
- Core democratic values
- Impact of character traits on individuals, school, and society
- The role of courage in demonstrating the character traits
- Warning signs of stress
- Resources for stress management
- Positive character in the school community

Skills
- Research the meanings of character traits and behaviors
- Analyze the impact of character traits on individuals, community and society
- Analyze situations and behaviors for character traits
- Make a self-assessment of character traits and develop a personal plan to demonstrate positive character
- Assess the character needs of the school, related to character
- Develop and implement a plan to build character at school

Grades 7-8 (Middle School)

Grades 9-12 (High School)

Table 3.4	Questions to Answer Before Preparing a Lesson Plan
Questions	**Notes**
1. What is the grade level, and what health knowledge will be addressed?	• Grades 1, 2, 3, etc.
2. What health content standard and benchmarks will be addressed?	• Selected from the National Health Education Standards
3. What should students be able to do at the end of the lesson?	• These should lead to attainment of the selected National Health Education Standard • What the student should know, value (feel), and do (behavior)
4. How will I know the student achieved the lesson objectives?	• Utilize assessment planning chart
5. What health knowledge will be included in this lesson?	• Information related to a health concept • Knowledge about skills (for example, using the POWER model for decision making, which is discussed in Chapter 4)
6. Which health skill(s) will be included in this lesson?	• What the student will know, value, and do as result of this instruction
7. Which health skill(s) will be utilized to teach the health knowledge?	• What you will be doing during the lesson • How students will be actively involved in learning
8. What teaching strategy(s) will be utilized for teaching health skills?	• What you will be doing during the lesson • What students will be doing during the lesson
9. How will I conclude each strategy and transition to the next strategy?	• Provide a statement that will transition from main concept/point to the next
10. What would be a motivating introduction to the lesson?	• Develop several focusing questions to help create interest (for example, "How many of you have ever felt like you were being bullied?")
11. How will the lesson conclusion return the focus to the learning objectives?	• What you will do to help the student fully realize the intent and important concepts of the lesson
12. What materials will be needed to teach the lesson?	• List everything needed and have it available prior to teaching the lesson

Source: Ferrara and McTighe 1992

Lohrmann's process for lesson planning is that the last three types of assessments (product, performance, and process) provide for better assessment of higher-order outcomes and require more than simple cognitive testing of information such as true-false or multiple-choice questions. (See the discussion on writing performance indicators.)

Because a prevailing philosophy for teaching health is to use the National Health Education Standards as the basis for curricular and lesson planning, the two lesson plan formats we provide samples of in this section make the most sense. Either format allows effective planning within the context of the National Health Education Standards. For either format, a logical starting point is to answer the twelve questions suggested in Lohrmann's format.

Deciding Student Outcomes

Keeping with the philosophy of focusing on individual health behaviors that represent at least half of the causes of premature death and illness, health educators have moved away from the traditional concept of behavioral objectives to what the Joint Committee on National Health Standards (1995) refers to as performance indicators. The National Health Education Standards were revised in 2005–2006. The original standards consisted of seven objectives, whereas the new standards consist of eight objectives. The current standards, as well as the predecessors, consist of a series of specific concepts and skills that students should know and be able to do in order to achieve each of the National Health Education Standards.

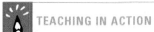 TEACHING IN ACTION | **Sample Daily Lesson Plan—Using National Standards Format**

Lesson Title: Do You Hear What I Hear?—Personal Hygiene

Date: February 19, 2012   **Time:** 10:00 A.M.   **Grade:** Three   **Teacher:** Avery

I. National Health Education Standards

Health Education Standard 7: Students will demonstrate the ability to practice health-enhancing behaviors and avoid or reduce risks.

II. National Health Education Standards Performance Indicator

7.5.1 identify responsible personal health behaviors.

III. Valued Outcomes

- Students will be able to identify basic parts of the ear.
- Students will be able to explain the process of hearing.
- Students will be able to identify ways to protect their hearing.

IV. Description of Strategy

1. Using a diagram of the ear, describe the parts of the ear and the process of hearing.
2. Blindfold five students and have other students make sounds using common objects, such as cans, glass, stones, and coins. Have blindfolded students identify the sounds.
3. Have five more students repeat the process in step 2, but they should wear earplugs as well. Ask students whether it was harder to hear with the earplugs, and explain why.
4. Have five more students come to the front. Repeat the process in step 2, but students should put an earplug only in the right ear. When finished, discuss the importance of having two ears for proper hearing.
5. Discuss with students ways in which their hearing may be damaged. Discuss how loud noises and diseases or conditions might damage hearing (ear infections, blows to the ears, and punctured eardrums).

V. Materials Needed

- Diagram of the ear and ear canal
- Various objects that have distinct sounds, such as coins, glass, and cans
- Five blindfolds and sets of earplugs

VI. Formative Evaluation

Benchmarks
- Level 1: Student was able to identify most of the parts of the ear.
- Level 2: Student was able to identify most of the parts of the ear, and described generally the process of hearing.
- Level 3: Student was able to identify nearly all parts of the ear. Student was able to describe mostly the process of hearing. Student was able to list some ways in which hearing might be damaged.
- Level 4: Student was able to identify all parts of the ear. Student was able to describe fully the process of hearing. Student was able to list ways in which hearing might be damaged.

VII. Points of Emphasis

1. Explain the importance of having two ears, not just one.
2. Explain how hearing works in relation to the ears and ear canals.
3. Explain the causes of hearing loss and how to protect against hearing loss.

Teacher Evaluation

1. Keep the lesson as taught?   yes _____ no _____

2. What I need to improve _____

3. Next time make sure _____

4. Strengths of lesson _____

Educational Objectives

From our perspective as health education writers, an excellent way to measure performance indicators is through developing sound instructional objectives. In particular, broad and measurable objectives are most helpful in assessing fulfillment. Performance indicators can help identify potential assessment areas, particularly when viewed within the three areas of framework found in Bloom's Taxonomies of Educational Objectives (Bloom 1956). The three domains are cognitive or knowledge; affective or attitudes/values; and behavioral, which focuses on skills or behavior. It is imperative in the teaching of health education to recognize that learning is reflected in ways other than simply recalling the content of health education. The ability to think, judge, evaluate, and act on the information is more important than simple recall of facts. What is important to remember is that students must not only have a correct knowledge base, but also must be able to evaluate and clarify their values/feelings if they are to select behaviors conducive to optimal health. Experiences must enable students to examine their beliefs and facilitate the skills of decision making, resulting in the potential for a positive lifestyle.

Writing Performance Objectives

To consider important only what can be measured results in the trivialization of instruction. What can be accomplished through well-planned instructional objectives is exposure to all three of Bloom's domains so that students can make decisions that enhance the overall quality of health throughout life. Students can be helped to internalize information so that it helps them make decisions that lead to positive health behaviors. The use of performance objectives is a start in the right direction. Performance objectives are brief, clear, and specific statements of what students will be able to perform at the conclusion of instructional activities. The learning objectives are predicated upon the performance indicators found in the National Health Education Standards.

It is useful to think of performance objectives as having three components. Definitions and examples of these components follow.

1. **Who**—the student or the individual who is to exhibit the knowledge, attitude, or behavior as the result of the teaching/learning process.
2. **Behavior expected**—what the student will do to show that learning has taken place. What is the student expected to know, feel, and do?
3. **Learning requirement**—what the student will know, feel, or do when the learning is completed. For example, "the student will label the diagram." It is generally a good idea to keep the verb as action-oriented as possible. However, the precision demanded by many educators has been replaced by the concept that the objective should be as broad in scope as possible, salient, and measurable

(Popham 1995). This concept builds nicely on Lohrmann's suggestions for choosing the methods of measurement before planning the instructional component. An example of a broad-scope objective might be as follows: "After reading a selected article on the social and physiological effects of alcohol, the student will compose a critical essay on the potential dangers of alcohol use associated with their personal use."

In using performance objectives, the teacher should strive to develop a reasonable number of manageable, broad, yet measurable statements that will help assess whether students have achieved the desired performance level. Attempting to become too precise in stating the objective may limit or obscure other valid indicators of a skill or ability. Teachers should view instructional objectives as starting points; they are not the totality of quality education. An alternate behavior exhibited by the student at the end of instruction may be an equally valid indicator that learning has taken place. With performance-based evaluation (see Chapter 5), the use of many different indicators of learning and behavior is now being fully recognized and appreciated.

In 2001, Anderson and Krathwohl changed the category names of the original Bloom's taxonomy (knowledge). The affective domain (valuing) remains the same as presented in the original writing. The psychomotor (behavioral) has been fine tuned by Davis (1970) and Harrow (1972). Figure 3.1 presents the cognitive, affective, and psychomotor domains, as well as the action verbs that can be used when writing each of the three types of performance objectives.

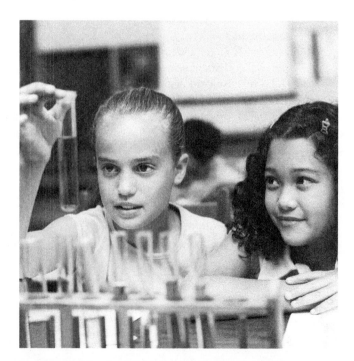

Learning activities help children internalize content and form concepts. The teacher must select activities that are best suited to each class.

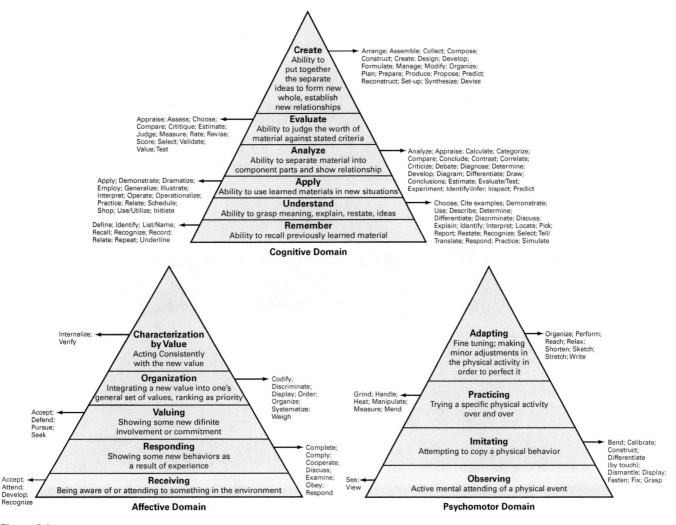

Figure 3.1
Taxonomic Domains and Action Verbs

Chapter In Review

Summary

- Teachers must recognize the complexity of life and seek to incorporate the dimensions of wellness into the teaching of health education.

- Content must be organized to ensure comprehensive coverage of grades K through 12.

- Scope and sequence must be considered when curriculum is developed.

- To help formulate scope and sequence for health education curriculum, the National Center for Chronic Disease Prevention and Health Promotion has developed the Health Education Curriculum Analysis Tool (HECAT).

- The National Health Education Standards provide the foundation for curriculum development and instruction.

- Health literacy is the ability of the student to obtain, interpret, and understand basic health information and services and the competence to use information and services in ways that enhance health.

- Effective health education requires a balance between factual information and the attitude or valuing component.

- Time must be allotted for examining values and for practicing critical thinking skills.

- The Michigan Model is an excellent example of a curriculum plan that used a coalition of state and voluntary agencies to develop a comprehensive approach to health education.

- Performance objectives based on the performance indicators found in the National Health Education Standards is the direction in which health education is currently moving.

Discussion Questions

1. What determines the nature of the content for a given grade level?

2. What is meant by the "scope and sequence" of health education?

3. Why are the National Health Education Standards important?

4. What are some barriers to quality health education?

5. Describe what is meant by the phrase "teaching for values."

6. What types of standards, curriculum guides, etc. are available from your state to help provide guidelines for teaching health education?

7. How does your state curriculum model for health education compare with the Michigan Model?

8. What purpose do objectives fulfill in the educational process?

9. What is outcome-based education?

Critical Thinking Question

1. Review the National Health Education Standards. Do they reflect what a "health-educated" child needs to know, value, and do to live a quality life that maximizes his or her potential? Are there modifications or additions you would make to better express the needs of students?

4 Strategies for Implementing Health Instruction

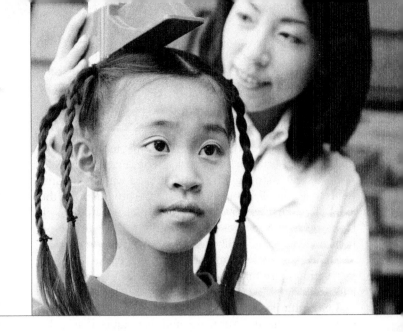

Valued Outcomes

After completion of this chapter, you should be able to:

- List the factors that affect the selection of teaching strategies.
- Discuss the elements of an effective decision making model.
- Describe reasons why teaching refusal skills is important.
- Discuss styles of learning.
- Select learning strategies that appeal to the various styles of learning.
- Describe how to effectively use various strategies for teaching.
- Discuss ways to use technology in the classroom.

Reflections

As you read through this chapter, try to think of situations in which students might use the various strategies. This helps students personalize the information and formulate their feelings about the material presented. Think in terms of what learning styles might be best suited to the plethora of possibilities for developing a knowledge base and for personalizing information. Develop several scenarios for and various strategies to address each learning style.

Each day, the nation's 132,700 schools provide an opportunity for 55 million students to learn about health and practice skills that promote healthy behaviors.

—*Division of Adolescent and School Health (2011)*

The Relationship of Strategies to Learning

A strategy is any activity or experience that teachers use to interpret, illustrate, or facilitate learning. Foder and Dalis (1989) view a strategy as anything used with or on students to accomplish the objectives of the program. For the most effective learning to take place, teachers should seek strategies that are student-centered and provide for group involvement. Additionally, teachers should use more than one strategy or activity for each major concept so that their instruction more fully encompasses the variety of student abilities and aptitudes.

Learning strategies make content and objectives come alive. Selecting strategies and techniques that make learning exciting and motivating is the direct responsibility of teachers, who, having established a working knowledge of the many strategies available in health education, are limited only by their own creativity.

The teacher must remember that selecting a variety of strategies does not ensure learning. Several other factors influence effective learning and must be considered, such as a relationship with the students that is conducive to learning. Treating students fairly is the first step in facilitating learning and creating a proper classroom atmosphere.

Many techniques to help promote creative learning are available. With proper preparation, the following strategies and equipment can be useful:

audio CDs and MP3s	newspapers
brainstorming	online activities
bulletin boards	panel discussion
buzz groups	peer helpers
case studies/committee work	puppet shows
CD-ROMs	resource speakers
charts/maps	role-playing
computers	self-appraisals
cooperative learning	slides
debates	social network
demonstrations/	specimens/models
experiments	storytelling
dramatization	tablets
DVDs	television
exhibits	transparencies
Facebook	values clarification
field trips	videotapes
magazines	word searches/crosswords
posters	

▪ Factors Affecting Strategies

When selecting strategies to provide learning experiences, keep the following criteria in mind:

- **Select strategies that contribute to total learning.** Some activities lend themselves to acquiring knowledge, whereas other activities are better suited to attitude assessment and decision making. Ideally, the strategies should help the student develop the ability to reason and assess the information being presented. Any strategy selected should involve the students as participants in the activity.

- **The more complex the concept, the more activities are needed to develop the concept.** As a general rule, for each concept, you should employ two strategies or activities. If the material is difficult, you may need more than two. Another reason for using more than one strategy is that students learn in a variety of ways and through different means. Thus, using a variety of strategies will help all students to grasp the concept under examination.

- **Begin with the simple and move to the more complex.** Once you have prepared the class for the activity through a proper introduction, the students should become part of the learning activity. With simple activities, students should be able to learn by means of group involvement, self-assessment, and class–teacher interaction. As the students become better able to deal with more difficult topics, more complex strategies can be used that require self-discovery or analysis of materials and conclusions.

- **Include audiovisual aids whenever possible.** These can include models, classroom exhibits, videos, Power Points, DVDs, CD-ROMs, online activities, and so forth. Audiovisual aids add another dimension to teaching concepts and are excellent for reinforcing learning.

Strategies can be classified into many different categories. Some authorities distinguish among strategies, media, and instructional materials, whereas other experts group all three into one category. Classification is unimportant as long as you can identify the strengths and weaknesses of each available technique. Your objective should be to select strategies that are appropriate and effective for your class and that are based on the learning styles of the students.

The strategy chapters that follow provide suggested grade levels for which the various activities are best suited. It is important to remember that with minor changes, most activities would be appropriate for other grade levels and can be used in combinations to optimize the desired mix of learning styles.

▪ Learning Styles and Strategies Selection

Having insight into the different types of learning styles is useful for many reasons. When you plan a health lesson, it is most important to employ a variety of strategies that appeal to the three basic learning styles: through sight (visual), sound (auditory), and touch/doing (kinesthetic).

It is impossible to address the many different theories of learning styles within the context of this book. Fortunately, most theories are similar in concept. Students—like all people—learn new information in different ways. If you use a strategy that does not fit with a particular student's learning style, the student will be unable to successfully process information. Thus, having a basic understanding of differences in learning styles and planning strategies can contribute to successful learning, assessment, and, ultimately, behavior change.

The **visual learner** may think in pictures and learn best from diagrams, PowerPoints, videos, and handouts. Visual learners often prefer to take detailed notes to absorb information and they generally do better on written tests than oral tests. When teaching from a PowerPoint or website, gain and maintain the focus of a visual learner by highlighting text, altering color scheme, or changing a font to indicate a change of topic. A teacher should encourage a visual learner to review notes often, use color-coded pens or highlighters on notes, make a mental picture of important words, and use memory devices (a mnemonic or acronym) to aid their learning.

The **auditory learner** learns best through lectures, discussions, and listening to what other students have to say. Written information may have little meaning until it is heard or spoken. To help this type of learner, teachers should use verbal direction and reinforcement, group discussion and activities, and even present information in a rhythmic pattern such as a poem or song. The auditory learner should be encouraged to record information and then listen to the recordings, rather than relying on notes or study guides. When studying, this type of learner can learn best through having another student or caregiver give the auditory learner an oral quiz. The auditory learner, when studying alone, should read aloud the new information to aid in memory and understanding.

The **kinesthetic learner** is one that learns best through doing, by touching an object, or replicating an action. They may struggle to learn by reading or listening, but will usually perform well in things such as experiments, physical activity, art, and acting. It is common for kinesthetic learners, also known as "doers," to focus on two different things at the same time (such as listening to music while learning or studying). They will remember things by going back in their minds to what their body was doing as they learned. In an elementary classroom setting, these students may stand out because of their constant need to move; their high levels of energy may cause them to be restless and impatient, but it's important for a teacher to recognize that kinesthetic learners' short- and long-term memory is strengthened by their use of their own body's movements.

It is important for teachers to build in various strategies that will appeal to the various learning styles. One problem is that teachers unconsciously tend to select the strategies that they use themselves. Teachers must constantly remind themselves to use a variety of approaches to facilitate knowledge assimilation, assessment of information, and influence behavior change.

An inventory developed by G. Price and R. Dunn (Table 4.1) was the first comprehensive approach to the assessment of student learning styles. The inventory, called the Learning Style Inventory (LSI), is designed for grades 3 through 12. The LSI seeks to provide those elements that are imperative to children learning. What is unique about the LSI is that it identifies the type of environment, instructional activities, social grouping(s), and motivating factors that maximize individual learning (Price and Dunn 1997, 5). The LSI surveys each student's preferences in each of twenty-two different areas, and it provides information as to how children prefer to function, learn, concentrate, and perform during educational strategies.

This scheme of learning may seem a bit overwhelming, but teachers must have a conceptualization of what strategies to employ in the classroom if their students are to learn best. Teachers can use the awareness provided by the LSI to build in a variety of learning situations and environments and thus enhance the learning potential of their students.

■ Multiple Intelligences—Implications for Health Education

Howard Gardner, a professor of psychology at Harvard University, defined seven types of intelligence. Since the definition of this initial group of seven intelligences, two other types of intelligence have been added for a total of nine types. The nine types of intelligence that have been identified are shown in the Health Highlight box on page 54.

According to multiple intelligences theory, all humans possess—in varying amounts—the nine identified intelligence types. Each person has different intellectual compositions. From the perspective of health education, the concept of multiple intelligences provides several thoughts concerning the planning of strategies for successful teaching. Many of these concepts have already been pointed out in the preceding sections of this chapter. However, the keys to multiple intelligences theory are successful strategy planning and effective implementation in the classroom. The guidelines below reflect the essential items for lesson planning that address multiple intelligences theory (Concept to Classroom: Tapping into Multiple Intelligence—Implementation 2002).

- **Teach subject matter through a variety of activities and projects.** The classroom should be filled with engaging activities that evoke a range of intelligences. Encourage students to work collaboratively as well as individually to support both their interpersonal and intrapersonal intelligences.

- **Integrate assessments into learning.** Students need to play an active role in their assessments. Offer students a number of choices for "showing what they know" about a topic. In addition to traditional paper-and-pencil tests, give the student opportunities to create meaningful projects and authentic presentations.

- **All students have all intelligences.** The intelligences should be nurtured throughout the whole spectrum of types to foster student learning and strengthen their entire intelligence.

Table 4.1   Environmental, Instructional, and Social Groupings and Motivating Factors That Maximize Individual Learning

Area	Student Preference
Noise level	Does the child prefer quiet or sound when learning?
Light	Does the student work best under bright lights, or does the student need dim or indirect light?
Temperature	Does the child concentrate best in a warm or cool environment?
Design	Does the student learn best in a formal environment, such as the classroom, or an informal environment, such as on a lounge chair, bed, or floor?
Unmotivated/self-motivated	Does the child do well to please himself or herself?
Not persistent/persistent	What is the student's inclination to complete tasks: to complete the task once begun or to take intermittent breaks?
Not responsible/responsible	What is the student's desire to do what he or she thinks ought to be done? Students who have low responsibility scores usually are nonconforming.
Structure	Does the student need specific directions or explanations when doing a task or prefer doing an assignment his or her own way?
Learning alone/peer-oriented learner	Does the student prefer to study alone or with a friend/group?
Authority figures present	Does the student feel more comfortable when someone who has authority or special knowledge is present?
Prefers learning in several ways	Does the child need a variety of learning situations as opposed to routines for learning?
Auditory preferences	Does the child learn best listening to verbal instructions?
Visual preferences	Does the child learn visually? An example is a child who can close his or her eyes and visually recall what he or she has read or seen earlier.
Tactile preferences	Does the student need to underline while reading, take notes when listening, or keep his or her hands busy?
Kinesthetic preferences	Does the child require whole-body movement and/or real-life experiences to best retain material?
Requires intake	Does the student seem to eat, drink, chew, or bite objects while concentrating, or does the student learn best with no such intake?
Functions best in evening/morning	What time of day does the student prefer to learn?
Functions best in late morning	Does the child prefer to learn during the late morning? The energy curve for these students is highest in late morning, around 10 A.M.
Functions best in afternoon	Does the child prefer to learn during the afternoon? Energy level is higher after lunch hour.
Mobility	How long can the child sit?
Parent figure-motivated	Does the individual want to do well to please the parent(s)?
Teacher-motivated	Does the student want to learn and complete tasks to please the teacher?

Source: Learning Style Inventory (LSI). Price Systems, 763 North 1750 Road, Lawrence, KS 66049, www.learningstyle.com. Reprinted by permission.

Decision Making and Health Strategies

As you have seen, it is important for students to have an opportunity to personalize information and make decisions relative to their health. They also must have a model that helps them assess the possibilities and consequences of their potential actions. If students are to make positive health decisions, the process of how to make intelligent decisions is crucial. These skills must be taught and utilized throughout the educational experience, and students must practice making decisions to enhance their decision-making skills. This practice goes beyond the model and helps them feel good about themselves (self-esteem), see that they can have control of their behavior (locus of control), and believe in their own decision-making skills (self-efficacy). See Chapter 6 for more information on self-esteem.

Several models can be utilized. A good model should have the characteristics described below.

1. It helps the student identify and define exactly what the problem/decision is.
2. It provides the opportunity to identify possible actions. It helps prepare the student to respond immediately to a situation and to formulate strategies for dealing with problems that do not require an immediate response.
3. It provides the opportunity to evaluate each of the possible actions the student might take to deal with the problem. Many alternative ways of dealing with the problem/situation should be identified; the more ideas, the better.
4. The model must also provide a way to assess the possible results of the various potential decisions previously identified. Questions that might be asked during this time include the following:
   - What has worked in a similar situation?
   - What might work that has not been tried before?
   - What does the law say concerning the potential solution?
   - Would my parents be proud of my decision?
   - What are the pros and cons of each alternative solution?
   - What are my fears concerning each alternative?
   - What are my feelings concerning each alternative?
5. It provides the opportunity to share the information with several people if time warrants. Make sure one of the people is a responsible adult—preferably a parent.
6. The model should help select the most appropriate action to be taken. Eliminate alternatives that are dangerous to oneself or others or that are illegal. The model should help determine the following questions:
   - Does my decision contribute to my health and welfare?
   - Does my decision contribute to other people's health and welfare?
   - Does my decision violate any laws or rules?
   - Does my decision show respect for myself?
   - Does my decision follow what responsible adults would do?
7. The model should help decide what steps must be taken to put the decision into action. Questions might include the following:
   - What do I need to do?
   - Where do I need help to enact my decision?
   - What is the timetable for enacting my decision?
8. Once the action has been taken, the model should help to reflect, evaluate, and revise the decision. Questions might include the following:
   - How do I feel about the decision?
   - Did it work out the way I wanted?
   - What would I do differently?
   - Would another alternative have worked better?

■ The POWER Model for Decision Making

Included in the Michigan Model for Comprehensive School Health Education is the POWER Model. It is an excellent example of a decision-making model that fulfills the above criteria. The POWER model, shown in the sample blank worksheet on pages 56–57, can be used at all grade levels with minor modifications. For students who have not yet developed their writing and reading skills, the teacher may have to read the headings and list the responses on an overhead or on the board. The important point is to introduce the steps for making wise decisions early in children's educational experience. As their skills improve, they can use the model in written form. Then they will have a framework for making decisions as their choices and consequences become more difficult. The model will probably have to be used in a group situation in early elementary grades but can be used in individual or group work for the later grades. An example demonstrating how the model works is given in the completed Worksheet on pages 58–59.

It is suggested that you take students through the other four options formulated as possible solutions and work through the potential good and bad results of these. What option are *you* most comfortable with?

■ Developing Refusal Skills

Refusal skills are part of good decision making. We need good refusal skills when it is necessary to say "No" to an action or to leave a potentially harmful situation. Any situation that threatens (emotionally or physically) personal safety or health, tempts students to break the law, detracts from personal character, asks students to disobey parental rules, or results in loss of self-respect calls for

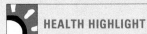

HEALTH HIGHLIGHT | **The Nine Multiple Intelligences**

1. **Verbal-Linguistic**—well-developed verbal skills and sensitivity to the sounds, meaning, and rhythms of words. A child whose strength is in this area enjoys language arts: speaking, writing, reading, and listening. This child will do well in the traditional classroom.

2. **Mathematical-Logical**—ability to think conceptually and abstractly and has the capacity to discern logical or numerical patterns. Children with this strength have an aptitude for numbers, reasoning, and problem solving. These children will also do well in the traditional classroom, in which teaching is logically sequenced and students are asked to conform.

3. **Rhythmic Intelligence**—ability to produce and appreciate rhythm, pitch, and timber. These children learn well through songs, patterns, rhythms, instruments, and musical expression.

4. **Visual-Spatial**—capacity to think in images and pictures and to visualize accurately and abstractly. These children learn best through visuals and spatial organization. They like to see what you are talking about in order to understand. They enjoy charts, graphs, maps, tables, illustrations, art, and puzzles.

5. **Bodily-Kinesthetic**—ability to control body movements and to handle objects skillfully. These children learn best through activities such as games, movement, and hands-on tasks (for example, building something). They may be labeled "overly active" in traditional classrooms, in which they are told to sit and be still.

6. **Interpersonal**—capacity to detect and respond appropriately to the moods, motivations, and desires of other people. This child is people-oriented and outgoing and does his or her learning cooperatively in groups or with a partner. He or she may be labeled as "talkative" or "too concerned about being social."

7. **Intrapersonal**—capacity to be self-aware and in tune with inner feelings, values, beliefs, and thinking processes. These children are especially in touch with their own feelings, values, and ideas. They may appear to be reserved but are quite intuitive about what they learn and how it relates to themselves.

8. **Naturalist**—ability to recognize and categorize plants, animals, and other objects in nature. These children love the outdoors, animals, and field trips. They also like to pick up on subtle differences in meanings.

9. **Existential**—sensitivity and capacity to tackle deep questions about human existence, such as what is the meaning of life, why do we die, and how did we get here. These children learn in the context of where humankind stands in the "big picture" of existence. They ask "Why are we here?" and "What is our role in the world?"

Source: Adapted from McKenzie 1999

strong refusal skills. The following rules teach students to develop good refusal skills.

- **Employ assertive behavior.** Students should recognize that acting assertively is being honest with what they are thinking and feeling. It lets others know that they are in control of their behavior and the situation. Teach them to say "No" clearly and firmly while looking directly at the person they are addressing.

- **Use body language that matches assertive verbal behavior.** Explain to students that body language must indicate that they are sincere without being aggressive or disrespectful. Students should also recognize that it is important to make sure that body language does not say "I would like to, but I don't think I can." Students should make it totally clear that they do not desire the drink, drug, or physical advances of the person with whom they are talking.

- **Don't get involved in potentially harmful/ dangerous situations.** Encourage students to think ahead concerning potentially dangerous situations. Tell students to avoid allowing themselves to be in a place where they might be pressured or tempted.

- **Be a positive role model.** Help students act and talk in a manner that commands respect and reflects their personal value system. They have a responsibility to protect themselves, obey the laws, and demonstrate good character. Explain to students that their reputation is important and that the people they associate with should be known for their own good character.

- **You don't have to say "No, thank you."** In a situation in which students are feeling pressured, there is no need to be polite. Teach students to tell a person that they do not appreciate his or her thought or action. Students should be very emphatic that they want no part.

Each of the strategies chapters includes opportunities for children to practice both the decision-making skills and refusal skills. Only through practice and being prepared can children make decisions and be prepared to resist the many pressures they face during the formative years.

A Positive Climate for Learning

Regardless of the strategy employed, the teacher must strive to create a classroom environment that is conducive to learning. Students should look forward to class, feel emotionally/intellectually unthreatened, and realize that they will be supported in their learning efforts. There are several things a teacher can do to facilitate a positive learning climate (Evertson et al. 2008, 123):

- Identify appropriate instructional goals and discuss them with students so that the intent is clear concerning what is expected.

- Insist that work be completed satisfactorily to mutually determined standards.

- Refuse to accept excuses for poor work.

- Communicate acceptance of imperfect initial performance when students struggle to achieve new learning.

- Convey confidence in the students' ability to do well.

- Display a "can do" attitude that generates student excitement and self-confidence.

- Avoid comparative evaluations, especially of lower-ability students, that might have them conclude they cannot meet expectations.

▪ Clarifying Activities

To personalize health concepts, students must relate to health instruction from the affective domain or attitudinal level. An excellent strategy for achieving this end is the use of valuing strategies activities. By examining and clarifying values, children can learn positive health behavior. As mentioned earlier, however, the use of values clarification techniques is not without some controversy. Values cannot and should not be avoided in health education, but the teacher must be adequately prepared to do the job correctly.

Begin by recognizing that values are relative, personal, and often situational. You should not attempt to teach your own personal values or the "correct" values; instead, your goal should be to help students assess and develop their own values so that these values lead to positive health behavior. It is essential that any value judgment made by the students be made through their own cognitive process. According to Hochbaum, Rosenstock, and Kegeles (1960), for a value judgment or health practice to evolve, the following criteria must apply:

- Students must perceive the issue as important.

- Students must believe that they are susceptible to the problem.

- Students must believe that the problem is serious.

- The intensity of the threat and resultant anxiety must not be so great as to paralyze the ability to act.

- There must be an action to take that the individual believes will be effective.

For students to function effectively when using clarifying strategies, they also must be prepared. Greenberg (1989, 43) states that the following are requisites of learner-centered instruction:

1. Familiarity with and trust of other program participants (students)
2. Friendship with at least one other participant
3. Listening skills
4. Knowledge of and experience with roles assumed by members and leaders of groups
5. Knowledge of and experience with the decision-making process
6. Cooperation and participation among all members of the program
7. An understanding and appreciation of both one's own feelings and the feelings of others
8. Open communication among disagreeing factions and empathy with those of opposing viewpoints
9. Recognition of unfulfilled needs of program participants and means of satisfying those needs
10. Appreciation of individual differences and unique potential

When engaging in any clarifying activity, the teacher must allot sufficient time for students to assess their own feelings about the issue under examination. Students must also feel free to assess their values without fear of being ridiculed or forced to pay lip service to the opinions of others, including the teacher. Keep in mind that clarifying activities do not lead to one "correct" solution to a problem; they are open-ended. (The purpose of these activities is to open the doors to additional assessment.) Also, as a teacher you are a participant in the activities and a role model for the students. Every student has the right to decline from speaking, without having to give a reason for declining. Respect individual feelings, and keep the activity nonthreatening.

Many instructional devices are available for incorporating clarification activities into the health curriculum. The ones you choose should be appropriate for the developmental level of the students. As already discussed, young children are not capable of dealing with highly abstract issues. Further, they do not have the experiential background to deal knowingly with topics far removed from their everyday world. Therefore, it is not realistic to attempt to grapple with such values-related issues as euthanasia or world hunger at the primary level.

▪ Simple Values-Related Strategies

One of the simplest and most appropriate activities for younger students involves what is known as a shield activity, which is an excellent tool for teaching children the ten prerequisites suggested by Greenberg. The major objective of this activity is to help children identify their values. The activity consists of filling in each segment of the shield with a values-related response, either in words or with drawings. A typical shield is illustrated in Worksheet 4.1 on page 478. Each child is given a copy of this worksheet to complete. For younger children, you should read the instructions aloud.

The following steps may be used to help children work through the activity.

1. After students have filled out the shield, ask them to cross out any area of the shield that they are unwilling to discuss.

The POWER Model

Name: _____

Date: _____

P: What's the PROBLEM?

The situation is: _____

The facts are: _____

My feelings are: _____

I think (concerning the situation): _____

My friends think/feel: _____

My problem is: _____

O: What are the OPTIONS?

The outcome I want is: _____

My options for reaching my outcome are:

1. _____

2. _____

3. _____

4. _____

5. _____

W: WHAT'S BEST to do?

Try out the three best options:

1. If I did this:	**Possible Good Results**	**Possible Bad Results**
_____	_____	_____
_____	_____	_____
_____	_____	_____

2. If I did this:	**Possible Good Results**	**Possible Bad Results**
_____	_____	_____
_____	_____	_____
_____	_____	_____

3. If I did this: **Possible Good Results**   **Posible Bad Results**

_____   _____   _____

_____   _____   _____

_____   _____   _____

The option I chose: _____

_____

E: ENACT your plan.

The steps I need to take are:

Task   **Who Does It**   **By When**

1. _____   _____   _____

2. _____   _____   _____

3. _____   _____   _____

4. _____   _____   _____

5. _____   _____   _____

I could get help from: _____

R: REFLECT on the outcome and REVISE your strategy (if necessary).

Now that the decision has been carried out:

I think _____

I feel _____

I achieved/did not achieve what I wanted because _____

It turned out _____

I learned I _____

I learned that others _____

Next time I'll _____

A The POWER Model

Name: *Daniela Ruiz*
Date: *February 19, 2012*

P: What's the PROBLEM?

The situation is: *My friend Beth borrowed my CD and hasn't returned it.*

The facts are: *I loaned it to her last week, and she keeps promising to return it but hasn't. I want my CD back*

My feelings are: *I'm angry because Beth keeps breaking her promise. I'm disappointed because I thought I could trust her.*

I think (concerning the situation): *I think I should not have loaned her the CD.*

My friends think/feel: *Some of my friends understand my feelings, but others think I'm being stingy.*

My problem is: *Beth has not returned my CD as she promised, and I want it back.*

O: What are the OPTIONS?

The outcome I want is: *For Beth to return my CD and to keep her friendship.*

My options for reaching my outcome are:

1. *Ask Beth again.*
2. *Tell Beth how important the CD is to me.*
3. *Tell Beth that she will not be my friend if she doesn't return the CD.*
4. *Talk to my parents.*
5. *Call Beth's parents.*

W: WHAT'S BEST to do?

Try out the three best options:

1. If I did this:	**Possible Good Results**	**Possible Bad Results**
Called Beth's parents	*Now: I'll get my CD back.*	*Beth could be in trouble.*
	Later: They might get Beth her own CD.	*Beth would not be my friend.*

2. If I did this:	**Possible Good Results**	**Possible Bad Results**
Told Beth how important the CD is to me	*Now: She might understand and give the CD back.*	*She'll just laugh at me.*

3. If I did this: | **Possible Good Results** | **Possible Bad Results**

Talked to my parents	Now. They would buy me a new CD.	My parents would be mad.

The option I chose: Tell Beth how important the CD is to me. I'll offer to call her in the morning to remind her to bring it to school.

E: ENACT your plan.

The steps I need to take are:

Task	Who Does It	By When
1. Find time to talk to Beth.	Me	After school
2. Ask Beth if I can talk with her.	Me	At lunch
3. Think about what I want to say.	Me	During study hall
4. Meet and talk with Beth.	Me	After school
5.		

I could get help from: My parents, my brother, and Beth's parents

R: REFLECT on the outcome and REVISE your strategy (if necessary).

Now that the decision has been carried out:

I think telling people the truth works.

I feel good that I confronted Beth.

I achieved/did not achieve what I wanted because I got my CD back, and I got it without hard feelings on the part of Beth.

It turned out well for me, and Beth was not mad at me.

I learned I do not have to allow a friend to take advantage of me.

I learned that others will respond to a reasonable request.

Next time I'll be more careful who I loan my things to and establish how long they can keep them.

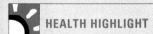

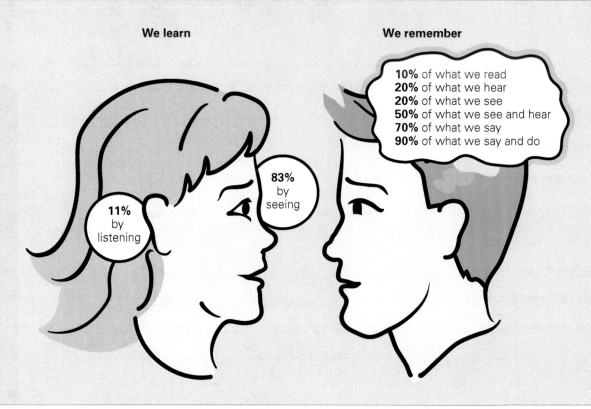

We learn

11% by listening

83% by seeing

We remember

10% of what we read
20% of what we hear
20% of what we see
50% of what we see and hear
70% of what we say
90% of what we say and do

2. Ask the students to move about the room in silence, holding the shield in front of themselves so other students can see the shields. Remind students that they should not talk.

3. After five to ten minutes, ask each student to select someone standing close by, or you may pair students. Tell students to sit together to discuss the shield. The process begins with the first student asking the other student a question concerning his or her shield. After answering the question, the second student asks a question. The process continues until all the areas in the shield have been covered. This usually takes five to ten minutes.

4. Ask the students in each pair to take turns introducing one another as each feels his or her partner would want to be introduced.

5. To bring closure, you might ask the children the following questions:

- How many of you knew the name of your partner before beginning the activity?
- Did you introduce yourself?
- Did you find some things that you shared with your partner?
- Did you find some things that were different from your partner?

- How did you feel about your introduction of your partner?
- What would you change about the introduction your partner made about you?
- Did you feel you were a good listener when your partner answered your questions?
- Can you write down one thing you learned about yourself?
- Can you write down one thing you learned about your partner?
- Can you write down one thing you learned about the entire class?

In presenting such an activity, it is essential that you thoroughly introduce, carry out, and summarize the experience. If this is not done, the activity becomes nothing more than a game. Through careful introduction, a psychological set is established so that the activity will be meaningful and the students will understand why they are doing it. By careful summation, you can help students assess their feelings and clarify existing values.

▪ Decision Stories

Decision stories are open-ended vignettes that describe a values-related dilemma and ask students to suggest a

In society today there is a wide diversity of people and cultures. These differences have fostered a need to accommodate unique physical, demographic, and economic situations (Garcia 1991). The elementary teacher must strive to view all children of various cultures from students' perspectives rather than from his or her own cultural perspective. This means that the classroom should facilitate a climate of understanding and sensitivity to diverse cultures, ethnicities, and races.

To understand multicultural sensitivity and diversity, a teacher must first be able to distinguish several terms. Page and Page (2006) define _culture_ as a set of values, attitudes, and practices held in common by a group of people, usually identified by ancestry, language, and geography. _Ethnicity_ refers to a portion of a population or subgroup having a common cultural heritage. _Race_ denotes a population distinguished by genetically determined physical traits, such as hair texture or color, skin color, eye shape, and body shape.

A teacher can develop multicultural sensitivity in several ways. He or she should strive to develop personal skills, such as showing warmth, respect, sincerity, concern, and caring for people of all cultures. It is imperative that the teacher understand the communities from which children come. In addition, the teacher must be culturally sensitive to how different ethnic groups learn and solve problems. Part of this involves understanding learning styles, communication patterns, and factors such as eye contact, body language, and physical closeness.

---

course of action. The stories should reflect real-life circumstances and should be appropriate to the age level of the children. No easy answer should suggest itself in the story, but viable courses of action must be possible for the activity to be meaningful. If only unacceptable or repugnant alternatives seem possible, children will be unable to incorporate positive decision-making skills into their own behavioral repertoires. A decision story children can identify with and relate to provides an excellent springboard for values discussion. A good decision story not only encourages students to sort out opinions, values, and feelings, but also requires students to think about them, test them, and try them out. The real test of the importance of values comes with application.

In preparing decision stories, keep in mind that the story should be between fifty and 150 words in length. It should include enough detail to establish realism and character, but it should not be so long as to obscure the central issue. Establish a focus on the main issue with relevant supportive facts and events. Be careful not to slant the story so that only one solution or course of action is implied. Remember to provide a descriptive title, and end with a focus question that asks each student to suggest a course of action. This question is also the basis for discussion of the issue (Hamrick, Anspaugh, and Smith 1980, 455). Following are examples of decision stories.

Pressure. Jim and Paul are fifth-graders in the same classroom. In the past few weeks, they have become friends. One day while walking home from school, Jim and Paul meet some of Paul's other friends by the park. Paul's friends are all smoking. They offer Paul a cigarette. He takes it and lights up. Paul's friends also offer Jim a cigarette, but he says no. The boys start to make fun of him and call him a chicken. Even Paul is laughing at his friend. **Focus Question:** What should Jim do?

Hot Spot. Mary's fourth-grade class is taking an important arithmetic test. Mary has studied hard for the test. In the seat next to her is her friend, Julia. Julia is worried that she will not pass the test. The teacher leaves the room for a minute. While she is gone, Julia asks Mary for some of the test answers. The other students see and hear this. The teacher will be back in the room soon. **Focus Question:** What should Mary do?

Students are an excellent source for developing such decision stories. After being exposed to a few models that you have written or located in values-clarification materials, students are usually eager to write vignettes of their own. This should be encouraged, because student-developed stories are highly relevant and motivating to the students themselves.

Presenting Decision Stories in Class. Begin by setting the stage for the story and motivating the class for the activity and the inquiry. Discuss the title of the story, and ask the children what it suggests to them. Stimulate the students' curiosity and get them involved from the start. For decision stories to be effective, students must be participants and not merely passive listeners. After a few minutes of this warm-up phase, present the story itself. Most of the stories can be read aloud. However, in some circumstances, it may help to give copies of the stories to the students so they can consider the details of the presentation.

Have the students offer individual responses to the focus question: "What course of action do you think is most appropriate?" Encourage thought and reflection on the matter, but do not force any student to respond unwillingly. A good way to get students thinking is to have each student write a response on paper. The writing process facilitates thinking through the situation that has been presented. This process could be structured in a manner that requires students to begin by defining the problem. Below the definition, the options or choices can be listed, along with the possible consequences of each action. Consequences can be either positive or negative or a combination of the two. Writing also requires each student to make a commitment based on the information presented. It should be made clear, however, that the written responses need not be shared with the class at this point.

Pooling Ideas.

Next, generate a list of all possible solutions to the decision story dilemma by asking students to share their responses with the class. This should be done on a volunteer basis. The teacher should not provide feedback to the students such as "That's good," or "I'm not sure that is such a good idea." Attempt to remain noncommittal. Respond with phrases such as "Thank you for sharing that idea with us," or by simply paraphrasing their responses. Then collect the responses and compile a list of solutions on the chalkboard without revealing which student offered any particular solution. You should also add possible solutions to the list that the students have overlooked.

Consider all the ideas put forth. Do not be judgmental, and do not reject any solution out of hand. Remember that the teacher's role is to help students clarify their own values, not to impose values on them.

Now divide the class into small groups and have each group discuss the possible solutions to the dilemma. Allow time for each group to reach a consensus on the preferred solution. Encourage the students to offer reasons for their choices.

Discussion and Reappraisal.

After each small group has come to some sort of agreement, have them present the results of their discussions to the whole class. Groups will probably opt for different solutions. Ask individual students why one solution seems better than another. Again, refrain from being judgmental, and display neutrality. Instead of commenting, "So you think that Mary should just pretend that she didn't hear Julia?" you might ask, "How could Mary have responded to Julia?" Finally, have each student reconsider the decision story in light of the class discussion (Smith, Hamrick, and Anspaugh 1981, 637). Some children will want to change their minds at this point. Others may modify their approach to the problem. Again, have each student write down his or her solution to the problem along with reasons why the solution seems best. Have the students reflect on the ramifications of their decisions. Without necessarily requiring verbal responses, ask questions such as the following:

- Have you ever been in a situation like the one in the story?
- Did you come to the same solution then?
- Did you or would you carry out your planned decision?
- What happened or what do you think would happen if you tried out this decision?

- How did this decision affect your own values?
- How were you affected by the decision?
- How were other people affected by your decision?
- Would you always make a similar decision?

Using this structured approach to decision stories will help students develop decision-making skills. It will also help them apply rational thought to everyday problems involving values.

▪ Role-Playing

Role-playing is an excellent strategy for helping establish what students are feeling, determining how others might feel in a given situation, or helping students to decide how they might handle a given situation or event. Students may either act out roles identified by the teacher or (after becoming comfortable with the technique) write their own roles. To facilitate an effective role-playing situation, give students a basic description of the situation and the role(s). The actual role-playing should be done with little or no rehearsal. A typical role-play should have a time limit of one to three minutes, followed by class discussion. Potential discussion questions include: Why did the role-players react to the situation in a particular way? What are some other potential solutions/suggestions for dealing with the situation? How might the role-play situation be done differently? Table 4.2 lists some guidelines for effective role-playing.

Other Verbal and Discussion-Oriented Strategies

Values clarification activities rely to a large extent on discussion, as do many other classroom strategies. Discussion is a useful technique, but it must be structured. Always keep in mind your objective in employing any particular discussion strategy so that you do not lose the focus. Several other discussion-oriented strategies

Table 4.2   Guidelines for Effective Role-Playing
Select role-players or ask for volunteers.
Set the scene. Describe the situation carefully but briefly.
Give brief, clear instructions.
End the situation if it becomes stalemated or repetitive.
Provide time to discuss: • What happened in the situation? • Why did the situation turn out the way it did? • Did the situation turn out as desired? • Who would have had to do what to make the situation turn out differently?

that have proven effective in health instruction are presented below.

Brainstorming

Like valuing strategies activities, brainstorming can be used to improve decision-making skills by having students generate many possible ideas concerning an issue. Freedom of expression and creativity are also encouraged. This strategy can be employed by all age groups and can foster a higher level of thinking. It is imperative that precise instructions be given about "how" and "what" is to be brainstormed. Possible topics for brainstorming sessions include the following:

- How can we get people to follow safety rules?
- How can we encourage people to eat nutritious snacks instead of junk food?
- How can we make our physical environment more healthful and more pleasant?

When you conduct a brainstorming session, it is very important to follow these four rules:

1. The problem to be brainstormed must be well defined.
2. Any and all ideas must be accepted.
3. Criticism of any idea put forth is not allowed.
4. All ideas should be evaluated objectively when the session is over.

Brainstorming can be used effectively in the lower as well as upper elementary grades. The biggest drawback is that, in a large class, not all children will have the opportunity to express their thoughts. Nonetheless, the activity can be quite productive. By encouraging and accepting all opinions, brainstorming may yield new or novel possible solutions to a problem. Even impractical suggestions can lead to new ways of thinking about an issue.

Follow-up is important. In the follow-up session, ask children to elaborate on their ideas. Present additional information that will be useful in making suggestions more practical or realistic. In doing so, emphasize to the class how the brainstorming session led to many approaches to the problem.

Buzz Groups

Akin to brainstorming, buzz groups are an effective strategy for examining a specific problem. Generally, this technique is productive if students are mature enough to use the format. It permits student participation in an atmosphere conducive to discussion. The buzz group strategy should not be overused, however, because too much small-group work can lessen student enthusiasm.

To use this approach, have students work in groups of three to five students. Avoid putting friends in the same group, or the discussion may tend to stray to issues aside from the assigned task. Have each group focus on a specific problem that you have introduced and discussed so that the children will have a knowledge base for their discussion. Each group should choose a chairperson and a recording secretary. The chairperson must keep the discussion on the topic, and the secretary records important points. Walk from group to group to help maintain the focus of each group.

Allow three to fifteen minutes for buzz group discussion. Examples of suitable topics for this strategy include how an accident victim should be handled, how children can get along better with brothers and sisters, what can be done to educate children about the dangers of smoking, and what can be done about vandalism.

After the discussion time is over, ask the recording secretary for each group to present the results of that group's discussion. The more controversial the topic, the more likely that many diverse opinions will be aired. In the summary discussion, encourage objective consideration of all approaches put forth.

Case Studies

Case studies are actual events that you can use in class for discussion. The decision story format (see pages 60–62) lends itself well to the case study strategy—just substitute the actual event for the hypothetical one. Good sources for case study materials are health journals, newspapers, news magazines, and television programs.

Cooperative Learning

An excellent strategy for fostering cohesiveness in the classroom is cooperative learning. This technique involves having students work together to solve an identified problem or to work toward some common goal. Have students work in small groups and instruct each group to arrive at a conclusion on a particular problem or situation. This strategy allows students to work together, and each child can provide input to the conclusions. Above all, do not allow one or two students to dominate any group. You may overcome this problem by listening carefully to the group discussions and refocusing them when needed. It is difficult to assign grades for cooperative learning because an individual's contribution to solving the problem or arriving at the solution is not easily determined. Topics such as those suggested for the brainstorming or buzz group activities lend themselves to cooperative learning.

Critical Essays

The teacher asks the students to write their evaluation or judgment concerning an issue, product, or concept. This strategy is an excellent way to help students determine their feelings, how they would react, or their perspective on a situation or issue. Critical essays allow the students to express their own personal learning experiences. You might ask the students to write why they feel a certain way, by what path they arrived at their feelings, or what effect the information, insight, or feeling will have on their behavior. This technique allows information gathered to be personalized in such a fashion that it has potential to develop attitudes and change/reinforce behavior.

▪ Debate

Debate focuses on the merits and problems associated with a proposed solution to an issue. Through the use of this technique, you can ensure that both sides of the issue are presented. Although debate can be used in the lower elementary grades, the strategy is more effective when used with older children, who are more articulate and better able to organize their thoughts for oral presentation. Students must also be able to work individually as well as cooperatively in groups.

Topics suitable for debate can include the use of nuclear power or its alternatives, organic foods versus genetically engineered foods, and the use of laboratory animals in medical experiments. Environmental issues are also good debate topics.

Thorough preparation for a debate is essential. Students who volunteer to be part of a debate team should be given ample time to become knowledgeable about the issue they will discuss. The whole class should engage in this preparation so that students who are not on the debate teams are prepared to deal with the pros and cons of the arguments objectively.

In selecting students for debate teams, be sure that both sides are well balanced in ability. The teacher's role is that of moderator. The moderator should keep both debate teams on the topic and also guard against emotions becoming too extreme during and after the debate.

▪ Committee Work

This technique allows small groups of children to research a topic of interest. Each group member has an opportunity to do in-depth research on the topic. For elementary school children, the work must be closely supervised and structured. It is very important that each member of the group contribute to the project if it is to be successful. Projects that lend themselves well to committee work include investigating different types of pollution, collecting newspaper and magazine articles on recent medical discoveries or health approaches, or researching types of foods used by different cultures as sources of essential nutrients.

Results of the committee work are presented orally. Encourage committee members to use exhibits and multimedia aids to reinforce their presentations. This strategy can also be used on an individual basis. In such an instance, each student makes a presentation of the research done.

▪ Lecture, Group, and Panel Discussion

Discussion in one form or another is probably the most common technique used in education. Lecture discussion is usually thought of as a lecture delivered by the teacher. However, this strategy should not be limited to one-way communication. Lecture discussion can be from teacher to student, student to teacher, or student to student. The technique should be a means for achieving two-way communication.

For group discussion to be effective, the teacher must develop an atmosphere of freedom in the classroom. Without this atmosphere, students will not state their true feelings. And the discussion must be kept on course. Curtis and Papenfuss (1980, 139) offer the following suggestions for conducting group discussion:

- Present a discussion topic or legitimize an appropriate student-formulated topic.

- Establish and maintain an atmosphere of thoughtful communication without injecting teacher value judgments.

- Make the ground rules for the discussion clear and enforce them.

- Try to understand what students are attempting to say, but do not badger or cross-examine students.

Panel discussion offers an opportunity for three to five students to investigate and report on a particular health topic. This strategy is similar to committee work, but it allows more give-and-take between the participating students. Usually fifteen minutes is sufficient time for a panel discussion. Adjust the time allotted to the attention span and developmental level of the class. When using this strategy, be sure that the students who will be panel members have a precise theme to explore. A prepared outline is also necessary so that the presentation is organized.

All three of these discussion techniques encourage the exchange of information and ideas between students. In this way, children are involved in the teaching/learning process. Discussion techniques also help students develop respect and understanding for the feelings and opinions of others.

To be successful, discussion must be guided. Stone, O'Reilley, and Brown (1980, 281) note six elements that must be addressed when preparing for a discussion:

1. Choose a topic that the students can discuss and have opinions on, such as violence.
2. Introduce the topic and motivate the class about it. For example, write the word *violence* on the board and ask the students, "What is this word? Can you give me some examples of violence? Where have you seen violence in your own life? Have you ever been in a fight? Have you ever hit anyone? Have you ever thrown something at someone with the intention of hitting them? All of these are acts of violence."
3. Prepare key questions that generate discussion. For example, ask students, "If you have been in a fight

or have ever hit someone, do you think it was appropriate or necessary? If someone hits you, should you hit that person back? If not, what should you do? Is it ever necessary or the best option to hit someone else? When might those times be? If not, what course of action can be followed?"

4. Provide structure to the discussion by keeping it going in a predetermined direction. For example, the focus of discussing violence is for each student to develop his or her own concept of the appropriateness or inappropriateness of violence. The emphasis needs to remain on these issues, even if the specifics are diverse.

5. Develop closure on the topic discussed. For the topic of violence, students can write a paragraph describing their personal outlook on violence.

6. Summarize and reinforce the key points. After writing paragraphs about violence, the class can review the issues discussed. For example, the teacher can write on the board, "We have decided that violence involves these kinds of activities…" and list them, along with "We think violence is appropriate/not appropriate in the following situations.…"

▪ Resource Speakers

Speakers can enrich many areas of health instruction. Possible resource speakers include doctors, nurses, police and fire department personnel, nutritionists, and health researchers. When contacting a resource speaker, be sure to provide that person with information about your class, including grade and developmental level. In this way, a speaker is less likely to talk down to or over the heads of the children. You should also politely emphasize that the speaker stick to the specific topic to be examined because some speakers are apt to digress to a favorite cause or concern not in keeping with your instructional objectives. Suggest that the speaker use multimedia aids if appropriate, as this will heighten student interest. Also, ask the speaker to allow time for a question-and-answer session.

Before the speaker addresses the class, ensure that adequate instruction has been provided so the students are not introduced to an unfamiliar topic. Also, provide information about the position and background of the resource speaker. For example, what exactly is a nutritionist? What does a nutritionist do, and for whom does the person work? Resource speakers can be very instructive, especially if the students are properly prepared and the speaker uses multimedia aids to keep the students' interest.

Action-Oriented Strategies

A variety of action-oriented or student-centered strategies can be used to enliven health instruction. These range from seatwork activities to field trips. Whenever possible, any strategy selected should help students discover concepts through action-oriented means. Strategies that incorporate at least two of the senses can greatly facilitate learning. Listening is fine, but listening plus seeing, tasting, smelling, touching, feeling, and doing is better.

▪ Dramatizations

Plays, skits, and puppet shows are all effective dramatization techniques. Each of these strategies is an excellent way of allowing students to express their feelings. Thorough preparation and follow-up are essential, however, lest these activities be seen merely as fun, with the point of the exercise being missed.

Presenting a play involves use of a script and props. You can use a commercial script or have students write their own script. A skit is much more informal. Only an outline for the story needs to be prepared, not an actual script. Each character speaks extemporaneously. Props are not required. Nonetheless, plays and skits are both quite time-consuming.

Puppet shows are great motivators for health behavior and attitude development. They are especially effective in the lower grades. Commercial puppets may be used, or children can make their own puppets. Puppets can be used for plays, skits, or role-playing (Timmreck 1978, 140).

▪ Storytelling

As a strategy, storytelling is similar to dramatization. However, the teacher is the active participant, and the children are onlookers. This is nonetheless an effective strategy for helping students identify positive health habits and for shaping attitudes. Using a flip chart or other visual aid can heighten the impact of storytelling, although props are not necessary for many stories.

▪ Flannel, Felt, and Magnetic Boards

Flannel or felt boards are made by stretching a piece of either aforementioned material over a large board or easel. Objects that will cling to the fabric can be placed on the board. Such boards are quite useful as aids in telling a story or developing a concept because objects can be added to the board or taken off during the presentation. These boards can also be used by the students in developing their own stories or presentations.

Magnetic boards serve the same purpose as flannel and felt boards. A magnetic board is simply a sheet of metal to which objects can be attached by means of small magnets. Chalk or special markers can also be used to write directly on many magnetic boards.

▪ Crossword Puzzles

Crossword puzzles are useful seatwork devices for building vocabulary and reinforcing concepts. They can be developed by the teacher, the students, or a computer program. Commercial crossword puzzles are also available. Crossword puzzles for younger children must be kept relatively simple. This technique is best employed with children in grade 3 and above. Some sample crossword puzzle worksheets are available at www.pearsonhighered.com/anspaugh.

Demonstrations and Experiments

Demonstrations and experiments help make verbal explanations more meaningful to students because they involve other senses, such as sight or touch. In a demonstration, the outcome should always be the same; in an experiment, the predicted outcome may vary. Otherwise, the two terms mean much the same. These techniques are especially useful with elementary school children. Students are always interested in demonstrations and experiments because these strategies help clarify what they have learned. Appropriate areas for demonstrations and experiments can include typing blood, feeding animals, determining the starch content of food, and brushing and flossing teeth.

When you consider either a demonstration or an experiment, careful planning is essential to make sure that it will actually work. All equipment should be set up ahead of time, and you should rehearse the demonstration or experiment before the class actually views the procedure. Introduce the procedure to the class and explain what you plan to do. All students should be able to see the activity. Encourage them to ask questions as you go, and be sure to explain what is happening at each stage. After the activity, reinforce the learning by writing important points on the chalkboard.

Exhibits

Exhibits allow students to view, examine, and touch health-related materials. Exhibits are most effective when the children help in the design and construction of exhibits. Careful planning is essential, as is a central theme. Always ask yourself: What is the point of the proposed exhibit? Your answer will provide a focus for the children, too.

Examples of appropriate exhibits include X-ray films of broken and healed bones, safety equipment used in different types of sports, dental instruments, and samples of raw foods, such as cereal grains. If the actual objects are unavailable or impractical for classroom display, pictures can be substituted, although they are not as effective.

Everything in an exhibit should be clearly labeled. Adding sound and motion, if feasible, will increase student interest. Use your imagination to make the exhibit as visually appealing and interest-provoking as you can.

Field Trips

Field trips can provide rich learning experiences. This strategy must be used sparingly, however, because field trips are time-consuming and often expensive. Further, parents and administrators must give their approval for any activity outside the school, and liability must be considered.

A field trip should always be a culminating activity rather than an introductory one. Children should be well prepared for the experience through prior classroom instruction. If the field trip is to be of value, the students must be able to understand what they will be seeing.

Good places for health-related field trips include the local health department, a dairy farm, a food-processing plant, or a sewage treatment facility. There are also many opportunities for field trips within the school grounds. On-site field trips are often quite effective as learning experiences for younger children. Although the places themselves are familiar, you can add a new dimension to them by explaining the structure and planning behind the area being explored. Examples of on-site field trips include visits to the school cafeteria, to a crosswalk area, or to the playground. For instance, at the crosswalk area you can ask children how the crosswalk is designed for safety. Are there school speed limit signs to slow traffic during school hours? Are crosswalk lines painted on the street? Do crossing guards supervise the crossing? These and other questions will help the students see the area in a new light.

Games

Games can stimulate interest while providing a review of concepts learned through other strategies. They are also sometimes a welcome relief from the normal classroom routine. In addition, games particularly help younger children understand the importance of following rules and provide useful experience in socialization. Many commercially available games, such as bingo, can be adapted to health-related topics, or you may wish to develop your own games if you have the time.

When using games as part of health instruction, be sure that the fun of the activity does not overshadow the health-related content of the game. Also, keep the game from becoming too competitive so that no player feels inferior.

Models and Specimens

Models and specimens allow students to have a multisensory experience of health-related topics. The value of models and specimens lies in their degree of accuracy. Many excellent models of body parts are available commercially. These include models of the human eye, heart, lungs, and other organs. Another useful model is a resuscitation practice dummy, a functional model that is used to teach mouth-to-mouth resuscitation.

Specimens can be obtained from biological supply houses. These include tissue samples, animal eyes, and so forth. Commercial slaughterhouses can also supply some of these items. Exercise discretion in the use of specimens. For some children such exhibits can be too grisly, so models are better employed.

▪ Peer Helpers

Peer-helper programs have proven successful in a number of informal settings. Peer helpers are children who have been trained to listen, support, offer assistance, and serve as models in a variety of roles, such as class monitors, tutors, big brothers/sisters, and playground helpers. Peer helpers can serve as excellent conduits between children and teachers.

The children selected to serve as peer helpers are usually a grade or two ahead of the groups they help. The key to a successful program is the training and supervision peer helpers receive. In the school setting, peer helpers can occasionally help to lead discussions or work one-on-one with other children. Peer helpers should be trained to help children think about a situation and develop a solution to or attitude about it. Peer helpers have been successful in helping to prevent smoking, drug and alcohol use, and eating disorders.

These ingredients must be present for a successful peer-helper program:

- **Well-qualified adult leaders**—Leaders must be knowledgeable in all aspects of program development, maintenance, and evaluation. National certifications and training workshops are available to help adults develop the skills for training the children.

- **Well-established goals**—An assessment must be done to determine what the needs are of the school, community, and children. The identified needs should be stated as goals, and the school and community should be made aware of the goals and purposes of the program.

- **Effective recruitment and selection processes**— Some programs will accept everyone who applies for training. Other programs may find it necessary to screen the students through interviews, letters of intent, and input from teachers. The peer-helper program should represent all the social and ethnic groups in the school community. If a child is not selected, he or she should be informed tactfully about the reasons for not having been selected as a peer helper and, whenever possible, the child should be engaged in some other aspect of the program.

- **Training**—Training should be adequate and appropriate. Typically training should include an introduction to the issue or topic based on the students' needs and should include a skill-building activity designed to help the peer helper practice, receive coaching, and build on his or her natural abilities. It is not unusual for the training to require a time framework of twenty-five to thirty hours.

- **Peer-helper involvement**—The ways that peer helpers become involved will depend on the needs of the school. Even if some of the peer helpers have no formal duties, they can act as natural helpers in their own classrooms. The school should have some way to recognize peer helpers.

- **Supervision**—A most critical element of an effective peer program is supervision. Weekly feedback and contact should be provided. Training should be a continuous process to help provide support and skill development for peer helpers. The ability of the supervisor(s) to model the use of skills in real-life situations is a crucial ingredient.

- **Evaluation**—Evaluation should be in terms of the program goals. It should describe how well the program has met its goals and point to possible changes (Carr 1992, 4).

▪ Self-Appraisals

There are many inventories that children can be given to help them assess their health status or feelings concerning an important issue. These instruments may be teacher developed or commercially prepared. Unfortunately, these assessments may not be appropriate for very young children or may provide a false sense of security. There is always the risk that children will not accurately report their true feelings. For example, a child may state that he does not smoke, realizing that to report correctly that he does indeed smoke would indicate a poor health habit. The strength of such inventories and assessments is that they help make children aware of potentially harmful behaviors and help to provide insight into positive health behaviors.

The Use of Media in Health Instruction

Educational media include everything from video to computers. For the present purposes, the term will be defined as any nonprint vehicle used for instructional intent. Such media include computers, television, DVDs, slides, overhead transparencies, animations, podcasts, and audio CDs.

▪ Computer-Assisted Instruction

Advances in technology and the decreased cost of computers in the last few years have led to more widespread use of computers in the classroom. In fact, many children today come from homes in which personal computers are used for a variety of purposes, from keeping business records to playing video games. The use of computers in health instruction has increased and will continue to increase.

Schools have access to a vast array of information through the Internet, a global network that can be linked to through the World Wide Web (WWW). The Web makes extensive use of multimedia, incorporating not only printed matter, but pictures, graphics, animation, and sound. Unfortunately, the Web has become host to much commercial advertising, but it remains a source of increasing health-related information that can be used in school.

The computer holds great potential for a variety of activities. Some suggestions for student use in the classroom include helping students manage and store large volumes of electronic information, developing skills that help students identify information that is essential and related to the task at hand, and developing information acquisition skills. In this regard the student should be able to analyze information, apply information gathered, and evaluate the information acquired (Rivard 1997, 21).

Further benefits of using the computer include active involvement of students and the capability for students both to see knowledge in relational ways to carry out higher-level thinking by selecting and evaluating information and to delve deeply into subjects and concepts while working either alone or in groups. The use of computers provides an excellent tie-in with outcome- or performance- based evaluation. For example, in both performance-based evaluation and in the use of computers the student must prepare, practice, experiment, and evaluate. As a result, students are expected to create a product and demonstrate competence before or among others. In addition, when there are several participants, performance can be interactive, enabling students to learn the impact of their actions through immediate feedback. Finally, outcome-based evaluation is promoted by the ability of peers to provide commentary on how to improve performance (Wagner et al. 1997).

As shown in Table 4.3, computer instructional programs tend to follow one of six types. Computers have great potential in the classroom. However, there are concerns teachers must be aware of. Obviously, the cost of purchasing sufficient quantities of computer hardware and software for the classroom, as well as the incompatibility of different systems, can be a problem. The use of computers also raises concerns about the security of information and the safety of students who have access to the Internet. Gold (1991) also expressed concern at the possibility of dehumanizing the health education process. However, with the advent of outcome-based evaluation, this seems less of a problem, because teachers must assist in developing objectives for the project, serve as overseer, and interact with the student as the work progresses. See the Health Highlight on page 70, Technology in the Classroom. The abundance of software programs makes choosing quality software more of a challenge, and because of limited school budgets, anything purchased generally must be used for a long time. Nevertheless, computer instruction is here to stay.

Television, Videotape, and DVD

It is probably safe to state that every school in the United States has access to television and VCRs (videocassettes recorders) or DVD (digital video disc) players. Many fine health-related video programs, designed with the elementary school child in mind, are available. Both the Public Broadcasting Service (PBS) and National Educational Television (NET) regularly provide programs that can be used in health education. The commercial networks also occasionally produce suitable programs. In addition to scheduled broadcasts, public and commercial agencies also make many programs available on videotape or DVD.

Making your own videotapes for health instruction is also a useful approach, although it can be an expensive task because of the equipment involved. If your school has the equipment, however, you should consider using it. Record class plays, skits, and sociodramas. For example, suggest that students produce their own health public service announcements or commercials for use in conjunction with consumer health discussions.

Choosing Videotapes, CD-Roms, or DVDs

In considering videotapes or DVDs as instructional devices, keep in mind that they should not serve as the sole basis of instruction and that every video must be carefully chosen and previewed. Consider the following questions when selecting either videotapes or DVDs for use in the classroom.

- Is the contained material interesting and appropriate to the age and grade level?
- Does the contained material convey the desired facts and concepts, and is it likely to contribute to the formation of positive health attitudes or behavior?
- Is the information accurate and up to date?
- Can the information be correlated with and integrated into the course of study at the required grade level?
- Is the language suited to the intended audience?
- Does it meet reasonable standards of technical excellence in terms of quality, sound, and acting?
- Is the videotape or disk of appropriate length?
- Are there commercial overtones that are distasteful and detract from the educational message?

Keep a file of all audiovisuals you preview. An example of a typical file entry is shown in the Teaching in Action box on page 71. Such recordkeeping will help you build an index of especially useful films and will alert you to inappropriate ones.

Slides and Digital Photographs

Another fairly inexpensive medium is 35-mm slides. These can be purchased from commercial sources, or you can make them yourself if you have a 35-mm camera and a bit of photographic skill. Depending on the kind of projector system you have, one slide tray will hold from 40 to more than 100 two-by-two-inch slides.

An even more convenient option is to create a digital photo slideshow to supplement your teaching. With the wide availability of digital cameras and the ease of transferring photos from a camera to a computer, this option can be a cost and time saver if you want to project a collection of images in class. If you create your own photos or slides, the

Table 4.3	Six Types of Computer Instructional Programs
1. Drill and practice	In drill and practice, students are presented a series of questions to answer or problems to solve. The computer immediately checks the responses and provides feedback to the student. Although drill-and-practice programs are one of the most common educational applications of computers, they can be unnecessarily boring for students and tend to promote rote learning. This strategy is most often used to reinforce or review material that is learned elsewhere.
2. Tutorial	The objective of the tutorial is to teach concrete concepts. The computer presents new information to the student, and then it poses a series of questions. Based on the responses provided by the student, the program either presents additional information or reviews the previous lesson. Users of this strategy should ensure that the software does not overwhelm the student with screen after screen of text. This repetition can quickly lead to learner fatigue.
3. Demonstrations	Demonstration programs allow students to observe a functioning model or situation. By observation, the student learns how systems work. For example, one commercial program demonstrates the effect of exercise on a graphic representation of a human heart, and another program illustrates how nerve impulses travel through the nervous system of a human body.
4. Simulations	Simulation programs imitate real or imaginary systems based on a modeler's theory of the operation of that system. Students test hypothetical courses of action by manipulating variables and observing the impact of these changes. This process allows the student to formulate realistic projections based on sound theory. Simulations can be used to make defined concepts more understandable. Programs currently available can simulate such things as a nuclear reactor, the human circulatory system, various ecosystems, and a malaria epidemic.
5. Instructional games	Games often use one or more of the strategies previously described. Instructional games are designed to meet well-defined instructional objectives. Instructional games have explicit rules and winners, but educational concepts and information must be mastered for the player to become successful. For example, one commercially available game requires knowledge of human anatomy and physiology to successfully complete a voyage through the human body.
6. Problem solving	Many advocates of computer-assisted instruction view the area of problem solving as one of the most powerful for the computer. Research has not indicated that using a computer is a significantly better way to teach problem solving than are other strategies, because the limited programming environment doesn't automatically guarantee transfer to real life. However, one problem-solving program confronts learners with original situations that require the use of already acquired knowledge in new circumstances. Because the computer provides both prompts as needed and immediate responses, the computer manages this type of activity well. Make sure that the educational strategy employed by the instructional program is appropriate for the content area and the students' abilities. Most important, consider whether the program being reviewed is superior to other strategies of teaching the same content.

subject matter could include class activities and field trips, health fairs, environmental problems in the community, and class projects. An advantage to using digital photos or slides is that you can delete or add to the sequence as you desire. In this way, you can keep your collection current.

▪ Overhead Transparencies

Used with an overhead projector, transparencies are extremely popular as teaching tools. Many health programs provide their own transparencies. Otherwise, you can make your own transparencies by photocopying your material onto acetate that is compatible with a photocopying machine. Transparencies can also be made on a computer utilizing an appropriate printer.

One unique feature of using a transparency is the ability to show a progression by using a series of overlays. Overlays can be employed to show the position of organs within the body or to add or remove captions for informal quizzes.

▪ Audio CDs, MP3s, and Podcasts

Selectively used, audio CDs, MP3s, and podcasts can be valuable teaching tools. They are typically inexpensive

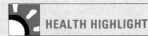

An excellent argument can be made for incorporating technology into the learning curriculum. The many benefits of technology include:

- Use of technology in the classroom can help to reach students of all learning styles.
- Increased interest and motivation by students often results from the use of technology.
- Students are better prepared for the future when using technology aimed at addressing each learning style; they can tailor their viewing and interactive activities based on their own method of learning and strengthen their ability to use alternate learning styles.

- Computers can be used to communicate with people all over the world.
- Computers can be used as tools to create instructional materials or as presentation devices to provide information in ways never before possible.
- Both students and teachers can examine issues almost immediately from multiple points of view and can learn how to deal with primary source documents that may not otherwise be available to them.
- As an instructional tool, technology helps all students—including poor students and students with disabilities—master basic and advanced skills required for future use (in higher education or the working world).

- As an assessment tool, technology yields meaningful information on demand about students' progress and accomplishments and provides a medium for storage of that information.
- As a motivational tool, technology can positively impact student attitudes toward learning, self-confidence, and self-esteem.

Source: Adapted from icdweb.cc.purdue.edu/~tituse/advantage.html, www.princeton.edu/~edutech/benefits/ben_level_1.html, www.ed.gov/Technology/Plan/NatTechPlan/benefits.html, www.electronic-school.com/0997f3.html, and www.globaled.org/curriculum/techintro.html.

(most podcasts are even free) and can be stopped as needed for discussion. Finding useful audio recordings may take some work on your part, however, because relatively few are available that relate directly to health instruction, although the number of relevant podcasts is growing quickly. For podcasts in particular, the main difficulty may lie in finding age-appropriate content.

Audio recordings are in some ways more versatile than visuals. You can easily make recordings of radio and television programs, for example, or of interviews with health officials, classroom guest speakers, and so forth. Recording commercials for classroom use can be useful when teaching consumer health.

▪ PowerPoint Presentations

Today many teachers are using computer presentation programs such as Microsoft PowerPoint to present content to their classes. PowerPoint is computer software that allows teachers to generate colorful slides that can be presented to the class using a projector and computer. The creative presentation capabilities of this software are limited only by the teacher's imagination and knowledge of the software. The biggest advantages of this software are that it is relatively inexpensive and it allows for both teacher- and student-generated presentations. In addition, there are many preexisting PowerPoint programs that can be found on the Internet. For example, the Centers for Disease Control and Prevention (CDC) provide many PowerPoint presentations to teachers free of charge.

▪ Selecting Appropriate Software

Initially, most educational software consisted of drill-and-practice exercises that were marginally useful in the classroom, and teachers were often disappointed with the results of using the software. Today, computers are no longer a novelty but an important part of the instructional strategies for promoting learning. The selection of software should be taken as seriously as the selection of any media, technology, or textbook. Several guidelines have been established to ensure a successful selection process (Komoski and Plotnick 1995):

- **Analyze needs**—Is the computer the most appropriate medium to satisfy the goals and objectives of the instructional process?
- **Specify requirements**—Factors to consider:
  - Will the school require multiple copies?
  - Will a site license be required?
  - Is the software compatible with the hardware available?
  - Is the software user friendly?
  - Is there technical support via a toll-free number?
  - Does the software meet the goals and objectives of the needs analysis?
- **Identify promising software**—Join an Internet listserv and read catalogs and reviews to find out what other teachers and professionals think of the software.
- **Preview software**—The most effective way to judge software is to personally review the material and to observe students as they utilize the program(s). If you cannot preview the software, do not use it in your classroom.

TEACHING IN ACTION | **A Checklist for Audiovisuals and Instructional Software**

Title _____ Date Reviewed _____

Distributor _____ Rent _____ Cost _____

Loan _____ Purchase _____ Cost _____

Media Type ☐ Audio ☐ CD-ROM ☐ Computer software ☐ DVD
 ☐ Slides/Photos ☐ Other

Evaluation Instructions

Below are criteria that can be used to rate audiovisuals, CD-ROMs, and other media. Not all sections are appropriate for all types of media. A four-point scale is provided for evaluating the various media.

  4 = Excellent 3 = Good 2 = Average 1 = Poor

Content/Format

___ 1. Technical/production accuracy   ___ 5. Viewer appeal   ___ 9. Music, background, dress
___ 2. Accuracy of content   ___ 6. Exude or elicit biases   ___ 10. Sound quality
___ 3. Grammar/spelling   ___ 7. Use of special effects   ___ 11. Creative production
___ 4. Multicultural inclusiveness   ___ 8. Length of production   ___ 12. Reference or user's guide

Overall Rating 48–43 = Excellent content/format 36–31 = Average content/format
 42–37 = Good content/format 30 and below = Poor content/format

Appropriate for intended audience(s)? ☐ Yes ☐ No   **Useful for special projects?** ☐ Yes ☐ No

Comments_____
_____
_____

Computer Software/CD-ROM Title _____

Distributor _____ Phone _____

License _____ Costs _____

Compatible with what hardware ☐ Mac ☐ Windows ☐ Other
 Version _____ ☐ Updates available

Needs for operation ☐ RAM ☐ Memory ☐ Modem ☐ CD-ROM ☐ Other

Grade level _____ **Computer skill level:** ☐ Beginner ☐ Intermediate ☐ Advanced

Technical information ☐ Graphics ☐ Help screens ☐ Personalize database
 ☐ Pulldown menu ☐ Information display Help hotline (   ) _____ - _____
 ☐ Assessments available

Output of individual student data ☐ Yes ☐ No   **Classroom data output** ☐ Yes ☐ No

Manuals provided ☐ Teacher ☐ Student ☐ Technical

Comments _____
_____
_____

Reviewed by _____ **Date** _____ **Recommended for purchase?** ☐ Yes ☐ No

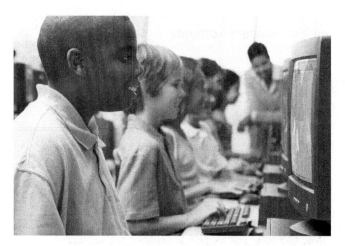

Computers can serve as excellent motivational tools for students.

- **Get post-use feedback**—Create a written record that has a quantitative scale for rating the software. After using the software, review this record to determine whether the software helped meet the goals and objectives of the instructional effort.

A Final Word

Strategies are just that—strategies. What makes health education come alive and generates the excitement that facilitates learning and, ultimately, positive health behaviors is quality teaching. We can complain that the emphasis on teaching students to pass state competency tests and that legislation such as No Child Left Behind are detrimental to the teaching of health education. However, if teachers can see the necessity of health education and can see past the curricular models, strategies, and debates, the bottom line lies with the ability of the teachers to deliver quality education.

What is quality teaching? In the text *What Great Teachers Do Differently*, the author states that great teachers make it "cool" to care (Whitaker 2004). Great teachers, regardless of what the next set of educational standards may be, help their students to succeed. The challenge is to first care yourself, then to get all students to care about what happens in the classroom. Once you, as the teacher, can accomplish this, anything is possible. Until you achieve this, any obstacle can seem insurmountable.

To be an effective teacher is both art and science. The science lies in learning how to construct lessons and an understanding of student growth and development, classroom organization, and classroom management. The art lies in learning to care for students, understanding student emotions, enjoying and expecting student success, and adding a touch of humor. Table 4.4 contains a list of positive teacher qualities (Strowage 2002). As you examine the list, ask yourself if you have these qualities.

It is important that each teacher pursue the abilities and qualities that make for teaching. The profession of teaching should be approached with the joy of a child. No set strategies can light the fire and create the passion for teaching health education—that comes from the depths of our being. When equipped with that desire, the strategies described in this chapter can help provide the impetus for successful teaching.

Table 4.4   Positive Qualities of Successful Teachers

• Assumes ownership for the classroom and the students' success	• Listens attentively to student questions and comments
• Uses personal experiences as examples in teaching	• Responds to students with respect, even in difficult situations
• Understands feelings of students	• Communicates high expectations consistently
• Communicates clearly	• Conducts one-on-one conversations with students
• Admits to mistakes and corrects them immediately	• Treats students equally and fairly
• Thinks about and reflects on practice	• Has positive dialogue and interactions with students outside the classroom
• Displays a sense of humor	• Invests time with single students or small groups of students outside the classroom
• Dresses appropriately for the position	• Maintains a professional manner at all times
• Maintains confidential trust and respect	• Addresses students by name
• Is structured, yet flexible and spontaneous	• Speaks in an appropriate tone and volume
• Is responsive to situations and students' needs	• Works actively with students
• Enjoys teaching and expects students to enjoy learning	
• Looks for the win-win solution in conflict situations	

Chapter In Review

Summary

- A strategy is an activity or experience that the teacher uses to interpret, illustrate, or facilitate learning.

- Proper selection of strategies helps provide interest, motivation, and reinforcement of learning.

- Strategies should contribute to total learning. More complex concepts should have several strategies, proceed from the simple to the complex, include audiovisual aids, and be based on the learning styles of the students.

- Regardless of the strategy, an environment that is conducive for learning must be developed and maintained.

- Clarifying activities help students to determine their feelings concerning issues and concepts.

- An effective model to facilitate good decision making must provide opportunities to practice decision-making skills.

- Learning styles are an important consideration in the choice of strategies.

- Multiple intelligences theory provides insight into why implementing a variety of strategies is essential to quality learning.

- Role-playing is an important tool that aids in decision making and helps determine feelings about situations or events.

- Verbal and discussion-oriented strategies include brainstorming, buzz groups, case studies, cooperative learning, critical essays, committee work, debates, panel discussion, and resource speakers.

- Action-oriented strategies include dramatizations; storytelling; flannel, felt, and magnetic boards; crossword puzzles; demonstrations/experiments; exhibits; field trips; games; and models/specimens.

- Peer-helper programs are an excellent strategy for offering other children assistance and serving as role models. Peer helpers must be trained.

- Instructional media are not strategies in themselves, but they do serve as valuable approaches for involving students in the learning process. Examples include computers, television, DVDs, slides and digital photographs, overhead transparencies, and audio recordings and podcasts.

- The decision to use any strategy should be based on how effective it will be in facilitating learning.

- A strategy should be chosen because it offers some teaching advantage, not simply novelty.

Discussion Questions

1. What factors should you keep in mind when selecting strategies for classroom use?

2. What elements should an effective decision-making model contain?

3. List and discuss the types of learning styles.

4. What is meant by the concept of multiple intelligences? What are the implications for health education?

5. Discuss the strengths and weaknesses of clarifying techniques.

6. What are the guidelines for developing effective role-playing situations?

7. Describe the process for using decision stories in the classroom, from preparation of the stories to discussion and follow-up activities.

8. Select three types of discussion-oriented strategies, such as brainstorming and debate, and discuss the strengths and weaknesses of each approach.

9. Select three types of action-oriented strategies, such as dramatizations and field trips, and discuss the strengths and weaknesses of each.

10. Why must discussion-oriented strategies be structured for greatest effectiveness?

11. What are the criteria for selecting software for the classroom?

12. Select three types of media, such as computers and television, and discuss the strengths and weaknesses of each.

Critical Thinking Questions

1. In the real-world classroom, how much consideration is given to attempting to incorporate some theory of learning style? What examples can you cite in relationship to your position? What do you think teachers could do to better incorporate learning-style theory into classroom instruction?

2. If you were given the chance to plan what you would consider the most exciting, motivating classroom for teaching health education, what would that class be like in terms of atmosphere, strategies, student involvement, and technology? Can your plan be implemented in today's schools? Why? Why not?

Access more material online at www.pearsonhighered.com/anspaugh. At this companion website for *Teaching Today's Health*, **you'll find chapter quizzes, web links, flashcards, a glossary, additional Worksheets, and more to help you succeed.**

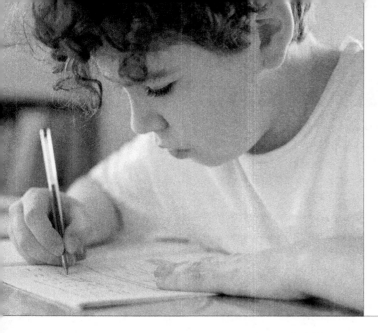

Measurement and Evaluation of Health Education

Understanding the differences between measurement, assessment, and evaluation is fundamental to the knowledge base of teaching, and certainly to the processes employed in the education of future teachers.

—*Robert Kizlik, Adprima (2008)*

Valued Outcomes

After completion of this chapter, you should be able to:

- Explain the difference between measurement and evaluation.
- List the skills needed to be competent in measuring and evaluating student progress.
- Discuss the steps necessary for developing a teacher-designed test.
- Describe how to write effective test items.
- Identify alternative methods of assessing student progress.
- Explain various grading strategies.
- Discuss the use of rubrics in grading.
- Discuss the use of benchmarks, standards, and performance indicators in assessment of learning.
- Explain how to assess students from a variety of cultures.
- Discuss how to assess students with different learning styles.

Reflections

The ultimate goal of measurement and evaluation is to determine how well the teacher has taught and how well the student has learned. As you read through this chapter, reflect on how you can most effectively use the concepts related to measurement and evaluation to enhance the success of your teaching and your students' learning.

Measurement and Evaluation

Every instructional effort should be evaluated to determine how successful it has been. Both student learning and teacher effectiveness must be determined. The emphasis in recent years on teacher accountability has made evaluation more important than ever.

In the education process, perhaps no terms are misused more often than *measurement* and *evaluation*. **Measurement** is the collection of information on which a decision is based. The purpose of measurement is to collect information for evaluation, such as tests. The measurement process is the first step in evaluation. The primary reasons for evaluating pupils are those reasons that are an essential part of a teacher's main responsibility: helping students improve in knowledge, skills, feelings, and attitudes, and helping students learn (Utah State Office of Education 2011). Measurement generally results in quantitative data in numerical form. The various types of tests, rating scales, attitude scales, checklists, and observation techniques used in the elementary school are all forms of measurement. The resulting raw data, however, must be evaluated before the effectiveness of the instruction can be assessed. Data are not information; they are only the basis for information. They answer the question "How much?"

Evaluation is the use of measurement in making decisions. It is also a process of comparing. For example, students are compared with other students or with a predetermined standard. Evaluation can be used to

- Improve instructional materials
- Improve student learning
- Determine content mastery
- Establish criteria or standards of performance for the course

Evaluation activities, if appropriately planned and used, can be powerful learning activities (Utah State Office of Education 2011).

Evaluation can be either objective or subjective. It is a judgment of what the numerical measurement data actually mean. For example, if all the students in a class get a perfect score on a test, has the instruction been successful? Perhaps not. The test might have simply measured what was known before any instruction. Or the test might have been so poorly constructed that the correct answers were obvious whether instruction had been provided or not.

More important, evaluation is now seeking to provide more than a score to determine successful learning. Techniques include performance-based evaluation, narrative grading, portfolio evaluation, group projects, individual exhibits, and critical thinking essays.

Two different forms of evaluation of student progress are formative and summative evaluation. **Formative evaluation** is gathering data for the purpose of improving specific aspects of a teaching/learning process. **Summative evaluation** is evaluation conducted at the end of a unit of instruction. An example is the use of a written test. Measurement and evaluation help teachers to:

- **Assess the effectiveness of the learning activities.** Measurement and evaluation will help determine whether learning activities have increased knowledge, helped clarify values or determined attitudes, and promoted decision-making skills. If not, the activities must be revised or replaced.

- **Motivate the student.** Tests help students recognize how much they have learned. Pretests are useful for introducing the scope of a topic and making students aware of the material that will be covered. Posttests then are used to chart actual student progress.

- **Help develop the scope and sequence of teaching.** Measurement and evaluation can help determine the level of teaching and the order in which it should occur. For example, if the knowledge level of a class is high, a simple review of the factual material may be all that is necessary before moving on to new subject matter. Or, if the students know the factual material, the teacher may decide to work next on developing attitudes toward this knowledge.

Assessment of learning in the classroom includes the use of standards, benchmarks, and performance indicators to evaluate each student's progress in learning and mastering tasks in specific content. Assessment also includes accountability—accountability of the students for meeting these standards, benchmarks, and indicators related to content, and accountability of the teachers based on students' scores on assessment tests. These types of assessment tell us how much students have learned, whether standards are being met, and whether educators have taught the material successfully.

Teacher Skills Needed for Competent Measurement and Evaluation

Becoming competent in measurement and evaluation does not happen overnight. Aspiring teachers develop these skills in education classes, in educational psychology classes, and during student teaching. As a teacher gains professional experience, these skills will be sharpened. The National Council on Measurement in Education (2002) notes that a teacher should be skilled in the eight areas described below.

1. **Choosing assessment strategies.** Teachers can describe the nature and use of different types of formal and informal assessments, including questionnaires, checklists, interviews, inventories, tests, observations, surveys, and performance assessments.

2. **Identifying, accessing, and evaluating the most commonly used assessment instruments.** Teachers know which assessment instruments are most commonly used in school settings to assess

achievement, including computer-assisted versions and other alternate formats.

3. **The techniques of administration and methods of scoring assessment instruments.** Teachers can implement appropriate administration procedures, including administration using computers. They can standardize administration of assessments when interpretation is in relation to external norms.

4. **Interpreting and reporting assessment results.** Teachers can explain scores that are commonly reported, such as percentile ranks, standard scores, and grade equivalents. They are skilled in communicating assessment information to others, including teachers, administrators, students, parents, and the community.

5. **Using assessment results in decision making.** Teachers recognize the limitations of using a single score in making an educational decision and know how to obtain multiple sources of information to improve such decisions.

6. **Interpreting and presenting statistical information about assessment results.** Teachers can describe data (for example, test scores, grades, and demographic information). They can compare a score from an assessment instrument with an existing distribution, describe the placement of a score within a normal distribution, and draw appropriate inferences.

7. **Conducting and interpreting evaluations of programs.** Teachers understand and appreciate the role that evaluation plays in the program development process throughout the life of a program. They can describe the purposes of an evaluation and the types of decisions that will be based on evaluation information. They can identify and evaluate possibilities for unintended outcomes and possible impacts of one program on other programs.

8. **Assessing students with diverse learning styles.** The teacher is able to design multiple forms of assessment that correspond to the student's learning style.

In health education, measurement and evaluation cannot be limited to the cognitive domain but must also be vitally concerned with the formation of attitudes and behavior patterns among students. Testing instruments emphasize quantitative measures, but these measures must also be employed to gain insight into qualitative areas. Selecting an instrument is not simply a matter of locating a test on specific content. It is important to select the best test available, *best* being defined in terms of most appropriate for specific objectives and for specific students. If one test fails to measure what the teacher wants it to measure, another test needs to be developed. Tests for assessing knowledge, attitudes, and practices are used to assess the impact of education on children.

Teacher-Designed Tests

Teacher-designed tests can be tailored to specific purposes and groups of students. This is a primary advantage. On the negative side, teacher-designed tests may lack validity and reliability. However, with experience, teachers should develop tests that are increasingly good indicators of student learning and change.

In constructing tests, teachers must include each of the following seven areas.

1. **Validity**—Does the test measure what it is supposed to measure? If the desire is to determine changes in student attitudes, for example, a test that asks students for factual information will not fulfill this intent. Validity is a matter of degree, not a characteristic that is absent or present. A test that is currently valid may not necessarily be valid in the future.

Because tests are designed for a variety of purposes and because validity can be viewed only in terms of purpose, it is not surprising that there are several types of validity. **Content validity** is defined as the degree to which a test measures an intended content area. **Construct validity** is the degree to which a test measures a hypothetical construct, such as intelligence.

2. **Concurrent validity**—This is the degree to which the scores on a given test are related to the scores on another test. **Predictive validity** is the degree to which a test can predict how well a student will do in a particular situation.

3. **Reliability**—This refers to the consistency of test results. For example, if a test gives the same results when measuring an individual or group on two different occasions then the scores can be considered reliable. Also, if different teachers rate the same essay on the same criteria and obtain the same score then we say the scores are reliable from one rater to another. In both cases, consistency and trustworthiness are considered in the reliability of the result (Utah State Office of Education 2011). Other factors that can affect the reliability of a test include the appropriateness of test items, the way the test is administered to the students, how the test is scored and interpreted, and the physical condition of the test environment.

4. **Objectivity**—Is the test fair to the students? For example, if the readability level of the test is too high, students may be unable to supply correct answers even if they understand the concept being tested. If there is more than one possible correct answer, students should not be penalized for providing reasonable alternatives.

5. **Discrimination**—Does the test differentiate among good, average, and poor students?

6. **Comprehensiveness**—Is the test long enough to cover the material? Keep in mind that a fifty-item test may be no more comprehensive than a ten-item test is if the items on the fifty-item test apply to only certain areas while neglecting others.

7. **Administration and scoring**. Is the test easy to give, use, and score? Keep in mind that the easiest test to administer and score may not be the best test for assessing the area. For example, an essay test, which is more difficult to score, may provide a better assessment of certain concepts than an easier-to-score true-false test.

Developing Tests

Developing good tests is a difficult task. The starting point is to establish a table of specifications. This table serves as the blueprint for the test. The purpose of the table of specifications is to ensure that all the objectives for a unit

Table 5.1 Specifications for Unit on Substance Abuse

Valued Outcome		
The learner will...	Content	Percentage of items
Define what constitutes substance abuse.	What substance abuse is; what can result from abuse; what some symptoms are	15%
List the various substances that can be abused.	Depressants (types); cocaine; marijuana; designer drugs; hallucinogens	35%
Discuss why people use drugs.	Reasons for drug use	15%
List where to get help for substance abuse.	Agencies; organizations; professionals	10%
Develop techniques for avoiding substance abuse.	How to say no to substance abuse	25%

or lesson are covered on the test. By developing the table, the teacher can ensure that the proper percentage of test items appears in relation to the emphasis placed on each objective (Table 5.1). The process of developing a test should involve the following steps:

- Prepare the table of specifications based on the unit objectives.
- Draft the test items.
- Decide on the length of the test.
- Select and edit the final test items.
- Rate the test items in terms of difficulty.
- Arrange the test items in order of difficulty from easiest to most difficult.
- Prepare the instructions for the test.
- Prepare the answer key and decide the rules for scoring.
- Produce the test.

The next area of concern is developing the various types of test items. Several types of test items can be used for assessment purposes. Some teachers may wish to use a variety of types, whereas other teachers may prefer one or two types. It is wise to employ at least two types of test items because some students don't always do well on a particular type of test item. For example, some students do well on essay tests, whereas other students do better on multiple-choice tests.

Another important consideration is the order in which the test items appear. Most important, all similar items should be grouped together. This helps to simplify directions, makes it easier for students to maintain the same psychological set throughout each section, and makes scoring the test easier. Test items should proceed from the simpler items to more complex ones.

Writing Effective Test Items

▪ True-False Tests

A **true-false test** consists of declaratory statements that are either true or false. Students must decide whether each test item is true or false and answer accordingly.

Advantages of the true-false test are as follows:

- Because it is so widely used, the true-false test is familiar to students.

- It is easy to construct, which is one reason why it is used extensively.

- It can be used to sample a wide range of subject matter. Because the items can be answered in a short time, a large number of test items can be included.

- It is easy to score, and the score is quite objective.

- It can be used effectively as an instructional test to promote interest and introduce points for discussion.

- It is versatile and can be employed for short quizzes, lesson reviews, end-of-chapter tests, and so forth.

- Items can be constructed either as simple factual statements or as questions that require reasoning.

- True-false items are especially useful when there are only two options concerning an issue.

Disadvantages of the true-false test are as follows:

- A simple true-false test is of doubtful value for measuring achievement.

- True-false tests often measure little more than a student's ability to memorize material. This is generally a lower-level difficulty of learning. One way to improve the difficulty of a true-false test is to have the students explain *why* a statement is true or false.

- It encourages guessing. Even without any knowledge of the subject matter, a student easily can pick correct answers by random choice.

- Constructing test items that are completely true or completely false without making the correct response choice obvious can be difficult.

- Avoiding ambiguities, irrelevant details, and clues is difficult.

- Unless the test consists of a large number of items, reliability is likely to be low.

- Items that test for minor details receive as much credit as items that test for major points do.

- If the material is in any way controversial, true-false items are difficult to construct. For example, the

following statement, although false, can give students a wrong perception: "Marijuana is not a harmful drug."

- If the relative degree of truth in an item is debatable. Such items should be avoided because students will try to guess what is in the teacher's mind instead of making their own decisions.

As long as you keep the disadvantages of true-false tests in mind, such tests can be helpful for assessing student performance. If used in testing, true-false questions are best for younger students. This type of question can be used as a discussion starter for older students. For example, ask older students, "True or False: If someone talks about suicide, they will not commit suicide." This type of framework for a question can encourage discussion and reflection.

Use the following guidelines when constructing true-false tests:

- Approximately 60 percent of the items on a true-false test should be true.

- Make the method for indicating responses as simple as possible. Usually, a blank to the left of the item in which the student must write "T" or "F" is the best format.

- Write original items. Do not lift statements directly from the textbook. (Using sample test questions from the teacher's guide is acceptable, however.)

- True statements should not be consistently longer than false statements are because this provides an obvious clue.

- Avoid ambiguous terms and qualifiers, such as *many* and *few*.

- Use specific determiners carefully. Whenever you employ such terms as *no, never, always, may, should, all*, and *only*, be sure that they do not make the correct answer obvious.

- Avoid the use of negatively stated items. For example, "Not eating balanced meals is not good for your health" is a confusing statement at best. Further, the second *not* can easily be overlooked in a quick reading.

- Make the items clear so that there is no doubt in the student's mind about what the item seeks to measure. One way to ensure clarity of purpose is to include the crucial element of the item at the end of the statement. Underlining the crucial element is another way to achieve this end, but too much underlining can be distracting and may signal statements that are obviously true or false.

- Avoid trick questions. Such items are poor measures of achievement and are not fair to the student. They measure general intelligence and alertness, not understanding of the concept. For example, "Coffee contains a drug called codeine" is a trick question. The student may know that the substance in coffee is caffeine, but may read caffeine for codeine.

Following are examples of properly developed true-false items:

_T_ 1. Drugs are harmful if they are abused.

_T_ 2. Brushing your teeth regularly can help prevent tooth decay.

_F_ 3. Meat is a good source of vitamin C.

_T_ 4. The heart and circulatory system move blood to all parts of the body.

_F_ 5. A burn on the skin should be treated with cold water.

■ Matching Tests

Matching tests call for the answers given in one column to be paired with a corresponding item in another column. This kind of test is in effect a form of multiple-choice test except that the number of answer choices is compounded.

Advantages of the matching test are as follows:

- This type of test is adaptable to many subject areas.
- It is especially useful for maps, charts, or pictorial representations.
- It is fairly quick to develop.
- The test format uses space economically.
- It is easy to score.

Just like true-false tests, matching tests measure little more than a student's ability to memorize material, making this also a lower level difficulty of learning. One way to improve the difficulty of a matching test is to increase the number of items to be matched. For example, if you have five items in the left column, place seven or eight items in the right column. This eliminates the student's ability to get a correct answer simply by guessing. Disadvantages of the matching test are as follows:

- This type of test does not assess the extent to which meaning has been grasped.
- It increases in difficulty as the number of items to be matched increases.
- It tests only factual information.
- It permits guessing.
- It is likely to include clues to the correct answers.

Use the following guidelines when developing matching test items:

- The test should cover only one subject area or topic.
- For younger children, include no more than ten items to be matched. For older children, fifteen items should be the maximum.
- Use the right-hand column for the response list.
- Ensure that there is only one possible correct response for each item.
- Arrange the responses in random order.

- Keep all items and responses on a single page.
- Include more response options than terms or statements to be matched.
- Clearly and precisely word each response option.
- Avoid providing clues to the correct matches.

Following are examples of properly developed matching items:

_a_ 1. compensation   a. covering faults by trying to excel in another area

_c_ 2. regression   b. creating make-believe events

_d_ 3. rationalization   c. acting in an immature way

     d. making an excuse for a mistake or failure

■ Multiple-Choice Tests

Items on **multiple-choice tests** require the student to recognize which of several suggested responses is the best answer. This kind of test provides an opportunity to develop thought-provoking questions while covering a great deal of material at the same time. It is considered the best short-answer test format. To increase the effectiveness of a multiple choice test question, each possible answer should be at least partially correct; at the very least, there should not be any possible answers that are obviously correct or incorrect.

Advantages of the multiple-choice test are as follows:

- Items can be written to measure inference, discrimination, and judgment.
- Items can be constructed to measure recall as well as recognition.
- Guessing is minimized when there are three to five potential answer choices.
- Sampling of material covered can be extensive. Many questions can be included on a test because a response can be made quickly.
- Scoring is objective. In a properly constructed item, only one possible response is correct.
- Scoring is rapid.

Disadvantages of the multiple-choice test are as follows:

- Developing a multiple-choice test is time-consuming.
- Items are too often factually based, unduly stressing memory.
- More than one response may be correct or nearly correct.
- It is difficult to exclude clues as to the correct response.
- Incorrect but plausible alternative answers are often difficult to develop.
- Items can take up a considerable amount of space.

- The students must do a lot of reading.
- The format does not allow students to express their own thoughts.

Use the following guidelines when developing multiple-choice tests:

- Express each item as clearly as possible, using words that have precise meanings.
- Make all choices plausible. When obviously incorrect options are included, the need to think is reduced accordingly.
- Be sure that only one response is correct.
- Keep the answer choices short whenever possible.
- The correct answer choice should be about the same length as the incorrect alternatives, not consistently longer or shorter than the incorrect answer choices are.
- For lower elementary school children, limit the answer choices to three. For upper elementary school children, use four answer choices.
- Between questions, scatter the position of the correct answer choices to avoid any set pattern.
- Avoid negatively worded items. If you must include negatives, underline, capitalize, or italicize the negative words so that they will not be missed.
- Use parallel construction in developing the answer choices. Avoid confusing and grammatically incorrect items such as this one:

____ 1. Shock can cause a person to pass out because not enough blood goes to
    a. the brain.
    b. is being pumped to the heart.
    c. the lungs slow down.
    d. stomach.

Instead, be consistent in construction as follows:

____ 1. Shock can cause a person to pass out because not enough blood goes to the
    a. stomach.
    b. brain.
    c. heart.
    d. lungs.

Following are examples of properly developed multiple-choice items:

_a_ 1. Which of the following nutrients helps repair the body?
    a. carbohydrates
    b. fats
    c. proteins
    d. vitamins

_b_ 2. Which of the following is not an inherited trait?
    a. shape of the nose
    b. tooth decay
    c. blood type
    d. skin color

Short-Answer Tests

Short-answer tests, also known as completion tests, consist of a number of statements that have certain key words or phrases omitted. Short-answer tests incude a variety of test item types, ranging from fill-in-the-blank to listing. This type of test measures the student's ability to select a word or phrase that is consistent in logic and style with the other elements in the statement. If students understand the implications of the sentence, they should be able to provide the answer that best fulfills the intent of the item.

Advantages of the short-answer test are as follows:

- This type of test is easy to construct.
- It has wide applications to testing situations that involve charts or diagrams.
- Guessing is minimized because the answer must come from the student.
- Student writing ability is not a major factor.
- Scoring is objective and fairly quick.

Disadvantages of the short-answer test are as follows:

- This type of test stresses factual information. The result may be a collection of items calling for unrelated facts or isolated bits of information.
- It places a premium on rote memory rather than on real understanding.
- Phrasing an item so that only one correct response is elicited is often difficult. Alternative answers provided by students may be very close to correct, making scoring problematic.
- In a poorly formatted short-answer test, answers may be scattered all over the page, as on a diagram, making scoring time-consuming.
- Clues within an item can allow students to respond correctly without understanding the concept being assessed.

Use the following guidelines when constructing short-answer test items:

- Be sure that short-answer items are phrased in language appropriate to the students' reading level.
- Avoid lifting items directly from the text and simply inserting blanks for key words or phrases. Try to create original items so that students' reliance on rote memory is minimized.
- Use blanks for significant words and phrases rather than for minor details.
- For younger children, indicate the number of words needed for the correct response by using spaces between the blanks.
- Whenever possible, avoid *a* or *an* before a blank.
- Don't begin an item with a blank if possible.
- Keep a high ratio of words supplied to words called for.
- When more than one correct answer is possible, put the alternatives in the scoring key if you are not scoring the test yourself.

Following are examples of properly developed short-answer test items.

1. List the four chambers of the heart.
   right atrium
   left atrium
   right ventricle
   left ventricle
2. The iris controls the amount of ___light___ going to the lens.
3. Light enters your eyeball through a clear tissue called the ___lens___.
4. The eyeball is filled with a fluid called _vitreous humor_.

Essay Question Tests

The **essay question test** requires the student to organize information in a systematic fashion. Use of essay questions allows you to gain insight into the amount of understanding students have developed from your instruction.

Advantages of the essay question test are as follows:

- This type of test is relatively easy to prepare.
- Essay questions can be written on a transparency or even dictated, thus eliminating the expense of photocopying materials.
- It encourages originality and creativity on the part of the student.
- Essay questions stimulate students to organize their thinking.
- Chances of cheating are minimized because of the amount of writing involved.
- Answers to essay questions help reveal the individuality of students. Questions can invoke a variety of responses that reflect personal attitudes, values, habits, and differences.
- Guessing at answers is reduced to a minimum.
- Essay questions are the best-known way of evaluating the qualitative aspects of verbal/written expression of thought.

Disadvantages of the essay question test are as follows:

- Determining reliability is difficult because different teachers will score essay answers in different ways.
- Scoring is rather subjective and is unconsciously influenced by such factors as legibility, neatness, grammar, spelling, word choice, and bluffing.
- Scoring is time-consuming. However, this task can be made somewhat easier with the development of a rubric for scoring the test (see the next section).
- Students who have poor writing or language skills are at a disadvantage.
- Write essay answers is time-consuming and students may feel pressured by this type of test. Slow writers are not necessarily slow thinkers, but this may be the impression given.

- Younger children have particular difficulty in formulating and writing answers to essay questions.
- An essay question test can sample only a limited amount of the material covered.

Use these guidelines when preparing an essay question test:

- Develop questions that will help you assess critical thinking skills rather than retention of facts.
- Begin with relatively easy questions. Placing difficult items at the beginning of the test discourages less able students.
- Phrase the questions specifically enough so that students know what kind of a response is being asked for. However, avoid focusing so narrowly that a mere listing of facts is called for.
- Limit the number of questions so that students do not feel overwhelmed, and give students adequate time to complete each answer.

Following are examples of properly developed essay questions:

1. In what ways do the eyes and hands work together as a team?
2. What advice would you give to a friend who has trouble getting along with a younger brother or sister?
3. How do television commercials try to get you to buy certain products? Pick one television commercial and tell how it tries to get you to buy a product.

Creativity in the Classroom

When giving tests to younger students, consider asking them to draw a picture or form a group and act out a skit in response to a question rather than requiring an essay or any other test with lengthy reading requirements. Tailor the type of test to best evaluate the learning of each particular group of students based on their attention spans and skill levels.

Measuring Health Attitudes

Because attitudes are so important in health behavior, they are frequently measured in health education and health promotion programs. Favorable attitudes toward health behavior typically lead to more positive health outcomes (Milwaukee County Nutrition and Physical Activity Coalition 2009). An attitude involves feelings, values, and appreciations. An attitude can also be described as a predisposition to certain actions.

Because one of the goals in teaching health is the development of positive health attitudes, it is essential to attempt to assess student attitudes. This is no easy matter, because attitudes are not within the cognitive domain and are not thus readily tapped by most kinds of tests. Many tests that attempt to measure attitudes are not constructed in a scientific manner and offer only limited information to the teacher (Morrow et al. 2005, 323). Even tests that

---

TEACHING IN ACTION | **Example of a Forced-Choice Attitude Scale**

Rating Myself: How I Feel

		Agree	Disagree
1.	My overall physical health is excellent.	_____	_____
2.	I have a positive attitude toward most things.	_____	_____
3.	I have the ability to make my life work.	_____	_____
4.	I relate well to other people.	_____	_____
5.	I have control of my life.	_____	_____

TEACHING IN ACTION | **A Likert Scale with a Five-Choice Spread**

How do you feel about members of diverse groups from other cultures? Answer the following. I would like a person from another cultural group:

		Strongly Agree	Agree	Not Sure	Disagree	Strongly Disagree
1.	As close kin by marriage.	_____	_____	_____	_____	_____
2.	As a personal friend.	_____	_____	_____	_____	_____
3.	On my street as neighbors.	_____	_____	_____	_____	_____
4.	Working alongside me in class.	_____	_____	_____	_____	_____
5.	As citizens of my country.	_____	_____	_____	_____	_____
6.	As visitors to my country.	_____	_____	_____	_____	_____
7.	Excluded from my country.	_____	_____	_____	_____	_____

Source: Adapted from Bogardus Scale of Social Distance and the Likert scale. Bogardus, Emory S., Social Distance in the City. *Proceedings and Publications of the American Sociological Society.* 20, 1926, 40–46; Likert, R. (1932). A Technique for the Measurement of Attitudes. *Archives of Psychology* 140: 1–55.

---

are designed for this purpose often lack validity, as students may respond with the answers that they think the teacher will favor rather than stating their true feelings or predispositions. Thus, it is important to supplement such testing instruments with other means of assessment, such as self-inventories, questionnaires, checklists, observation, informal conferences, small-group discussion, and anecdotal recordkeeping. These strategies produce subjective indications of what the child's attitudes may be. With these limitations in mind, we now examine some of the more common written measures for assessing student attitudes.

▪ Attitude Scales

A scale is a testing instrument that requires the student to choose between alternatives on a continuum. Two polar choices, such as yes/no or agree/disagree, may be offered, or a range of choices may be provided.

The Teaching in Action box above shows a **forced-choice scale,** a scale that provides only two options about each statement being considered. This kind of **attitude scale** is appropriate for use with younger children, who lack the developmental ability to handle more complicated attitude scales.

The major disadvantage of the forced-choice scale test is that students can readily perceive what the "correct"

response should be. They will respond accordingly, even if the answer does not reflect their actual attitude toward the issue. This problem can be overcome to a certain degree by establishing an atmosphere in the classroom of warmth, trust, and rapport.

A **Likert scale** is a more sophisticated attitude scale that provides a range of choices about each attitudinal issue. The more choices that are offered, the more discrimination a student must have to complete the scale. The second Teaching in Action box above provides an example of a Likert scale.

Scoring may be done in a variety of ways, depending on how the statements in the scale are phrased. For example, the continuum of responses may be weighted from 1 to 5, with the lowest score for a *strongly disagree* statement and the highest score for a *strongly agree* statement. Thus, if a student checks *strongly agree* to the statement, "Being stoned all the time is no way to live," the score would be a 5. An *undecided* response would rate a 3, and a *strongly disagree* would rate a 1. Note that the scoring rank must be reversed for oppositely worded statements, such as "Experimenting with drugs is not really very risky." In this case, a *strongly disagree* response would score as a 5.

The total numerical score derived from adding the individual response scores offers a measure of how firmly opinions and attitudes are held about the issues examined in the scale. However, this measure, despite its seeming quantitative preciseness, is only a rough indicator of attitude. Bear in mind that the scoring system is arbitrary; that even with five options, students are still making forced choices; and that students may respond with "correct" answers that do not actually reflect their true attitudes. Instruments used for attitude assessment should not be used for purposes of grading, because this will further bias the students' responses.

■ Observation

As mentioned earlier, the use of attitude scales to assess children's feelings and values has its limitations. The results of such scales are often inconclusive. Scales or other measurement devices, such as checklists or student surveys, should be augmented with other techniques, including observation and anecdotal recordkeeping.

Observation is an excellent way of assessing behavior. Because observation can be done on an ongoing, daily basis, it can provide important clues as to attitude and predisposition to action. A major disadvantage of observation is that it is time-consuming. Further, discretion must be exercised so as not to violate student and parent privacy.

Teachers can structure activities in order to observe students' attitudes toward various health issues. For example, the teacher can mark several spots throughout the classroom with *strongly agree* and *strongly disagree* labels. As a teacher calls out a specific issue, for example, "A family member should always tell a terminal patient about his or her illness," the students can walk to the spot that best reflects their attitude toward the statement. This type of activity enables the students to take a public stand regarding the issue. However, the teacher should use caution in including controversial issues in such a public forum. Also, some students might be too embarrassed to declare their values publicly and might go to the spot occupied by friends or the majority of the class.

In assessing student health attitudes, an attempt to remain neutral in observations should be made. Variations in personal health attitudes and behaviors are not necessarily a cause for concern. Children are still forming their attitudes about health-related issues. They should not be expected to have completely made up their minds about

health practices. If they have, there would be far less point to the job of teaching.

Further, attitude formation is a gradual process. Instant changes in behavior patterns are not necessarily going to occur. The teacher's efforts can make a difference. With these thoughts in mind, one method to use in assessing attitudes is the checklist. The checklist allows the observer to note quickly and effectively whether a trait or characteristic is present. Checklists can be useful in evaluating learning activities or some aspects of personal-social interaction. The Teaching in Action box below is a sample checklist for evaluating student behavior after a unit on respect for others.

As has been noted, measuring attitudes is difficult. Any technique used to measure and evaluate attitudes or health practices should be done carefully and with student input if it is to be part of the grading process. If this is done, students will be more likely to reveal their true feelings or their actual practices. Alternatively, the evaluation can be used to plan for future instruction and to help students understand their current level of development. The more aware students become about themselves, the more likely it is that they will use this awareness to make conscious decisions about future behavior.

Traditional Grading Strategies

Grades serve to inform students, parents, teachers, and administrators about the progress and work efficiency of the student. Ideally, grades should not be an end in themselves. Instead, they should act as motivators for students to do their best and as guides for the students to future courses of study. For parents, student grades identify the child's strengths and weaknesses and also help clarify the goals of the school. If parents gain insight through grades as to what the school is attempting to accomplish, parents will be in a better position to cooperate with the teacher in enhancing the child's education. Administrators can use grades to see how effective the curriculum is and to step in to provide extra help, such as special programs, counseling, and so forth, for students who need it.

Each school district has its own approach to grading. Teachers should become familiar with the system used in

---

TEACHING IN ACTION | **Observation Checklist for Assessing Respect for Others**

Name _____ Date of Assessment _____

Observation _____

Observer _____

Directions: Listed below are characteristics related to "Respect for Others." For the student listed, check those characteristics that are appropriate.

_____ Respects views and opinions of others   _____ Respects the property of others

_____ Is sensitive to needs of others   _____ Works cooperatively with others

_____ Is sensitive to problems of others   _____ Addresses others in a respectful manner

their district in order to apply the district's standards objectively and fairly.

The Percentage Method

This grading method is based on 100 percent. It assumes more precision than can actually exist and essentially reduces the range of scores that might fall between 70 and 100 percent if other grading methods are used. Any student falling below 70 percent correct responses on a given test fails. Many school districts that employ this method use a scale similar to the following:

A = 93–100 percent
B = 85–92 percent
C = 78–84 percent
D = 70–77 percent
F = Below 70 percent

The A to F Combination Method

The A to F combination method system of grading is a combination of the percentage method and other descriptors that indicate student performance. With this method, students can be rated in relation to both the group norm and personal development. The A to F combination method better enables students and parents to know whether learning and work are being accomplished at peak capacity. For example, it is possible for students to make a C grade and still have students and parents appreciate that students are working near maximum effort. A typical example of how this method is structured is as follows:

A = excellent work and working at or near capacity; 93–100 percent
B = good work and working at or near capacity; 85–92 percent
C = average work or all that should be expected; 78–84 percent
D = much less than should be expected; 70–77 percent
F = no noticeable progress; less than 70 percent
1 = above grade level
2 = at grade level
3 = below grade level

The numbers can be used in conjunction with the letter grades. For example, a child who receives a grade of B-2 is performing near capacity at grade level, whereas a child who receives a grade of B-3 is performing near capacity but below grade level.

Pass/Fail

Some of the symbols used to indicate achievement are O, S, and U for *outstanding*, *satisfactory*, and *unsatisfactory*. The symbols P and F are also used to indicate *pass* or *fail*. Other teachers may use E, S, N, or U for *excellent*, *satisfactory*, *not satisfactory*, and *unsatisfactory*.

Unfortunately, any course using these symbols may be viewed as less important than those courses receiving the traditional A to F grades. Certainly, in the case of health education, this connotation must be avoided because the knowledge, attitudes, and behaviors developed have the potential to be life enhancing, and, in some cases, lifesaving.

There are no easy answers in choosing a grading system. The best method is really a combination of systems. Each teacher and school system must weigh the advantages of each type of grading strategy and select the one that best informs students and parents of progress.

Performance-Based Evaluation

In addition to traditional cognitive testing, which generally involves the use of paper-and-pencil tests, teachers must now be able to evaluate students' attitudes and values about health behaviors. Also, as the Indiana Department of Education states in their standards, teachers must understand the individual differences among adolescents and young adults and the influence of these differences on their behavior and learning. Obviously, this includes the diverse values from different cultures and how those values and cultures impact health behaviors and learning in the classroom (Indiana Department of Education Licensing Rules 2011). Most evaluation specialists refer to these types of evaluation as **performance-based evaluation** (Table 5.2). Performance-based evaluation is not contingent on what the students recall, but on how they show what they have learned. Several techniques lend to this type of evaluation. Examples include portfolios, exhibitions, group projects, and critical thinking essays.

Portfolios are defined as a purposeful collection of student work that exhibits effort, progress, and achievement. To ensure that portfolios will serve as useful tools, the following guidelines should be kept in mind:

1. There must be student involvement in selecting the components that will constitute the portfolio.
2. Students should include information that allows them to self-reflect and self-criticize.
3. Student activities should be reflected in projects, writing, and drawings, and result from the student's learning goals.
4. The portfolio should reflect the growth of the student in progress toward achieving insight and attitude/behavior development. It should reflect the feelings and thinking of the student.
5. Evaluation should be based on each student's established standards, not on comparisons with other students in the class.

Exhibitions are considered valid performance-based measures to show initial mastery of a subject as well as various levels of proficiency (Rhode Island Department of Elementary and Secondary Education 2008). Examples of exhibits might include developing displays, writing skits or plays, or designing bulletin boards. The use of exhibitions to

Table 5.2	**Performance-Based Assessments**	
Performance assessment is used to evaluate higher-order thinking and the acquisition of knowledge, concepts, and skills required for students to succeed in the 21st-century workplace.		
Assessment Activity	Selecting a response	Performing a task
Nature of Activity	Contrived activity	Activity emulates real life
Cognitive Level	Knowledge/comprehension	Application/analysis/synthesis
Development of Solution	Teacher-structured	Student-structured
Objectivity of Scoring	Easily achieved	Difficult to achieve
Evidence of Mastery	Indirect evidence	Direct evidence

Source: Liskin-Gasparro, J. (1997) and Mueller (2008). *Comparing Traditional and Performance-Based Assessment.* Paper presented at the Symposium on Spanish Second Language Acquisition, Austin, TX. Used by permission.

assess learning provides opportunities for students to learn from their peers or to practice presenting their work to others.

Critical thinking essays can be defined as a cognitive writing activity that allows the student to analyze or synthesize information in order to make a decision (McCown, Driscoll, and Roop 1996, 382). The teacher can have students write critical thinking essays to develop their higher level thinking by evaluating a health-related topic. For example, have older students research a topic like passive euthanasia. Then, guide the students through a series of learning activities on the same topic. Following these teaching procedures, the students would write a critical thinking essay in which they evaluate arguments or debate points on the topic under study. This type of strategy requires more thought than rote memorization or merely rephrasing what someone else has stated, and therefore helps the student learn the material better.

Performance-based evaluation is a very important concept in health education, because attitude and ultimately behavior are the culminating factors. Obviously, in the case of both portfolios and exhibitions, group work and critical essays may be an extensive part of the process. Certainly when using this type of evaluation, it is difficult to tell where instruction stops and assessment starts because of the interwoven nature of the two in performance-based evaluation. The goal should be to help students focus on what they have learned, how they have changed, and what they have achieved as a result of the process. What better way to do this than to allow the student to have input on what will constitute learning and evaluation? Perhaps the greatest advantage of performance-based evaluation is that, if done properly, children can learn, achieve, and progress in a fashion that does not label or negatively affect their self-esteem.

▪ Peer Evaluation

A trend in the current rethinking of how evaluation should occur is to involve students in the process. One strategy for accomplishing this is through peer evaluation. Peer evaluation occurs when students evaluate each other's work (McCown, Driscoll, and Roop 1996, 457).

Peer evaluation happens all the time on an informal basis when students look at one another's work for comparison with their own efforts. For peer evaluation to be effective, students should work together to establish the criteria or standards used for judging their work. By setting the standards for judgment, students have established their own goals, which they expect their work to reflect. Assessment can be done through the use of checklists or questionnaires.

▪ Narrative Grading

Narrative grading has been defined as "serious dialogue between student and teacher about the quality of the work" (Shor 1992). The dialogue should be student generated and should reflect creative options as well as critical thinking. The facts should not be isolated from the student's experience. Effort should be made to help the student personalize the information to ensure positive health-related behavior. The advantage of this type of grading is that, once the student verbalizes a concept, he or she is more likely to take ownership of it. This strategy also enables students to assess their feelings on particular topics. The biggest disadvantage is that the process can be very time-consuming when the group is large.

Narrative grading is a performance-based evaluation that teachers can use to assess students' work. Instead of merely assigning a number, percentage, or letter grade to a student's work, the teacher writes the evaluation in narrative form (e.g., paragraph style). Of course, this type of evaluation can be combined with the other forms of evaluations, like letter grades. Ideally, a narrative evaluation should briefly describe the course and evaluate the strengths and weaknesses of the student's performance in the various areas of class activity including discussion, coursework, homework, tests, and general understanding of the course content (UC Santa Cruz 2011). Some of the benefits of narrative grading are:

- It provides the student and transcript evaluators with significantly more information about the student's academic performance than does a traditional letter grade.

- A narrative allows the teacher to recognize exceptional or noteworthy performance.
- Teachers observe individual students more closely to personalize their descriptions of student performance.
- Evaluators are encouraged to study a student's entire performance record rather than focusing on a single summary measure.

National Health Education Standards and Grading

Many states use the Health Education Assessment Project (HEAP) State Collaborative on Assessment and Student Standards (SCASS) to assess their health education programs. This is an effective health education assessment resource that helps schools to align curriculum, instruction, and assessment with the National Health Education Standards, helping to improve student health behaviors through health education (Council of Chief State School Officers 2011). HEAP has developed a bank of resources designed to promote professional development in assessment for school health education; these HEAP Assessment Items are used by HEAP member states to improve accountability at all levels (state, district, and local).

Presenting health education that is aligned with the NHES and performance indicators is important for a number of reasons. These reasons, as identified by Tappe (2010), include the following:

> Standards-based health education is important because it supports health literacy and healthy behaviors among students, it provides guidance for health instruction in schools, it sets expectations for student achievement in health education and for the evaluation of health education programs, it provides direction for developing policy in support of comprehensive school health education, and it provides insight for developing health education curricula and providing professional preparation and development. Standards-based health education is an integral component of an overall school health program and is critical to promoting the learning and health of students, families, schools, and communities.

The performance criteria and standards are used so that students, teachers, parents, community members, and employers are aware of the nature of excellence and what it takes to succeed. Students can see where they are, and teachers can tell parents how their children are progressing toward proficiency (Table 5.3).

Health curricula used today should reflect current research and standards. Reviews of effective programs and input from health education specialists have identified characteristics of an effective health education curriculum (CDC 2011); these state that an effective curriculum:

- Focuses on clear health goals and related behavioral outcomes.
- Is research-based and theory-driven.

Table 5.3 Curriculum Planning
Stage 1: Establish Desired Results • What long-term goals are sought? • How will students arrive at important understandings? • What essential questions will students explore? • What knowledge and skills will students acquire? • What established goals or standards are targeted?
Stage 2: Track Evidence • What performances and products will reveal evidence of understanding of important concepts? • By what criteria will performance be assessed? • What additional evidence will be collected for all Stage 1 Desired Results?
Stage 3: Finalize Learning Plan • What activities, experiences, and lessons will lead to the desired results and success in assessment? • How will the learning plan help students in acquiring, understanding, and internalizing information? • How will the unit be organized to optimize achievement for all learners? • Are all three stages properly aligned?

Source: From *Understanding by Design*, 2nd Edition, (pp. 17–19), by Grant Wiggins and Jay McTighe, Alexandria, VA: ASCD. © 2005 by ASCD, www.ascd.org. Adapted with permission.

- Addresses individual values and group norms that support health-enhancing behaviors.
- Focuses on increasing personal perceptions of risk and harmfulness of engaging in specific health risk behaviors and reinforcing protective factors.
- Addresses social pressures and influences.
- Builds personal competence, social competence, and self efficacy by addressing skills.
- Provides functional health knowledge that is basic, accurate, and directly contributes to health-promoting decisions and behaviors.
- Uses strategies designed to personalize information and engage students.
- Provides age- and developmentally-appropriate information, learning strategies, teaching methods, and materials.
- Incorporates learning strategies, teaching methods, and materials that are culturally inclusive.
- Provides adequate time for instruction and learning.
- Provides opportunities to reinforce skills and positive health behaviors and to make positive connections with influential others.
- Includes teacher information and plans for professional development and training that enhance effectiveness of instruction and student learning.

The Development of Rubrics

Rubrics are the criteria that will be utilized to assess and evaluate how the student performs in the health education instructional process. Rubrics describe a set of fixed measurements and criteria, which are accompanied by examples of products that represent different levels of accomplishment or skill acquisition.

The rubric is an authentic assessment tool that is particularly useful in assessing complex and subjective criteria. Table 5.4 provides an example of a scoring rubric.

Authentic assessment is geared toward assessment methods that closely correspond to real-world experience and applies such evaluations to all areas of the curriculum. It was originally developed in the arts and apprenticeship systems, where assessment has always been based on performance. The instructor observes the student in the process of working on real-life problems, provides feedback, monitors the student's use of the feedback, and adjusts instruction and evaluation accordingly.

The rubric is a formative type of assessment because it becomes an ongoing part of the teaching and learning process. Students are involved in the assessment process through both peer evaluation and self-assessment. As students become familiar with rubrics, they can assist in the rubric design process. This involvement empowers the students and, as a result, their learning becomes more focused and self-directed. Authentic assessment, therefore, blurs the lines between teaching, learning, and assessment.

The advantages of using rubrics in assessment are that they allow assessment to be more objective and consistent; focus the teacher to clarify his or her criteria in specific terms; clearly show the student how his or her work will be evaluated and what is expected; promote student awareness of which criteria to use in assessing peer performance; provide useful feedback regarding the effectiveness of the instruction; and provide benchmarks against which to measure and document progress.

Rubrics can be created in a variety of forms and levels of complexity; however, they all contain common features that focus on measuring a stated objective (performance, behavior, or quality), use a range to rate performance, and contain specific performance characteristics arranged in levels indicating the degree to which a standard has been met.

Some states are working together currently to develop the actual assessment standards and measures related to the National Health Education Standards. States are invited to join one or more of the projects that develop standards and student assessments through pooled resources and effort. (These projects will be linked to the emerging national health standards and new ideas about appropriate assessment methods.) One such project is the Health Education Assessment Project (HEAP), in which the group has developed assessment measures, performance tasks, and performance events, plus a portfolio assessment model to measure this area. Member states will have sufficient assessment resources to conduct assessment at the state and local levels. Professional development materials have also been developed (HEAP 2006).

Table 5.4 Scoring Rubrics			
The completion of this form will result in a total core concepts score and clearly delineated actions or goals.			
NHES #1: Students will comprehend concepts related to health promotion and disease prevention to enhance health.			
Connections	**Score**	**Comprehensiveness**	**Score**
Completely and accurately describes relationships between behavior and health. Draws logical conclusion(s) about the connection between behavior and health.	4	Thoroughly covers health topic, showing both breadth (wide *range* of facts and ideas) and depth (*details* about facts and ideas). Response is completely accurate.	4
Describes relationships between behavior and health with some minor inaccuracies or omissions. Draws plausible conclusion(s) about the connection between behavior and health.	3	Mostly covers health topic, showing breadth and depth, but one or both less fully. Response is mostly accurate, but may have minor inaccuracies.	3
Description of relationship(s) between behavior and health is incomplete and/or contains significant inaccuracies. Attempts to draw a conclusion about the connection between behavior and health, but conclusion is incomplete or flawed.	2	Minimal coverage of health topic, lacking breadth or showing little to no depth. Response may show some inaccuracies.	2
Inaccurate or no description of relationship(s) between behavior and health. Inaccurate OR no conclusion drawn about the connection between behavior and health.	1	No coverage of health topic information. Little or no accurate information.	1
Source: From *RMC Analytic Rubrics for National Health Education Standards,* © 2007. Used by permission of Rocky Mountain Center for Health Promotion and Education.			

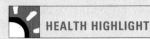

HEALTH HIGHLIGHT | Example of Health Curriculum Guide from Tennessee Department of Education

Standards for Healthful Living

Personal Health and Wellness: K–2

Domain Description: Personal health and wellness is influenced by individual heredity and involves a lifelong process of choices and behaviors that lead to healthful living and disease prevention.

Standard 2: The student will understand the importance of personal hygiene practices as related to healthful living.

Learning Expectations:

The student will:

2.1 demonstrate essential personal hygiene practices;

2.2 identify the importance of good versus poor personal hygiene practices;

2.3 explain the importance of not sharing personal hygiene items (toothbrush, combs, brushes);

2.4 describe physical/emotional/social health implications of personal hygiene.

Performance Indicators:

At Level 1, the student will be able to:
- identify proper hygiene skills (e.g., handwashing, shampooing, flossing, toothbrushing, and bathing);
- list healthy outcomes from using proper personal hygiene habits;
- list the consequences of not using proper personal hygiene habits.

At Level 2, the student will be able to:
- apply proper hygiene practices (e.g., handwashing, shampooing, flossing, toothbrushing, bathing);
- identify consequences of poor oral hygiene (e.g., cavities, gum disease, and tooth loss);
- identify consequences of poor personal hygiene (e.g., body odor, illness, and poor self-image);
- describe healthy outcomes from using proper personal hygiene habits.

At Level 3, the student will be able to:
- demonstrate proper hygiene practices;
- explain the importance of proper hygiene practices;
- compare and contrast the difference between the practice of good and poor personal hygiene habits;
- describe how good personal hygiene relates to a positive outlook and self image;
- analyze the affect of personal hygiene on social relationships.

Teacher Assessment Indicators (examples):

The teacher may:
- apply cooking oil and ground cinnamon to the students' hands. Students rub their own hands together, see the sediment and think it is dirt, wash hands as normally do. Observe that oil and cinnamon are still evident. Students then apply soap and use proper handwashing techniques as taught by the teacher;
- provide a dental mold for students to demonstrate proper toothbrushing techniques (invite dental professional if needed);
- role play with discussion on the topic of social/emotional/physical implications of poor personal hygiene practices (e.g. puppets, books, videos).

Source: Tennessee Health Curriculum Guide, Tennessee.gov

An excellent program in performance-based education is *Assessment Tools for School Health Education*. This work provides a foundation for assessment in health education, and it provides a framework for performance-based education. The manual provides a complete description of assessment in health education, including examples of scored student work and a lesson that demonstrates the use of the assessment system (HEAP 2006).

Using Benchmarks and Standards to Assess Student Progress

Standards and benchmarks are used to help the teacher understand what students are expected to know and to be able to do in each subject. These methods are used in assessing the students' progress in learning and as an attempt to raise the performance of all students.

▪ Content Standards

Content standards describe the knowledge and skills expected of students at certain stages in their education. Implementing content standards means that every school in a particular school system has the same expectations for all students in key subjects, although there is enough flexibility to allow individual schools and teachers to help students meet the standards in different ways. For example, schools may use various materials, and teachers may teach differently. But the goal is the same: clear learning expectations and high levels of achievement for all.

Often, a school system will create **performance tasks** that determine whether a student has reached the content standards. These tasks include hands-on demonstrations, written projects, and portfolios, as discussed earlier in this chapter. Typically, these methods of assessing student work supplement traditional methods. Teachers often use these performance tasks and scoring guides to describe a student's expected level of performance. Because not all students test well, a well-rounded series of assessments will give students a variety of opportunities to demonstrate what they have learned.

▪ Benchmarks

Benchmarks are set at various grade levels (similar to the National Health Education Standards described in Chapter 3—i.e., grades 2, 5, 8, and 12). Benchmarks are used to ensure that students are progressing appropriately. For example, National Health Standard 3 says that "Students will demonstrate the ability to access valid information and products and services to enhance health." The benchmarks for that standard would be more specific. A grade 5 benchmark, for example, might say that students must recall main ideas and details, put events in order, predict outcomes, and draw conclusions. By grade 8, students must be able to understand the techniques used by the author and the author's purpose. By grade 12, students must read to determine goals and beliefs and to take positions on issues. Not all students will reach benchmarks at the same time. Some students may need more assistance. For example, a school system might provide before- and after-school tutoring, summer school, or Saturday school as opportunities for students. You can see an example of state-specific standards and benchmarks in the Health Highlight.

Shorts tests that teachers administer periodically during the school year can be used as benchmark assessments. These assessments allow teachers to see immediate feedback on how well students are meeting the outlined academic standards. Regular use of these assessments can be used as a tool to measure student growth and design curriculum to meet the learning needs of each individual student (Coffey 2011).

Chapter In Review

Summary

- The purpose of measurement and evaluation is to determine whether instructional objectives have been fulfilled.
- Measurement involves the construction, administration, and scoring of tests.
- Evaluation is the process of interpreting, analyzing, and assessing the data gathered.
- Newer methods used for evaluation include performance-based evaluation, narrative grading, portfolios, group projects, individual exhibits, and critical thinking essays.
- The purposes of assessment are to reveal how much students have learned, whether standards are being met, and whether educators have taught the material successfully.
- Tests should be valid, reliable, objective, able to discriminate, comprehensive, and easy to give, use, and score.
- Typical test question types are true-false, matching, multiple choice, short answer, and essay.
- Measuring attitudes is difficult; examples of useful tools include attitude scales, checklists, and critical thinking essays.
- Traditional grading strategies include the percentage method, the A to F combination, and the pass/fail or satisfactory/unsatisfactory method.
- Newer assessment methods include performance-based evaluation, critical thinking essays, peer review, and group projects.
- Rubrics are important tools for facilitating personal achievement.
- Benchmarks and standards are now used to guide teaching and learning.

Discussion Questions

1. Differentiate measurement from evaluation.
2. Discuss the purposes of measurement and evaluation, and explain how you can achieve these purposes.
3. Why is a table of specifications necessary when developing a test?
4. Discuss some of the techniques used to assess attitudes in health education. What are the shortcomings of these techniques?
5. What purposes do assessment and grading serve in health education?
6. Discuss some of the common methods of grading used in the elementary school.
7. What are the advantages/disadvantages of utilizing rubrics for evaluation purposes?
8. Explain what content standards and benchmarks are, and describe the implications of their use in schools throughout the country.

Critical Thinking Questions

1. In what ways can you as a teacher reduce the "adversarial relationship" between student and teacher that is sometimes caused by the grading process?
2. How can you as a teacher help your students enjoy learning for the sake of learning instead of learning just to make a grade?
3. What skills do you possess that will enable you to be a competent evaluator of student progress? What skills do you need to develop?
4. Explain your feelings about the relative importance of measuring attitudes in a health education class.
5. Your principal has suggested to you that health education should be graded on a pass/fail basis. How would you justify using a grading scale similar to other core subjects?

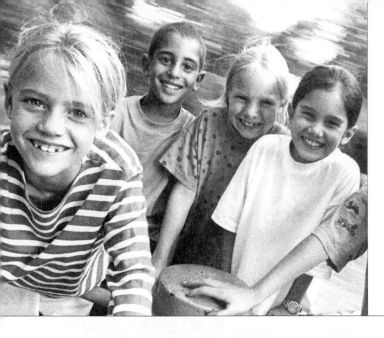

Mental Health and Stress Reduction

6

Dwell upon the brightest parts in every prospect... and strive to be pleased with the present circumstance.

—*Abraham Tucker (1774)*

Valued Outcomes

After completion of this chapter, you should be able to:

- Define mental health.
- Identify the characteristics of emotionally healthy students.
- Describe how psychosocial factors contribute to mental health.
- Describe the importance of self-esteem in fostering mental health.
- Discuss strategies for enhancing self-esteem of students.
- Discuss the characteristics of students with learning disabilities.
- Discuss the indicators of psychiatric problems in students.
- Identify the potential problems associated with latchkey children or children from separated/divorced families.
- Identify the means of dealing with students who have experienced the death of a pet, friend, grandparent, parent, or sibling.
- Define the terms stress and stressor.
- List the detrimental health effects of prolonged stress.
- Identify strategies for dealing with stress.
- Discuss the role of the family in maintaining and influencing the emotional health of students.
- Discuss the effects of bullying on students.

Reflections

There was a folk singer by the name of Jimmie Rodgers who recorded a song called "Child of Clay." One of the lines in that recording was "bended, molded, and shaped into what we are today." As you read this chapter, reflect on the many factors that influence students' perceptions of self and ultimately their mental health. What are significant influences in children's lives? What potential impacts (both negative and positive) do these events, people, and institutions have? What can teachers do to positively influence the children under their tutelage?

The Importance of Mental Health

There is probably no area more vital than that of helping students to develop sound mental health practices. We need only look at the rates of alcohol and drug use among our nation's youth, the suicide rates for adolescents, the reported depression among youth, the number of school-aged children who run away from home each year, and the violence that occurs in our schools to realize the importance of helping students achieve and maintain good mental and emotional health. Without the sense of inner peace and balance that comes with good mental health, no individual can be considered completely healthy. The links between mental and physical health are clear. Yet the goal of good mental health is in many ways more elusive than the goal of good physical health. If an individual receives proper nutrition, exercises on a regular basis, gets plenty of relaxation and sleep, and follows good personal health practices, he or she has a high probability of remaining physically fit. Unfortunately, there is no easy prescription for good mental health. There are, however, identifiable characteristics of people who are mentally healthy. Experts have defined **mental health** as the ability to perceive reality as it is, to respond to its challenges, and to develop rational strategies for living (Hales 2011, 25).

Implied in this definition is the concept that emotionally healthy people are in touch with their feelings and can express those feelings in a proper fashion. This chapter provides information about mental health principles that will help your students develop sound mental health. Topics discussed include human needs and the development of self-esteem, behavior and the expression of emotions, stress and its relationship to mental health, values and patterns of decision making, and the role of the family in the development of mental health.

Characteristics of the Emotionally Healthy Individual

If mental health is defined as the ability to perceive reality and to respond to the challenges of life, then what are the characteristics of an emotionally healthy individual? Maslow has conceptualized emotional happiness in what he calls self-actualized people. There are individuals who seem to live, or be living, at their fullest. Maslow goes on to suggest that a self-actualized person has five important qualities (Maslow 1983):

1. **A sense of realism**—the ability to deal with the world as it is and not demand that it be otherwise.
2. **A sense of acceptance**—the ability to accept themselves and others.
3. **A sense of autonomy**—the ability to direct themselves, acting independently of their environments. They are not afraid to be themselves. They are inner-directed people who find guidance from within their own values and feelings.
4. **A sense of creativity**—a sense of appreciation for what goes on around them. They are open to new experiences and do not fear the unknown.
5. **A capacity for intimacy**—the ability to be open to the pleasure of intimate physical contact and the risks/satisfaction of being close to others in a caring, sensitive way.

Payne and Hahn (2010) expand upon the concept of an emotionally healthy person by listing the following characteristics. Healthy people

- Feel comfortable about themselves.
- Are capable of experiencing the full range of human emotions.
- Are not overwhelmed by their emotions—either negative or positive.
- Accept life's disappointments.
- Feel comfortable with others.
- Receive and give love easily.
- Feel concern for others when appropriate.
- Establish short-term and long-term goals.
- Function autonomously where and when appropriate.
- Generally trust others.
- Lead a health-enhancing lifestyle that includes regular exercise, sound nutrition, and adequate sleep.

There is no one ideal for emotional health. Certainly the lack of any one characteristic does not indicate an emotionally unhealthy person. Probably no one has all these characteristics, and most of us fall short at some time, but the lists can provide a benchmark for how well we are achieving or moving toward being emotionally healthy.

This process of achieving mental wellness is a lifelong process and begins the moment we are born. How we interact with our siblings, how our parents relate and interact with us, and our perceptions throughout life influence our mental wellness. The experiences each child undergoes while in the elementary school are very important. The perceptions of success, feelings of acceptance by peers and teachers, and the supportive emotional climate in the classroom all contribute to the emotional well-being and development of the child's self-esteem. The process begins when the child enters school each morning and continues until he or she leaves in the afternoon. The information learned each day, each year, and year after year eventually shapes self-perception and molds us into what we perceive ourselves to be. The home, family, and other institutions also help develop our perceptions, but none impacts as strongly as each teacher with whom we have contact during our elementary school years. The elementary teacher can provide confidence, appreciation, praise, fairness, security, approval, friendship, and acceptance. Through modeling, developing decision-making skills, and being in a success-oriented situation, children learn to accept themselves and others.

What Children Need to Achieve Emotional Health

The fulfillment of basic emotional needs such as love, affection, acceptance, and a feeling of importance are essential to children developing a self-identity and their self-esteem. All people need to receive love and affection. Everyone needs to feel a sense of acceptance and importance from others. If these basic needs can be fostered, the child's potential for successfully interacting with others, meeting individual needs for independence and self-expression, and resolving personal and social conflicts are clearly enhanced. The child is freer to pursue higher human goals, culminating with what Maslow calls *self-actualization needs* (Hamrick, Anspaugh, and Ezell 1986). Maslow's hierarchy of human needs (Figure 6.1) applies throughout our lives and certainly in the early developmental years of the elementary child.

W. Edwards Deming, noted statistician and the father of quality management, offered the following points in an essay titled "A System of Profound Knowledge" (Deming 1994). These points seem most relevant to keep in mind when discussing the mental health of children. (In this excerpt, we have substituted the term *children* for *people*, which was originally used in the essay.) Deming stated:

- Children are different from one another.
- Children learn in different ways and at different speeds.

- Children are born with a need for relationships with other people and with the need to be loved and esteemed by others. There is an innate need for self-esteem and respect.
- Circumstances provide some children with dignity and self-esteem. Circumstances deny other children these advantages.
- No one can enjoy learning if he or she must constantly be concerned about grades and receiving gold stars for performance.
- Extrinsic motivation is submission to external forces that neutralize intrinsic motivation.
- Under extrinsic motivation children are ruled by external forces.
- Leaders (teachers), by virtue of their authority, have an obligation to make changes in the system of management that will bring improvement. (The authors believe that Deming means teachers should be prepared to facilitate within the school and in each individual classroom an atmosphere that helps each child feel respected and successful.)

Elementary aged children with unmet emotional needs tend to demonstrate poor decision-making and problem-solvings kills, poor self-image and low self-confidence, inability to resolve interpersonal conflicts, inability to concentrate, and poor refusal skills (Goodwin, Goodwin & Cantrell 1986). Schools, teachers, and parents need to give mental health a high priority to jointly address these behaviors.

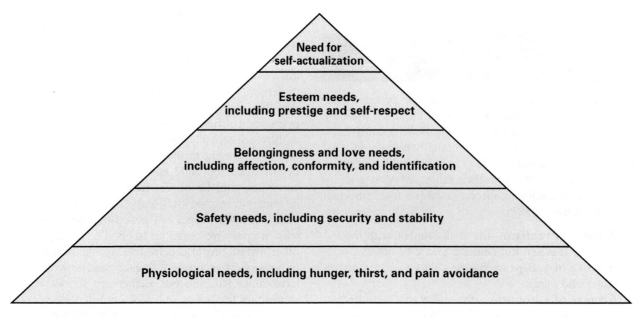

Figure 6.1

Maslow's Hierarchy of Basic Human Needs

Source: Abraham H. Maslow, *Motivation and Personality*, 1954 Harper and Row, p. 236.

1. Teach children to like themselves. Help them discover their unique qualities, skills, and talents, and help them be proud of who they are.

2. Teach children to be good to themselves. Encourage them to reward themselves periodically with emotional or material favors.

3. Help children learn to be introspective, to examine motives for behavior, and to be insightful about their own conduct.

4. Help each child accept her or his limitations. Think in terms of competency levels rather than in terms of success or failure.

5. Help children deal with a problem or crisis as it arises rather than allowing them to let pressures mount as they worry about "what ifs."

6. Help each child establish realistic goals, both short term and long term, and help children work toward accomplishing their goals.

7. Help children express their emotions in terms of how the emotion makes them feel rather than in terms of how other people make them feel. "I feel angry for having to do a homework assignment over the weekend" is healthier than "Ms. Barnes, you make me angry. You shouldn't assign a homework assignment over the weekend."

8. Encourage children to involve themselves in diversified activities and cultivate many interests. Encourage them to not center their life around one person, place, or activity.

9. Encourage children to develop a sense of humor. Help them learn to laugh and enjoy life.

10. Teach children to be optimistic.

Self-Esteem and the Development of Emotional Health

Many health educators and mental health authorities believe that self-esteem is the foundation of emotional health. **Self-esteem** can be defined as a combination of self-confidence and self-respect—the feeling that one is capable of coping with life's challenges and is worthy of happiness. In other words, self-esteem is how people perceive themselves. People who have high self-esteem have confidence in themselves, have the ability to solve problems rather than just worry about them, have the ability to confront or eliminate the things that frighten them, have the ability to take reasonable risks, and are able to nurture themselves (Martin and Martin 2002).

In the early years of children's lives, self-esteem is based largely on their perceptions of how the important adults in their lives judge them. The extent to which children believe that they have the characteristics valued by the adults and peers in their lives determines greatly their perception of self. Families, communities, and ethnic groups may vary in the criteria on which self-esteem is based. Some groups may emphasize athletic ability, others physical appearance; others evaluate boys and girls differently. Factors such as stereotyping, prejudice, and discrimination may also contribute to low self-esteem among children (Katz 2002).

Bean (1992) maintains that four conditions are important if children are to develop and maintain high self-esteem:

1. **A sense of connectiveness**—children must feel a part of something; feel related in important ways to specific people, places, or things; identify with a group of people; feel something important belongs to them (a sense of ownership); and feel they belong to something or someone.

2. **A sense of uniqueness**—children must feel that they have special qualities, are valued for who they are, and can do things that no one else knows or can do. They must feel that they can express themselves in their own unique way, feel creative and imaginative, feel respect for themselves, feel enjoyment for their differences or uniqueness, and feel that they are affirmed for what they are rather than what they are not.

3. **A sense of power**—children must believe in themselves, feel competent, feel comfortable with responsibility, feel in control of themselves despite pressures experienced, feel comfortable when they have responsibility to fulfill, feel confident they can make decisions to solve problems, be able to use skills they have learned, be comfortable with learning new skills, and feel others can't make them do things they really don't want to do.

4. **A sense of models**—children have the ability to tell right from wrong, have people in their lives who are worthy of being emulated, have a consistent set of values and beliefs to guide their actions, can depend on past experiences to help avoid problems or avoid being intimidated by new ones, have a sense of purpose, are able to make sense of their lives and of the circumstances in which they live, know the standards being used to judge them, are able to organize their environment to accomplish tasks, and experience satisfaction from learning.

Rinholm (1999) suggests some general ways to improve self-esteem in the classroom:

1. **Build a sense of security**—children need to feel safe and know what is expected. Discuss the rules with the class and the advantages of having rules,

follow predictable routines, make the class a safe environment (emotionally and physically), and make the classroom a positive and comfortable place to be.

2. **Build the child's sense of identity**—this concept refers to helping students recognize their uniqueness as well as their strengths/weaknesses. Activities include collages, pictures, and reports on their interests, likes, dislikes, and experiences.

3. **Enhance the child's sense of belonging**—it is important for children to feel part of a larger group and that they are accepted. Activities include those that help the students learn about one another, opportunities for group work, and how to handle social situations—such as dealing with conflict or knowing what to do or say when given a compliment.

4. **Build a child's sense of purpose**—children must have goals and be actively working toward them. Activities that support this notion include helping children set their daily/weekly goals and helping them identify individuals they admire.

5. **Build a child's sense of competence**—help children to develop the belief that they can meet goals and achieve success. Help children see their strengths and the progress they have made; teach children to praise themselves for their successes.

A most important point for teachers to keep in mind is the axiom from medical practice that states "First, do no harm." The words of a teacher can weigh heavily on children. As a teacher, you serve as role model, parent, and authority figure, and children pay close attention to your attitudes and interactions with them. Every day you should find something positive to say to each child and give each child a special moment in the classroom. See the Health Highlight box for more ways to foster positive self-esteem.

Self-esteem is necessary for developing self-expression and independence. A person who has a feeling of self-worth is also better equipped emotionally to show concern for others. As the individual begins to develop meaningful relationships with others who recognize and reward his or her unique qualities of expression, independent thinking flourishes. A strong sense of self-worth permits open and honest communication with others because rejection and disapproval are not feared as great risks. The establishment of self-esteem is a lifelong process. This lifelong quest is more easily attainable if the nurturing of emotional and social well-being has been emphasized in infancy and childhood, thus promoting a sense of security, identity, autonomy, and intimacy early in life.

Self-esteem is the result of three factors: (1) how children perceive themselves, (2) how they want to be, and (3) what expectations they perceive others have for them. The foundation of positive self-esteem is shaped in early childhood, primarily by interactions with parents and other family members. Positive comments and attitudes toward the child contribute to his or her sense of competency and shape the perception of self.

Kuersten has stated "We all know that social and emotional factors affect learning and preparedness to learn. If a kid is feeling unhappy, it's hard for him or her to focus on school work. If a kid is feeling stressed, or is pressured by peers not to perform well, this can reduce academic learning" (Kuersten 1999). Kuersten goes on to say that there are many ways that schools can address children's emotional needs. They can offer a coordinated, systematic social and emotional education curriculum and a supportive, safe environment in which the teacher nurtures students' personal development; schools also can do much to establish a network of supportive programs and individuals in the community. In essence what Kuersten is suggesting is the necessity of a coordinated school health program (see Chapter 1).

When children enter school, teachers should help them to develop positive self-esteem by providing a positive emotional climate in the classroom. Teachers also can help children view themselves realistically and as being unique and lovable. Children need to know they are valued and accepted regardless of intellect, appearance, dress, or other social criteria.

When considering self-esteem, there are several areas related to learning conditions of which the teacher must remain aware. Some of those issues are outlined in the remainder of this section and are followed by guidelines that can help teachers deal with children in the various situations. As with all conditions that potentially affect children, the actual diagnosis must be left to psychological and medical professionals.

▪ Learning Disabilities

A **learning disability (LD)** is a neurological disorder that affects a child's ability to receive, process, store, and respond to information (National Center for Learning Disabilities 2006). LD is not a single disease but rather a group of disorders. The United States Department of Education has indicated that 5 percent of public school students have some type of learning disability (National Institute of Mental Health 2006).

Learning disabilities do not include mental retardation, autism, behavioral disorders, or laziness. Children who have LDs cut across all economic, cultural, and environmental levels. Generally, most experts state that there seems to be no apparent cause, but LDs tend to occur in families. Further, some LDs occur when there are complications associated with pregnancy or childbirth. The Individuals with Disabilities Act (IDEA), passed in 1997, and the Americans with Disabilities Act (ADA), passed in 1990, ensure that children who have learning disabilities have a right to different forms of assistance. The type of assistance varies with the type of LD. Table 6.1 lists some types of learning disabilities and provides indicators of that particular LD.

Table 6.1 Learning Disabilities and Related Symptoms

Disability	Area of Difficulty	Symptoms	Examples
Dyslexia	Processing language	Reading, writing	Letters, numbers, words written or pronounced backwards
Dyscalculia	Math skills	Computation, unable to remember math facts, concepts of time, and money	Difficulty learning to count by 2s, 3s, and 4s
Dyspraxia	Fine motor skills	Coordination, manual dexterity	Trouble with scissors, drawing
Dysgraphia	Written expression	Handwriting, spelling, composition	Illegible handwriting, difficulty organizing ideas
Auditory processing disorder	Interpreting auditory information	Language development, reading	Difficulty anticipating how a speaker will end a sentence
Visual processing disorder	Interpreting visual information	Reading, writing, math	Difficulty distinguishing letters such as "h" and "n"

Source: Adapted from the National Center for Learning Disabilities 2006

▪ Attention Deficit Hyperactivity Disorder

Attention deficit hyperactivity disorder (ADHD) is one of the most common psychiatric disorders that appear in childhood. Children who have the disorder cannot stay focused on a task or activity, demonstrate impulsive behavior, and experience difficulty with finishing a task. ADHD is most often diagnosed in children between ages 6 and 12. Most research suggests ADHD is diagnosed four to nine times more often in boys than in girls (Bender 1997).

Individuals with ADHD exhibit a combination of behaviors: They fidget with hands or feet or squirm in their seat; experience difficulty remaining seated and difficulty sustaining attention and waiting for a turn in tasks, games, or group situations; blurt out answers to questions before the questions have been completed; have difficulty following through on instructions and in organizing tasks; shift from one unfinished activity to another; fail to pay close attention to details and make careless mistakes; lose things necessary for tasks or activities; show difficulty in listening to others without being distracted or interrupting; exhibit wide ranges in mood swings; and have great difficulty in delaying gratification.

After a child starts school, the symptoms of ADHD become more noticeable. During this period, ADHD can disrupt many aspects of a child's life. Learning and academic performance, adjusting to change, sleeping, and getting along with others are all potential problem areas. It is estimated that between 3 and 5 percent of children have ADHD, or approximately 2 million children in the United States. This means that a class of 25 to 30 children is likely to have at least one child who has ADHD (National Institute of Mental Health 2011).

There are three patterns of behavior that indicate ADHD. People who have ADHD may be consistently inattentive, may be hyperactive, and may be impulsive. They may exhibit all three types of behavior or only one or two of the three behaviors. There are three recognized subtypes of ADHD. The **predominantly hyperactive-impulsive type** does not show significant inattention; the **predominantly inattentive type** does not show significant hyperactive and impulsive behaviors; and the **combined type** displays inattentive and hyperactive and/or impulsive symptoms. Whether a child has ADHD must be determined by a variety of professionals. Child psychiatrists can diagnose ADHD, provide therapy, and prescribe any needed medications. Child psychologists are also qualified to diagnose and treat ADHD. They can provide therapy for the child and help the family develop ways to deal with the disorder. But psychologists are not medical doctors and must rely on the child's physician for medical exams and prescriptions (National Institute of Mental Health 2011).

No two children with ADHD are alike, and it's important to keep in mind that no single educational program, practice, or setting will be best for all children. Teachers who are successful in educating children with ADHD focus on a three-pronged strategy. (1) They identify the unique needs of the child. For example, the teacher determines how, when, and why the child is inattentive and hyperactive. (2) The teacher selects appropriate educational practices associated with academic instruction, behavioral interventions, and classroom accommodations. (3) The teacher combines these practices into an individualized educational program (IEP) or other individualized plan and integrates this program with educational activities provided to other children in the class. Teachers should keep in mind that transitions from one lesson or class to another are particularly difficult for students with ADHD. When they are prepared for transitions, these children are more likely to respond and to stay on task (United States Department of Education 2011).

Some basic strategies outlined by the United States Department of Education may assist teachers in conducting effective lessons in classrooms that include students with ADHD:

- **Be predictable.** Minimal rules and minimal choices are best for children with ADHD.

- **Support the student's participation in the classroom.** Provide students with private, discreet cues to stay on task and advanced warning when they will be called upon.

- **Use assistive technology and audiovisual materials.** Use a variety of technologies to present academic lessons, making instruction more visual and allowing students to actively participate.

- **Check student performance.** Question individual students to assess their mastery of the lesson.

- **Ask probing questions.** Allow a child sufficient time to work out an answer to a problem you've posed; wait a period of time before giving the answer or calling on another student. Ask follow-up questions that give children an opportunity to demonstrate what they know.

- **Perform ongoing student evaluation.** Watch for signs of lack of comprehension (daydreaming or visual or verbal indications of frustration).

- **Help students correct their own mistakes.**

- **Help students focus.** Offer follow-up directions or assign learning partners.

- **Provide additional oral or written directions.**

- **Lower noise level.** Remind students about the behavioral rules stated at the beginning of the lesson.

- **Break down assignments into smaller, less complex tasks.**

- **Highlight key points.** Highlight key words in the instructions on worksheets before the lesson begins. Show children how to identify and highlight a key sentence and important facts and operations.

- **Eliminate or reduce frequency of timed tests.**

- **Use cooperative learning strategies.** Have students work together in small groups to maximize their own and each other's learning. Use strategies such as Think-Pair-Share, where teachers ask students to think about a topic, pair with a partner to discuss it, and share ideas with the group (Slavin 2002).

Professionals currently feel that ADHD medications, mostly stimulants, accompanied by behavioral therapy can help children control their hyperactivity, pay attention better, and focus on tasks at an effective level. The use of drugs should be carefully monitored by the physician and behavioral specialist working with the child. Problems that teachers must be vigilant for in the ADHD child include depression, anxiety disorders, inappropriate conduct, drug abuse, antisocial behavior, and poor self-esteem.

▪ The Impact on Self-Esteem

It should be pointed out that not all children with ADHD and a learning disability have self-esteem problems. Unfortunately many do, and educators have the responsibility to help ensure that enthusiasm and confidence are not eroded because of treatment or occurrences in a child's life. The National Center for Learning Disabilities has the following recommendations for dealing with these children (2008):

- Be empathetic. See the world through the child's eyes.

- Communicate with respect. Don't interrupt or put children down.

- Give undivided attention. Children feel loved when we spend one-on-one time with them.

- Accept and love children for who they are. Allow them to feel more secure in reaching out to others.

- Treat mistakes as learning experiences.

- Emphasize children's strengths.

- Allow children to solve problems and make decisions.

- Discipline to teach. Do not discipline in a way that intimidates or humiliates the child.

▪ Values and Patterns of Decision Making

Central to the establishment of self-esteem, the expression of emotions and resulting behavior, and the ability to cope effectively with distress are the decision-making patterns that children learn in order to make life adjustments in harmony with their value system. When decisions about a particular issue reflect actions and attitudes that are in agreement with strongly held values, a person is left intact emotionally because personal behaviors and values remain compatible. If decisions produce behaviors that contradict a person's value system, self-esteem is diminished, emotions are exhibited in an unhealthy fashion resulting from lack of resolution over inner conflicts, and stress increases. Decision-making patterns can serve as valuable clues to the way individuals perceive themselves, their relationships with others, and the world around them. Children's actions tell much about their underlying value system, which in turn mediates many of the decisions made about life adjustments. Learning to make decisions following clarification and consideration of values can help each child sustain and enhance self-esteem and the emotional balance crucial to good mental health.

Behavior and the Expression of Emotions

The most obvious indicator of a child's emotional health is behavior. Psychologists state that there is always a reason for behavior. The reasons may not be immediately apparent either to the child or to others; nevertheless, there are underlying motives for all behavior. Much of a child's conscious and subconscious behavior is centered around fulfilling basic emotional needs. Such behavior patterns are often shaped by the ways in which these needs were satisfied or reinforced early in life. Thus, if a change in behavior is desired, the child must learn new, and perhaps healthier, ways of fulfilling basic needs. Everyone experiences feelings of sadness, anger, joy, fear, depression, and apprehension, but the way in which these emotions are expressed varies from person to person. Usually the emotional expression of these feelings becomes labeled as the individual's "behavior." Therefore, a better understanding of emotions may lead to greater understanding of a child's behavior and overall emotional health.

The way in which a child expresses his or her feelings is largely determined by the way the child perceives, either consciously or subconsciously, the situation that triggers the feeling. In other words, two students who are exposed to the same situation—say, disagreement with a teacher over an answer to a test question—may react quite differently, based on different individual assessments of the situation. Such assessments are based in part on how the situation affects fulfillment of basic needs or efforts aimed at attaining autonomy, identity, or other personal goals. In many cases, the situation is perceived as having little impact and therefore elicits minimal emotional expression. Situations that are perceived as having great influence tend to elicit stronger, more overt expression. Thus, emotions are displayed in varying modes of expression as well as varying degrees of intensity. A child is considered more emotionally healthy when emotions are exhibited in a positive way and with an intensity proportional to the situation's impact. Children who consistently display either inimal emotional expression about circumstances generally viewed as having major importance (for example, intimacy with others, successful completion of a difficult task, and death of a family member or pet) or intense emotional expression about events that are not generally viewed as having major importance (for example, having to redo a homework assignment, misplacing an article of clothing, and losing a football game) are considered less emotionally well adjusted.

Emotion itself does not determine mentally healthy or unhealthy behavior, but rather the degree and frequency of the emotion expressed makes this determination. All children on occasion have allowed their emotions to run out of control or be expressed in ways that were not as appropriate, positive, or desirable as they could have been. This type of behavior is a problem only when it becomes a consistent pattern. Often such a pattern of emotional outburst is a result of inner anxiety due to stress originating from conflicts between unconscious drives or needs and conscious values that have been imposed. All people (adults as well as children) share the same emotions. A feeling or emotion is not inherently "good" or "bad," but can be expressed in ways that either promote well-being or detract from it. Mentally healthy behavior largely stems from an individual's ability to recognize, analyze, interpret, and communicate feelings in a consistent, balanced, and positive manner.

▪ Defense Mechanisms

A **defense mechanism** is any behavior a person uses to avoid confronting a situation or problem. Children learn and use various mechanisms early in their elementary school years. Although defense mechanisms can be helpful in dealing with the stresses of life, some children can use them to the extreme. When defense mechanisms are used inappropriately, they can hinder a child's emotional health. Examples of common defense mechanisms are provided in Table 6.2.

Children and Major Psychiatric Disorders

A child who has a major psychiatric disorder has a very serious illness that may affect the life of the child for many years. Some of the signs that a child may need to be examined by a psychiatrist include the following:

- Failure to look or smile at parents or other caregivers
- Very strange actions or appearance
- Lack of movement or facial expression
- Odd way of speaking or use of private language that no one else understands
- Strange conversations with self
- Strange, odd, or repetitive movements such as spinning, hand-flapping, or head banging
- Panic in response to a change in surroundings

Teachers and parents should remain alert to any of these behaviors. A comprehensive evaluation will involve a psychiatrist, parents, teachers, pediatricians, and neurologists and the administration of a broad array of developmental and psychological tests. Partly because of the tremendous changes that occur in children as they grow, diagnosis of major psychiatric disorders in children is one of the most

---

TEACHING TIP

Good mental health involves insight into one's attitudes and feelings. An excellent way to help students get in touch with their feelings and attitudes is to involve them in art projects. For example, you might ask them to draw/paint what they are feeling about topics associated with mental health.

Table 6.2 Common Defense Mechanisms

Defense Mechanism	Definition
Compensation	Making up for weakness in one area by emphasizing strengths in another area *Example*: A child is unsuccessful as an athlete but is a musician; consequently, emphasis is placed on music.
Daydreaming	Escaping from frustrations, boredom, or unpleasant situations through fantasy *Example*: Faced with a divorce of the father and mother, a child creates a mental image of the perfect family.
Displacement	Transferring feelings concerning one situation or person to another object, situation, or person *Example*: Unable to respond with anger toward a parent, the child goes home and abuses a younger child.
Idealization	Holding someone or something in such high esteem that it becomes perfect or godlike in the eyes of the child *Example*: A star athlete who is held in such high regard that his or her human characteristics or shortcomings are overlooked.
Identification	Taking on the quality of someone who is admired *Example*: Performers are often so admired that children attempt to talk, walk, and act as they perceive their idol to do.
Projection	Shifting the responsibility of one's behavior onto someone else *Example*: The child blames the teacher because a test grade was poor rather than accepting the responsibility for not studying sufficiently.
Rationalization	Providing plausible reasons for behavior that are not the real reasons *Example*: A child states she does not like birthday parties and refuses to attend when she really just feels insecure.
Regression	Childish, inappropriate behavior by an adult or a return to former, less mature behavior when under stress *Example*: A child becomes extremely angry when unable to attend a movie or social event. A regressive response may be to cry or throw something.
Repression	Attempting to bury or repress unpleasant or upsetting thoughts *Example*: The child is unable to remember a psychologically painful event, such as the death of a grandparent.
Sublimation	Turning unacceptable thoughts or actions into socially acceptable behaviors *Example*: An aggressive child turns to athletics to redirect his or her energies.

difficult areas of medicine. According to the American Academy of Child and Adolescent Psychiatry (AACAP), no sign should be ignored—the earlier severe mental problems can be identified, the better the prognosis (AACAP 2002).

▪ Obsessive-Compulsive Disorder in Children

As many as 1 in 200 children and adolescents may have **obsessive-compulsive disorder (OCD)**. OCD is characterized by recurrent obsessions or compulsions, impulses, or images that are unwanted. They are not simple worries or preoccupations. The obsessions and compulsions cause significant distress and anxiety and interfere with daily routine, relationships, social functioning, and academic performance.

A younger child who has OCD may fear that harm can occur as a result of an intruder entering an unlocked door or window. As a result, the child may check all doors and windows in an attempt to relieve anxiety. Children may develop rituals, such as compulsive handwashing.

Researchers have demonstrated that OCD is a brain disorder and tends to run in families, although this does not mean a child will automatically develop symptoms. Studies have shown that OCD may develop or worsen after a strep infection. A child may develop OCD even if there is no previous family history (AACAP 1999a). Most children can be treated with a combination of psychotherapy and medications such as the serotonin reuptake inhibitors. Family, school, and teacher cooperation are central to successful treatment.

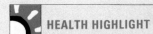

HEALTH HIGHLIGHT | **Dealing with Terrorism**

In the wake of the terrorist attacks on the World Trade Center in New York City and the Pentagon in Washington, DC, our lives and those of our children changed forever. The Psychological Trauma Center has identified several important issues to be aware of when helping children cope with the magnitude of the events of September 11, 2001, and the events that have followed and may occur in the future as the result of the actions of extremist groups throughout the world.

The Issue of War

Children will not understand the War on Terrorism. Children need to have this very different kind of war explained to them. They will see pictures of the military and military action taking place on television. They will see the devastation of suicide bombers and the carnage of the war. Some students may have a family member called to serve his or her country. Children must be given an opportunity to talk about what they are seeing, hearing, and feeling concerning the threat(s) to our country.

Expressing Anger Toward a Different Culture or Ethnic Group

Children must realize that the terrorists who attacked the World Trade Center and the Pentagon were a group of people who have very different ideas about the world in which we live. These individuals performed an evil act. This does not mean that other people of the same cultural background share the same beliefs. Rather, they too may be feeling angry and sad about what has happened.

All Questions May Not Be Answerable

Children want their questions answered. The Psychological Trauma Center suggests that we answer the question of "why" by explaining, *"Bad people in this world who wanted to make a statement are behind the events of September 11 (and the events that will occur in the future). The way they went about making their statement was hurtful to many people. The government is looking for them for the bad things they did."* It is fine to say we don't have an answer. It may be necessary to say, "I don't know," or "I'll try to find out."

Blaming

Some children may express fear and anxiety toward children of other nationalities, feeling someone from their country was responsible for acts of terrorism. Children need to be taught how to deal with their feelings without blaming others.

Source: Adapted from Psychological Trauma Center 2002

▪ Panic Disorder in Children

Children who have **panic disorder** have unexpected and repeated periods of intense fear or discomfort, accompanied by racing heartbeat and shortness of breath. General panic disorders typically begin in adolescence, although they may begin in childhood.

A panic attack may last from a few minutes to hours. They occur without warning, and the symptoms include intense fearfulness, racing or pounding of the heart, dizziness/lightheadedness, trembling or shaking, sense of unreality, and fear of dying, losing control, or going crazy (AACAP 1999d). In severe cases, the child may be afraid to leave home and may become depressed, at risk for use of drugs and alcohol, or even prone to suicidal behavior. Treatments for the disorder are quite effective. Psychotherapy can help the child and family learn ways to reduce stress or conflict that cause an attack. Medications stop the panic attacks.

▪ Depression and Children

Depression in children parallels that in adults with minor differences due to developmental considerations (Magg and Forness 1991). A condition characterized by loss of interest and feelings of extreme or overwhelming sorrow, sadness, and debility, **depression** is a symptom of underlying conflict, tension, or anxiety and may be exhibited in varying degrees for varying lengths of time. The same criteria used to identify depression in adults are used for diagnosing the condition in children. The American Psychiatric Association (APA) and AACAP have stated the following criteria that need to be present for a diagnosis of depression (APA 1999; AACAP 1999c). According to the APA, at least five of these criteria must be present for a diagnosis of depression to be made (APA 1987):

- Depressed mood
- Loss of interest or pleasure in all or almost all activities
- Significant weight loss or weight gain
- Insomnia or excessive sleeping
- Psychomotor agitation or retardation
- Fatigue or loss of energy
- Feelings of worthlessness or excessive or inappropriate guilt
- Diminished ability to think or concentrate; indecisiveness
- Thoughts of suicide or suicide attempts

The Causes of Depression. There are no simple answers to why children become depressed. The APA (1999) estimates that three to six million children and adolescents suffer from depression in the United States. They also state that most children with depression go untreated. Most experts now believe there are multiple reasons for depression. Obviously, not all the reasons apply to children, but some of the situations presented hold implications for the development of depression in children. Some possible factors include the following (Chandler and Kolander 1989, 4–5; APA 1999):

- **Heredity**—Studies show some depressive disorders are hereditary. For example, bipolar disorder has been linked in some cases to a genetic defect.

- **Environment**—Research has shown that stressful life events, especially those involving a loss or threatened loss, often precede episodes of depressive illness. Examples include the death of a loved one, a move to a new home, or physical illness. In most instances the loss induces feelings of sadness and anxiety and often guilt or shame.

- **Background and personality**—People who have certain psychological backgrounds or personality characteristics appear to be more vulnerable to depression. Many specialists believe that some depressive disorders can be traced to a troubled childhood; they attach particular importance to disturbed relationships between a child and his or her parents. Also, people who have low self-esteem, who consistently view themselves and the world with pessimism, or who become easily overwhelmed by stress tend to be more prone to depression.

- **Biochemical factors**—Some types of depression may result from abnormal chemical activity within the brain. These chemicals play a role in the transmission of electrical impulses from one nerve cell (neuron) to another. These chemical messengers, called *neurotransmitters*, set in motion the complex interactions that control moods, feelings, and behaviors. Research suggests that episodes of depression or mania may be related to an improper balance of neurotransmitters. Do biochemical factors cause depression, or does depression cause the biochemical disturbance? No one knows with certainty.

- **Physical illness**—People who have chronic medical illnesses are at high risk of psychiatric illness, especially depression. Some diseases, such as hypothyroidism, (underactive thyroid gland) can bring on a depressive reaction. Depression also may be an early sign of a serious underlying disease, or an undesirable side effect of certain prescription medications.

As stated previously, not all of the above causes are considerations for depression in children. However, Patros and Shamoo (1989) have identified several indicators of childhood depression, as shown in Table 6.3.

Suicide in Children and Adolescents

Each year, more than 4,000 young people between the ages of 15 and 24 kill themselves. In 2009, suicide accounted for 10.1 percent of all deaths among 15- to 24-years-olds

Table 6.3   Indicators of Childhood Depression

Indicator	Response in Child
Lack of interest	Daydreams, withdrawn, poor schoolwork, disruptive
Change in appetite	Picks at food, gives away food, increase in appetite
Changes in sleep pattern	Falls asleep in class, listless, tardy, poor attention in class
Loss of energy	Tired or restless behavior
Blaming self inappropriately	Self-critical, cries quickly, upset by surprises or changes
Negative feelings of self-worth	Critical of others, socially withdrawn, doesn't stand up for herself/himself
Feelings of sadness, hopelessness, and worry	Sad, unhappy, feels defeated, withdrawn, acts frightened, poor peer relationships
Morbid thoughts	Talks or writes about death, overreacts to someone's death
Aggressive or negative behavior	Picks on others, talks back, easily frustrated
Increased agitation	Cannot sit still, short attention span, makes noise, talks under breath
Increased psychosomatic complaints	Frequently complains of headaches, stomachaches, or vague physical symptoms
Decreased academic performance	Drop in grades, poor concentration, messy work area, poor test performance
Poor attention and concentration	Cannot stay on task, frequently interrupts, disruptive behavior, appears not to listen

(CDC 2009). In 2005, 16.9 percent of U.S. high school students reported they had considered attempting suicide during the twelve months preceding the survey (Eaton et al. 2006). Each day, over 1,000 people in this age group attempt suicide. Suicide is the fifth leading cause of death for children 5 to 14 years of age (AACAP 2009). Children and adolescents who commit suicide feel cut off, alienated, and isolated. They truly believe that living is useless and more than they can tolerate.

Although the overall rate of suicide in the United States has remained fairly constant in recent years, the rate of suicide among young children has increased. The numbers might even be higher if the current social stigma against

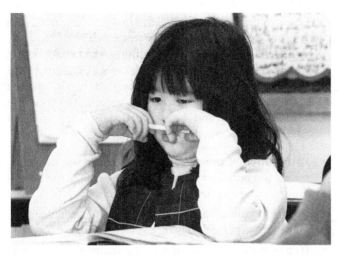

Teachers must be aware of possible depression in children.

suicide did not cause many adolescent suicide cases to go unreported. Adolescents are most likely to commit suicide when they experience overcrowded conditions, a broken family, or feelings of rejection, hopelessness, or loss. Some wish to escape from a difficult situation, gain attention, or punish people who caused them to have negative feelings; therefore, they may view death as an acceptable alternative. Further, an adolescent is at higher risk for suicide if a significant adult role model attempts or commits suicide or if violence is commonplace in the child's environment, either in the home or through the media (DeSpelder and Strickland 1987).

Nelson and Crawford (1991) found that elementary students who experienced thoughts of suicide reported that family problems were significant contributors. Such factors as divorce, separation, and parental alcoholism were the main factors. Peer acceptance and academic pressures also contribute to elementary children's suicide attempts.

Most childhood suicides are preceded by changes in behavior, some subtle and some more overt. Children may lose interest in school and friends, experience an increase of illnesses, become very sad for increasing periods of time, quit eating, or have trouble sleeping. Other observable signs of suicidal behavior include the following:

- Saying such things as, "I wish I were dead," or "I'd be better off dead"
- Giving away prized objects
- Lacking direction or goal-setting behavior
- Exhibiting depression, withdrawal, weight loss, or apathy
- Showing a sudden lack of academic progress
- Communicating feelings of hopelessness
- Using drugs and alcohol
- Withdrawing from friends, family, and normal activities
- Undergoing a radical personality change

- Exhibiting violent, hostile, or rebellious behavior
- Revealing a preoccupation with death through a school composition
- Cutting and other types of self-mutilation
- Running away from home

Other signs could probably be added to this list. Every teacher must be cognizant of these signs and symptoms if suicide is to be prevented. It is imperative that children suspected of suicidal thoughts receive help from professionals trained to deal with the situation.

Latchkey Children

The term **latchkey child** describes any child who is regularly left without direct adult supervision before or after school. Indications are that over seven million children under age 13 are either left to go to school or return home without adult supervision. These situations may result from both parents working or from divorce. The end result is that many children leave home without breakfast or return home to care for themselves, with the possible consequences of fear of someone breaking into their home, fear of being alone, fear of older siblings, and greater likelihood of being lonely and bored (Stroher 1986). Fear and boredom can lead to involvement with gangs or to a greater chance of trouble resulting from the lack of adult supervision. Undersupervised children may experience significantly more personality problems and a higher incidence of depression in adolescence and adulthood (Page and Page 2006).

Obviously, latchkey children are expected to assume a great deal of responsibility for their own welfare. Stroher (1986, 16) has suggested that teachers can help latchkey children by carefully structuring homework assignments because these children do not have adults around to help them complete assignments correctly. Consider the possibility of establishing a telephone hotline to help students with homework. During the school day, allow time for children to discuss their personal concerns with the teacher. Latchkey children particularly need time to discuss or talk with adults. Also establish streamlined, workable procedures for contacting the parents in emergency situations involving the child, and develop both before- and after-school day care programs. Children do better with continuous adult supervision in school-based programs than when left to their own resources.

Divorce and Separation: The Effects on Children

More than half the children in the United States will spend some portion of their childhood in a single-parent situation. Almost one million divorces occur each year; over 49 percent of second marriages result in divorce. In 2010,

12 percent of children lived only with their mothers, and 2 percent lived only with their fathers (U.S. Department of Health and Human Services 2010). The net result is that teachers are having to deal with more emotional/psychological problems than ever before. These problems are represented by delinquency, psychological disturbance, hostility, low self-esteem, low evaluation of the family, and poor self-restraint and social adjustment.

The reactions of children may depend on age. Preschoolers may become frightened about separation or divorce because they see themselves as being abandoned. A child of this age may not want to attend or may fear attending school. Such children may regress in their behavior, with lapses in toilet training or their ability to dress themselves (Ricci 1982). They may use dolls, teddy bears, and blankets as security objects. Among children six to eight years of age, the most common feeling is sadness. This is manifested through crying, sobbing, and a desire to be with the missing parent. Children nine to twelve years of age are likely to respond with vigorous activity. Older children may align themselves with one parent and want little or nothing to do with the other parent (Wallerstein and Kelly 1981). School-aged children may blame themselves for causing the divorce. Parents' ongoing commitment to the child's well-being is vital. Children do best if they understand that their mother and father will still be their parents and remain involved with them even though the marriage is ending. Long custody fights and pressure to choose one parent over the other only add to the damage the child suffers as a result of divorce. Psychotherapy for the children and divorcing parents can be helpful to all concerned (AACAP 1999b).

The teacher may be the one source of stability and security the child has in a divorce or separation. This can be emphasized by the fact that "only 45 percent of children do well after divorce; 41 percent are doing poorly, worried, underachieving, self-deprecating, and often angry; and 14 percent are strikingly uneven [in their emotional functioning]. Girls consistently adjust better to divorce than boys, both socially and academically. This would imply that boys may be suffering more from the absence of their fathers" (Stepfamily Foundation 2003). The teacher may be able to assure such children that the separation/divorce was not their fault and that they are still loved, and help them discuss their feelings of fear, anger, and guilt. Encourage the child to be honest about his or her feelings. In addition, be watchful for signs of academic failure, overaggressiveness, lack of concentration, nervousness, or becoming isolated from peers, which may require informing the parent or the school counselor.

Bullying and Student Health

Bullying is repeatedly carrying out an act or verbalizing an action to attempt to dominate or intimidate another person. This is a type of abuse that can take the form of emotional, verbal, and physical acts. Bullying is a widespread and serious problem that can happen anywhere, in any school and in any grade. It is an occurrence that is increasingly being recognized in our school culture. Most children and teenagers have experienced some form of bullying. It is not a phase children have to go through, it is not "kidding around," and it is not something to grow out of. Bullying can cause serious and lasting harm. Bullying involves (Department of Human Resources 2011):

- **Imbalance of power**: people who bully use their power to control or harm, and the people being bullied may have a hard time defending themselves
- **Intent to cause harm**: actions done by accident are not bullying; the person bullying has a goal to cause harm
- **Repetition**: incidents of bullying happen to the same person over and over by the same person or group

Bullying can take many forms. **Verbal bullying** can include name-calling and teasing. **Social bullying** involves spreading rumors, leaving people out on purpose, and breaking up friendships. **Physical bullying** can escalate to hitting, punching, and shoving. A more recent addition to the bullying sphere is **cyber bullying**. Cyber bullies use the Internet, mobile phones, or other digital technologies to intimidate and harm others. See the Health Highlight: Cyber Bullying for a more in-depth examination of this phenomenon.

Bullying has consequences for all who are involved in the act. The act of bullying, being bullied, and witnessing the actual act of bullying all can have serious and lasting effects. Those who are bullied face higher risks of depression and anxiety and increased thoughts of suicide (these can persist into their adult lives); decreased academic achievement (GPA and standardized test scores) and school participation; greater likeliness to skip or drop out of school; and greater likeliness to retaliate through extremely violent measures. In twelve of fifteen school shootings in the 1990s, it's been determined that the shooter had a history of being bullied. Bullies have higher risks of abusing alcohol and/or drugs in adolescence and as adults and are more likely to engage in early sexual activity than those who do not bully. As adults, they are also more likely to have criminal convictions and traffic citations, and to be abusive toward their romantic partners, spouses, or children. Those who witness bullying tend to have increased use of tobacco, alcohol, or other drugs, increased likelihood of mental health problems (including depression and anxiety), and are more likely to miss or skip school.

When dealing with bullying, the self-esteem of the student seems to play a significant role. Students with higher self-esteem have an easier time handling conflict and resisting the negative pressures involved with bullying, having better abilities to ward off and deal with those who are cruel or mean natured. Further, they seem to smile more readily, enjoy life, are realistic, and generally more optimistic than those who have low self-esteem. Contrasting these characteristic with students with low self-esteem, the low self-esteem student finds it more difficult to deal with major anxiety and frustration, thus

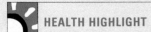 **HEALTH HIGHLIGHT** | **Cyber Bullying**

Cyber bullying is using technology (the Internet, interactive and digital technologies, PDAs or mobile phones) to harass or bully another person. A cyber bully uses cruel or embarrassing rumors, threats, harassment, or stalking to intimidate their target. The pressures of cyber bullying have led some students to commit or attempt suicide. It is very difficult to trace a cyber bully.

Statistics

- 42 percent of kids have been bullied while online
- 35 percent of kids have been threatened online
- 58 percent of kids admit someone has said mean or hurtful things to them online

- 53 percent of kids admit having said something mean/hurtful online to another person
- 58 percent have not told their parents or adult about something mean or hurtful said to them online

Types of Cyber Bullying

Direct attacks: Messages are sent directly to the victim. Examples include instant messaging and text messaging; stealing passwords to access online profiles; posting to blogs or websites; sending pictures, pornography, or other junk messages via e-mail or cell phones, and impersonation in an online environment.

Cyber bullying by proxy: Using others to help cyber bully the victim. Bullying by proxy can be done without the knowledge of the accomplice or in a way that causes a group to bully the victim. The proxy may access the victim's online accounts or may change passwords so the victim cannot access their own accounts without the knowledge that it is done with the intention of bullying.

The cyber bully may pose as the victim on hate group chat rooms, post on child molester sites, or advertise for sex on behalf of the victim. The cyber bully will then wait for friends or others to attack the victim online or offline.

---

finding it difficult to deal with the tactics of a bully. The student lacking self-esteem buys into the tactics and actions of the bully. Those who think poorly of themselves and find themselves being bullied may become passive, withdrawn, or depressed. Students with low self-esteem see temporary setbacks as permanent and intolerable, and will have difficulty using appropriate coping mechanisms in response to bullying tactics.

Death and Children

In today's society, most children do not directly experience the trauma of death. The concept of death is alien to many children. Most children develop a sequence of understanding concerning death, beginning with total unawareness in early childhood to a developmental point in which death is conceptualized as final and universal (Fredlund 1984). For many children, initial contact with death may occur when a pet dies. Children feel significant pain and need extra support to deal with their feelings of loss and grief, even for the death of a pet. (The effects of death on children and adolescents are discussed in greater detail in Chapter 23.)

Rules for Developing and Maintaining Mental Health

Children should be encouraged to practice positive mental health habits in the same way they are taught to practice sound personal health habits. Just as children can take responsibility

for their own physical well-being by following health "rules," they can also foster high levels of emotional well-being by following similar mental health "rules." By internalizing certain guidelines and incorporating them into daily living, each individual can promote good mental health and effective life adjustment. Positive mental health can be taught each day of every school year. Teachers must realize that they are directly responsible for establishing the emotional tone of their classrooms, as well as the foundation of students' self-worth. When each child leaves elementary school, she or he needs to have developed positive self-esteem and perceptions of living.

The Role of the Teacher in Promoting Mental Health

There are many other ways in which the teacher can promote positive emotional characteristics. Each child should be treated as a unique individual. It is important for the teacher to offer personal observations or words of praise that let a child know he or she is performing well or progressing well on a given task. Encourage children to hone their individual talents by providing opportunities for them to do so during the normal course of classroom activity. The chance to work on a special project of personal interest or to contribute ideas and opinions without being ridiculed or rejected may enhance autonomy and initiative. Learning experiences that both challenge and provide success will reinforce children's feelings of competency and mastery.

HEALTH HIGHLIGHT | **Fostering a Positive Classroom Atmosphere**

Here are several guidelines developed by Page and Page (2003) for fostering an emotional climate conducive to mental wellness.

1. Quickly learn the names of students, call them by name, become familiar with their interests and talents, and show respect for each student.
2. Be prepared and enthusiastic. Make learning fun and subject matter relevant and challenging to students.
3. Begin each class promptly. Develop and maintain routines for taking attendance, opening class, and so on.
4. Remember the three Fs of good discipline: *firm*, *fair*, and *friendly*.
5. Expect no problems—don't be looking for them. Expect students to be competent, capable, and eager to learn. It is better to be proven wrong than to have students live up to negative expectations.
6. When problems arise, handle them immediately and consistently before they escalate into larger ones. Don't use "major artillery" for minor infractions.
7. Avoid sarcasm, ridicule, and belittling remarks, and help students to do likewise.
8. Avoid all suggestions of criticism, anger, or frustration. It is better to make personal corrections in private conferences with students.
9. Be alert for indications of latent skills and interests in students and encourage them in their development.
10. Listen nonjudgmentally to student comments, and create an atmosphere in which students feel at ease.
11. Arrange for a high ratio of successes to failures in academic tasks.
12. Involve students in the setting of individual academic goals.
13. Avoid encouraging competitiveness between students in your grading practices and learning activities.
14. Demonstrate the characteristics of effective teachers: warmth, friendliness, fairness, a good sense of humor, enthusiasm, empathy, openness, spontaneity, adaptability, and a governing style that is more democratic than autocratic.

Teachers can provide activities that help students consider how they want to live their lives and what their goals should be. For example, a teacher can ask students to write down what they hope to accomplish in the near and in the distant future and then help students develop ways of achieving these goals. This method of clarifying important goals will help students keep minor problems in perspective (Olsen, Redican, and Baffi 1986). Furthermore, teachers need to help students place their inability to meet goals in the proper perspective, so that feelings of doubt, embarrassment, or inadequacy do not result.

It is important for a teacher to become an effective listener and a skilled observer. Children regularly need opportunities that let them express their feelings and thoughts openly. A teacher can become an active listener by paraphrasing the student's comments to let the child know the message was understood. Such active listening will demonstrate to children that the teacher genuinely cares about them.

The role of the teacher in promoting student mental health is crucial. The attitudes teachers demonstrate during their daily interactions with students affect the emotional climate of the classroom. One of the best things a teacher can do to promote emotional health in students is to help them learn to accept responsibility for their own behavior. A common mistake we all make is to try to shift the blame for something we did onto someone else. Students must be taught that a crucial element of emotional development is the ability to accept responsibility and live with mistakes. Further, the type of rapport that is established between teacher and student conveys many messages that influence children's perceptions about acceptance, trust, support, self-esteem, competency, and independence. See the Health Highlight box above for more suggestions on how to foster an emotional climate conducive to mental wellness.

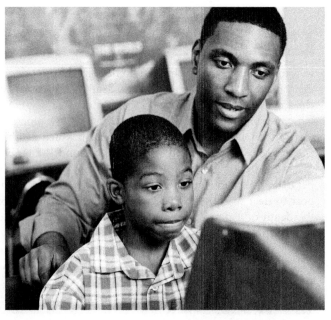

The teacher plays an important role in establishing a positive classroom atmosphere.

The Role of the Family in Developing Emotional Health

An individual's emotional health status can be gauged by assessing how much the basic emotional needs for love, acceptance, and support from others contribute to the individual's feelings of self-worth. It is helpful also to determine the degree of balance with which behaviors are expressed and the ways in which people face and resolve situations through decisions that are compatible with personal values. All these foundations of positive mental health are first learned and cultivated within the family. As a result, it is crucial that all teachers have some notion of how family structure, interaction, and values influence the behavior and attitudes of students in the classroom.

Single-parent families may greatly affect a child's view of self as well as the world in general. Some children also face the task of having to be incorporated into two different family structures that produce different sets of stepparents and stepsiblings. Teachers must be sensitive to these differences in living arrangements and family structure.

Family interaction also contributes greatly to the development of children's mental health. Communication patterns between parents, parents and their children, and between siblings are all important factors. Communication should allow for intimacy—that is, sharing of one's innermost fears and concerns—without reprisal or rejection. Interaction patterns between family members set the tone for all other social interaction. Within the family, children develop a sense about what they can do or accomplish, what their roles in life should be, and what types of behaviors are appropriate, acceptable, and desirable. Criteria for sharing, completing expected tasks, being praised or punished, and many other things are learned through family modeling and values. The family sets guidelines for all behavior by means ranging from types of discipline to ways of expressing love and affection. As a result, attitudes, habits, and emotions reflect family attitudes, habits, and emotions.

Stress and Its Relationship to Mental Health

Because of its influence on behavior and the expression of emotions that may result, the topic of stress should be included in any discussion of mental health. Everyone, young and old, is exposed to daily stress that must be accommodated to ensure emotional stability. Therefore, people of all ages must realize that many situations produce feelings of anxiety or apprehension that cause the same fluctuation in levels of mental wellness as those experienced in physical wellness. The key is to learn to reduce anxiety and tension as they arise so that levels of stress are more easily managed.

Stress is the nonspecific response of the body to an unanticipated or stimulating event. Stress can accompany a pleasant or an unpleasant event. Hans Selye has described stress resulting from a pleasant event as **eustress**. This type of stress comes from events, such as getting something new or being selected as a class officer. Although anxiety is produced, this type of stress helps us be more effective in physical, social, and psychological functioning. **Distress** is stress generated from a negative or unpleasant event. Prolonged distress can have a negative or debilitative effect on health. Unchecked distress interferes with physiological and psychological functioning (Selye 1975).

Anything that elicits a stress response is called a stressor. A stressor can be an event or situation. What one person may perceive as stress may not be stressful to someone else. For example, skydiving would be terrifying for many people, yet other people may view it as a relaxing recreational activity. Possible sources of stress in children include the following:

- Death of a parent or grandparent
- Death of a brother or sister
- Marital separation of parents
- Divorce of parents
- Hospitalization of a parent
- Remarriage of a parent to a stepparent
- Birth of a brother or sister
- Loss of job by father or mother
- Moving to a new city

It is both impossible and undesirable to live in a stress-free environment. Stress cannot be totally avoided. From a positive perspective, stress can enhance ability, act as a motivator, and be a means of self-protection. Unfortunately many children live in highly stressful situations. Factors such as poverty, crowding, and exposure to drugs, abuse, and violence can all contribute to stress.

▪ The General Adaptation Syndrome

Any event or circumstance that upsets the body's physiological balance is a stressor. The body is constantly striving to maintain a physiological balance, or **homeostasis**. Regardless of the type of stress that occurs, eustress or distress, when an individual perceives a stressor, the body automatically responds with a three-stage process known as the **general adaptation syndrome (GAS)** (Selye 1975), shown in Figure 6.2.

The first phase of the general adaptation syndrome is referred to as the *alarm phase*. The brain interprets an event or situation as a stressor and immediately prepares the body to deal with it. Sometimes this initial response is called the fight-or-flight syndrome because the body literally reacts as if it is either going to stand and fight or run away. The emotional response causes physical reactions such as muscle tenseness, increased heart rate, dry mouth,

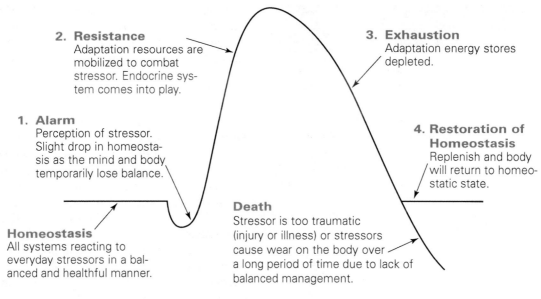

Figure 6.2
The General Adaptation Syndrome

or sweaty palms. The second stage of the GAS is *resistance*. During this phase the perceived stressor is dealt with through increased strength and sensory capacity. Only after meeting the demands of the stressful event can the body return to normal.

When stress is chronic, sufficiently pervasive, or traumatic enough, the third stage of *exhaustion* is reached. At this point the body must restore itself and rest or serious health problems are potentially possible. Adverse effects of mismanaged or long-term stress include heart problems, stomach problems, high blood pressure, and/or achy muscles and joints.

All the stages in the GAS are the result of chemical messages in the form of hormones. For example, during the alarm phase the pituitary gland releases a hormone (adrenocorticotropic hormone, or ACTH) that stimulates other endocrine glands to also release hormones, resulting in the fight-or-flight response. Hormonal messages cause an increase in blood volume and blood pressure. The hormones epinephrine and norepinephrine initiate a variety of physiological responses, including increased heart rate and increased metabolic rate. They also stimulate the release of other hormones called **endorphins**, which serve to diminish pain.

Obviously, the continual hormonal stimulation caused by chronic stress doesn't let the body return to homeostasis. Fortunately, the effects of most stressors can be partially or completely reversed with adequate stress management techniques. Early use of these techniques can reduce the adverse effects of stress.

▪ Effects of Chronic Stress

Chronic stress can cause problems in several areas of a child's life. Psychosomatic illnesses, such as headaches and physical injuries, may result from an abnormal response to stress. A child may withdraw emotionally from other people and experience feelings of worthlessness, apathy, loneliness, anger, hostility, and low self-esteem. Behavior problems such as hyperactivity, accident susceptibility, truancy, substance abuse, and low academic achievement may also result from stress. Low self-esteem and anxiety may lead to a lack of concentration and a disrupted capacity to process information (Jones 1985).

Other behaviors that could indicate that children are under too much stress include the following:

- Frequent headaches
- Sighing
- Diarrhea/constipation
- Nausea
- Faintness
- Hair twirling
- Clenched fists
- Nervous cough
- Fast or excessive talking
- Fingernail biting
- Back-and-forth rocking
- Depression
- Anger
- Continual boredom
- Lip biting
- Crying
- Proneness to errors
- Nightmares
- Persistent (compulsive) itching

▪ Dealing with Stress

It is important to determine which sources of stress arise from intrinsic stimuli, such as being inwardly driven to reach a goal, and which sources of stress arise from extrinsic stimuli, such as pressure from a teacher to turn in a homework assignment, parental separation, or death of a grandparent. It is also beneficial to attempt to determine whether the source is regular, routine, or consistent, as in the case of a daily conflict or being self-conscious with peers. Sources of stress that are regular, routine, or consistent generally have a greater potential for creating long-term negative effects because they wear on the individual constantly and may therefore demand more time to resolve. Sudden, isolated sources of stress tend to be crisis situations that first require a return to some degree of normalcy and may later involve a more lengthy process of conflict resolution.

Putting the stress-producing situation in realistic perspective is helpful in objectively evaluating its impact. To do this, the teacher should help the student mentally classify events as they arise and decide which situations can be personally handled after careful consideration of the possible alternatives. Those events involving either deeper inner conflict or interaction with others may require the assistance of a third party or outside expert. After putting the cause of the stress into perspective and outlining possible courses of action, students should be helped to select the course of action that seems likely to produce the most healthful, positive, or desirable results. The student should then be aided in carrying out the course of action and evaluating its effectiveness to determine whether similar courses of action should be repeated for similar circumstances or whether modifications need to be considered.

> **Creativity in the Classroom**
>
> Demonstrate for students what different types of *stress* can do. *Stress* on a pencil causes it to break. *Stress* on a spoon causes it to bend. Relate this to the influence of *stress* on their own health and well-being.

■ Stress Management in Children

Stress management and stress reduction skills can help children cope with life's stresses and increase their potential for reaching and maintaining high levels of emotional health throughout life. There are a variety of healthful ways to reduce the adverse effects of stress. Examples include exercise, relaxation techniques, and deep-breathing exercises. Some children can use hobbies, arts and crafts, and reading activities as alternative forms of stress reduction.

Exercise. One of the most natural methods of relieving stress is exercise. Aerobic exercise activates hormones, fatigues tense muscles, and allows the stressed student to attain a pleasantly tired but relaxed state. Activities such as walking, jogging, cycling, and swimming all directly reduce adverse symptoms of stress.

Relaxation Techniques. Several kinds of relaxation techniques may be used to combat the ill effects associated with stress. These techniques include, but are not limited to, progressive relaxation, meditation, and creative visualization. A child who is able to relax under very trying circumstances will experience fewer of the physical symptoms associated with poor stress management.

Progressive relaxation is one method that is especially useful for children. Progressive relaxation requires a quiet room and the space to assume a comfortable position. Instructions can be given on an audiotape or verbally by a teacher/facilitator in a classroom situation.

The key to progressive relaxation is to tense each muscle group as the command is given (typically for about ten to fifteen seconds); then when the signal is given, relax that muscle group immediately and completely (for approximately ten to fifteen seconds). This is a procedure that needs to be practiced, but once the method is learned, it can certainly help to reduce stress.

Deep-breathing exercises are very similar to natural relaxation. In fact, deep breathing uses the body's natural relaxation response. Students can be reminded that they often use deep breathing (sighing) when under stress without being aware of it. Deep-breathing exercises done in regular patterns can further help the student relax when experiencing stress.

Meditation can be approached from several perspectives. The purpose of the technique is to help the student temporarily "tune out" the world while evoking the relaxation response. During a meditation session, a word or phrase is concentrated on to help eliminate all outside distractions. While in a comfortable position the participant breathes deeply, slowly inhaling and exhaling. The participants focus on the word or phrase with each breath. This format can best be learned from an instructor or tape that can provide instruction.

Visualization (creative imagery) is a form of relaxation that makes use of the imagination. This is an excellent method to teach students. To use this technique, a comfortable position is assumed, the eyes are closed, and several deep breaths are taken. There are several variations of visualization. For example, a tranquil scene such as a beach or forest can serve as the focal point for the visualization. Visualization can be used to envision a goal or behavior change. There are a variety of tapes available that can aid the teaching of this technique.

Biofeedback is based on scientific principles designed to enhance awareness of body functioning. Sensory equipment is used to create awareness of subtle body changes such as increases or decreases in body temperature, muscle contractions, or brain wave variations. As people become more sensitive to fluctuations in functioning, they can learn to evoke the relaxation response by countering their automatic stress response as it occurs. A few sessions are usually required to recognize differences and then alter physiological responses. Equipment for biofeedback ranges from relatively inexpensive to quite costly.

Other Relaxation Techniques. Other techniques that require no special equipment or training but serve to help dissipate stress symptoms are humor, music, and effective time management.

Laughing is a powerful stress-reducing agent. Laughing or humor helps us to keep things in perspective, maintain a positive attitude, and realize that life is seldom perfect. It has been found that blood pressure and heart rate can actually decrease after a good laugh. Laughing or even smiling are excellent ways to alter a negative mood. Certainly one of the things that can be promoted in a healthy classroom environment is laughter. The laughter should not be based on racial or ethnic factors or at the expense of a student, but rather based on the funny things that occur during the school day.

Quiet music serves to soothe the autonomic nervous system by easing tensions and lessening strong emotions. It is difficult to invoke the relaxation response if the music is inappropriate or irritating to the listener. Classical music affords exposure to the artistic beauty of life as well as evoking the relaxation response.

A perceived or actual lack of time is a major contributor to the stress response. In children, effective time management can be fostered by helping them to establish goals and priorities in their daily lives. By learning effective time management at an early age, children can eliminate a great deal of stress as they mature. Some suggestions for effective time management include teaching children not to procrastinate, to set realistic goals, to establish priorities and write them down, to learn to say no when necessary, to build in relaxation time every day, and to visualize themselves completing their priorities.

The Role of Effective Communication in Reducing Stress

People often experience a tremendous amount of stress when they feel that others are controlling their lives. Anxiety results when a person feels exploited, humiliated, and/or a lack of respect. This anxiety and the accompanying stress can be reduced through a change in attitude toward oneself and through the use of effective communication skills.

Many times stress will result from children's inability to express feelings to others honestly. Individuals often refuse to express their feelings to others because they want to avoid confrontation or because they do not feel as important as the other person is. Some children do not wish to hurt anyone's feelings, yet this type of passive behavior causes a child to think less of himself and to be angry at the other person. Such a lack of respect for self increases stress because the person tends to store the anger internally. Conversely, aggressive behavior, in which a person physically abuses, insults, or criticizes the other person, can ruin relationships and thus increase stress.

Assertive communication—the type that communicates a respect for self as well as the other person—permits individuals to stand up for their rights without ignoring the rights of others. An important part of assertive behavior is a healthy self-concept in which people believe they are worthy individuals and capable of having their own feelings and beliefs. It also implies that people have a right to speak up if they have been treated unfairly, and they have a right to say no. Assertiveness involves making "I" statements; for example, "I feel" and "I think," which imply that a person takes full responsibility for his or her feelings. Assertive people are able to clearly and confidently say no and tell others what they think and feel without hurting others or putting them down. Teachers can help children learn how to communicate and be good listeners. Children can learn to speak with positive verbal and body language and be polite. Such communication is very effective in improving self-image and relationships with others and in dealing with stress.

Emotionally intimate communication with others also helps lessen the effects of life's stressors. This type of communication is more than just discussing the weather or other superficial topics. Teachers can facilitate such communication by allowing children to share their innermost feelings. Children should not be afraid to share their feelings with others for fear of being rejected. If a child bares his or her soul to the teacher, the teacher must sympathize with the situation and provide emotional support. If the teacher demonstrates through words or behavior an unwillingness to give emotional support, anxiety, loneliness, and rejection can result. However, if children learn they are safe in sharing their intimacies, teacher–child relationships can become much stronger. Such intimate relationships add greatly to the child's quality of life, whereas the lack of such relationships contributes to discontentment, anxiety, and stress.

Chapter In Review

Summary

- The characteristics of the emotionally healthy child include positive self-esteem, a positive sense of self-worth, a concern for others, the ability to develop meaningful relationships, and the ability to make decisions.

- Unexpressed emotions can lead to frustration, hostility, and resentment.

- Mechanisms used to deal with feelings include compensation, daydreaming, idealization, projection, rationalization, regression, and sublimation.

- Depression is the most frequently occurring emotional disorder and is a symptom of underlying conflict or tension.

- Depression can be the result of heredity, personal background, personality, biochemical factors, or physical illness.

- Depression can be a major cause of adolescent suicide.

- Students should be helped to like themselves, be good to themselves, accept their personal limitations, deal with their problems, establish realistic goals, express emotions properly, develop their sense of humor, and cultivate an optimistic attitude.

- Teachers must recognize the impact of familial socializations on the child entering the classroom and attempt to relate equally and objectively to children from diverse backgrounds and living arrangements.

- Students with special emotional health needs include the latchkey child; children of separation, divorce, or single parents; or a child experiencing loss in the form of death of a parent, grandparent, sibling, or pet.

- How students relate to emotional situations and crisis tends to depend on their age.

- Bullying is a significant problem in schools.

- Teachers need to listen and show their acceptance, support, encouragement, and concern for all children, especially for those experiencing special situations or crises.

- Stress is defined as the body's physical and/or psychological response to an unanticipated event.

- Stress can be pleasant (eustress) or unpleasant (distress); prolonged distress has a debilitating health effect.

- Anything that causes stress is called a *stressor*.

- The body goes through three stages (collectively called the general adaptation syndrome) in response to a stressful event—alarm, resistance, and exhaustion.

- Students can be taught techniques for dealing with stress, such as exercising, deep breathing, meditation, visualization, biofeedback, humor, and effective time management.

- Learning effective communication patterns is one of the best methods of protecting against negative stressful responses.

Discussion Questions

1. Identify the characteristics of good emotional health.
2. Why is self-esteem so important in the development of mental health?
3. How can the teacher enhance self-esteem in the classroom?
4. What are some major concerns for severe psychiatric disorders in children?
5. Describe obsessive-compulsive disorder.
6. What can be some long-term consequences of panic attacks?
7. What are some possible signs of depression in children?
8. What is the general adaptation syndrome (GAS)?
9. What is the difference between eustress and distress?
10. How can good decision-making skills help the child deal with distress?
11. What should teachers strive to teach students to promote emotional health?
12. What are the implications of divorce for children?
13. What potential problems may arise for latchkey children?

Critical Thinking Questions

1. It has been said, "Our histories form our perceptions, which are realities of how we perceive life." What are some reasons that one's perceptions may not be accurate?

2. Think about fostering a classroom that promotes optimum opportunity to facilitate learning and promotes the health and welfare of the student. Develop a written statement that reflects your basic beliefs about what type of atmosphere must exist and teacher attributes that would be conducive to facilitation of your philosophy.

3. Develop a statement regarding bullying that would provide guidelines for schools and teachers to follow if they observed or become aware of bullying of any form.

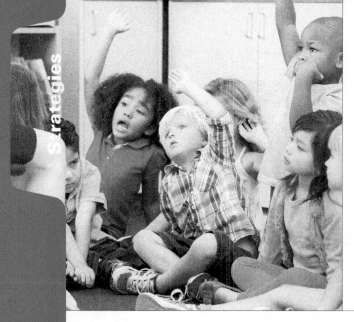

Strategies for Teaching Mental Health and Stress Reduction

We are nothing more than a product of the decisions we choose to make.

—*Author Unknown*

NATIONAL HEALTH EDUCATION STANDARDS

1. Students will comprehend concepts related to health promotion and disease prevention to enhance health.

2. Students will analyze the influence of family, peers, culture, media, technology, and other factors on health behaviors.

3. Students will demonstrate the ability to access valid information and products and services to enhance health.

4. Students will demonstrate the ability to use interpersonal communication skills to enhance health and avoid or reduce health risks.

5. Students will demonstrate the ability to use decision-making skills to enhance health.

6. Students will demonstrate the ability to use goal-setting skills to enhance health.

7. Students will demonstrate the ability to practice health-enhancing behaviors and avoid or reduce risks.

8. Students will demonstrate the ability to advocate for personal, family, and community health.

Valued Outcomes

After completion of this chapter, you should be able to:

- Realize every person is unique and special with many good qualities.

- Understand that all people share basic human needs for physical safety, love, security, emotional support, and acceptance from others.

- Discuss how personality development is affected by one's self-concept and acceptance from others.

- Develop strategies that illustrate the expression of emotions in mentally and emotionally healthy ways.

- Discuss why open and honest communication is an essential part of good mental health.

- Develop and utilize strategies to identify stressors and effectively deal with stressful situations.

- Help students learn personal responsibility in their conduct and interactions with others.

Reflections

As you review the activities in this chapter, select a strategy for grades K through 8 from the text or develop a new strategy that would demonstrate a personalization of the topic chosen. Be prepared to discuss how your strategies at each grade level would enhance the conceptualization of the topic at each grade level.

Mental Health: An Integral Part of Life

Mental health is a very significant part of our overall health. Sometimes our mental health is more difficult to maintain than our physical health is. As teachers, we can enhance our students' mental health through the ways in which we interact with them. An open, accepting demeanor on the part of the teacher in a classroom can determine the effectiveness of the learning environment. Conversely, a regimented, pressure-filled atmosphere in the classroom will stifle students' creativity and interfere with their ability to learn. One of the most important aspects of mental health that should be taught to elementary students is the acceptance of others. Teachers should emphasize that each individual is unique and that differences among individuals make life more interesting, not more difficult. This concept of uniqueness is especially important to teach when a greater number of special students are mainstreamed into the "normal" classroom.

Another vital lesson to be taught in emotional health is the relationship between freedom and responsibilities. Elementary children struggle with ambivalent feelings toward dependence and independence. Sometimes they get angry when their parents treat them like little children, yet they are reluctant to accept the additional chores and responsibilities that accompany growing older. Students need to understand that growing older can mean greater freedom in that they are allowed to do things younger children cannot do, but with the additional freedom comes the expectation to act prudently and responsibly.

Good relationships with others often begin with a healthy image of ourselves; therefore, a major goal in teaching mental health and stress reduction should be to foster self-esteem in children and to help them understand that in order to love others, they must accept themselves. Healthy self-esteem can enhance effective communication with others, which in turn helps build good relationships and resolve conflicts with family and friends. Further, an important part of a relationship is being able to communicate assertively and listen effectively. Building good mental health must begin in infancy and early childhood. By the time children enter school, their mental health has been strongly influenced by family and peers. But effective learning strategies are also a powerful shaping influence. By helping children build feelings of positive self-esteem, develop good decision-making skills in harmony with their values, and learn to cope with the stressors in life, the teacher can guide children toward emotional well-being.

Shown to the right of each activity in this chapter is the suggested grade level(s) for which the activity might be appropriate. However, many of the suggested activities could be modified for use at various grade levels.

Information Assessment Activities

Information assessment activities are designed to help children develop their critical thinking skills, personalize information, and establish concepts conducive to high-quality wellness. Teachers can design a variety of activities that are value based, depending on the content being discussed. Some suggestions follow.

Special Me
Grades PK–3

Valued Outcome: Students will realize they are special and unique at all stages of their lives.

National Health Education Standards: 1, 2

Description of Strategy: This strategy is designed to help students feel good about themselves and to enhance their self-esteem. Ask students to list five things they are good at or that they have accomplished. Have students draw, color, and label each event or accomplishment. Compile the drawings in a folder and have students decorate the front of the folder (some students may choose to use photographs). Emphasize that everyone has special talents and abilities, with different accomplishments throughout their lifetimes.

Materials Needed: construction paper or colored paper, glue or tape, markers or crayons, folders, photographs (optional)

Processing Questions:

1. What are the things that make you feel good about yourself?
2. What are your talents?
3. How can we help other people feel good about themselves?
4. Should we always believe everything someone says about our performance or actions? Why or why not?

○ **Integration:** Art

✓ **Assessment:** Students can list five things they like about themselves.

Happy or Sad?
Grades PK–3

Valued Outcome: Students will be able to associate the emotions "happy" and "sad" with positive and negative situations.

National Health Education Standards: 1, 4

Description of Strategy: Let each child draw a happy face and a sad face on a paper plate. Attach these to craft sticks. As you give examples of positive and negative situations, students will hold up the face that indicates how they would feel in each situation.

Materials Needed: paper plates, crayons, craft sticks

Processing Questions:

1. Can you give an example of a situation that made you feel happy?
2. Can you give an example of a situation that made you feel sad?
3. Happy and sad are two common emotions. What are some other emotions you have felt today?

○ **Integration:** Art

✓ **Assessment:** Students can correctly associate the emotions "happy" and "sad" with positive and negative situations and can provide their own examples of other positive and negative situations.

Helping Others   Grades K–6

Valued Outcome: Students will realize that they can help others feel good about themselves through encouragement and kindness.

National Health Education Standards: 2, 8

Description of Strategy: Have students work in small groups. Have students share ways that others make them feel good about themselves (compliments, encouraging words, and so on). Following the small-group discussion, ask each group to share their thoughts with the class. Write the class responses on a large sheet of paper. Ask each person in the various small groups to provide a compliment to every person in his or her group. Make sure the comments are sincere and that everyone has nice things said about him or her. Emphasize that in order to feel good about ourselves, it is important to not always think about ourselves, but to encourage others and be kind in our comments to each other.

Materials Needed: markers, butcher paper

Processing Questions:

1. Can we help others feel good about themselves?
2. How do we sometimes make others feel bad about themselves?
3. Why is it important to consider others' feelings and not always our own?

✓ **Assessment:** Students can list five things they can do to help others feel good about themselves.

Looking at Me   Grades 4–6

Valued Outcome: Students will be able to understand that everyone has strengths and weaknesses.

National Health Education Standards: 1, 2, 5, 7

Description of Strategy: Have students make a list of five to ten things that they consider to be their strengths and weaknesses. Compiling a personal list of your own to share

with the class is also helpful. Allow time for discussion and sharing so students will realize that nobody is perfect. Follow up the discussion by having students select a famous person and research what they think are that person's strengths and weaknesses. After reviewing the famous people, ask students to describe how that person could have improved his or her weaknesses. Emphasize that no one is perfect.

Materials Needed: pen or pencil, paper, references on famous people

Processing Questions:

1. What strengths did you identify?
2. What weaknesses did you identify?
3. Does everyone have strengths and weaknesses?
4. Do people who are famous or whom you admire have some weaknesses? What are some examples?
5. Is it okay that we are not always perfect?

✓ **Assessment:** Students can identify weaknesses in themselves and list ways to overcome or deal with what they consider their weaknesses.

Voting Questions   Grades 4–6

Valued Outcome: Students will examine their feelings for the various topics presented.

National Health Education Standards: 2, 5, 8

Description of Strategy: Voting questions are another way to help students establish their feelings on various topics. The teacher can develop a variety of questions that lend themselves to a particular topic. The questions should be read aloud. Ask students to raise their thumbs up if they agree with the question, to point their thumbs down if they disagree, and to fold their arms if they are unsure or undecided. Some examples of potential questions: Do you find it difficult to talk with your parents? Do you feel scared to speak in a large group? Do you have a friend with whom you can discuss problems? Do you wish others would listen to you better?

Materials Needed: teacher- or student-prepared voting questions

Processing Questions:

1. What seem to be the areas that represent the biggest problems?
2. What are some ways we can deal with these problems?

✓ **Assessment:** Students can identify problems and potential solutions for dealing with those problems.

Name Tag Descriptors   Grades 4–6

Valued Outcome: Students will be able to name ways in which they are unique.

National Health Education Standard: 1

| TEACHING IN ACTION | **Daily Lesson Plan** |

Lesson Title: Setting My Sails

Date: January 8, 2012   **Time:** 9:00 a.m.   **Grade:** Four   **Teacher:** Robertson

I. National Health Education Standards

Health Education Standard 6: Students will demonstrate the ability to use goal-setting skills to enhance health.

II. National Health Education Standards Performance Indicator

6.5.1 set a personal health goal and track progress toward its achievement.

III. Valued Outcomes

- Students will explain what goals are and the difference between long- and short-term goals.
- Students will realize that setting realistic goals can help them have higher self-esteem.
- Students will realize the importance of accomplishing goals.

IV. Description of Strategy

1. Explain what goals are, different types of goals that can be made (long- or short-term), and the importance of setting S.M.A.R.T. (specific, measurable, attainable, realistic, time-sensitive) goals.
2. Have students write down two short-term and two long-term goals.
3. Have students list things they need to do in order to accomplish their goals. Let students know that they will be asked in two weeks about what they have done to accomplish their short-term goals.
4. In a couple of weeks, have students write down things they did or did not do to accomplish their goals. Ask students how they felt when they accomplished their goals and when they didn't.
5. Discuss benefits of setting and accomplishing goals. Have students give examples of things that get in the way of accomplishing goals. Discuss how it is okay to not reach every goal they set. Explain that a way we can enhance our mental health is by setting realistic goals.

V. Materials Needed

- Pen/pencil
- Paper

VI. Formative Evaluation

Benchmarks
- Level 1: Student was able to identify different types of goals.
- Level 2: Student was able to identify different types of goals and explain what must be done to accomplish different goals.
- Level 3: Student was able to identify different types of goals. Student was able to explain what must be done to accomplish goals and recognizes roadblocks to achieving goals.
- Level 4: Student was able to identify different types of goals. Student was able to explain what must be done to accomplish goals and recognizes roadblocks to achieving goals. Student was able to describe how accomplishing goals can lead to higher self-esteem.

VII. Points of Emphasis

1. Explain the difference between long-term and short-term goals.
2. Explain the importance of setting realistic goals and keeping focused.
3. Explain how accomplishing goals makes us feel good and not doing so makes us feel bad.

Teacher Evaluation

1. Keep the lesson as taught?   yes _____   no _____

2. What I need to improve _____

3. Next time make sure _____

4. Strengths of lesson _____

☀ TEACHING IN ACTION | **Daily Lesson Plan**

Lesson Title: Coping with Stress

Date: January 16, 2012   **Time:** 10:00 a.m.   **Grade:** Eight   **Teacher:** Stone

I. National Health Education Standards

Health Education Standard 7: Students will demonstrate the ability to practice health-enhancing behaviors and avoid or reduce health risks.

II. National Health Education Standards Performance Indicator

7.8.2 demonstrate healthy practices and behaviors that will maintain or improve the health of self and others.

III. Valued Outcomes

* Students will identify possible sources of stress.
* Students will identify the effects that stress can have.
* Students will identify positive ways to reduce stress.

IV. Description of Strategy

1. Talk with students about sources of stress and the effects of stress on health. Describe what might happen to someone who is under too much stress. Have students list positive and negative ways to reduce stress. Practice some relaxation techniques in class (e.g., deep breathing or visualization) so they can understand what the techniques look and feel like.
2. Divide the class into four groups and assign each group a stressful situation. Ask each group to create a bulletin board that focuses on stress responses to the situation. The board should indicate positive ways to reduce stress in the given situation. Provide various art materials and magazines for students to cut out pictures. Each group will present their bulletin board in class.
3. Discuss how too much stress can lead to poor health. Managing stress takes practice. Explain that properly handling stress can lead to better mental health and decision-making capabilities.
4. Review stress-reduction techniques (e.g., exercise, relaxation, and effective communication) and when they should be used. Tell students that different techniques work for different people.

V. Materials Needed

* Construction paper/magazines/stencils
* Scissors
* Bulletin boards

VI. Formative Evaluation

Benchmarks

* Level 1: Student was able to define stress.
* Level 2: Student was able to define stress and identify possible sources of stress.
* Level 3: Student was able to define stress. Student was able to identify possible sources of stress and describe some stress management techniques.
* Level 4: Student was able to define stress. Student was able to identify possible sources of stress and describe various positive and negative stress management techniques.

VII. Points of Emphasis

1. Explain ways to recognize stress and the different forms in which it can present itself.
2. Explain ways of coping with stress and how different stressors require different coping mechanisms.
3. Explain how effective stress management can improve overall health and well-being.

Teacher Evaluation

1. Keep the lesson as taught?   yes _____   no _____

2. What I need to improve _____

3. Next time make sure _____

4. Strengths of lesson _____

Description of Strategy: Each student should be provided with a piece of paper and crayons. Discuss how each person is unique. Instruct the student to make a name tag with a drawing that shows one of his or her interests. Cut the name tag out and write the child's name on the tag. The class can then guess each person's interests.

Materials Needed: paper or name tags, crayons or colored pencils

Processing Questions:

1. How do the activities we like to do differ?
2. Is it okay that we all like different activities?
3. What are some ways that all of us are alike?
4. What are really important characteristics that we should all have?

✔ **Assessment:** Students can identify at least three ways they are each unique.

Using Technology to Understand Mental Health and Stress   Grades 4–8

Valued Outcome: Students will utilize technology to develop information and present the findings for the selected topic.

National Health Education Standards: 3, 5

Description of Strategy: Each student should select a topic that was discussed in class concerning mental health. Topics could include: learning disabilities, self-esteem, defense mechanisms, obsessive compulsive disorders, depression, stress, suicide, and bullying. Each student should investigate their chosen (or assigned) topic using online resources. These sources should include trusted, reliable web sites like www.nimh.nih.gov. After gathering information, each student should then write an essay about their topic. The essay should cover the facts they have assembled, and also a critical evaluation of how they perceive the topic based on the additional information.

Materials Needed: computers, Internet, word processing program or pencils and paper

Processing Questions:

1. What were the most important facts learned from the investigation?
2. What are the implications of the information for you personally?
3. What information you found did you agree with? Disagree with? Question?

◯ **Integration:** Computer technology, Language arts

✔ **Assessment:** Students will write an essay listing the most important facts of their research and why the information was important/unimportant to them.

Friends Should Be...   Grades 4–8

Valued Outcome: Students will be able to identify characteristics of a good friend.

National Health Education Standards: 1, 2

Description of Strategy: Using the following list, ask each student to rank-order within each grouping the characteristics most important to look for in a friend. Then group students by gender and ask them to decide, by consensus, characteristics that are the most important.

A	B	C
____ Smart	____ Honest	____ Loyal
____ Popular	____ Dependable	____ Conscientious
____ Funny	____ Dedicated	____ Trustworthy
D	**E**	**F**
____ Open	____ Quiet	____ Healthy
____ Discreet	____ Bubbly	____ Happy
____ Closed	____ Talkative	____ Successful

Materials Needed: above list (may be expanded), pencils

Processing Questions:

1. What common characteristics did the various groups identify?
2. Were there differences between the boys' and the girls' choices of important characteristics?
3. What other characteristics would be important to you in a friend?
4. Of the important characteristics identified, do you feel you portray those characteristics?

✔ **Assessment:** Students can list what characteristics they feel are most important in a good friend.

Relationship Collage   Grades 4–8

Valued Outcome: Students will develop insight into the many people who influence their lives.

National Health Education Standards: 2, 3

Description of Strategy: This activity is designed to help students see the influence of relationships they have with peers, family, teachers, coaches, and so on. Have students make a collage of their relationships. A picture of the student should be in the center of a piece of posterboard. Around his or her picture, the student puts other pictures or drawings that represent the many people with whom he or she associates.

Materials Needed: paper, colored pencils, pictures or drawings of students and individuals with whom they interact

Processing Questions:

1. Who are the most important people in your life?
2. What do these people do for you?

3. How do they influence you and your behavior?
4. Are there any negative influences from these people?
5. What can you do about the negative influences?

◯ **Integration:** Art

✓ **Assessment:** Students can identify the people who influence them and describe how those influences can be positive or negative.

The Time of My Life   Grades 7–8

Valued Outcome: Students will be able to identify how they spend the hours of each day.

National Health Education Standard: 1

Description of Strategy: For this activity, have each student draw a circle and divide it into four sections on a piece of paper (Figure 7.1). The circle represents a twenty-four-hour time span, with each quadrant equaling approximately six hours. From the categories shown, ask each student to divide the circle according to the amount of time that he or she thinks should be spent on the following activities: spending time with friends, spending time with family, learning at school, working on homework, and sleeping.

Materials Needed: paper to draw circle (or a prepared form), pencils

Processing Questions:

1. How do you like your time schedule?
2. Is there anything you need to change?
3. Why is how we use our time important?
4. Why do we tend to do those things we like best?

◯ **Integration:** Math

✓ **Assessment:** Students can identify how many hours per day they spend on each activity and can assess whether they think their use of time is effective.

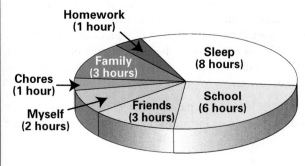

Figure 7.1
Time Circle

Decision Stories

Follow the decision stories procedure (discussed in Chapter 4, pages 60–62) for presenting decision stories such as the following. For each of the decision stories, write a list on the board of ideas generated by the class for how to deal with each situation. Ask the students to discuss the merits of the methods suggested.

✓ **Assessment:** Students can identify health-enhancing behaviors and exhibit positive decision-making skills.

Handling Stress   Grades K–3

José has just invited his friend, Leroy, to play, but Leroy replied, "I don't want to play with you anymore." José feels angry, frustrated, and rejected.

Focus Question: How can José handle the stress caused by this situation?

National Health Education Standards: 5, 7

Where Did I Put Them?   Grades 4–6

Sally is getting ready for school. She cannot remember where she put her shoes. She looked under the bed, under the chair, and behind the door. Sally begins to cry because she thinks she will be late.

Focus Questions: What could have been done to keep Sally from getting upset? What should Sally do now?

National Health Education Standards: 5, 7

I Dare You   Grades 4–6

Ling is new in her neighborhood and wants to make new friends. Jill asks her to take an unsafe dare in order to be accepted by the others in the neighborhood.

Focus Questions: What should Ling do? Is it worth placing yourself at risk to be accepted? How can Ling decide whether she should take a risk to be accepted?

National Health Education Standards: 2, 4, 5, 7

New Girl in School   Grades 4–6

Betty notices that the new student in class is being ridiculed by two of Betty's friends because the new student is the only one in class wearing glasses. They are talking with other girls and writing notes.

Focus Question: What should Betty do?

National Health Education Standards: 5, 8

A Nasty Note   Grades 7–8

Juan was going to the lunchroom when he saw Fred sticking something in Peggy's locker. Later, Juan sees Peggy crying because she found the note, which made fun of her family.

Focus Questions: What should Juan do to help? How does Peggy feel?

National Health Education Standards: 5, 8

Dramatizations

Appropriate Personality Traits   Grades K–3

Valued Outcome: Students will be able to demonstrate healthy ways to react to specific feelings.

National Health Education Standards: 1, 4

Description of Strategy: Have class members role-play the following situations to illustrate healthy personality traits appropriate to the situation.

1. getting a poor grade on a test
2. losing your favorite toy
3. accidentally damaging someone else's property

Processing Questions:

1. Is it okay to get angry? Why or why not?
2. What is one good way to handle anger?
3. Think of a situation in which you got angry. What did you do? How could you have reacted differently?

✔ **Assessment:** Students can identify, suggest, and demonstrate healthy ways to react to negative situations.

Guess My Trait   Grades 4–6

Valued Outcome: Students will be able to express a specific personality trait through role-play.

National Health Education Standards: 1, 2

Description of Strategy: Ask several children to role-play a personality trait that you have whispered to them. One child will act out the personality trait, and the rest of the class will guess the personality trait. Both positive and negative traits can be role-played.

Processing Questions:

1. What is one of your own personality traits?
2. Were all the traits demonstrated in the role-play situations desirable ones?
3. Differentiate between the desirable and the undesirable personality traits.

✔ **Assessment:** Students can differentiate desirable from undesirable personality traits and can name several of their own desirable personality traits.

Truth and Consequences   Grades 4–6

Valued Outcome: Students will observe, discuss, and role-play consequences that result from taking specific actions.

National Health Education Standards: 4, 5

Description of Strategy: Have a small group of volunteer students role-play the following situations and the resulting consequences:

1. A student decides not to do his homework.
2. A man speeds on the highway because he is late.
3. A girl receives a birthday gift and refuses to thank the person she received it from.

Afterward, discuss the following questions: Did the person accept responsibility for his or her actions? What results would occur if he or she had acted differently?

Processing Questions:

1. What are the consequences of not doing your homework?
2. What are the consequences of disobeying laws or rules?
3. What action would you expect the girl who received a birthday gift to demonstrate?

✔ **Assessment:** Students can correlate positive and negative behaviors with positive and negative consequences and demonstrate good decision-making skills by suggesting alternative behaviors to avoid the negative consequences discussed.

Body Language   Grades 4–6

Valued Outcome: Students will be able to express emotions in both verbal and nonverbal ways.

National Health Education Standard: 4

Description of Strategy: Role-play how you can communicate the same thing with or without words. Have students use body language to express an emotion, and then have them verbally demonstrate the same emotion.

Processing Questions:

1. Give an example of a verbal statement to let someone know you care about them.
2. Name a nonverbal way to let someone know you care about them.
3. Give an example of a nonverbal expression of anger.

✔ **Assessment:** Students can identify and demonstrate both verbal and nonverbal expressions of various positive and negative emotions.

Emotional Reactions   Grades 4–8

Valued Outcome: Students will be able to explain how the same emotion can be expressed in different ways.

National Health Education Standard: 4

Description of Strategy: Have students role-play how they would act if they felt good about themselves or if they did not feel good about themselves, for example, after being disciplined in public by parents for inappropriate behavior. Discuss with the class how differently students role-play these emotions.

Processing Questions:

1. Give an example of a wrong way to handle a specific emotion.
2. What might the consequences be of handling an emotion a wrong way?
3. Which way seemed to be the best way of dealing with the emotion and why?

✓ **Assessment:** Students can identify positive ways to deal with negative emotions.

Hidden Messages   Grades 4–8

Valued Outcome: Students will be able to communicate in both verbal and nonverbal ways, identifying advantages and disadvantages to both ways.

National Health Education Standard: 4

Description of Strategy: Have students work in small groups. Ask half the groups to use dialog to present a play that has a hidden message or moral, and ask the remaining groups to present their plays nonverbally. After all groups have finished, ask for identification and interpretation of the messages, and discuss the advantages and disadvantages of verbal and nonverbal communication.

Processing Questions:

1. Name one disadvantage of nonverbal communication.
2. Name one advantage of nonverbal communication.
3. Name one disadvantage of verbal communication.
4. Name one advantage of verbal communication.

✓ **Assessment:** Students can name two advantages and two disadvantages of both verbal and nonverbal communication.

The Decision   Grades 4–8

Valued Outcome: Students will be able to demonstrate ways to handle emotions associated with rejection and family crisis situations.

National Health Education Standards: 2, 4, 5

Description of Strategy: Provide an open-ended hypothetical situation appropriate for the grade level that involves either rejection by a peer group or a family crisis. Then divide the class into three groups. Supply two of the

groups with the ending they will enact. Ask the third group to devise their own scenario. Let each group dramatize its ideas and compare differences. If time and attention allow, provide additional situations and rotate tasks.

Processing Questions:

1. What is one good way to handle rejection?
2. What is one bad way to handle rejection?
3. What is a helpful thing to do in a family crisis?

✓ **Assessment:** Students can identify several positive ways to deal with crises and rejection situations discussed.

Giving and Gaining   Grades 4–8

Valued Outcome: Students will be able to demonstrate an understanding of the necessity for compromise in specific situations.

National Health Education Standards: 4, 5

Description of Strategy: Have several students role-play a situation in which an individual's personal values must be compromised for the good of the group. Examples might include the mayor allowing an individual to make an unpopular speech or a police officer enforcing a law that he or she does not agree with. Follow with a discussion of why the person made the compromise.

Processing Questions:

1. What is a situation in which it would not be good to compromise? Why?
2. Why is compromise necessary in some situations?
3. What might happen if no one ever compromised?

✓ **Assessment:** Students can explain when compromise is and is not appropriate.

Refusal Skills   Grades 4–8

Valued Outcome: Students will be able to identify refusal skills to use when responding to peer pressure.

National Health Education Standards: 2, 4, 5, 7

Description of Strategy: Students will discuss the definition of peer pressure and how peer pressure is used by friends and others to influence their behavior. Specific techniques used by peers and others will be identified: name calling, acceptance, and so on. The teacher will solicit responses regarding the results of using poor judgment and giving in to peer pressure. The following questions will be asked:

- How will you feel about yourself if you use poor judgment?
- What kinds of trouble could you encounter as a result of your actions?
- What physical effects will your action cause?

Explain and cite examples of the following refusal steps:

1. Ask questions.
2. Name the trouble.
3. Identify consequences.
4. Suggest alternatives.
5. Leave.

Have students practice refusal steps in an activity called "The Pressure Seat." Students sit in a circle with one student in the center of the group. The student chooses a peer pressure situation strip from the can. Have the student read the situation aloud, and give him or her one minute to respond to the situation. Then have the group discuss the situation and tell if it agrees or disagrees with the decision made by the student. Have the student in the pressure seat choose another student to take his or her place, and continue until each group member has had a chance to sit in the pressure seat.

Materials Needed: chairs to form a circle, strips of paper listing different peer pressure situations, can

Processing Questions:

1. What are the five refusal steps?
2. What are some things that might occur if you are unable to effectively deal with peer pressure?
3. How did you feel about the decisions you made in the pressure seat?

✓ **Assessment:** Students can name the five refusal skills to use when responding to peer pressure.

Discussion and Report Techniques

Ups and Downs   Grades PK–3

Valued Outcome: Students will be able to identify uplifting emotions and depressing emotions and associate them with specific circumstances.

National Health Education Standards: 1, 4

Description of Strategy: Discuss emotions in terms of "ups" and "downs." What emotions make us feel up or down? Ask volunteers if they are feeling up or down today and what circumstances led to their feeling this way.

Materials Needed: none

Processing Questions:

1. Name two emotions that make you feel "up."
2. Name two emotions that make you feel "down."
3. Give an example of an event that caused you to experience emotions that made you feel "down."

✓ **Assessment:** Students demonstrate awareness of their own uplifting and depressing emotions and are able to identify circumstances that influence their emotions.

Emotions and Me   Grades K–3

Valued Outcome: Students will be able to match facial expressions with emotions, identify emotions associated with specific situations, and discuss reasons for having specific feelings.

National Health Education Standards: 1, 4

Description of Strategy: Ask who in the class is happy, sad, or angry, and why. Explain the importance of expressing emotions and understanding behaviors associated with specific emotions. Give students a worksheet showing different faces with different expressions (see Worksheet 7.1 on page 479). The worksheet will ask students to match a word from the top of the sheet with its expression. Help students with this, asking what types of situations made the student feel each emotion.

Materials Needed: worksheet with faces and emotions

Processing Questions:

1. What feelings make us feel good inside?
2. What feelings make us feel bad inside?
3. Why is it important to be able to express your feelings?

✓ **Assessment:** Students can correctly correlate facial expressions and emotions on the worksheet and can suggest situations that match each emotion.

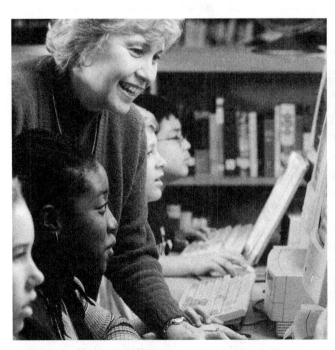

The teacher can do much to foster each student's mental health by reinforcing special talents and allowing expression of feelings.

Caring
Grades K–6

Valued Outcome: Students will be able to discuss ways in which they can help meet the needs of others by caring.

National Health Education Standard: 8

Description of Strategy: Discuss the different needs of a pet dog or cat. When the animal is hungry, we feed it. When it is lonely, we play with it and talk to it. When it is sleeping, we don't disturb it. People have needs that have to be met as well. Discuss how we can help meet the needs of others by caring.

Processing Questions:

1. How could you help meet the needs of a sick parent?
2. How could you help meet the needs of an infant?
3. How could you help meet the needs of a grandparent in a nursing home?

✔ **Assessment:** Students can list ways they can demonstrate care for another person.

Getting to Know You
Grades 4–6

Valued Outcome: Students will be able to describe and discuss various aspects of their personalities.

National Health Education Standard: 1

Description of Strategy: Ask students to print the word *personality* as the heading on a sheet of notebook paper and have them write several phrases that describe their own personalities. Let volunteers share their papers with the class.

Materials Needed: paper, pencils or pens

Processing Questions:

1. What do you think is one of your most important personality traits, and why do you think it is important?
2. What personality trait do you find to be your least desirable?
3. If you could have any personality trait you wanted, what would you choose and why?

✔ **Assessment:** Students can identify several of their own personality traits and discuss personality traits that they might like to change or obtain in the future.

Who Can I Turn To?
Grades 4–6

Valued Outcome: Students will be able to identify sources of help for specific situations.

National Health Education Standards: 3, 4, 5

Description of Strategy: Ask students to think about whom they can talk to when they need advice. Give the class a situation (e.g., "a friend is making fun of you"). Let students decide to whom they would go for help in the situation.

Processing Questions:

1. Whom do you feel you can go to about a problem you are having with peer pressure?
2. Whom do you feel you can go to about a problem you are having with a friend?
3. Whom do you feel you can go to about a family crisis?

✔ **Assessment:** Students can list several appropriate resources they can go to for help in dealing with problems.

We Are Different People
Grades 4–6

Valued Outcome: Students will be able to describe how they behave differently in various relationships.

National Health Education Standard: 2

Description of Strategy: Brainstorm examples of how one person can function in several relationships at one time, such as friend, sibling, child, and student. Emphasize how we behave differently in various relationships.

Processing Questions:

1. What is different about how you express anger at a parent and at a teacher?
2. What is different about the way you express love for a friend and for a sibling?
3. Do you think we hurt the people we care about the most? Why or why not?

✔ **Assessment:** Students can write a brief essay describing how they behave differently in their various relationships.

Picture the Emotion
Grades 4–6

Valued Outcome: Students will be able to identify expressions of emotions.

National Health Education Standards: 1, 2, 4

Description of Strategy: Post photographs on a bulletin board showing a variety of people in different situations and ask students to comment on the emotions being expressed in the photographs, such as happiness, love, sorrow, fear, and anxiety.

Materials Needed: bulletin board, photographs

Processing Questions:

1. What is the most common emotion depicted on the bulletin board?
2. Whose facial expression shows the most pain, and what are the circumstances surrounding this emotion?

3. Whose facial expression shows the most joy, and what are the circumstances surrounding this emotion?

✓ **Assessment:** Students can write a brief essay describing one of the emotions depicted in one of the photographs and identifying related circumstances from the photo that prompt the emotion.

Living by the Rules   Grades 4–6

Valued Outcome: Students will be able to identify reasons for rules.

National Health Education Standard: 7

Description of Strategy: Sometimes it is hard for young children to understand why it is necessary to follow directions or obey rules. Discuss several rules or laws and the reasons for each. For example, a traffic speed limit helps to prevent accidents, injuries, and deaths. It also helps to conserve fuel. Rules for a game help make the activity fair and fun. Discuss what happens when someone doesn't follow the rules of a game.

Processing Questions:

1. Why are traffic laws necessary?
2. Why are rules necessary in games?
3. What are some possible dangers associated with not following parents' rules?

✓ **Assessment:** Students can identify reasons for rules in a variety of health-related situations and can suggest other rules they have experienced and reasons for them.

Cartoon Personalities   Grades 4–6

Valued Outcome: Students will be able to identify personality traits of a cartoon character.

National Health Education Standard: 1

Description of Strategy: The teacher will ask students to determine the personality traits of cartoon characters. The teacher will hold up a picture of a cartoon character and have students describe the character's personality.

Materials Needed: pictures of cartoon characters

Processing Questions:

1. Which cartoon characters had undesirable personality traits, and what are these traits?
2. Which cartoon characters had desirable personality traits, and what are these traits?
3. Do you have any of the same personality traits as the cartoon characters? Which traits?

✓ **Assessment:** Students can identify which cartoon characters are most like them and why.

Who Am I? Stories   Grades 4–6

Valued Outcome: Students will be able to recognize the different and unique qualities of every individual.

National Health Education Standards: 1, 2, 4

Description of Strategy: Have students write a story and make a drawing about themselves. After they have completed the stories and drawings, collect them and read the papers aloud. Have students guess whose paper is being read.

Materials Needed: paper, pencils, crayons or markers

Processing Questions:

1. Name as many favorite animals as you can remember that were mentioned by your classmates.
2. Name as many different hobbies as you can that were mentioned by your classmates.
3. What other interesting qualities were mentioned in your classmates' stories?

◯ **Integration:** Art, Writing

✓ **Assessment:** Students can name positive and unique qualities of their classmates.

Who Am I? Worksheets   Grades 4–6

Valued Outcome: Each student will be able to identify and discuss his or her unique qualities and those of others.

National Health Education Standard: 4

Description of Strategy: Lead a discussion emphasizing the uniqueness of every individual. Students will receive a worksheet to fill out about themselves. The teacher will then read several aloud, and students will guess who they are about.

Materials Needed: "Who Am I?" worksheet (see Worksheet 7.2 on page 480)

Processing Questions:

1. What does it mean to have a unique quality?
2. Will people have some different qualities even if they seem just alike? Explain.
3. What makes each person different?

◯ **Integration:** Writing

✓ **Assessment:** Students can fill out their worksheet describing themselves and discuss the traits of their classmates in a positive way.

State of Mind   Grades 4–6

Valued Outcome: Students will be able to differentiate between positive and negative ways to express emotions.

National Health Education Standard: 4

Description of Strategy: Ask students to share with the class specific times when they felt happy, sad, mad, or some other strong emotion. Ask students to also share how they acted when they felt these emotions. Obtain copies of "Goofus and Gallant®"—the cartoon series that depicts two young boys, one who displays bad behavior and one good, from *Highlights* magazines. Hand them out to the class. Have the class discuss why they think Goofus and Gallant acted as they did. Ask, "What will be the consequences of the good action?" Also call for a discussion of consequences of the bad action.

Materials Needed: the cartoon "Goofus and Gallant®" from *Highlights* magazine

Processing Questions:

1. Why is sharing our emotions with others so important?
2. Give an example of healthy ways to handle anger.
3. Give an example of unhealthy ways to handle anger.

✓ **Assessment:** Students can identify positive and negative ways to express emotions and describe the consequences of each choice.

"Me" Poster   Grades 4–6

Valued Outcome: Each student will be able to identify personal interests, characteristics, relationships, goals, and other important aspects of his or her life.

National Health Education Standards: 2, 4, 6

Description of Strategy: Students will draw, bring in pictures, or write about their lives. They will then place items—possibly including baby pictures, birthday pictures, a list of future goals, family members' pictures, or other important mementos—on a poster to be displayed in the classroom. Set aside class time for the children to tell about their posters.

Materials Needed: glue, scissors, poster boards, essays, drawings, magazines, personal mementos, photographs

Processing Questions:

1. Which things in your life make you feel most proud?
2. What has been the most important event in your life and why?
3. Who are the most important people in your life and why?

○ **Integration:** Writing, Art

✓ **Assessment:** Students can identify three key events, relationships, and goals that are most important to them.

Question Box   Grades 4–8

Valued Outcome: Students will be able to identify personal fears, worries, or dilemmas.

National Health Education Standards: 3, 4

Description of Strategy: Supply a large, colorful box, and encourage students to anonymously submit questions that they want to discuss regarding personal fears, worries, or dilemmas. Set aside about 30 minutes each week to discuss as many of these as possible.

Materials Needed: question box

Processing Questions:

1. What is your worst fear and why?
2. What specific things cause you to worry?
3. Who are some people you could talk to about your worries and fears?

✓ **Assessment:** Students can identify and discuss fears, worries, and dilemmas and name several solutions or resources for dealing with problems.

Steps to the Top   Grades 4–8

Valued Outcome: Students will be able to name qualities or rules for building mental health.

National Health Education Standards: 2, 4, 5

Description of Strategy: Have students trace one of their feet on construction paper. Inside the foot outline, ask each student to write a quality or rule for building mental health. These qualities can include self-love, self-respect, consideration of others, open communication, honesty, practicing what you preach, or sound decision making. Tack the footprints on a bulletin board in ascending steps to good mental health.

Materials Needed: construction paper, scissors, markers or pens, bulletin board

Processing Questions:

1. Explain how your footprint relates to building mental health.
2. Why is it important to have good mental heath?
3. What are some characteristics of poor mental health?

✓ **Assessment:** Students can explain why each of the qualities chosen by their classmates is conducive to good mental health.

Coping with Stress   Grades 4–8

Valued Outcome: Students will be able to identify positive ways to reduce stress.

National Health Education Standard: 7

Description of Strategy: Divide the class into four groups. Ask each group to create a bulletin board that focuses on positive ways to reduce stress. Bulletin boards should be redone each week for a month so that each group's message can be seen and discussed.

Materials Needed: construction paper, scissors, stencils, bulletin board

Processing Questions:

1. Name three positive ways to reduce stress.
2. What might happen to someone who is under too much stress?
3. How often should stress reduction techniques be used and why?

✔ **Assessment:** Students can identify three positive ways to reduce stress and can explain why stress reduction techniques are important.

How to Handle Peer Pressure   Grades 4–8

Valued Outcome: Students will be able to identify positive and negative ways they are influenced by their peers.

National Health Education Standards: 2, 4, 5, 7

Description of Strategy: Solicit responses to the following questions:

1. Name a situation in which you were influenced by your friends in a decision you made.
2. Why do you think friends are able to persuade you to do things you know are wrong?
3. Why is it important to avoid the negative influence of your friends?
4. How can being influenced by your friends be dangerous to yourself and others? Give specific examples.
5. What are some positive ways peers can influence one another?
6. What is unique about you?
7. List four characteristics of your two closest friends.
8. List two physical and two personality characteristics of your two closest friends, and discuss these characteristics.

Emphasize to students the need for accepting who they are and being proud of their decisions.

Processing Questions:

1. Why do we sometimes give in to peer pressure?
2. How is each of us different?
3. What are some dangers of peer pressure?

TEACHING TIP

Have students determine stressful events that occur during the week by keeping a journal. Students should record stressful events and how they coped with the events for one week. This will help them identify the coping mechanisms they are using, and will also allow them to identify their physical and emotional reactions. Let students share their journals with each other and discuss the different ways they reacted.

✔ **Assessment:** Students can name three ways they are influenced by their peers and explain how negative peer pressure can undermine their own unique qualities.

Musical Compliments   Grades 4–8

Valued Outcome: Each student will be able to write positive statements about other students and will describe feelings in response to positive statements made about her or him.

National Health Education Standard: 8

Description of Strategy: Lead a discussion about self-esteem, asking the following questions:

1. How does it make you feel when someone says something nice about you?
2. Do you make it a point to compliment people when they do something good?
3. Do you try to note the good things about a person, even when there are things about them that you dislike?
4. Have you ever thought about your own good qualities and why people like to be around you?

Give each student a piece of paper cut into one of various shapes, such as a child, a musical note, or a heart. Have students write their names on the cutout they receive and pass them around the room while you play music. When the music stops, each child will write something positive about the person whose cutout they receive. Continue this until students have written on several different cutouts. Give students a few minutes to sit quietly and read the comments written about them. Then ask students to write a paragraph telling how this activity made them feel.

Materials Needed: cutouts, markers, music player, music, paper, pens or pencils

Processing Questions:

1. Which comment on your card made you feel particularly special, and why?
2. How did it make you feel to write something nice about someone else?
3. Give an example of a compliment.

○ **Integration:** Writing

✔ **Assessment:** Students' written responses will describe their feelings about the positive statements others made about them. Students will be able to describe how paying compliments to others can make both others and themselves feel good.

Understanding Bullying I   Grades 5–8

Valued Outcome: Students will be able to discuss what bullying is and the ramifications thereof.

National Health Education Standards: 2, 4, 5

Description of Strategy: The purpose of this strategy is to help students understand what bullying is, the types of bullying, and how to deal with the situation when being bullied. Introduce the lesson by asking the students if they know what is met by the term "bullying." Use either an overhead projector or write on poster board/chalk board the main concepts identified. Ask "why" someone would want to bully another person. Explain that the class will explore not only what bullying is but what happens to students who witness bullying and the person who is the victim of bullying.

1. Ask students to find terms on the Internet. Have the student write the definitions they find. Words to be defined would include bullying, relentless, empathy, ridicule, ethics, alternative, intervention, victim, taunting, verbal bullying, physical bullying, and cyber bullying.
2. Discuss with the class each of the terms and relate them to how they relate to bullying.
3. Have students list on poster board a description of bullying, the characteristics of bullying, and effects of bullying on the victim, witnesses, and the bully.

Materials Needed: computer, Internet, poster board

Processing Questions:

1. Can words/actions hurt someone emotionally? Physically?
2. Have you or has someone you know been bullied?
3. Why do you think a person bullies another?
4. How should you deal with someone who bullies you?
5. What should you do if you witness someone bullying another student?

○ **Integration:** Social studies

✓ **Assessment:** Students should be able to define the words related to bullying and state the effects of bullying upon the victim and those who witness the act.

Understanding Bullying II   Grades 5–8

Valued Outcome: The students will realize how bullying affects the bully, those who witness bullying, and the victim.

National Health Education Standards: 2, 4, 5

Description of Strategy: This activity is a follow-up to the Bullying I strategy. The concept is for students to develop insight into the effects of bullying and how to deal with and prevent such acts. Have students review websites (selected by teacher) to investigate the statistics on bullying, the types of bullying, the effects of bullying on all involved, and the effects of bullying on self-esteem. After receiving the information found on the selected websites, have the students report on their findings for each of the topics investigated. The information may be shared through PowerPoint slides, on poster board, or by listing items on the chalk board. Discuss each of the topics, emphasizing the effects of bullying, how bullying can be prevented, and what to do if being bullied or witnessing someone being bullied.

Processing Questions:

1. What are the statistics concerning the various types of student bullying?
2. What are the results of bullying on those involved—victim, witnesses, bully?
3. How does bullying make the victim and witness feel when observing or being bullied?
4. What can you do if you are being bullied?
5. What can you do if you witness someone being bullied?

Materials Needed: computer, Internet, poster board

○ **Integration:** Computer technology, Language arts

✓ **Assessment:** Have students summarize each discussion by listing at least five rational answers to each question.

Coping with and Controlling Stress   Grades 7–8

Valued Outcome: Students will be able to assess their stress level and use relaxation and self-management techniques in response to stressful situations.

National Health Education Standards: 5, 7

Description of Strategy: Ask students to list three things they find stressful and want to discuss. List the responses on the board. Ask, "Why are peer pressure, grades, and the need for acceptance such common stressors?" Lead a discussion on effectively dealing with these stressors, and explain the following techniques for handling stressful situations: quiet reflection, biofeedback, progressive muscle relaxation, and visualization. Obtain a copy of a stress test, and have students take it to determine their current level of stress. Explain to students that they are to maintain a daily journal listing all stressful situations they encounter, how they react, and if there could be a better way to handle the stressor.

Materials Needed: stress test, paper and pencils for journal

Processing Questions:

1. What areas of your life create the most stress for you?
2. Describe one effective way of handling a stressor.
3. What are some advantages and disadvantages of stress?

○ **Integration:** Writing, Science

✓ **Assessment:** In their journals, students can identify several stressors in their lives and explain how the stress management techniques discussed could be applied in those situations.

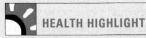

HEALTH HIGHLIGHT | **Deep Diaphragmatic Breathing for Relaxation**

Deep breathing is the most basic technique used in relaxation and is often the foundation for other methods of relaxation and stress reduction. The primary benefit of this technique is that it can be done anywhere and anytime. The method consists of completely filling the lungs when breathing and exhaling very slowly. This type of breathing necessitates a conscious decision to redirect attention to the basic physiological function of breathing. There are four phases to the process.

- Phase I: Inspiration—Taking the air into your lungs through your mouth. Completely fill your lungs.
- Phase II: Slight pause before exhaling.
- Phase III: Exhalation—Release the air from the lungs very slowly through the mouth.

- Phase IV: Another very slight pause after completely releasing all air in the lungs, and then begin the next inhalation.

Focus on your breathing, and notice how relaxed your whole body becomes during the breathing exercise, especially the chest, shoulders, and abdominal areas. Consider ways you can effectively teach this concept to your students.

Stress Feelings
Grades 7–8

Valued Outcomes: Students will understand the relationship between stress, feelings and physical symptoms, and situations in their lives and can use a breathing exercise to reduce stress.

National Health Education Standards: 5, 7

Description of Strategy: Define stress, and lead students to think of times when stress has affected them. Discuss the advantages and disadvantages of stress. Students will list times when they have felt stress. Ask students to discuss the feelings and physical symptoms they have had in association with stressors. Demonstrate a breathing exercise effective in reducing stress. Hand out copies of the stress worksheet (see Worksheet 7.3 on page 481). Have students keep a record of stressful events that occur at home and bring them back to class for discussion.

Materials Needed: poster showing common symptoms of stress, paper and pencils, stress worksheets

Processing Questions:

1. Name two physical symptoms of stress.
2. Name two feelings that might be associated with stress.
3. Why do you think the breathing exercise demonstrated in class helps to reduce stress?

✓ **Assessment:** Students will be able to define stress, identify five feelings they have that cause stress, and be able to use one breathing exercise to reduce stress.

Experiments and Demonstrations

Unique! That's Me!
Grades K–3

Valued Outcome: Each student will be able to identify two ways in which he or she is unique in relationship to his or her classmates.

National Health Education Standard: 4

Description of Strategy: Ask students to discuss ways in which individuals are unique. Students will play a voice-guessing game to show how everything about a person, even their voice, is unique and special. Have a student sing the words, "Voices never are the same. Can you guess what is my name?" to the tune of "Twinkle, Twinkle, Little Star." Have the rest of the class, with eyes closed, raise their hands to guess the voice. Repeat the activity until everyone has had a turn to sing, with students relocating around the room after each turn. Then have students examine their fingers and those of their classmates with a magnifying glass. Use fingerpaints or fingerprint ink and have students make a thumb print on a paper star to be worn on their clothing.

Materials Needed: poster with song words, magnifying glasses, fingerpaints or ink, paper stars, safety pins for name tags

Processing Questions:

1. What does the word *unique* mean?
2. Is it good or bad to be unique? Explain.
3. In what ways are you a unique person?

○ **Integration:** Music, Science

✓ **Assessment:** Students can explain what it means to be unique and describe their own unique qualities with a positive attitude.

Costume Party
Grades 4–6

Valued Outcome: Students will be able to express personality traits through costume.

National Health Education Standards: 1, 4

Description of Strategy: Ask each student to come to class in a costume that depicts as many of his or her personality traits as possible. The class as a whole lists what traits students think are revealed. A secret ballot vote is cast for costumes that are the most accurate, inaccurate, humorous, puzzling, and eye catching.

Materials Needed: costumes from students' homes, materials for casting secret ballot (pencils, paper, box, etc.)

Processing Questions:

1. Explain why you chose the costume you were wearing.
2. Describe the costume and personality traits of your closest classmate.
3. Which classmate had the most humorous costume? Why?

✓ **Assessment:** Students can identify why their costume depicted their personality.

Mental Health in Music   Grades 4–8

Valued Outcome: Students will be able to describe characteristics of healthy living.

National Health Education Standards: 1, 2

Description of Strategy: Have students compose songs that describe healthy living. They can bring in CDs that describe a human relationship. Discuss the feelings depicted in the music. Pay attention to the tone of the music as well as the words of the song.

Materials Needed: students' CDs, CD player

Processing Questions:

1. Can you name one characteristic of a healthy relationship?
2. What feelings are mentioned in the song you wrote?
3. Besides having healthy relationships, what are some other characteristics of healthy living?

○ **Integration:** Music

✓ **Assessment:** Students can name five characteristics of healthy relationships and explain the importance of these characteristics as components of healthy living.

Human Scavenger Hunt   Grades 4–8

Valued Outcome: Students will be able to identify human qualities that emphasize individual uniqueness.

National Health Education Standard: 1

Description of Strategy: Have students simulate a scavenger hunt, but have them look for various unique human qualities, such as red hair, green eyes, friendliness, or quick-temperedness. Suggest students write the names of classmates on their paper next to the appropriate quality.

Materials Needed: list of human qualities to seek, paper, pencils

Processing Questions:

1. What did you think was the most interesting quality you found in your scavenger hunt?

2. How many different qualities might one person have?
3. Do any two people have the same qualities? Why or why not?

✓ **Assessment:** Students can identify positive characteristics in each of their classmates.

Hearing Is Not Always Listening   Grades 7–8

Valued Outcome: Students will be able to demonstrate and discuss listening and observation skills.

National Health Education Standard: 4

Description of Strategy: Set up several listening and observing demonstrations to emphasize that these are learned skills. Here are some possible examples.

- Prearrange with several students to get "lost" during recess. (Have them go to the library or other supervised area.) When the rest of the class returns, ask them to help with descriptions of each missing person. Also have them indicate anything they might have overheard during recess that might give a clue to why these students are gone. After the missing students return, discuss implications of the activity.
- Tell students you are going to read a story and you want them to listen carefully. Read aloud a short story that has several specific details about a main character's problem or situation and the succeeding events. Immediately following the story, ask each student to write a brief summary of the story, being as specific and accurate as possible. Let volunteers share their versions. Then read the original again. Compare listening skills.

Materials Needed: story, paper, pencils

Processing Questions:

1. What is the difference between hearing and listening?
2. How did the versions of the student responses differ, and why do you think this occurred?
3. What is the advantage of being a good listener?

○ **Integration:** Literature, Writing

✓ **Assessment:** Students can explain the difference between hearing and listening and can name several advantages of being a good listener.

Puzzles and Games

Emotional Musical Chairs   Grades K–6

Valued Outcome: Students will be able to associate emotions with facial expressions.

National Health Education Standards: 1, 4

Description of Strategy: Students will discuss specific feelings they have had on specific occasions. Tell students that everyone's feelings are important and should be respected. Have students participate in a game of musical chairs. Chairs are arranged in the same way as for the traditional game; however, no additional chairs are removed during the game. Before starting, place pictures, each with a face showing a different emotion, in a box. Students move around the chairs as the music plays and try to find a place to sit when the music stops. The student without a chair draws a picture out of the box and shows it to the other students. The student then tells what emotion he or she thinks the person in the picture is feeling. All of the remaining students then tell what emotion they think the person in the picture is feeling. Have students make faces and act out the emotion until the music starts again. The game continues until all the emotions in the box have been acted out.

Materials Needed: chairs, pictures of faces showing different emotions, box, music player, music

Processing Questions:

1. What are some of the ways you express your emotions?
2. When do you share your feelings or emotions with others?
3. Discuss a time when you made someone else happy, sad, angry, and so on.

✓ **Assessment:** Students can describe how body language and facial expressions are associated with emotions.

Silent Steps   Grades 7–8

Valued Outcome: Students will be able to identify feelings experienced through a nonverbal group effort to reconstruct a jigsaw puzzle.

National Health Education Standard: 4

Description of Strategy: Have students work in groups of five to seven. Provide each group with a sealed manila envelope that contains a sheet of colored construction paper cut into five to seven shuffled jigsaw pieces. Each group should receive a different colored puzzle with differently shaped pieces of equal difficulty. Instruct each group member to randomly select a puzzle piece from the envelope. When you give the signal to start, students must reconstruct the pieces without saying a word. As each group completes the puzzle, have them raise their hands—they still cannot talk. When all groups have finished, allow students to discuss their feelings during this activity.

Materials Needed: construction paper, manila envelopes

Processing Questions:

1. What feelings can result from nonverbal communication?

2. Discuss how the puzzle would have been solved if verbal communication had been used.
3. What are the advantages to verbal communication?

✓ **Assessment:** Students can name several advantages and disadvantages of nonverbal communication and ways in which nonverbal communication can incite emotions.

Other Ideas

Facial Forecasts   Grades PK–3

Valued Outcome: Students will be able to draw a facial expression depicting a specific emotion.

National Health Education Standards: 1, 4

Description of Strategy: Assign each student an emotion. Provide students with paper plates and crayons, and ask them to draw their own faces indicating the emotion. Have students use mirrors if necessary. The plates may be used for a colorful wall display.

Materials Needed: paper plates, crayons, mirrors

Processing Questions:

1. How did your face look when you expressed anger?
2. How did your face look when you expressed happiness?
3. Do people's facial expressions always indicate how they feel? Why or why not?

○ **Integration:** Art

✓ **Assessment:** Students can describe how their drawing matches the emotion they were assigned.

How Do I See Myself?   Grades K–6

Valued Outcome: Each student will be able to describe and discuss differences and similarities between herself or himself and others.

National Health Education Standards: 2, 4

Description of Strategy: Lead a discussion regarding differences and similarities among individuals, pointing out that many things that are similar have different qualities. For example, "fruit" includes all fruit, but a pear is not like an apple. Animals have many varieties, as do plants. Give students paper and crayons and ask them to make their own name tags with drawings of things that describe them.

Materials Needed: visual aids of different fruits, animals, and plants; construction paper; crayons; safety pins for name tags

Processing Questions:

1. What are some positive aspects of individual differences?
2. What type of attitude should we have regarding other peoples' differences?
3. In what ways do you treat others the way you would like to be treated?

✓ **Assessment:** Students can identify and describe differences and similarities between themselves and their classmates in a positive way.

Stress Facial Forecasts   Grades K–6

Valued Outcome: Students will be able to identify signs, symptoms, and causes of stress and be able to describe effective coping mechanisms and resources for dealing with stress.

National Health Education Standards: 2, 3, 4, 5

Description of Strategy: Lead a discussion about stress, including information dealing with signs, symptoms, and causes of stress. Students will use a mirror to observe their own facial expressions when they are under stress. Pass out paper plates and markers or crayons so students can draw their impressions of themselves under stress.

Materials Needed: photocopied pages of common stressors among children, danger signs of stress, ways of coping with stress, mirror, paper plates, markers, crayons

Processing Questions:

1. What are some signs of stress?
2. What is one thing you can do when faced with a stressor?

3. Who are people you can talk to about stressful events in your life?

◯ **Integration:** Art

✓ **Assessment:** Students can describe what stress is and identify how it affects them. Students can list ways to deal with stress and name resources that are available to them for dealing with stress in their lives.

Emotions Bag   Grades 7–8

Valued Outcome: Students will be able to describe personal emotional experiences as well as reactions in those situations.

National Health Education Standard: 4

Description of Strategy: Give each student a paper bag to keep for two days. Students should keep track of their emotions for that time period by writing a description about their emotional experiences and their reactions to those situations as they happen. Students will keep each description in their bag and then share them with the class.

Materials Needed: paper bags, paper, pencils

Processing Questions:

1. What was an emotion you described that made you feel bad inside? What caused this emotion?
2. What was an emotion you described that made you feel good inside? What caused this emotion?
3. Did you experience the emotion of anger? If so, how did you react?

◯ **Integration:** Writing

✓ **Assessment:** Students can describe three different emotional experiences, their causes, and their reactions.

Access more material online at www.pearsonhighered.com/anspaugh. At this companion website for *Teaching Today's Health*, you'll find chapter quizzes, web links, flashcards, a glossary, additional Worksheets, and more to help you succeed.

8 | Body Systems

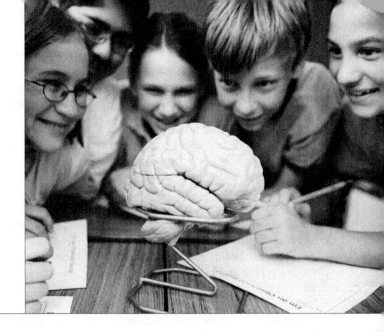

Valued Outcomes

After completion of this chapter, you should be able to:

- Describe the function and structure of skin, hair, and nails.
- Explain the different roles of the brain.
- Discuss the function of selected components (structures) of the nervous system.
- Describe the functions of selected glands and hormones associated with the endocrine system.
- Discuss the role of each component of the respiratory system in the breathing process.
- Trace a drop of blood through the circulatory and pulmonary systems.
- Describe the major function of red blood cells.
- Explain the function of white blood corpuscles in fighting off infection.
- Describe how food travels through the body.
- Describe the function of the skeletal system.
- Describe how liquid and solid wastes are filtered in the body.
- Differentiate between voluntary and involuntary muscles.

The human body is the most remarkable machine in existence. There is no computer that surpasses its capability. There is no mind brilliant enough to synthetically make a human.

—Beverly Lutz Sr. (2008)

NATIONAL HEALTH EDUCATION STANDARDS

1. Students will comprehend concepts related to health promotion and disease prevention to enhance health.

Reflections

All the organs and systems of the body depend on each other. When one part is not functioning properly, it sometimes affects several other parts. As you read this chapter, note the many ways in which the various body systems are interdependent.

A Unique Machine

The human body is an efficient functional organism—an amazing and well-organized machine. If cared for properly, it will generally perform well.

At conception, individuals are given the capacity for growth, development, and functioning through genetic factors. However, environmental factors—especially health-related behaviors—determine what actually occurs as an individual matures.

Health and health enhancement cannot be achieved without keeping the body and its systems in good condition. This chapter and the next will provide you with information you can use to help children learn about their bodies and how to care for them. A brief outline and description of several of the major systems of the body are presented here with a discussion of how these systems function. (The reproductive system will be discussed in Chapter 11.)

The Integumentary System

The largest human organ is skin, which is part of the **integumentary system**. If the skin from a 150-pound person were stretched flat, it would cover almost two square meters. Among its many functions, skin protects the muscles, bones, and other body organs. Skin forms a protective barrier that prevents the entry of pathogens. In addition, skin helps to regulate body temperature by means of perspiration, and melanin in skin helps protect the body from harmful ultraviolet light. Skin also contains nerve cells that enable people to feel warmth, cold, pain, touch, and other sensations.

Skin is made up of three layers, which contain thousands of hair follicles, oil glands, and sweat glands as well as nerve endings (Figure 8.1). The outermost layer of skin is the *epidermis*. These cells of the epidermis are replaced every twenty-eight days, thus allowing cuts and bruises to heal quickly. The middle layer of skin is the *dermis*. This layer of skin contains the sebaceous glands. These glands are sometimes referred to as oil glands and produce a substance called sebum, which lubricates skin and hair. In the teenage years these glands may make more sebum than necessary, which can contribute to acne, a skin disorder that results when bacteria infect clogged pores. The innermost layer of the skin, the *subcutaneous tissue*, is made up of connective tissue, sweat glands, blood vessels, and fat cells. This subcutaneous layer protects the other organs from injury and aids in maintaining body heat.

For most people, the body is covered with hair, another component of the integumentary system. Hair often serves as an insulator. For example, the hair on the head helps retain heat because people lose as much as 90 percent of their body heat through the head. Hair also can be found in or around our nose, ears, and eyes. These small hairs help keep pathogens, dust, and other particles from entering the body. A hair consists of the hair shaft, or the part of the hair above the skin surface, and a root, or the soft, bulblike structure of hair that is embedded in the skin (see Figure 8.1). The root is located in a saclike follicle from which the hair grows.

Another component of the integumentary system is nails. Nails protect the tips of the fingers and toes and provide support to each. Nails are made up of epidermal cells that are transformed into a thin nail plate—the part of the nail that is visible—by a process called *keratinization*. When nail cells accumulate, they are pushed forward, causing nails to grow.

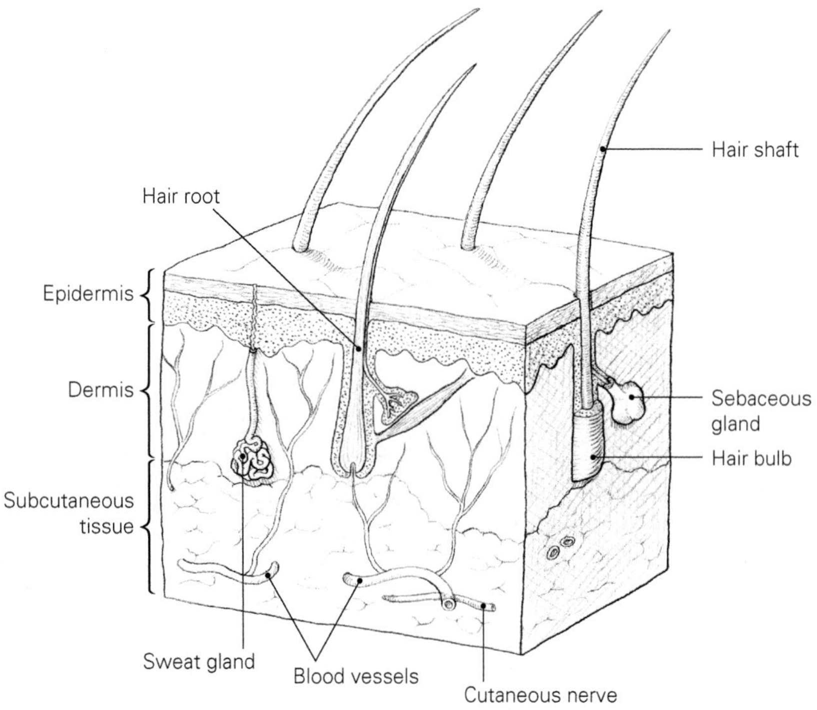

Figure 8.1
Skin and Hair

The Nervous System

All physiological functions and many psychological ones are controlled in one way or another by the nervous system. The nervous system is composed of two parts—the central nervous system and the peripheral nervous system. The central nervous system includes the brain and the spinal cord. The peripheral nervous system includes the outlying nerves and nerve pathways that are not part of the brain or the spinal cord.

The Central Nervous System

The central nervous system is composed of the brain and the spinal cord (Figure 8.2). The brain contains about 100 billion nerve cells (*neurons*) and trillions of support cells called *glia*. The spinal cord is 42–45 cm long, and it weighs about 35–40 g. The vertebral column, the collection of articulated bones that houses and protects the spinal cord (the backbone), is about 61–71 cm long—much longer than the spinal cord.

The Brain: An Overview.

The average human brain weighs about 1,400 g (3 lb). When the brain is removed from the skull, it looks a bit like a large pinkish gray walnut. The brain is composed of four parts: the cerebrum (seat of consciousness), the diencephalon, the cerebellum, and the brain stem.

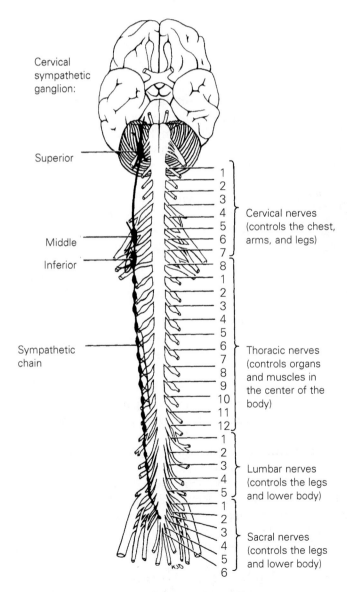

Cervical sympathetic ganglion:

Superior

Middle

Inferior

Sympathetic chain

1
2
3
4
5
6
7
Cervical nerves (controls the chest, arms, and legs)

8
1
2
3
4
5
6
7
8
9
10
11
12
Thoracic nerves (controls organs and muscles in the center of the body)

1
2
3
4
5
Lumbar nerves (controls the legs and lower body)

1
2
3
4
5
6
Sacral nerves (controls the legs and lower body)

Figure 8.2
The Brain and Spinal Cord

The *cerebrum* governs intelligence and reasoning, learning, and memory. Within the cells of the cerebrum, learning involves change in gene regulation and increased ability to secrete transmitters.

The *diencephalon* includes the hypothalamus and thalamus. The *hypothalamus* regulates homeostasis. It has regulatory areas for thirst, hunger, body temperature, water balance, and blood pressure and links the nervous system to the endocrine system. The *thalamus* serves as a central relay point for incoming nerve messages.

The *cerebellum* is the second largest part of the brain, after the cerebrum. It functions in muscle coordination and maintains normal muscle tone and posture. The cerebellum coordinates balance.

The *brain stem* has three parts: the medulla oblongata, pons, and midbrain. The *medulla oblongata* is closest to the spinal cord and is involved with the regulation of heartbeat; breathing; vasoconstriction (blood pressure); and reflex centers for vomiting, coughing, sneezing, swallowing, and hiccupping. The *midbrain* and *pons* are also part of the unconscious brain and largely act as relay stations for neural information.

The Cerebrum and Lobes of the Brain.

The cerebrum, the largest part of the human brain, is divided into left and right cerebral hemispheres that are connected to each other by bundles of nerve fibers, the largest and most obvious of which is the corpus callosum. The cerebral hemispheres are covered by a thin layer of gray matter known as the cerebral cortex. The word *cortex* comes from the Latin word that means "bark"; thus, the cortex is a sheet of tissue that makes up the outer layer of the brain. The cortex in each hemisphere of the cerebrum is between 2 and 4 mm thick.

The surface of the cerebral cortex is covered with bumps, or bulges, called *gyri* (singular *gyrus*), and grooves called *sulci* (singular *sulcus*). In higher mammals, such as humans, there are many gyri and sulci; lower mammals, such as rats and mice, have very few gyri and sulci.

The folding of the cerebral cortex into gyri and sulci increases the amount of cerebral cortex that can fit in the skull. In fact, the total surface area of the human cerebral cortex is about 324 square inches—about the size of a page of newspaper! Although most people have the same patterns of gyri and sulci on the cerebral cortex, no two brains are exactly alike.

The various sulci and gyri divide each hemisphere of the cerebral cortex into four lobes: occipital, temporal, parietal, and frontal (Figure 8.3). A fifth lobe called the insula is located within the cortex. No region of the brain functions alone, although major functions of various parts of the lobes have been determined.

The frontal lobe is located in front of the central sulcus and is concerned with reasoning, planning, parts of speech, movement (motor cortex), emotions, and problem solving. The temporal lobe is located below the lateral fissure and is concerned with hearing, processing of language, and memory. The parietal lobe is located behind the central sulcus

HEALTH HIGHLIGHT | **Indelible Learning**

In order for students' brains to retain what they have learned, three criteria must be met:

1. The learning is meaningful to the student.
2. The student experiences strong emotions about the learning.
3. The student applies the learning within twenty-four hours.

These are the three principles of permanent or indelible learning.

Health educators, as well as psychologists, have long emphasized the need for "active learning" during a teaching/learning session. If a student does not apply the learning to some meaningful link in the brain, the learning is lost rapidly. Under brain theory, active learning builds patterns and programs in the brain and provides feedback loops.

The emotional, or value, attachment to the information is important in order for the student to respond to the learning challenge. This is considered the *motivating force* to learn. Educational theorists believe that it activates the "mid-brain," a control center for emotions that catalyzes thorough and deep learning through imagery.

Brain-compatible education means that what occurs in schools is consistent with how the brain is designed and operates. All three learning principles must be present in the learning process, otherwise learning will not take place. The lesson must be *meaningful* in content, material, and delivery to be clearly understood, and motivational to maintain an adequate attention span. The lesson must provide for meaningful *application* to be better understood. The lesson must have *emotional* communication to keep the learning alive. With these three principles governing the learning plan, motivation to learn flourishes.

Source: Excerpted and adapted from "Indelible Learning" by Wayne B. Jennings and Gary Philips, http://braincompatiblelearning.org, © 2008. Used by permission.

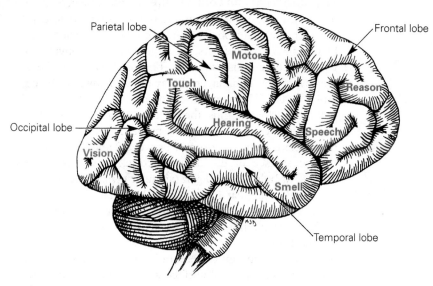

Figure 8.3
The Control Centers and Lobes of the Brain

and is concerned with perception of stimuli related to touch, taste, pressure, temperature, and pain. The occipital lobe is at the base of the skull and processes visual information.

The Diencephalon.

Two major structures of the diencephalon are the thalamus and hypothalamus. The thalamus acts as a switching center for nerve messages. The thalamus receives sensory information and relays this information to the cerebral cortex. The cerebral cortex also sends information to the thalamus, which then transmits this information to other areas of the brain and spinal cord. The hypothalamus is a major homeostatic center, having both nervous and endocrine functions.

The Cerebellum.

The cerebellum, along with the pons and medulla, is part of the hindbrain, but it is not considered part of the brain stem. The word *cerebellum* comes from the Latin word for "little brain." The cerebellum is located behind the brain stem. In some ways, the cerebellum is a bit like the cerebral cortex; the cerebellum is divided into hemispheres and has a cortex that surrounds these hemispheres. Functions of the cerebellum include fine motor coordination and body movement, posture, and balance.

The Brain Stem.

The brain stem is a general term for the area of the brain between the thalamus and spinal cord. Structures within the brain stem include the midbrain, pons, and medulla oblongata, which is continuous with the spinal cord. The brain stem is the smallest and most primitive part of the brain, so it controls the most basic bodily functions. For example, the medulla oblongata and pons control heart rate, constriction of blood vessels (and thereby blood pressure), digestion, and respiration; the reticular formation, which runs through the entire brain stem, controls level of consciousness; and the colliculi of the midbrain are involved with reflexes that coordinate head and eye movements and mediate the startle reflex (turning the head toward a sound).

The Spinal Cord.

The spinal cord is the main pathway for the delivery of information between the brain and peripheral nervous system (where information is received by specialized receptors and sent out to muscles and glands).

The spinal cord runs along the dorsal side of the body and links the brain to the rest of the body. The gray matter of the spinal cord consists mostly of cell bodies and dendrites. The surrounding white matter is made up of bundles of interneuronal axons (tracts). Some tracts are ascending (carrying messages to the brain), others are descending (carrying messages from the brain). The spinal cord is also involved in reflexes that do not involve the brain.

The spinal cord of vertebrates is encased in a series of (usually) bony vertebrae that comprise the vertebral, or spinal, column. Although the vertebral column is somewhat flexible, some of the vertebrae in the lower parts of the vertebral column become fused as the sacrum and coccyx (tailbone). The spinal cord is located within the *vertebral foramen* (central holes in the vertebrae).

■ How the Parts of the Brain Work Together

The various parts of our brain work together in order for us to function. As an example, let's follow the different processes of the brain as they relate to taking a drug. The cerebral cortex helps with cognitive functions, like speaking and making decisions; we speak about taking drugs and make a decision whether or not to use a drug. The cerebellum plays a vital role in coordinating our muscles and joints; in our example, our cerebellum would assist us in picking up the drug and administering the drug (i.e., putting it in our mouths, injecting it, etc.). The brain stem controls the functions that happen automatically that are crucial to survival. So, again in our example, once the drug is taken, the brain stem will send out information from the brain and spinal cord to the muscles, skin, and other organs to control the changes the drug causes to our heart rate, blood pressure, and breathing (National Institutes of Health 2011).

■ The Peripheral Nervous System

The peripheral nervous system connects the central nervous system with sensory receptors and organs, muscles, and glands. Twelve pairs of cranial nerves extend from various brain regions; thirty pairs of spinal nerves (eight cervical, twelve thoracic, five lumbar, and five sacral) and one coccygeal nerve arise from the spinal cord. The peripheral nervous system has two components: the somatic nervous system and the autonomic nervous system. The *somatic nervous system* controls skeletal muscles and voluntary movements of the body (see the section on muscles, page 141). The *autonomic nervous system (ANS)*, also called the involuntary or visceral motor system, innervates cardiac (heart) muscles and smooth muscles of the various organs and glands.

The Autonomic Nervous System (ANS). The organs (*viscera*) inside our body, such as the heart, stomach, and intestines, are regulated by the ANS, the part of the peripheral nervous system that controls smooth muscle. In most situations, we are unaware of the workings of the ANS because it functions in an involuntary, reflexive manner. For example, we do not control when blood vessels change size.

The ANS regulates muscles in several parts of the body—for example, in the skin (smooth muscle around hair follicles and blood vessels); around blood vessels (smooth muscle); in the eye (smooth muscle controlling pupil size and lens shape); in the stomach, intestines, and bladder (smooth muscle of organ walls); and in the heart (cardiac muscle).

The autonomic nervous system is divided into two parts: the sympathetic division and the parasympathetic division. The sympathetic division activates the body's fight-or-flight response and prepares the individual to deal with stress. The parasympathetic division of the ANS has the opposite effect—it promotes calming and digestion and restores the body to its resting state.

The Endocrine System

Closely associated with the nervous system is the endocrine system. Both systems provide means of communication within the body, but the endocrine system is the slower of the two. This section describes some of the glands associated with the endocrine system. Figure 8.4 shows the endocrine glands.

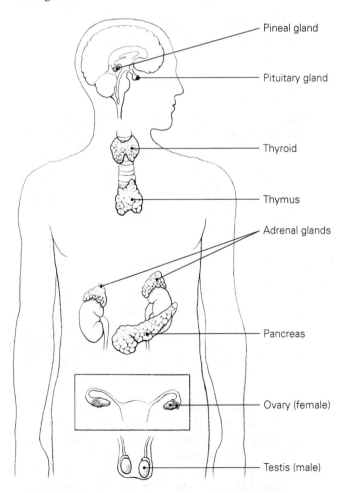

Figure 8.4

Major Structures of the Endocrine System

The endocrine system's role is that of a regulator. Through the production and secretion of chemical-signaling substances called *hormones* from glands dispersed throughout the body, the endocrine system keeps other body systems and metabolic processes in balanced operation. The two "controller" glands of the endocrine system are the hypothalamus and the pituitary gland. They secrete hormones that in turn signal other endocrine glands to activate. The hypothalamus and the posterior lobe of the pituitary gland contain neural tissue, thus establishing the close relationship between the endocrine system and the nervous system.

▪ The Hypothalamus

The hypothalamus is composed of several different areas and is located at the base of the brain. It is about the size of a pea (about $1/300$ of the total brain weight), but it is responsible for some very important behaviors. One important function of the hypothalamus is the control of body temperature. The hypothalamus acts like a thermostat by sensing changes in body temperature and then sending out signals to smooth muscle of blood vessel walls to adjust the temperature. For example, if you are too hot, the hypothalamus detects this and then sends out a signal to expand the capillaries in your skin. This causes blood to be cooled faster. The hypothalamus also controls the pituitary gland.

▪ The Pituitary Gland

The pituitary gland is composed of two lobes and is located in a small bony cavity at the base of the brain. The anterior lobe is made of glandular tissue and produces and secretes a number of hormones. The posterior lobe is made of neural tissue and acts as a storage unit for hormones produced by the hypothalamus. A stalk links the posterior pituitary to the hypothalamus, which controls release of pituitary hormones.

Anterior Pituitary Lobe. The anterior lobe (often called the master gland) is connected to the hypothalamus through a network of specialized vessels. It secretes six different hormones. These hormones influence various structures and functions, such as skin pigmentation, activating the reproductive glands, regulating human growth and development as a whole, and regulating adrenal secretions.

Posterior Pituitary Lobe. The posterior pituitary stores and releases hormones into the blood. Antidiuretic hormone (ADH) and oxytocin are produced in the hypothalamus and transported by axons to the posterior pituitary, where they are dumped into the blood. ADH controls water balance in the body and blood pressure. Oxytocin is a small peptide hormone that stimulates uterine contractions during childbirth.

▪ The Thyroid Gland

The thyroid gland is located in the neck. Follicles in the thyroid secrete thyroglobulin, a storage form of thyroid hormone. Thyroid-stimulating hormone (TSH) from the anterior pituitary causes conversion of thyroglobulin into thyroid hormones T4 and T3. Almost all body cells are targets of thyroid hormones.

Thyroid hormone increases the overall metabolic rate and regulates growth and development as well as the onset of sexual maturity. Calcitonin is also secreted by large cells in the thyroid; it plays a role in the regulation of calcium.

▪ The Adrenal Glands

The adrenal glands are located above the kidneys. Each gland is divided into an inner medulla and an outer cortex. The medulla synthesizes amine hormones; the cortex secretes steroid hormones. The adrenal medulla consists of modified neurons that secrete two hormones; epinephrine (sometimes called adrenaline) and norepinephrine. Stimulation of the medulla by the sympathetic division of the ANS causes release of hormones (especially epinephrine) into the blood to initiate the short-term fight-or-flight response to stress. The adrenal cortex produces several steroid hormones in three classes: mineralocorticoids, glucocorticoids, and sex hormones. Mineralocorticoids maintain the electrolyte balance critical for proper bodily functions. Glucocorticoids produce a long-term, slow response to stress by raising blood glucose levels through the breakdown of fats and proteins; they also suppress the immune response and inhibit the inflammatory response. The sex hormones (especially testosterone) produced by the adrenal cortex are important mostly during the fetal stage and early puberty; these sex hormones decline in significance when compared to sex hormones produced by the gonads (ovaries and testes).

▪ The Pancreas

The pancreas contains exocrine cells that secrete digestive enzymes into the small intestine and endocrine cell clusters (the pancreatic islets) that secrete the hormones insulin and glucagon. The balance between insulin and glucagon levels regulates blood glucose levels. After a meal, blood glucose levels rise, prompting the release of insulin, which causes cells to take up glucose and causes liver and skeletal muscle cells to form the carbohydrate glycogen. As glucose levels in the blood fall, insulin production is inhibited. If blood glucose levels fall too far, glucagon causes the breakdown of glycogen into glucose. In turn, the glucose is released into the blood to return glucose levels to within a homeostatic range. Glucagon production is inhibited when blood glucose levels rise.

▪ The Health of the Endocrine System and the Body

The parts of the endocrine system must function properly as a part of the body or problems can arise. To examine this relationship, let's look at diabetes. Insulin is a hormone produced by the pancreas (part of the endocrine system) to control blood sugar; diabetes can be the result of too little insulin, resistance to insulin, or both. The development of diabetes can negatively affect the overall functioning of the body. To understand diabetes, it is important to first understand the normal process by which food is broken down and used by the body for energy. Several things happen when food is digested: Glucose, a sugar that is a source of fuel for the body, enters the bloodstream. The pancreas makes the insulin that moves glucose from the bloodstream into muscle, fat, and liver cells, where it can be used as fuel. People with diabetes have high blood sugar because their pancreas does not make enough insulin and/or their muscle, fat, and liver cells do not respond to insulin normally.

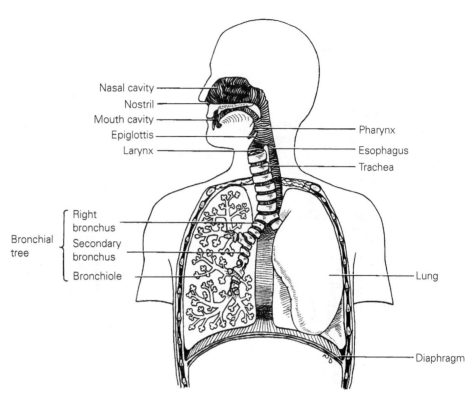

Figure 8.5
The Respiratory System

This disruption of the normal functioning of the endocrine system can lead to low level symptoms like fatigue, thirst, and blurry vision. The more extreme complications of diabetes can include hypertension, coronary artery disease, coma, and stroke (National Institutes of Health 2011).

The Respiratory System

Air enters the body through the nose and is then warmed, filtered, and passed through the nasal cavity. Air moves through the pharynx, then the epiglottis (a flap that prevents food from entering the trachea), and into the trachea, or windpipe. The upper part of the trachea contains the larynx. The vocal cords are two bands of tissue that extend across the opening of the larynx. After passing the larynx, the air moves into the bronchi that carry air in and out of the lungs. Figure 8.5 illustrates the respiratory system.

The trachea and bronchi are reinforced with cartilage to prevent their collapse, and they are lined with ciliated epithelium and mucus-producing cells. Bronchi branch into smaller and smaller tubes known as bronchioles, which terminate in grapelike sac clusters known as alveoli. Alveoli are surrounded by a network of thin-walled capillaries. Only about 0.2 mm separate the alveoli from the capillaries due to the extremely thin walls of both structures.

The lungs are large, lobed, paired organs in the chest (also known as the thoracic cavity). Thin sheets of epithelium

(pleura) separate the inside of the chest cavity from the outer surface of the lungs. The pleura reduce friction as the chest expands during breathing. The bottom of the thoracic cavity is formed by the diaphragm.

Ventilation is the process of breathing in and out. When you inhale, muscles in the chest wall contract, lifting the ribs and pulling them outward. The diaphragm moves downward, enlarging the chest cavity. Reduced air pressure in the lungs causes air to enter the lungs. Exhaling reverses these steps.

The cause of improper functioning of the respiratory system is often determined by a **chest x-ray**. The test may be performed in the cases of a persistent cough, difficulty breathing, or chest pain, and is often used to diagnose or check the progress of tuberculosis, lung cancer, or other chest or lung disease (National Institutes of Health, Chest X-Ray, 2011).

The Circulatory System

The heart is a four-chambered structure—two atria and two ventricles—with muscular walls that contract in a rhythmic pattern to pump blood. An *atrioventricular (AV) valve* separates each atrium from each ventricle. A *semilunar (SL, also known as arterial) valve* separates each ventricle from its connecting artery. Figure 8.6 on page 136 illustrates the heart and the circulatory system. (For a discussion on the diseases that affect the cardiovascular system, see Chapter 15.)

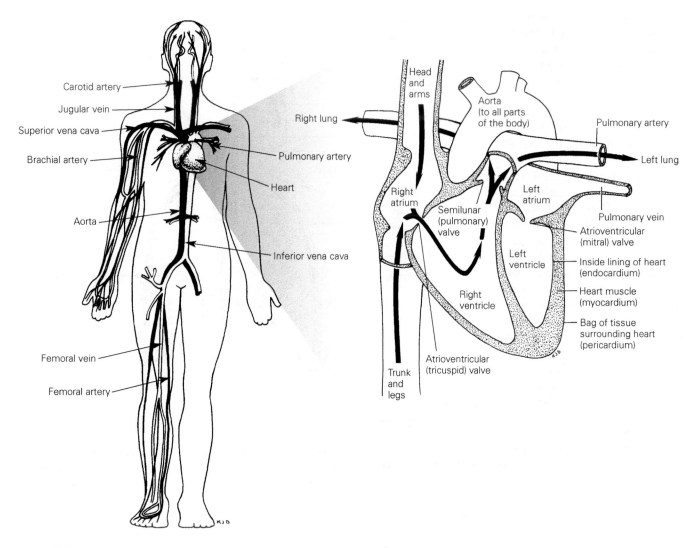

Figure 8.6
The Circulatory System

■ The Heart

For most people, the heart beats (or contracts) about seventy times per minute. The human heart will undergo more than three billion contraction cycles during a normal lifetime. The cardiac cycle consists of two parts: *systole* (contraction of the heart muscle) and *diastole* (relaxation of the heart muscle). Atria contract while ventricles relax. The pulse is a wave of contraction transmitted along the arteries. Valves in the heart open and close during the cardiac cycle. Heart muscle contraction is due to the presence of nodal tissue in two regions of the heart: the *sinoatrial (SA) node* initiates heartbeat, and the *AV node* causes ventricles to contract. The AV node is sometimes called the pacemaker because it keeps the heartbeat regular. Heartbeat is also controlled by the ANS.

Blood flows through the heart from veins to atria to ventricles and then out by arteries (see Figure 8.6). Heart valves limit flow to a single direction. One heartbeat, or cardiac cycle, includes atrial contraction and relaxation, ventricular contraction and relaxation, and a short pause. Normal cardiac cycles (at rest) take about 0.8 seconds. Blood from the body flows into the venae cavae, which empty into the right atrium. At the same time, oxygenated blood from the lungs flows from the pulmonary vein into the left atrium. Seventy percent of the blood from the atria passively flows into the ventricles, then the muscles of both atria contract, forcing additional blood through each AV valve.

Diastole is the filling of the ventricles with blood. Ventricular systole opens the SL valves, forcing blood out of the ventricles through the pulmonary artery and aorta. The sound of the heart contracting and the valves opening and closing produces a characteristic "lub-dub" sound. Lub is associated with closure of the AV valves; dub is the closing of the SL valves.

Human heartbeats originate from the SA node near the right atrium. Modified muscle cells contract, sending a signal to other muscle cells in the heart to contract. The signal spreads to the AV node, where it is relayed to cause the ventricles to contract simultaneously.

The two main routes for circulation are the pulmonary circuit (to and from the lungs) and the systemic circuit (to and from the body). Pulmonary arteries carry blood from the heart to the lungs. Pulmonary veins carry blood from the lungs to the heart. Blood in the pulmonary arteries is low in oxygen and high in carbon dioxide, whereas blood in the pulmonary veins is high in oxygen and low in carbon dioxide. In the lungs gas exchange occurs: oxygen diffuses into the blood, and carbon dioxide (a waste product of cellular metabolism) diffuses out of the blood. The *aorta* (carries blood from the heart to the body) is the main artery of the systemic circuit. The *venae cavae* (carry blood from the body to the heart) are the main veins of the systemic circuit. Coronary arteries deliver oxygenated blood, food, and so on to the heart.

Take Steps for a Healthy Heart Given how critical the heart is to the functioning of the circulatory system, it's important to take care of this vital muscle. The National Heart, Lung, and Blood Institute (2011) suggests some basic steps you can take to address your own heart health:

- Learn about the risk factors for heart disease and the symptoms of a heart attack.
- Eat heart-healthy foods.
- Be physically active on most days of the week.
- Stop smoking.
- Have your weight and waist measured.

As can be seen by the basic nature of these steps, it is helpful for your young students to develop healthy habits early in life to avoid some long-term health issues.

▪ Blood

Mammalian blood consists of a liquid (plasma) and a number of cellular and cell fragment components. *Plasma* is the liquid component of the blood. Plasma makes up about 55 percent of blood; cells and fragments make up about 45 percent of blood. Plasma is 90 percent water and 10 percent dissolved materials, including proteins, glucose, ions, hormones, and gases. Plasma also contains other nutrients, wastes, and salts. Proteins in the blood aid in transport of large organic molecules, such as cholesterol.

Red blood cells, also known as *erythrocytes*, are flattened, biconcave cells that carry oxygen. The molecule hemoglobin, which is part of red blood cells, makes it possible for the cell to carry oxygen. Mature erythrocytes lack a nucleus. They are small—four to six million cells are found in a cubic millimeter of blood—and each cell has 200 million hemoglobin molecules. Humans have a total of twenty-five trillion erythrocytes, which is about a third of all the cells in the body. Red blood cells are continuously manufactured in the red marrow of long bones, ribs, the skull, and vertebrae. The life of an erythrocyte is only 120 days, after which it is destroyed in the liver and spleen. Iron from hemoglobin is recovered and reused in erythrocyte synthesis. Each second, two million red blood cells are produced to replace those taken out of circulation.

White blood cells, also known as *leukocytes*, are larger than erythrocytes, have a nucleus, and lack hemoglobin. Leukocytes make up less than 1 percent of the blood's volume. They are made from stem cells in bone marrow and function in the cellular immune response. There are five types of leukocytes (neutrophils, eosinophils, basophils, lymphocytes, and monocytes—one form of which is the macrophage), each with a different role in the immune system. The functions of the various leukocytes include releasing histamine, an inflammatory chemical that dilates blood vessels and attracts other leukocytes to the inflamed site; producing antibodies to aid in protecting against infection; attacking and scavenging foreign proteins and bacteria, some fungi, viruses, parasitic worms, and antigen-antibody complexes; and moving out of the capillaries to fight infectious diseases in interstitial areas (regions between cells). Some leukocytes inactivate inflammatory chemicals that are released during allergic reactions and attack the antigen-antibody complexes involved in allergy attacks.

Platelets result from cell fragmentation and are involved in blood clotting. They carry chemicals essential to the blood clotting process. Platelets survive for ten days before being removed by the liver and spleen. There are 150,000 to 300,000 platelets in each milliliter of blood. Platelets adhere to tears in blood vessels to temporarily plug the gap until a series of chemical events causes blood to coagulate (clot) in the area. For most people, this clotting action is normal. However, a hemophiliac's blood cannot clot without treatment that includes proteins called clotting factors.

What Is High Blood Pressure? **High blood pressure** is an abnormal condition in which the force of the blood pushing against the sides of the arteries is consistently in the high range. Two numbers represent blood pressure. The higher (*systolic*) number, always listed first in a blood pressure reading, shows the pressure while the heart is beating. The lower (*diastolic*) number shows the pressure when the heart is resting between beats. Normal blood pressure for adults is less than 120 (systolic) over 80 (diastolic). A blood pressure reading equal to or higher than 140 over 90 is high, and a reading between 120–139/80–89 requires lifestyle modifications to reduce the risk of cardiovascular disease. High blood pressure can lead to stroke, heart attack, heart failure, and kidney failure (American Heart Association 2008).

▪ The Lymphatic System

Water and plasma are forced from the capillaries into intracellular spaces. This interstitial fluid transports materials between cells. Most of this fluid is collected in the capillaries of a secondary circulatory system called the *lymphatic system*. Fluid in this system is known as lymph. Lymph flows from small lymph capillaries into lymph vessels (which are similar to veins in that they have valves that prevent backflow) and is filtered through lymph nodes and lymph organs. Lymph nodes are small irregularly shaped masses that are clustered in the armpits, groin, and neck. Lymph nodes are critical for your body's immune response, and many of your immune reactions begin there. When you have an infection, your lymph nodes can get larger and feel tender or sore (U.S. Department of Health and Human Services 2011). Cells of the immune system line channels through the nodes and attack bacteria and viruses that are traveling in the lymph. Lymph is then returned to the cardiovascular system through the thoracic duct and right lymphatic duct.

The Digestive and Excretory Systems

The *digestive system* contains organs for breaking down food so it can be absorbed and used by cells. The digestive system is responsible for processing food and breaking it down into usable proteins, minerals, carbohydrates, fats, and other substances. Figure 8.7 illustrates the digestive system.

Digestion includes both mechanical and chemical processes. The mechanical processes include chewing food to reduce it to small particles, the churning action of the

stomach, and intestinal peristaltic (wavelike) action. Three chemical reactions take place during digestion: conversion of carbohydrates into the simple sugar glucose, breaking down of protein into amino acids, and conversion of fats into fatty acids and glycerol. These processes are accomplished by specific digestive enzymes.

The digestive process begins in your mouth, when you start eating. The salivary glands produce secretions that are mixed with the food. The saliva begins to break down starches into dextrin and maltose. Then, the chewed food goes down your esophagus to the stomach by means of peristalsis. This only takes a matter of seconds. The stomach contains gastric secretions that include chemicals such as hydrochloric acid and some enzymes, including pepsin. Pepsin breaks proteins into peptones and proteoses.

The food is churned in the stomach and enters the small intestine. The partially digested food (*chyme*) is gradually released through the pyloric sphincter into the upper small intestine, where the majority of chemical digestion occurs. Two intestinal enzymes are renin (found in children) and lipase; renin separates chyme into liquid and solid portions, and lipase acts on fat. The small intestine absorbs almost all the nutrients from the chyme into the bloodstream, leaving unusable residue and some water. This waste passes through the colon (or large intestine) to the rectum, and some of the water is absorbed by the body. The resulting solid waste, called feces, passes out of the body through the anal canal and the anus.

▪ How to Take Care of the Digestive System

Eating the proper foods is probably the best way to take care of your digestive system. That means not only eating the right foods (making sure you're eating enough fruits and vegetables and fiber), but also eating those foods in the appropriate quantities. It is beneficial for your digestive system if you follow a schedule when you eat. You don't have to eat the same foods at the same time every day, but following a fairly normal schedule can positively impact your digestive system. Drinking plenty of water is also very helpful, and any alcohol should be consumed in moderation.

Exercise is very beneficial for every system in the body, including the digestive system. Exercise can encourage peristalsis, the movement of the solid wastes through the intestines, for elimination. Also, a lack of physical activity may increase the risk of stomach cancer (National Institutes of Health 2009).

If you consistently or constantly have an upset stomach, like heartburn or constipation, a health care provider should be consulted to determine the cause. Although smoking is most often linked to heart disease and lung cancer, smoking can also cause detrimental effects to the digestive system (including the development of ulcers and gallstones) (NIH 2009).

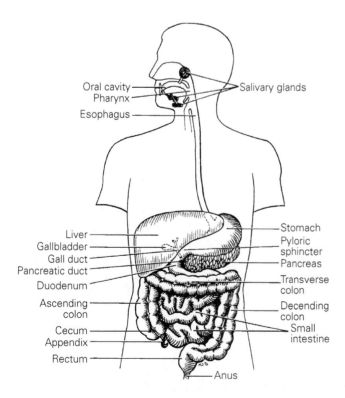

Oral cavity
Pharynx
Esophagus
Salivary glands

Liver
Gallbladder
Gall duct
Pancreatic duct
Duodenum
Ascending colon
Cecum
Appendix
Rectum

Stomach
Pyloric sphincter
Pancreas
Transverse colon
Decending colon
Small intestine
Anus

Figure 8.7
The Digestive System

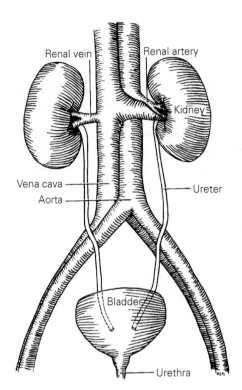

Figure 8.8
The Excretory System

The Kidneys

The *excretory system* includes the kidneys. The major function of the kidneys is to regulate the water content, electrolyte concentration, and acidity of the body by excreting each substance in an amount adequate to achieve balance and maintain normal concentrations in the extracellular fluid. The kidneys remove substances from blood and, sometimes, add substances to it. Also, the kidneys are responsible for the removal of metabolic waste products from the blood and the excretion of these wastes in the urine.

Nephrons, the microscopic functional units within kidneys, collect and filter waste products that have been delivered to the kidneys by the circulatory system through the renal artery, a major artery that leads directly from the aorta to each kidney. The ureters collect the filtered fluid (urine) and pass it to the urinary bladder, where it is stored and then excreted through the urethra (Figure 8.8).

The Skeletal and Muscular Systems

The body and all its organs and systems are given support, protection, and mobility by the skeletal and muscular systems. More than 200 bones make up the human skeleton, and the more than 600 muscles attached to these bones and extending across joints allow body movement and act as a protective covering. Red blood cells are produced in the long bones of the body and in such places as the sternum (breastbone) and pelvis (hip bones), shown in Figure 8.9.

Bones are composed of a porous, inner layer of spongy tissue surrounded by compact and hardened outer material. In infancy, bones are elastic, flexible, and soft. Through the maturation process and with the ingestion of vitamin D and minerals (primarily calcium and phosphorus), bones become more rigid and grow thicker and longer. Throughout life, regions of bones may become thicker and stronger or thinner and weaker, depending on various conditions, such as the degree to which the attached muscles are used. For example, a baseball pitcher may have thicker bone where the muscles most frequently used to throw the baseball are attached.

The skeletal and muscular systems give overall form and shape to the human body. A characteristic feature of humans is the upright walking posture, which relies on a

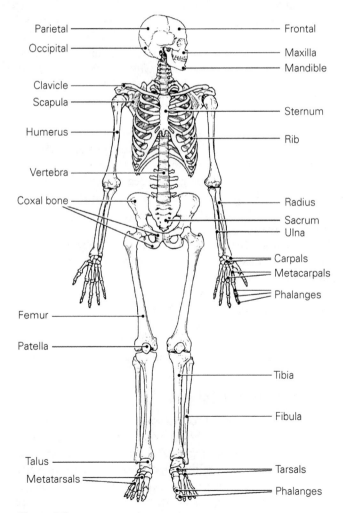

Figure 8.9
The Skeletal System

strong vertebral column and pelvis for support. Other major human bone structures are the skull, sternum and rib cage, pectoral girdle (shoulder), and limb bones (including the hands and feet).

The places where bones meet are called joints, the degree of mobility of which depends on the physical needs of the location of the joint. There are three broad structural categories of joints. **Synovial joints** have a fluid-filled cavity and are the most flexible type of joint. Examples of synovial joints include the hip and shoulder joints (*ball-and-socket joints*, which rotate through a wide range of motion), the junction of the skull with the top of the vertebral column, wrist and hand bones (*plane* or *condyloid joints*, in which bones slide across each other), and the elbow and knee joints (*hinge joints*, which allow motion in only one plane).

Cartilaginous joints have articulating surfaces that are covered with cartilage and permit a moderate amount of flexibility. The junctions between the ribs and vertebrae are an example of cartilaginous joints, as are the epiphyseal plates (cartilaginous growth regions that connect the ends of the long limb bones to the central shaft and that elongate and eventually convert to bone as a child reaches physical maturity).

Fibrous joints provide the least flexibility because the joints are joined together with fibrous tissue, such as that found between the teeth and their bony sockets. The sutures of the skull are fibrous joints. The sutures of the skull are relatively loose when a baby is born, which makes it easier for the baby to move through the birth canal, but the sutures will fuse together as the individual ages. Eventually, the skull plates function as a single unit to protect the brain.

▪ The Vertebral Column

Composed of thirty-three *vertebrae*, the vertebral column (spinal column or backbone) extends from the base of the head down to the hip region and allows bending, twisting, and turning motions of the upper body. Because the vertebrae encase the delicate spinal cord that conducts all nervous system messages to the brain, any injury along the spinal column is extremely serious and may lead to paralysis.

There are five divisions, or groupings, of bones in the spinal column. The first seven vertebrae are called the *cervical vertebrae* and comprise the neck. These are followed by twelve *thoracic vertebrae*, which support the upper trunk region. The five *lumbar vertebrae* extend to the waist and are followed by five fused *sacral vertebrae* in the lower back. The *coccyx*—four relatively small bones—marks the end of the spinal column and is commonly referred to as the *tailbone*. The cervical, thoracic, and lumbar vertebrae are more flexible structures than the sacral vertebrae and coccyx are because they are joined by separate disks of cartilage that cushion the impact of walking, running, jumping, and similar movements.

▪ The Skull

The human skull, situated above the vertebral column, includes the cranium and the bones of the face. The cranium is a group of sixteen large, flat, hard bones that form a domelike structure that surrounds and protects the brain. The *facial bones* provide protection for the eyes, nasal passages, and the cheeks. These bones also make up the hinged upper and lower jawbones, the maxilla and the mandible, respectively.

▪ Sternum and Rib Cage

The sternum is a thick, flat, elongated rigid bone that overlies the heart. Attached by cartilage to both the sternum in the front and the thoracic vertebrae in the back are ten pairs of ribs that form the *rib cage*. Two other pairs of ribs are attached to the thoracic vertebrae but are not attached to the sternum and are thus referred to as *floating ribs*. The rib cage and sternum protect the lungs and heart.

▪ The Pelvis

The pelvis is formed by connections of the sacral vertebrae and coccyx of the vertebral column with the hip bones in the side and front portions of the body. When joined together, these bones form a large, bowl-like structure. The pelvis helps to protect some of the organs of the reproductive system and the excretory system, as well as to support the upper part of the body and to stabilize leg motions during walking and running. The pelvis, with its ability to rotate, also aids in twisting, turning, and sitting motions.

▪ Bones of the Legs and Feet

Extending from each side of the hip is the upper leg bone, or *femur*. It is the largest bone in the body. The femur is attached at the knee to the shin (*tibia*), which is the largest bone in the lower leg. The knee is protected by a small bony kneecap, the *patella*. To the outward side of the tibia lies the *fibula*, the other lower leg bone. Because the leg bones are porous—they are made up mostly of spongy bone rather than compact bone—they are well adapted for supporting body weight and providing mobility. Heavier, solid bones would not be suitable for these functions.

The tibia and fibula are joined to the bones of the feet at the ankles, or *tarsals*. Extending from the tarsals are the five long bones of the upper foot, which are called the *metatarsals* and which are arched and joined to the fourteen bones of the toes, the *phalanges*. Because these bones are arched, they provide further support and stability for maintaining the body in an upright position.

Bones of the Arms and Hands

Joined to the flat, triangular shoulder blade (*scapula*) is the upper arm bone (*humerus*), which hangs below the collarbone (*clavicle*). The humerus attaches at the elbow to the *ulna*, the longer lower-arm bone, and the *radius*, the shorter lower-arm bone (on the thumb side). These bones in turn connect with eight wrist bones, or *carpal bones*, which provide flexibility and rotation for the hands. Attached to the carpals are the five *metacarpals* that form the palm of the hand. These are then joined to the fourteen phalanges, the bones of the fingers. Because of the multiple joints in the fingers, the hands are ideal for performing clutching and grasping motions.

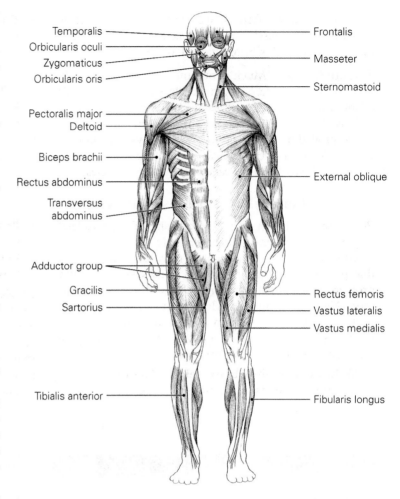

Figure 8.10
The Muscular System

The Muscles

The human body contains more than 650 individual muscles—most of which are attached to the skeleton—that make it possible for us to move around. In fact, the main function of the muscular system is motion. The muscular system consists of three different types of muscle: skeletal, cardiac, and smooth. Each of these different muscle types has the ability to contract, which allows for body movements and functions. Figure 8.10 shows many of the skeletal muscles of the muscular system.

Muscles can be involuntary or voluntary. The muscles that we control consciously are called the voluntary muscles, and the muscles that we cannot control consciously are the involuntary muscles. The heart (made largely of cardiac muscle) is an example of involuntary muscle. Some muscles, such as the muscles that cause blinking, can be controlled consciously or unconsciously.

Skeletal Muscle. Skeletal muscle makes up about 40 percent of an adult's body weight. It has stripelike markings, or striations. Skeletal muscles are composed of long muscle fibers that slide against each other during contractions. The nervous system controls the contraction of the muscle fibers. Many skeletal muscle contractions are automatic—for example, they help maintain body posture and keep the muscles toned and ready for voluntary contractions. Many actions of the muscles are consciously controlled, so skeletal muscle is often called voluntary muscle.

Cardiac Muscle. Cardiac muscle is found only in the heart. Cardiac muscle makes up the wall of the heart, called the myocardium. Like skeletal muscle, cardiac muscle is striated and contracts in much the same way that skeletal muscle does. However, cardiac muscle is different from other types

TEACHING TIP

Integrate health lessons about the body systems into other subject areas. During a math lesson have the students count the number of muscles in the human arm and leg and use this information in an addition, subtraction, or ratio problem.

of muscle because it forms branching fibers. Unlike skeletal muscle, cardiac muscle cells are attached to other cardiac muscle cells instead of being attached to a bone.

Smooth Muscle. Much of our internal organs are made up of smooth muscle. Smooth muscle is found in the walls of the urinary bladder, gallbladder, arteries, and veins as well as the digestive tract. Smooth muscle contractions are controlled by the autonomic nervous system and hormones. We cannot consciously control the smooth muscle, which is why they are called involuntary muscles.

▪ Care for the Skeletal and Muscular Systems

People often take for granted the health of their skeletal and muscular systems. Often it is only when people are faced with a broken bone, muscle tear, or a skin blemish that people think about these vital body systems. Health problems that affect bone, muscle, and skin are common (National Institutes of Health 2011). J. M. Hootman (2007) suggests that many potential musculoskeletal problems can be minimized or avoided through good general health practices. These practices include:

- **Maintain a healthy body weight**. This results in less stress on joints and muscles.

- **Engage in regular physical activity**. A well-rounded regimen of aerobic, flexibility, and muscle-strengthening activities is necessary for normal bone and joint health.

- **Don't smoke**. A nonsmoking lifestyle may be linked to lower rates of some musculoskeletal conditions (including low back pain, traumatic injury).

- **Protect yourself from injury**. Be aware of musculoskeletal disease risk factors associated with sports and occupational injuries, as well as general risk-taking behaviors (i.e., wear a helmet when riding a bicycle).

- **See your health care provider regularly**. Regular checkups can help recognize early symptoms of deteriorating musculoskeletal health. Early identification and treatment can potentially delay disability.

It's also important to eat properly to obtain vital nutrients the body needs to sustain musculoskeletal health. Eating appropriate amounts of protein, vitamin D, and calcium can help muscles and bones remain strong. Resistance training and stretching can help increase muscle strength and bone density and help keep muscles, tendons, and ligaments limber (Wittman 2011).

Chapter In Review

Summary

- Almost every individual begins life with a sound, healthy body that requires care and maintenance.

- Knowledge of body systems and how they interact with one another is important in building and promoting personal health and well-being.

- Each body system has special roles and functions that directly or indirectly affect all other body systems.

- The integumentary system includes skin, hair, and nails.

- The brain and nervous system receive messages from all other parts of the body and act to keep both an internal and external balance (homeostasis).

- The body's internal balance depends greatly on the release and regulation of hormones from the endocrine system, which strongly influences growth, development, and reproduction.

- Oxygen, essential to all cells, is channeled into the body by the respiratory system and delivered to all tissues through the actions of the circulatory system; carbon dioxide waste is removed along the same pathway.

- The circulatory system acts as a delivery and removal system for nutrients and wastes and works with the lymphatic system to mediate the immune response.

- Chemicals and nutrients are ingested as food, broken down, and made usable for cells and tissues by the digestive system.

- The excretory system removes wastes from the body.

- The skeletal and muscular systems provide physical shape and structure for the body, protect organs, and enable movement.

Discussion Questions

1. Compare the functions of the central and peripheral nervous systems, then compare the somatic and autonomic divisions of the peripheral nervous system.

2. How are the glands in the body dependent on the hypothalamus?

3. Explain the interactive functioning of the cerebrum, the cerebellum, and the brain stem.

4. Compare the functions of the atria and ventricles.

5. Describe the connection between the kidneys and the digestive system.

6. Compare voluntary and involuntary muscles.

Critical Thinking Questions

1. Explain the interaction of genetics, socioeconomic status, and illness with regard to their influences on personal health.

2. Using what you know about the nervous system, describe the connection between eye problems and learning.

3. Explain the interdependence among the muscular, skeletal, and nervous systems.

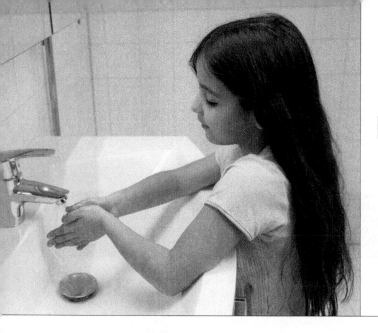

Personal Health

It is essential that personal health habits be learned at an early age.

Valued Outcomes

After completion of this chapter, you should be able to:

- Discuss the proper care of the skin, nails, and hair.

- Define *posture*, and explain its importance to personal health.

- Describe the function of the five major senses, and discuss their possible impairments and care.

- List the behavioral indications of vision and hearing problems.

- Describe how to maintain good dental health.

- Define *fitness*, and name its five components.

- Discuss the importance and appropriate amounts of physical activity, relaxation, and sleep for children.

- Discuss the *Healthy People 2020* objectives that are related to fitness and physical activity.

Reflections

There are several issues related to personal health that affect not only one's physical health, but also one's emotional health. As you read this chapter, reflect on the emotional aspects of personal health and how this can affect a student's capacity to learn.

Developing Good Habits Early

It is not enough to know about the structure and function of the human body. The human body must be given daily attention to ensure its continued performance. This attention is the responsibility of the individual. Thus, it is essential to learn personal health habits at an early age. Inattention to personal health practices in childhood has consequences in later life.

This chapter focuses on the areas of personal health that are considered the most crucial for the elementary school child. These areas include personal appearance, care of the senses, dental health, fitness, relaxation, and sleep; disease control and prevention are described for selected topics.

Personal Appearance

A multitude of factors can influence personal appearance, including genetics, socioeconomic status, illness, and so forth. However, in this section of the chapter, only care of the skin, care of the nails, care of the hair, and the importance of posture are discussed. Because of its far-reaching effects on almost all other areas of health, nutrition is presented in a separate chapter (Chapter 17).

▪ Skin

Skin is the outside covering of body tissue that protects inner cells and organs from the outside environment. The skin is the largest organ of the body, and its cells are continuously replaced as they are lost to normal wear and tear. The skin covers between 12 and 20 square feet in area and accounts for 12 percent of body weight. The outer two layers of skin are the **epidermis** (outermost layer of the skin) and the **dermis**. The thickness of the epidermis and the dermis varies over different parts of the body. These layers are thickest on the palms of the hands and feet, where friction is needed for gripping, and they are thinnest on the eyelids, which must be light and flexible. The layers also produce fingernails, toenails, and hair. The dermis, or inner layer of skin directly under the epidermis, is thick, sturdy, and rich in nerves, blood vessels, hair follicles, and sweat glands. It shields and repairs injured tissue. This layer consists mostly of **collagen**, which originates from cells called fibroblasts and is one of the strongest proteins found in nature. It gives skin its durability and resilience. Subcutaneous tissue lies beneath the dermis and contains **lipocytes**, cells which store lipids to form a fatty layer that cushions muscles, bones, and inner organs against shocks and acts as an insulator and source of energy during lean times. The skin registers sensation constantly and supports a teeming, unseen population of tiny organisms.

Skin Conditions and Diseases.

Acne. Acne is caused by inflammation of the oil glands in the skin and at the base of strands of hair. In the teenage years, hormones stimulate the growth of body hair, and the oil glands secrete more oil. The skin pores become clogged, and bacteria grow in the clogged pores. If a sebaceous gland becomes clogged, a whitehead appears; if the material oxidizes, it darkens to form a blackhead.

Body odor. One of the mechanisms the body has for cooling is the ability to perspire. Humans have two types of sweat glands. The first type is eccrine glands, which produce a clear, odorless sweat that appears all over our bodies and helps to regulate body temperature. The second type of sweat gland is apocrine glands, which produce a thicker sweat and are located in the underarm and groin areas. Proteins and lipids in the sweat produced by apocrine glands are metabolized by bacteria on the skin's surface, causing the rather distinct odor associated with body odor. Body odor can be particularly distinctive during adolescence because apocrine glands begin to function during puberty. The problem usually can be dealt with by washing with a deodorant soap, and washing clothes with deodorizing detergent. Deodorants or antiperspirants may be used to combat body odor. A body deodorant allows the person's sweat to release from the skin, but uses antiseptic agents (like those found in soaps) to kill odor-causing bacteria. Antiperspirants contain chemicals like aluminum that block the pores of the skin and prevent the perspiration from releasing. Some persons will have allergies to deodorants and/or antiperspirants.

Ringworm (tinea). Ringworm is an infection of the skin, hair, or nails. It gets its name from its appearance on the skin—it often looks like a ring-shaped rash. Ringworm is caused by several different types of fungi. Other names for ringworm include tinea, dermatophytosis, athlete's foot (ringworm of the feet), and jock itch (ringworm of the groin).

Make it clear to students that ringworm is not caused by a worm! People can get ringworm from other people, animals, or places. People can get it through contact with a person who has ringworm or by using items such as clothes, towels, or hairbrushes that were used by someone who has a ringworm infection. Animals can carry some types of fungi on their fur or skin without showing signs of ringworm infection. Sick or carrier animals can transmit fungi to people by direct or indirect contact. Places such as gyms, shower stalls, and floors can transmit the fungus if used by someone with ringworm. Other people can catch the fungus if exposed to these places. Ringworm is easily diagnosed and treated. A doctor can do some simple tests to determine whether a rash is caused by a fungus. Treatment is usually an antifungal cream, which is applied to the site of infection, or pills taken by mouth.

If you have ringworm, you can avoid spreading it to others by following your doctor's advice for proper treatment;

keeping your skin, hair, and nails clean and dry; washing towels and clothing in hot water and soap to destroy the fungus; and staying away from common areas such as community pools and gyms until your infection goes away.

Ringworm can be prevented by keeping common-use areas clean; using a floor and bath cleaner that contains a fungus-killing (fungicidal) agent; avoiding physical contact with a person or animal who has ringworm; and not sharing clothing, towels, hairbrushes, or other personal items.

Impetigo. Impetigo is a common skin infection in young children caused by streptococcal or staphylococcal bacteria. A rash appears four to ten days after exposure. The rash looks red and round and may be oozing. It can occur as small blisters that contain puslike material and that may break and form a flat, honey-colored crust. The rash is most commonly seen on the face and around the mouth but can occur any place on the skin and is often itchy. Impetigo is spread through direct contact with infected skin. Less commonly, it can be spread through touching articles (such as clothing, bedding, and towels) contaminated by the blisters. Topical treatments and/or antibiotics are available.

A person with impetigo should

- Wash the rash with soap and water and cover it loosely with gauze, a bandage, or clothing.
- Wash hands thoroughly, especially after touching an infected area of the body.
- Use separate towels and washcloths.
- Avoid contact with newborn babies.
- Be excluded from school or day care until twenty-four hours after the start of treatment.
- Avoid handling food until twenty-four hours after the start of treatment.

Pediculosis. Lice infestation, or pediculosis, arises when head or body lice—extremely small, parasitic insects—attach to hair shafts. They are passed from infested people through either direct contact or contact with an article of clothing or object used by the infested individual. The lice live and lay eggs in seams of clothing and suck blood from the skin. Lice were formerly responsible for the spread of typhus fever. Also, lice infestation is the major reason for physical inspections of schoolchildren during the earliest years of formal health education.

Itching results from the blood-sucking action of the lice, and a secondary infection may occur. Application of an appropriate insecticide can destroy the lice. To prevent widespread outbreaks, schoolchildren should be thoroughly inspected for lice.

Sunburn. People who have fair or light complexions do not have as much protective pigment in their skin as people who have darker skin do. Lighter-skinned people should not stay in the sun for extended periods because they are more vulnerable to sunburn than darker-skinned people are, but all people should avoid overexposure to the sun. Overexposure to the sun has been linked with skin cancer. (See Chapter 15 for more information about cancer, including skin cancer.) People who must be in the sun for a long time during work or exercise should cover the exposed areas of the skin with clothing or a good sunscreen. For best protection, sunscreen should be reapplied regularly.

> **Creativity in the Classroom**
>
> To help your students remember sun safety tips, as you mention each tip put on your sun hat, dab sun block on your nose, and slip on sunglasses and a long sleeve shirt.

Care of the Skin. Daily personal cleanliness is the best means of caring for the skin. Washing the hands, feet, and face a few times each day with warm water and soap helps remove dirt, bacteria, and oil. Although a daily shower or bath is not necessary, it is a good practice to encourage. Also, emphasize the need to wear proper clothing to suit temperature variations and to protect the skin. Be sure to provide instruction concerning general skin care principles as well as information about special needs. Different skin types may require different kinds of daily care; for example, people who have oily skin may need to clean their faces and wash their hair more often than people with dry skin do. Allergic skin reactions to certain soaps, lotions, or creams may result, so nonallergenic preparations may be necessary. In the event a problem arises, children need to know that a dermatologist is a physician who specializes in care of the skin and skin disorders.

▪ Fingernails and Toenails

Nails grow from the epidermal layers of the matrix (nail base). As older cells grow out and are replaced by newer ones, they are compacted and take on a dead and hardened (keratinized) form that can be cut painlessly. The average growth rate for nails is 0.1 mm each day, but individual rates depend on age, time of year, activity level, and heredity. Disease, hormone imbalance, and the aging process also affect nail growth. Fingernails grow faster than toenails do. Nails grow more rapidly in the summer than in the winter. Nails on a person's dominant hand (right versus left) usually grow faster, and men's nails grow more quickly than women's do, except possibly during pregnancy and old age (American Academy of Dermatology 2011).

Cuticles—softer than nails but nevertheless hardened skin tissue—surround fingernails and toenails and sometimes break or crack because little oil reaches them. Both the nails and cuticles protect the fingers and toes.

Care of the Nails. Because of their exposed location, nails take a lot of abuse. Nail disorders comprise about 10 percent of all skin conditions. Most of us, at one time or another, have closed fingers in doors, suffered from ingrown toenails, or endured minor nail infections. Most minor nail injuries heal on their own, although they may be unsightly for a while due to the nail's slow growth rate. More serious injuries or disorders may require professional treatment. Symptoms that could signal nail (or other health) problems include color or shape changes, swelling of the skin around the nails, and pain. Additionally, the persistence of white or black lines, dents, or ridges in the nail should be reported to a dermatologist.

White spots on the nails are very common and usually recur. These small spots result from injury to the matrix of the nail, where nail cells are produced. They typically are not a cause for concern and will eventually grow out.

Nail biting is a common problem, especially among young children. Although the habit typically disappears with age, it has been linked to anxiety with older children and adults. Nail biting not only ruins the look of the nails, but also is a good way to transfer infectious organisms from the fingers to the mouth and vice versa. Nail biting can also damage the skin surrounding the nails, allowing infections to enter and spread. Some nail-biters are cured by applying bad-tasting nail polishes or liquids to the nail.

Many nail problems are due to poor nail care. To maintain nail health, keep nails clean and dry to keep bacteria and other infectious organisms from collecting under the nails; cut nails straight across with only slight rounding at the tip; use a fine-textured file to keep nails free of snags; and avoid nail-biting. Ingrown toenails should not be "dug out," especially if they are sore; instead, a physician should provide treatment. Nail changes, swelling, and pain can signal serious problems that should be reported to a health care provider (MedicineNet.com 2011).

Hair

Hair grows on almost all regions of our bodies. Males and females have the same amount of hair in the concentrated areas (such as under the arm and on the scalp), but they differ in the amount of hair on other parts of the body (such as the face). Hair growth, color, and coarseness are determined by heredity and pigment. People who have less pigment usually develop blonde or light brown hair, while those who have the most pigment have black hair. Red hair typically has the coarsest texture, while blonde hair is the least coarse.

Like the nails, hair is an outgrowth of the skin itself. It originates from hair follicles in the dermis. The hair root within the follicle is composed of living cells that are nourished by blood vessels. As a result, removal of hair by its roots is painful. However, as is the case with nails, the visible hair shafts themselves are dead, keratinized tissue that can be cut painlessly. Hair shafts on the head grow from about two to six inches before they begin to fall out naturally when combed or brushed. Except in cases of inherited male pattern baldness, rare illness, or as a result of some forms of chemotherapy, hair that falls out is continually being replaced.

Hair serves a protective role. Hair on the head guards against excessive exposure of the underlying scalp to solar radiation, as does body hair to some degree. Denser growths of hair also act as a covering that helps regulate body temperature—a tremendous amount of body heat is lost when the head is uncovered in cold temperatures. The eyelashes shield the eyes from dust and other irritants.

Care of the Hair. Hair need not be washed or shampooed daily. Sebum, or oil, comes to the surface of the scalp through the hair follicle. Some people secrete more sebum than others do and therefore should wash their hair more often. Hair should not be washed with extremely hot water, because this makes hair dry and brittle. Hair should be cleaned often and brushed or combed regularly.

Avoid unnecessary combing, teasing, bleaching, and heat exposure. Because dull, brittle hair, like the nails, may be a signal of underlying health problems, pay close attention to changes in its growth patterns and texture.

Posture

Posture is more than just standing or sitting straight up. The term **posture** refers to graceful, efficient movement of the body, whether walking, standing, or performing any type of motion. All parts of the body should be used correctly to maintain balance. When a person has poor posture, the muscles, instead of the bones, bear the burden of the off-center weight, and the person becomes fatigued more quickly.

Poor posture may be caused by a number of problems, including weak muscles, chronic fatigue, bone deformities, and careless habits of walking, sitting, and standing. Because students spend so much time during the school day sitting at a desk, it is important to encourage the students to sit properly. Each desk should be at an appropriate height for the individual to allow both feet to touch the floor without straining. The seat of the desk should allow the knees to be higher than the hips are to remove stress from the lower back. The back of the chair should encourage the proper spinal curve when the child is seated. The tray of the desk should be slanted sufficiently so the student need not lean forward to write and read.

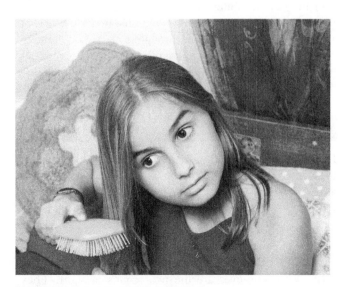

Hair should be brushed only when it is dry.

HEALTH HIGHLIGHT | **Make Vision a Health Priority**

The CDC and the National Eye Institute are encouraging all Americans to make vision a health priority. The loss of vision is associated with falls, depression, social isolation, and overall poorer health. People with vision loss may have difficulties with activities such as reading, meal preparation, and driving a car, which can compromise quality of life (CDC 2011). According to the CDC:

- Vision impairment becomes more common as people age.
- Women, minority groups, and people with chronic diseases like diabetes may be at higher risk for vision impairment.
- While some eye conditions (cataract, glaucoma, diabetic retinopathy, and age-related macular degeneration) can cause vision loss and even blindness, other problems can be easily corrected with glasses or contact lenses.

Eye Care

Many common vision problems and eye diseases have no early warning signs. Visiting an eye care professional for a comprehensive exam can help identify future problems and possibly correct current vision issues. Early detection, timely treatment, and appropriate follow-up may prevent vision loss and blindness. People with certain diseases, such as those with diabetes, may need more frequent and comprehensive eye exams.

Protect Your Vision

1. Get a comprehensive dilated eye exam.
2. Know your family's eye health history.
3. Eat right to protect your sight— particularly dark leafy greens and fish high in omega-3 fatty acids.
4. Maintain a healthy weight.
5. Wear protective eyewear when playing sports or doing activities around the home.
6. Quit smoking or never start.
7. Wear sunglasses that block out 99 to 100 percent of both UV-A and UV-B radiation.
8. Clean your hands and your contact lenses properly to avoid the risk of infection.

Source: Centers for Disease Control and Prevention. May 17, 2010. *Your Eyes are the Windows to Your Health: Schedule an Eye Exam Today.* Available at: www.cdc.gov/Features/HealthyVision/

Posture can be positively influenced through proper nutrition for proper bone growth, exercise to tone the muscles, properly fitting clothing and shoes, well-designed furniture (including desks, chairs, and beds), lifting and carrying objects properly, and proper education.

Poor posture is most often seen in junior high and senior high school students who are self-conscious about height or breast development. However, some postural defects are skeletal in nature. For example, scoliosis, or curvature of the spine, may produce postural defects. Sometimes after an illness, injury, or infection, poor muscle tone may cause slouching or slumping. In most instances, however, these types of postural defects can be corrected under the care of an orthopedic surgeon either through surgery, body braces, various exercises, orthotic lifts in the shoes, or a combination of surgery and exercise. Ideally, these defects are discovered very early in life, when correction is much easier.

The Senses

By conveying a myriad of messages to the brain each day, the sensory organs keep us in touch with our physical and emotional environments. Five major senses keep us informed about the world around us. These are vision, hearing, touch, taste, and smell.

The Sense of Vision

The Eye. The eyes are the two organs of sight. They are located in the front upper part of the skull and consist of structures that focus an image onto the retina at the back of the eye; the retina is a network of nerves that converts this image into electrical impulses that are sent to the brain. The eyeball lies in pads of fat within the orbit, a bony socket that provides protection from injury. Each eyeball is moved by six delicate muscles, which are activated and coordinated by nerves in the brain stem.

The eyeball has a tough, outer coat called the **sclera**, or white part of the eye. The front, circular part of the eye is the **cornea** and is transparent. The cornea performs most of the light refraction (bending) that directs light toward the retina. Behind the cornea is a shallow chamber full of watery fluid, at the back of which is the **iris** (colored part) and the **pupil** (hole at the center of the iris). The pupil appears black, and its diameter changes in response to light intensity to control the amount of light that enters the eye. Immediately behind the iris and in contact with it is the crystalline **lens**, which contracts to alter its shape and permit fine focusing of an image on the retina. Behind the lens is the main cavity of the eye, filled with a clear gel. On the inside of the back of the eye is the **retina**, a structure of nerve tissue on which the images are focused by the cornea and the lens. The retina needs a constant supply of oxygen and sugar, which are supplied by a thin network of branching blood vessels just under it called the **choroid plexus**. The eyeball is sealed off from the outside by a flexible membrane called the **conjunctiva**, which is attached to the skin at the corners of the eye and forms the inner lining of the lids. The conjunctiva's primary function is to secrete mucus that protects the eyes from damage due to dryness.

Visual Defects. The retina functions similarly to film in a camera. If light is not perfectly focused on the retina, vision will be blurred.

Astigmatism. *Stigma* means "point." *Astigma* means "without a point." Astigmatism occurs when light entering the eye is "split" into two separate parts instead of focusing to one precise point on the retina. Astigmatism usually occurs because the eye's front window, the cornea, is irregularly curved. Symptoms of astigmatism include blurred vision, squinting, eyestrain, blurring of fine detail, and headache. Treatments of astigmatism may include use of corrective lenses (glasses or contact lenses) and/or refractive surgery.

Hyperopia (Farsightedness). To see clearly, light must enter the eye and come to a precise focus on the retina. Hyperopia occurs when light entering the eye is brought to a focus behind the retina. Generally most people are born farsighted, so hyperopia does not tend to develop later in life as nearsightedness often does. Symptoms of hyperopia include clearer far vision, blurred near vision, frontal headaches, and eyestrain with near work. Treatment includes glasses, contact lenses, or refractive surgery. Lenses used to correct hyperopia are called plus lenses; they are thickest in the center and get thinner toward the edge (convex lenses). These lenses "pull" the eye's focus forward until it falls directly on the retina, producing clear vision. Both glasses and contact lenses use this same optical design.

Myopia (Nearsightedness). Myopia occurs when light entering the eye is focused before it reaches the retina. Symptoms of myopia include blurred distance vision, clear near vision, squinting, and poorer night vision. Treatment includes glasses, corrective lenses, contact lenses, and refractive surgery. Lenses used to correct myopia are concave, so they are thinner in the center and thicker toward the edges in order to diverge the light before it enters the eye, focusing the image backward onto the retina.

Strabismus (Crossed Eyes). Strabismus results any time the eyes are not pointed at the same point in space. Strabismus is seen most commonly in children, where it represents a muscular misalignment between the eyes. (A total of twelve eye muscles are used to keep the eyes aligned with each other.) Contrary to popular belief, most children will not outgrow a crossed eye. In fact, more damage will usually result if treatment is not initiated early. Failure to treat a constantly crossed eye can lead to lazy eye, or poor vision in the affected eye (amblyopia). Crossed eyes that occur suddenly in adults usually result in double vision and should be promptly evaluated; they are most often the result of head injury, stroke, or aneurysm. Any form of crossed eyes should be evaluated by an eye health professional. A thorough vision examination can determine the proper diagnosis and treatment plan needed to ensure a good outcome.

Care of the Eyes. The eyes are among the most sensitive and delicate organs in the body. Because they work together, an injury, infection, or impairment to one eye may result in damage to the other. Therefore, any visual abnormality should be dealt with either by a physician or an optometrist.

In your instruction, emphasize individual responsibility for protecting the eyes from harmful chemicals such as dyes, bleaches, cleansing products, insecticides, and cosmetic irritants. Also stress the potential danger of playing with objects that could penetrate or damage the eye, such as air rifles, fireworks, and slingshots. Teach children to keep dirty hands, fingers, and soiled materials away from the eyes and to alert adults to any eye discomfort or visual problem. Students should never self-medicate the eyes with drops, ointments, or creams.

Eye examinations should be given at birth, followed by additional testing around the age of five, during adolescence, and every two years thereafter. More frequent eye examinations may be needed after the age of forty because the aging process usually affects vision. In addition, eye examinations often uncover many underlying health problems such as diabetes, glaucoma, high blood pressure, and systemic infections.

The teacher should make adjustments in the classroom to help alleviate some problems of students who have poor vision. Have the students sit toward the front of the class so they can see the board more clearly. Some students might need a written handout if they have tremendous difficulty seeing the board.

▪ The Sense of Hearing

The sense of hearing greatly assists communication with others. It provides information about the environment in the form of sounds, both those that are innocuous and those that signal danger. The ears also contain structures that help an individual maintain a sense of balance.

The Ear. The ear is an organ for hearing and balance. It consists of three parts: the outer ear, the middle ear, and the inner ear. The outer and middle ear mostly collect and transmit sound. The inner ear converts sound waves to electrical (nervous) signals and contains an apparatus that maintains the body's balance. The outer ear is the part of the ear that is visible and is made of folds of skin and cartilage. It leads into the auditory canal, which is about one inch long in adults and is separated from the middle ear by the eardrum. The **eardrum** is a thin, fibrous circular membrane covered with a thin layer of skin; it vibrates in response to the changes in the air pressure that constitute sound. The middle ear is a small cavity that conducts sound from the eardrum to the inner ear by means of three tiny, linked, movable bones called **ossicles**. These are the smallest bones in the human body and are named for their shape: The **hammer (malleus)** connects the eardrum to the **anvil (incus)** with a broad joint; a very delicate joint connects the anvil to the **stirrup (stapes)**. The base of the stirrup fills the oval window, which leads to the inner ear. The inner ear (**labyrinth**) is a very delicate series of structures deep within the bones of the skull. The front (the **cochlea**) is a tube resembling a snail's shell and is concerned with hearing. The rear part (the **semicircular canals**) is concerned with balance.

Hearing Impairments. The inability to hear can arise from a variety of causes, including congenital defects, illness, and injury. The most common hearing disability is conductive hearing loss, which can occur for a variety of reasons and is characterized by some sort of blockage or structural defect in the auditory canal or middle ear that warps or muffles the vibrations. Some conditions of conductive deafness can be corrected, and most are amenable to treatment.

Care of the Ears. The ears should be protected from loud noises, blasts, or other environmental hazards that can cause damage to the eardrum or affect frequency detection. Teach children to recognize the dangers of inserting anything into their ears as well as the importance of informing an adult of any ear discomfort. Children who continually pull on their ears or seem to have trouble with balance and equilibrium should be referred to an otologist or an otolaryngologist, physicians specializing in care of the ears. Hearing tests should be administered at the preschool level as well as periodically throughout the school years.

Pay close attention to children who seem inattentive or unresponsive; these behaviors may signal hearing impairment rather than intellectual or emotional difficulties. The teacher should watch students for the following indications of hearing problems:

- Chronic nose and throat trouble
- Runny ear
- Complaints of pressure, ringing, or buzzing in the ear
- Frowning when trying to listen
- Leaning forward or turning the head while listening
- Good written work, but poor oral work

The best thing to do for a child who has hearing loss is to detect the condition early and get medical attention. In the classroom, the teacher should place the child near the front of the room, look directly at the student, and speak clearly and slowly. Provide the student with a written handout to help the student keep up with any lesson that is presented orally. For more information about accommodating hearing-impaired children in the classroom, go to the book website (www.pearsonhighered.com/anspaugh).

The Sense of Touch

Numerous sensory receptor cells in the skin provide the body with the sensations of pain, heat, cold, and touch (pressure). A different type of sensory receptor cell detects each of these stimuli. Heat receptors obviously trigger sensations very different from those triggered by touch receptors, for example, even though all skin sensory cells send comparable signals through the central nervous system. The difference in sensations occurs because the message from each type of receptor cell is sent to a particular region of the brain. That is, heat receptors send electrical impulses to the heat centers in the brain, whereas touch receptors send their messages to the touch centers of the brain. Different areas of the skin vary in their degree of sensitivity, with the fingers being among the most sensitive due to the high concentration of receptor cells. The sense of touch arises when unequal pressure occurs between the skin and an object or material in contact with it. This unequal pressure produces a depression in the skin or moves hair follicles, and thus touch is perceived.

Care of the Sense of Touch. Problems associated with loss of sensation are neurological in nature and, as a result, are complex and varied. Therefore, very little can be done by the individual to affect the sense of touch. However, children should be aware of diminished sensation in any part of the body and should report such an occurrence.

The Senses of Taste and Smell

The senses of taste and smell are closely aligned because they each enhance and are enhanced by the other. These senses can affect health in many ways—for example, influencing choices of food.

Taste buds are the sensory receptor cells within the visible papillae, or bumps on the tongue. Hairlike projections on the taste buds are stimulated by food dissolving in saliva and send impulses to the brain from connecting nerves. The taste buds detect sweet, salty, bitter, and sour flavors as well as a flavor called umami, which pertains to glutamic salts such as monosodium glutamate (MSG). In addition, the tongue differentiates temperature as well as texture of foods, adding greater variety to the sense of taste.

Food is not easily tasted if nasal passages are blocked, as in the case of a head cold. Food in the mouth produces odors in the form of vapors that travel through the nasal passages, where they stimulate receptor cells in the upper nasal region. If the passages are blocked, the odors do not reach these cells, and the sense of taste/smell is diminished accordingly. Nerve endings attached to these cells join to form the olfactory nerve (first cranial nerve), the nerve that sends messages concerning smell to the cerebral cortex.

Care of the Senses of Taste and Smell. As with the sense of touch, not much can be done personally to maintain the senses of taste and smell. Impairment because of blockage of the nasal cavity due to colds or infection is temporary and will abate. Impairment due to nerve damage, although rare, cannot be reversed, so loss of taste and smell may be permanent.

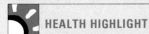

A comprehensive school physical activity program (CSPAP) coordinates physical education, physical activity during school, physical activity before and after school, staff involvement, and community involvement in order to allow students to take advantage of all opportunities for school-based physical activity. It is hoped that this approach will develop physically active students who engage in at least sixty minutes of daily physical activity. Students within a CSPAP are also expected to develop the knowledge, skills, and confidence to be physically active for a lifetime.

Physical education is the foundation of a CSPAP. A formal PE program provides standards-based instruction on motor/movement knowledge and skills, physical activity and fitness knowledge and skills, personal and social responsibility, and valuing physical activity for its many benefits. A properly coordinated CSPAP program will integrate various elements to allow students to maximize understanding, application, and practice of the knowledge and skills learned in PE. Students become physically educated and willing to take advantage of a variety of opportunities to practice and enjoy physical activity both within and outside of school.

A CSPAP is part of Coordinated School Health (CSH), a larger school health framework that encompasses health education, physical education, health services, mental health and social services, nutrition services, a healthy and safe environment, and family and community involvement. These are all elements to be considered with the implementation of a comprehensive school health program.

Source: American Alliance for Health, Physical Education, Recreation and Dance. April 2011. *Overview of a Comprehensive School Physical Activity Program.* Available at www.aahperd.org/letsmoveinschool/about/overview.cfm

Dental Health

Dental Problems

Most oral health problems are related to dental plaque. If plaque is not removed, it begins to harden and turn into a calcified mass that is known as tartar. Plaque interacts with the foods we eat and produces acids that erode enamel and cause tooth decay (caries). Tooth decay is one of the most common human diseases. Early loss of calcium is countered by the natural tendency of saliva (which is calcium rich) to replace calcium in the enamel.

The first indications of tooth decay are white spots on the enamel caused by the loss of calcium. Bacteria may invade the pulp of the tooth, causing a constant tooth pain, especially during the night. The bacteria may also produce an abscess, and eventually the tooth may need to be extracted by the dentist.

When dental plaque grows, it releases toxins that irritate the gums, causing gingivitis. If left untreated it may lead to a more serious form of gum disease (periodontitis). Long-term gingivitis can cause gum recession, which exposes tooth roots and makes teeth hypersensitive. Metabolic processes of plaque bacteria can produce organic compounds that are responsible for bad breath (halitosis). The tooth surface is susceptible to picking up stains from our diet (for example, tea) and habits (such as smoking) that cause discoloration. Problems related to the correct positioning of teeth are called orthodontic problems. These problems may be corrected by orthodontists and some dentists.

Care of the Teeth

Daily flossing and brushing of the teeth, preferably after each meal but at least once a day, is the best way to maintain good dental health. Flossing should be done before brushing because it removes plaque from between teeth, which can then be eliminated completely by the toothbrush. Flossing should be done using about 18 inches of floss wound around the middle fingers until only a few inches are left. The ends of the remaining floss section are then grasped between each thumb and forefinger and eased between the gum and tooth so that a scraping motion against the side of the tooth can occur. This procedure should be repeated with each tooth, using a new section of floss each time. Brushing removes plaque from tooth surfaces and is best accomplished by angling the brush against the gumline, applying a back-and-forth (side-to-side) motion using gentle strokes on the outside, inside, and biting surfaces of the teeth. Fluoridated toothpaste is recommended. Avoid brushing too hard; this may also cause gums to recede.

In addition to daily flossing and brushing, particular attention should be paid to diet. Avoidance of sweets is recommended, and the intake of foods high in vitamin D will help the child develop strong teeth. Regular dental examinations, preferably twice a year, from childhood throughout adulthood will also do much to ensure good dental health.

Fitness, Relaxation, and Sleep

Fitness

Today, there is a growing emphasis on looking good, feeling well, and living longer. Substantial health benefits are gained by following basic guidelines for recommended physical activity. Children and adolescents (ages six through seventeen) should do one hour (sixty minutes) or

| **HEALTH HIGHLIGHT** | **Appropriate Physical Activity for Pre-Adolescent Children** |

The following are the summary guidelines from the National Association for Pre-Adolescent Children:

- Children should accumulate at least sixty minutes, and up to several hours, of age-appropriate physical activity on all or most days of the week.
- Children should participate in several bouts of physical activity lasting fifteen minutes or more each day.

- Children should participate each day in a variety of age-appropriate physical activities designed to achieve optimal health, wellness, fitness, and performance benefits.
- Extended periods (periods of two hours or more) of inactivity are discouraged for children, especially during the daytime hours.
- Expose youngsters to a wide variety of physical activities.

- Teach physical skills to help maintain lifetime health and fitness.
- Encourage self-monitoring so youngsters can see how active they are and set their own goals.
- Individualize intensity of activities.
- Focus feedback on the process of doing your best rather than on product.
- Be active role models.

Source: NASPE 2006.

---

more of physical activity every day, and most of the hour should be either moderate- or vigorous-intensity aerobic physical activity; at least three days per week they should be participating in vigorous-intensity activity. They also should do muscle-strengthening and bone-strengthening activity at least three days per week (U.S. Department of Health and Human Services 2008). For all individuals, some activity is better than none. Physical activity is safe for almost everyone, and the health benefits of physical activity far outweigh the risks.

Fitness can be described as a condition that helps us look, feel, and do our best. More specifically, it is "…the ability to perform daily tasks vigorously and alertly, with energy left over for enjoying leisure-time activities and meeting emergency demands. It is the ability to endure, to bear up, to withstand stress, to carry on in circumstances where an unfit person could not continue, and is a major basis for good health and well-being" (President's Council on Physical Fitness and Sports 2002).

▪ Physical Activity in School

Physical activity that takes places within school hours or on school grounds can open up opportunities for all students to meet their daily and weekly goals for physical activity. Participating in the nationally-recommended sixty minutes of daily moderate- or vigorous-intensity physical activity can help prepare the brain for learning and aid in student concentration in the classroom. The American Alliance for Health, Physical Education, Recreation and Dance (AAHPERD 2001) recommends that schools encourage:

- Integration of physical activity into classroom lessons
- Physical activity breaks in the classroom
- Recess (at the elementary school level) and drop-in physical activity, e.g., after eating lunch (at the middle and high school levels)

There are many national programs available to help students reach their goals for daily physical activity. For example, the goal of the Let's Move in School program is to ensure that every school provides a comprehensive school physical activity program that will help children and adolescents develop the knowledge, skills, and confidence to be physically active for a lifetime (AAHPERD 2011).

▪ Relaxation

Relaxation is one of the body's most useful tools in combating fatigue, either physical or mental, or both. By learning how to relax during the day so that alert and conscious functioning continues, a person can reduce feelings of listlessness, tiredness, apathy, tension, and aches and pains.

Fatigue may be due solely to physical overexertion or to a drain of mental capabilities after engaging in such chores as reading, writing, problem solving, or studying in general. Fatigue can also be produced by adverse environmental conditions, such as improper ventilation or lighting, or by emotional stress.

Relaxation involves the releasing of physical and mental tension through varied and diverse means that can include doing nothing, meditating, watching television, listening to music, taking a hot bath, or relaxing the muscles with a massage. The ways in which an individual chooses to relax should be based on personal interests, environment, or setting, and comfort with the procedure or technique. Regardless of how it is achieved, relaxation needs to be

TEACHING TIP

Try integrating some physical activity and fitness lessons into normally sedentary classroom time. For example, create an age-appropriate math problem that asks students to measure and calculate their resting pulse, workout pulse, and recovery pulse.

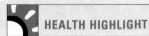 **HEALTH HIGHLIGHT** | *Healthy People 2020* **Objectives Related to Fitness and Physical Activity**

The following are *Healthy People 2020* objectives related to fitness and physical activity:

1. Reduce the proportion of adults who engage in no leisure-time physical activity by 10 percent.

2. Increase the proportion of adults who meet current federal physical activity guidelines for aerobic physical activity and for muscle-strengthening activity by 10 percent. This objective includes increasing the proportion of adults who engage in aerobic physical activity of at least moderate intensity for at least 150 minutes/week or of vigorous intensity for 75 minutes/week, or an equivalent combination, AND the proportion of adults who engage in aerobic physical activity of at least moderate intensity for more than 300 minutes/week or of vigorous intensity for more than 150 minutes/week, or an equivalent combination. Further, it includes increasing the proportion of adults who perform muscle-strengthening activities on two or more days of the week.

3. Increase the proportion of adolescents who meet current federal physical activity guidelines for aerobic physical activity and for muscle-strengthening activity by 10 percent.

4. Increase the proportion of the nation's public and private schools that require daily physical education for all students, with a 10 percent improvement.

5. Increase the proportion of adolescents who participate in daily school physical education by 10 percent.

6. Increase regularly scheduled elementary school recess in the United States by one state per year through 2020.

7. Increase the proportion of school districts that require or recommend elementary school recess for an appropriate period of time, with a 10 percent improvement.

8. Increase the proportion of children and adolescents who do not exceed recommended limits for screen (television) time by 10 percent.

   8.1 Increase the proportion of children aged zero to two years who view no television or videos on an average weekday.

   8.2 Increase the proportion of children and adolescents aged two years through 12th grade who view television, videos, or play video games for no more than two hours a day by 10 percent.

9. Increase the number of states with licensing regulations for physical activity provided in child care by one state per year. This includes activity programs providing large muscle or gross motor activity, development, and/or equipment.

10. Increase the proportion of the nation's public and private schools that provide access to their physical activity spaces and facilities for all persons outside of normal school hours (that is, before and after the school day, on weekends, and during summer and other vacations) by 10 percent.

11. Increase the proportion of physician office visits that include counseling or education related to physical activity, with a 10 percent improvement.

12. Increase the proportion of employed adults who have access to and participate in employer-based exercise facilities and exercise programs.

13. Increase the proportion of trips made by walking. This includes adults aged eighteen years and older and trips of one mile or less.

14. Increase the proportion of trips made by bicycling. This includes adults aged eighteen years and older, and trips of five miles or less.

15. Increase legislative policies for the built environment that enhance access to and availability of physical activity opportunities.

Source: U.S. Department of Health and Human Services. May 2011. Healthy People 2020: Physical Activity. Full text available at http://healthypeople.gov/2020/topicsobjectives2020/pdfs/PhysicalActivity.pdf

incorporated into every individual's lifestyle, just as exercise does, so the stress reaction can be minimized and personal health and well-being can be maximized.

Sleep

The body's need for sleep must be met consistently in order to maintain good health. Unlike exercise and relaxation, sleep is an involuntary process that does not require a planned or prescribed regimen that must be purposely enacted by the individual. In fact, scientists still cannot fully explain all the mysteries associated with sleep, including its cause and why it is needed.

Although individuals vary in the amount of sleep they need, the National Sleep Foundation has noted that the need for sleep changes with age. As shown in Table 9.1, children aged three to five years (preschool) typically require from eleven to thirteen hours sleep, whereas children aged five to twelve years (elementary and middle school) require from nine to eleven hours of sleep.

Table 9.1	**Recommended Hours of Sleep per Day**	
Infants	0–2 months	10.5–18 hours*
	2–12 months	14–15 hours*
Children	12–18 months	13–15 hours*
	18 months–3 years	12–14 hours*
	3–5 years	11–13 hours*
	5–12 years	9–11 hours
Adolescents		8.5–9.5 hours
Adults		7–9 hours

(*including naps)
Source: National Sleep Foundation 2007

Chapter In Review

Summary

- Almost every individual begins life with a sound, healthy body that requires care and maintenance.

- Personal health is of concern to everyone.

- Without good health, the quality of life is diminished considerably and day-to-day existence becomes a burden instead of a joy.

- To ensure good personal health, each individual must assume responsibility for taking care of his or her own body to keep it in good condition.

- Learning to maintain and enhance one's health and well-being in early childhood through sound health practices is crucial for sustaining high levels of personal health in later life.

- It is important to teach children the elements of personal health, including an appreciation for personal appearance, the senses that allow them to relate to their environments, and good dental health.

- Children must be taught to exert purposeful, conscious action in incorporating and integrating regular intervals of exercise, relaxation, and sleep into their living patterns.

Discussion Questions

1. Discuss the hazards of overexposing the skin to the sun.

2. Describe the proper posture while sitting at a desk, walking, bending, and lifting.

3. What are some methods that teachers can use to accommodate visually impaired or hearing-impaired students in the classroom?

4. Discuss the *Healthy People 2020* objectives that are related to fitness and physical activity.

Critical Thinking Questions

1. Explain the interaction of genetics, socioeconomic status, and illness with regard to their influence on personal health.

2. Describe the connection between eye problems and learning.

3. Explain the interdependence of the senses of taste and smell.

4. Why is sleep so important to elementary and middle school children?

5. How can lessons about personal health be integrated into other curricular areas, such as science, art, math, and physical education?

Access more material online at www.pearsonhighered.com/anspaugh. At this companion website for *Teaching Today's Health*, you'll find chapter quizzes, web links, flashcards, a glossary, additional Worksheets, and more to help you succeed.

10 Strategies for Teaching Body Systems and Personal Health

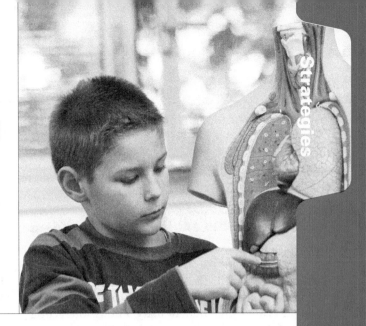

After completion of this chapter, you should be able to explain the following statements:

Valued Outcomes: Body Systems

- Daily care and maintenance of the human body and an understanding of how its systems operate serve as the foundation for personal health and well-being.

- The integumentary system is the first line of defense for the body and functions to help maintain body temperature.

- The nervous system receives, interprets, and sends messages that help direct and guide all other body systems.

- The endocrine system helps maintain balance among all body systems through the secretion of hormones.

- The reproductive system is activated in puberty and creates and perpetuates human life.

- The respiratory system provides the pathway and mechanics for oxygen to enter the body and carbon dioxide to leave it.

- The circulatory system, through the heart's pumping of blood, delivers oxygen and other essential chemicals to the body.

- The digestive and excretory systems break down food so that it can be used for all body processes. Substances that cannot be used are eliminated from the body as waste products.

- The skeletal/muscular system provides the body and its parts with shape, support, protection, and movement.

Valued Outcomes: Personal Health

- Adequate dental care and regular visits to health care professionals are important in maintaining personal health.

- Consistent, routinely scheduled, prescribed exercise programs promote personal health and well-being.

- Relaxation and sleep allow bodily processes and functions to renew their energy sources.

A sound, healthy body is the basis for optimal personal health and well-being.

NATIONAL HEALTH EDUCATION STANDARDS

1. Students will comprehend concepts related to health promotion and disease prevention to enhance health.

2. Students will demonstrate the ability to access valid information and products and services to enhance health.

3. Students will demonstrate the ability to use interpersonal communication skills to enhance health and avoid or reduce health risks.

4. Students will demonstrate the ability to use decision-making skills to enhance health.

5. Students will demonstrate the ability to practice health-enhancing behaviors and avoid or reduce risks.

6. Students will demonstrate the ability to advocate for personal, family, and community health.

Reflections

As you read through this chapter, consider the interaction of the several body systems. For example, how would it affect your sense of sight if your hearing were damaged? What precautions would you have to take if a part of your endocrine system was malfunctioning?

Planning Learning Activities

A sound, healthy body is the basis for optimal personal health and well-being. From the instant of birth and throughout life, an individual strives first to meet basic physiological needs. As a result, instruction about the function and care of the human body and its interacting systems is of the utmost importance to children, especially at the elementary school level. Learning opportunities should demonstrate and emphasize health practices that ensure maintenance of body systems so that students develop positive health habits that will enhance their physiological growth and development.

Because children generally enjoy and are interested in participating in physical activity and discovering the unseen mysteries of their own body actions, teaching about body systems should be an exhilarating and challenging experience for you. Throughout instruction, students should be made aware of the interrelationships between all body systems and should develop a sense of ownership with regard to their own bodies so that personal commitment to their upkeep is fostered.

Teaching the Concepts of Body Systems and of Personal Health

Health education was formerly limited to hygienic practices. Since those days, health education has branched out to include concepts from sociology, psychology, and other disciplines. However, we must not overlook the importance of teaching children about taking care of their bodies. In teaching personal health, emphasize to your students that enhancing well-being is largely an individual responsibility. The concept of personal health is an abstract idea that young children need to learn; yet many of the practices associated with health maintenance are already familiar to children and can be used as a base for building understanding of the concept. To do this, relate daily health practices to overall well-being. In this way, students will begin to see that discrete practices, such as face washing or tooth brushing, are components of an overall approach to optimum health. That is, a person does not wash simply to clean a part of the body, and tooth brushing and flossing are not done simply to help prevent tooth decay. Rather, these and other personal health practices are parts of an overall maintenance and health enhancement program. To bring this point home, note that personal body cleanliness plays an important role in the prevention of disease, just as proper dental care contributes to overall health. It is also important that students understand how the body works and why maintenance activities help ensure better overall physical health.

The strategies described in this chapter are designed not only to teach specific health practices, but also to foster good personal health habits. Knowing how to brush one's teeth properly is of little value unless tooth brushing and allied dental care are performed on a regular basis. For this to occur, students must personalize the information you present and make decisions to develop good habits. Continually emphasize that personal health is a matter of personal accountability.

Information Assessment Activities: Body Systems

Values Voting · Grades K–3

Valued Outcome: Students will be able to clarify values regarding activities related to personal health.

National Health Education Standards: 1, 4

Description of Strategy: The following questions can be posed by the instructor, with the students voting yes or no on each. Discussion should be allowed to interrupt the voting at any time.

How many of you...
  use good posture when you sit, stand, and walk?
  eat foods that lead to good health?
  get regular physical examinations?

Processing Question: What health habits most affect the health of your body systems?

✔ **Assessment:** Students can identify healthy habits and values.

Sun Safety Art Project · Grades: K–3

Valued Outcome: Student's will be able to list tips for protecting the skin while out in the sun.

National Health Education Standard: 1

Description of Strategy: After teaching a unit on sun safety, form the students into groups of three or four. Provide each group with a large poster board and markers. Each group will be asked to come up with four tips per group (and create a poster) for how to stay safe while exposed to sunlight. You may decide to remind students of standard sun safety tips before beginning the activity (limit time in the sun, use sunscreen, wear protective clothing, avoid tanning), or let them be creative with their safety recommendations.

TEACHING IN ACTION | **Daily Lesson Plan**

Lesson Title: Body Systems Position Statement

Date: January 29, 2012   **Time:** 1:00 P.M.   **Grade:** Five   **Teacher:** Baba

I. National Health Education Standards

Health Education Standard 8: Students will demonstrate the ability to advocate for personal, family, and community health.

II. National Health Education Standards Performance Indicator

8.5.1 express opinions and give accurate information about health issues.

III. Valued Outcomes

- Students will be able to identify each body system.
- Students will be able to explain the importance of each body system.
- Students will able to weigh the importance of one body system versus another.

IV. Description of Strategy

1. Divide the class into six groups, and assign one of the following body systems to each group: nervous system, endocrine system, respiratory system, circulatory system, digestive/excretory systems, and skeletal/muscular system.
2. Have each group research their body system. Students should identify the function and possible problems associated with the system. Finally, students should develop a five-minute statement that attempts to convince class members that the system is the most important body system.
3. After all groups have presented their statements, have the students vote (heads down, arms raised) to determine which system is the winner. Students cannot vote for their own body system.
4. Follow with a discussion asking if one system is really more important than the other body systems and how the systems affect each other. Explain why each of the body systems is needed to keep the body healthy.

V. Materials Needed

- none

VI. Formative Evaluation

Benchmarks

- Level 1: Student was able to identify some body systems.
- Level 2: Student was able to identify all body systems and describe some of their functions.
- Level 3: Student was able to identify all body systems and fully describe the function of each. Student was able to list some things that might go wrong if certain body systems are not properly functioning.
- Level 4: Student was able to identify all body systems and fully describe the function of each. Student was able to list things that might go wrong if each of the body systems was not properly functioning.

VII. Points of Emphasis

1. Explain the role that each body system plays in maintaining proper health.
2. Explain the importance of all body systems working together.
3. Explain what the students can do to ensure that each of their body systems stays healthy.

Teacher Evaluation

1. Keep the lesson as taught?   yes _____ no _____

2. What I need to improve _____

3. Next time make sure _____

4. Strengths of lesson _____

| **Daily Lesson Plan**

Lesson Title: Flossing Teeth

Date: January 22, 2012   **Time:** 11:00 A.M.   **Grade:** Two   **Teacher:** Coletta

I. National Health Education Standards

Health Education Standard 7: Students will demonstrate the ability to practice health-enhancing behaviors and avoid or reduce health risks.

II. National Health Education Standards Performance Indicator

7.2.1 demonstrate healthy practices and behaviors to maintain or improve personal health.

III. Valued Outcomes

- Students will be able to explain common dental problems.
- Students will be able to explain why flossing is important in the care of their teeth.
- Students will be able to demonstrate how to hold dental floss while pretending to floss their teeth.

IV. Description of Strategy

1. Show students pictures of healthy teeth. Explain and show pictures of common dental problems.
2. Describe how flossing teeth once each day can prevent many dental problems. Show students the different types of floss, let them handle the floss, and have them compare the flosses.
3. Explain the process of flossing and how it is important to keep gums and teeth healthy and to remove food that gets trapped between the teeth.
4. Give each student a piece of yarn, and have them compare yarn and dental floss.
5. Use a model to demonstrate proper flossing. Show students the proper way to wrap the yarn around their fingers, and have them pretend they are flossing their teeth. Remind students that an adult should supervise when they floss at home.

V. Materials Needed

- pictures of healthy and damaged teeth/gums
- different kinds of floss
- yarn cut into twelve- to fourteen-inch lengths

VI. Formative Evaluation

Benchmarks

- Level 1: Student was able to differentiate between healthy and damaged teeth.
- Level 2: Student was able to differentiate between healthy and damaged teeth. Student was able to identify some common dental problems.
- Level 3: Student was able to differentiate between healthy and damaged teeth. Student was able to identify common dental problems and explain how flossing is important in preventing these problems.
- Level 4: Student was able to differentiate between healthy and damaged teeth. Student was able to identify common dental problems. Student was able to explain and demonstrate how flossing is important in preventing these problems.

VII. Points of Emphasis

1. Explain the cause of most oral health problems.
2. Explain how neglecting care for teeth has a direct unhealthy impact on teeth and gums.
3. Explain how often to floss and the importance of proper flossing.

Teacher Evaluation

1. Keep the lesson as taught?   yes _____ no _____

2. What I need to improve _____

3. Next time make sure _____

4. Strengths of lesson _____

Materials Needed: poster board and markers for each group of students

Processing Question: What safe behaviors can each person practice while out in the sun, especially in the summer or at a pool or beach?

○ **Integration:** Art

✓ **Assessment:** After the lesson, each student will be able to list four "sun safety" tips.

Being Good to Me   Grades 3–5

Valued Outcome: Students will be able to discuss habits they perform to care for the body.

National Health Education Standard: 7

Description of Strategy: Have students work in small groups, and ask each group to list five routine things they do for themselves that they consider beneficial. Compare group lists to see how many items relate to care of the body. Then write on the board each item relating to body care, and ask the groups to rank them in terms of importance in maintaining body functioning. Follow with general discussion.

Processing Question: What are the most important personal health habits necessary to maintain proper body functioning?

✓ **Assessment:** Students can write five habits they use to enhance their personal health.

Rank-Ordering Health Practices   Grades 4–5

Valued Outcome: Students will be able to list in order of priority (rank-order) practices that affect each body system.

National Health Education Standards: 4, 7

Description of Strategy: Prepare a handout from the list below that lists each body system and three health practices that affect it. Ask students to rank the practices on a five-point scale according to the positive influence each practice has on that system, 1 being the most positive and 5 being most negative.

Examples:

Digestive/Excretory System	Skeletal/Muscular System
___ eating fresh fruits and vegetables	___ sitting and standing straight
___ eating foods high in fiber	___ getting plenty of exercise
___ limiting sweet snacks	___ relaxing during the day

In the class discussion that follows, indicate that all the practices are important but that some directly influence specific body systems more than others.

Materials Needed: paper and pencil, handout

Processing Question: What practices are significant in affecting the body systems?

✓ **Assessment:** Students can correctly rank the influences on the body systems.

Body Image Sentence Completion   Grades 4–5

Valued Outcome: Students will be able to complete sentences with their own thoughts about several statements related to body image.

National Health Education Standard: 4

Description of Strategy: Provide students with handouts containing incomplete statements such as those listed below. Have students complete the statements. Then have them share their answers with a partner.

My body is…

I like my body because…

I take good care of my body by…

The bones of my body are…

I help my muscles by…

When I breathe, I…

When I eat,…

Materials Needed: pencils, handouts

Processing Question: What do you feel are the strengths and weaknesses about your body shape?

✓ **Assessment:** Students can support their statements regarding their body shape.

Information Assessment Activities: Personal Health

Smiley/Sad Face   Grades K–2

Valued Outcome: Students will be able to differentiate between fitness activities they like and dislike.

National Health Education Standard: 4

Description of Strategy: Give your students cards that have a yellow "smiley face" on one side and a blue "sad face" on the other. Ask volunteer students to describe to the class an exercise they do for fun and fitness. After the student describes the exercise, have the other students hold up a smiley face if they would like to try that exercise, or a sad face if they would not. Explain that it is all right to have different preferences for exercises.

Materials Needed: cards for each student with a yellow smiley face on one side and a blue sad face on the other side

Processing Question: In what fitness activities do you most like to participate?

✓ **Assessment:** Students can name three forms of exercise they like or would like to try.

Good Health/Bad Health   Grades K–3

Valued Outcome: Students will be able to differentiate healthy from unhealthy behaviors.

National Health Education Standard: 7

Description of Strategy: Divide the class into small groups. Distribute magazines, glue, and scissors. Each group receives a sheet of paper divided in two. One part is headed "Good Health" and the other "Poor Health." Instruct the students to look through the magazines and find pictures that show people involved in healthy and unhealthy behaviors, and then paste the pictures under the appropriate heading. This is a team activity, and the students will have to discuss among themselves which heading would be appropriate for the behaviors.

Materials Needed: magazines, glue, paper, scissors

Processing Question: What variables make a behavior healthy or unhealthy?

✓ **Assessment:** Students can correctly identify behaviors as healthy and unhealthy.

Personal Health Voting   Grades K–5

Valued Outcome: Students will be able to clarify their values regarding personal health habits.

National Health Education Standards: 1, 4

Description of Strategy: Give each student a card that is green on one side and red on the other side. Explain to the students that the green is for "agree" and the red is for "disagree." Remember that there are no right or wrong answers. When you ask a question, the students hold up green cards if they agree with the question (or would answer yes) and hold up red cards if they disagree with the question (or would answer no). Ask the following questions:

How many of you . . .

would rather go to a birthday party than keep your dental appointment?

would encourage your brother or sister to clean his or her teeth?

it is funny to bump someone at the drinking tain?

feel that brushing your teeth is necessary to prevent cavities?

feel that eating snacks is harmful to your teeth?

would rather eat a sweet snack than fruit or a raw vegetable?

go to sleep when you are very tired without brushing your teeth?

Materials Needed: cards for each student with red on one side and green on the other

Processing Question: How important are personal health habits to you?

✓ **Assessment:** Students demonstrate awareness of their own values about dental health.

Exercise and Sleep Attitude Scale   Grades 3–5

Valued Outcome: Students will be able to clarify their attitudes toward exercise, relaxation, and sleep.

National Health Education Standards: 1, 4

Description of Strategy: Create a handout listing the following forced-choice attitude scale to discover the students' attitudes about the concepts of exercise, relaxation, and sleep. Tell students to choose Agree or Disagree.

	Agree	Disagree
1. Exercise makes me feel good.	____	____
2. Sleep is important to my health.	____	____
3. I take time during the day to do something I enjoy.	____	____
4. I sleep eight or nine hours a night.	____	____
5. Exercise can be fun.	____	____
6. Taking time during the day to do something enjoyable keeps me healthy.	____	____
7. My body can benefit from exercise all my life.	____	____
8. I often feel tired when I awake in the morning.	____	____

After students have completed the activity, have them share their answers in a large-group discussion.

Materials Needed: pencils, handout

Processing Question: How are sleep, relaxation, and exercise beneficial to you?

✓ **Assessment:** Students can name five ways that exercise, relaxation, and sleep are beneficial to personal health.

Dental Health/Self-Confidence　　Grades 3–5

Valued Outcome: Students will be able to differentiate between good and bad dental care.

National Health Education Standard: 7

Description of Strategy: On a piece of paper, have students make two columns, one with the heading "Good Dental Care" and the other with the heading "Bad Dental Care." Under each heading, the students should list different ways that dental care can affect self-confidence. Example:

Good Dental Care	**Bad Dental Care**
Smiles frequently	Negative self-image
Good first impression	Covers smile
Positive self-image	Poor first impression

This activity could be repeated with other personal health behaviors.

Materials Needed: paper and pencils

Processing Question: In what ways can practicing good dental health make you feel better about yourself?

✓ **Assessment:** Students can list at least two positive effects of good dental care and two negative effects of bad dental care.

Relaxation Ranking　　Grades 3–5

Valued Outcome: Students will be able to list ways to relax.

National Health Education Standard: 7

Description of Strategy: Prepare a list of ten ways people can relax during the day. Ask each student to rank-order the measures from most effective to least effective. Have students work in small groups, and indicate that each group must come to a consensus ranking. Record each group's ranking on the board and allow time for explanations, questions, and summarization.

Materials Needed: chalk, chalkboard, pencils, paper

Processing Question: What are the most effective ways to relax?

✓ **Assessment:** Students can list at least five ways to relax.

What Sleep Means to Me　　Grades 4–5

Valued Outcome: Students will be able to interpret the value of sleep.

National Health Education Standard: 1

Description of Strategy: Have students sketch or paint a picture showing their interpretation of the value of sleep. Have them write a statement about their picture, such as

I smile more when I get enough sleep.

I can run faster when I get my sleep regularly.

I am always tired, but I hate to go to bed.

I get sleepy in school when I stay up too late.

Materials Needed: crayons or paints, paper, pencils

Processing Question: How important is sleep to one's personal health?

○ **Integration:** Art

✓ **Assessment:** Students' interpretive statements express the value of sleep to their personal health.

Self-Portrait　　Grades 4–5

Valued Outcome: Students will be able to describe their strengths in narrative and pictorial form.

National Health Education Standard: 4

Description of Strategy: Provide large pieces of paper and crayons to each student. Ask the students to draw a picture of themselves. (This may best be done at home where a mirror is available and time constraints are removed.) On the reverse side, have students list what they perceive to be their positive attributes. Also have them describe the measures they take to promote personal health.

Materials Needed: large pieces of paper, crayons

Processing Question: What are your positive attributes?

✓ **Assessment:** Students can clearly illustrate their own strengths and weaknesses in pictorial form.

Personal Health Sentence Completion　　Grades 4–5

Valued Outcome: Students will be able to verbalize their feelings regarding several personal health habits.

National Health Education Standard: 4

Description of Strategy: Have students provide endings to statements such as the following:

I like the way I look because…

Sleep is…

I take care of my eyes by…

If I lost my sense of hearing,…

Sitting, standing, and walking with good posture help to…

Lack of exercise makes me…

Processing Question: How important do you think it is to take care of your personal health?

✓**Assessment:** Students can describe their feelings towards several personal health habits.

Decision Stories: Body Systems

Present decision stories such as the following to the class. (Follow the procedure discussed in Chapter 4, pages 60–62, for using the stories as a values clarification activity.)

For each of the decision stories, write a list on the board of ideas generated by the class for how each situation should be dealt with. Ask the students to discuss the merits of the methods suggested.

✓**Assessment for Decision Stories** Students can identify health-enhancing behaviors and exhibit positive decision-making skills.

Mary's Father   Grades K–3

Mary's father smokes cigarettes. Mary has just learned how important the heart and lungs are for the proper functioning of the body.

Focus Question: How can Mary tell her father about the bad effects on her father's and her own body from his smoking cigarettes?

National Health Education Standards: 5, 8

Rita's Dilemma   Grades 5–6

Rita comes from a large, loving family. She has three brothers and four sisters. Her family is poor, but her parents do the best they can. After studying about body systems in class, Rita is aware that it is important to have regular physical exams to make sure that the body is functioning properly. She is now in the fifth grade but hasn't seen a doctor since kindergarten. Rita knows her parents are having a hard time taking care of all the children. There never seems to be enough money to live on. Rita is feeling fine and has only missed one day of school this year (because of a cold).

Focus Question: Should she mention anything to her parents about getting a checkup?

National Health Education Standards: 7, 8

Decision Stories: Personal Health

Vision Problems   Grades K–2

Kathy is the youngest member in her family. She has two older brothers. Both her parents and her brothers wear eyeglasses. Kathy has felt sorry for them because she thinks that glasses make people look funny, and they seem to be such a nuisance. Her brothers can't run or play games as easily because their glasses are always falling off. Kathy has just found out that she needs glasses, too, and she is having trouble getting used to the idea.

You are a good friend of Kathy's. You have perfect vision and don't wear eyeglasses. You sense that Kathy is feeling sorry for herself and feeling jealous of your good vision.

Focus Question: What would you say to Kathy?

National Health Education Standards: 5, 8

Teeth and Truth   Grades K–2

It's been over a year since Danny has been to the dentist. Danny knows that his mother forgot about his regularly scheduled dental appointment because he answered the phone when the hygienist called to remind them about the appointment. He didn't tell his mother because he didn't want to go back, but, for the last few weeks, one area of Danny's mouth has been feeling funny every time he eats. Danny hates going to the dentist. He is also afraid that he will be punished if he tells his mother what he did.

Focus Question: What should Danny do? Why?

National Health Education Standards: 7, 8

Fitness Decision Story   Grades 3–5

You have been invited to spend the afternoon with two different friends. You like both friends equally. One friend wants to spend the afternoon playing his new video game. The other friend wants to go rollerblading in the park.

Focus Question: Which activity do you do, and why?

National Health Education Standards: 5, 7

The Christmas Party   Grades 4–5

Elizabeth's teacher has asked her to be in charge of the fifth-grade Christmas party in her classroom this year. This is really an honor for Elizabeth, and she wants to do everything just right—but Elizabeth cannot eat sugar, and most of the holiday treats are loaded with it. Elizabeth thought of maybe having a sugarless Christmas party, with lots of vegetables and dips and other foods without sugar, but she is really worried that the other students would turn up their noses at this idea. She certainly doesn't want the party to be a flop.

Focus Question: What do you think she should do?

National Health Education Standard: 5

Dramatizations: Body Systems

Have students dramatize different body systems as if they actually were the body system in question. Be creative in developing these activities. The following examples may be helpful.

Circulatory System   Grades 3–5

Valued Outcome: Students will identify the major organs of the circulatory system.

National Health Education Standard: 1

Description of Strategy: Introduce the organs of the circulatory system by showing an overhead transparency from an anatomy book and briefly describing what each one does. Divide the class by eye color and reassemble students in the form of the circulatory system of a person (lying down) using the different groups as different organs. Using red and blue beanbags to represent oxygenated and deoxygenated blood, respectively, start a rotation of the beanbags through the different groups or organs. During this process explain how each organ does its job. Rotate the groups until everyone has played all the organs of the circulatory system. Reassemble the students into their regular class formation, and ask questions about each organ and its function. Use the transparency as a guide. Make sure that everyone has answered at least one question.

Materials Needed: overhead transparency of circulatory system organs, red and blue beanbags

Processing Question: Do the organs of the circulatory system clean the blood that circulates through the human body?

○ **Integration:** Science

✓ **Assessment:** Students can correctly identify the organs of the circulatory system and their functions.

Source: South Carolina State University 2002

Digestive System   Grades 3–5

Valued Outcome: Students will identify the major organs of the digestive system.

National Health Education Standard: 1

Description of Strategy: Introduce the organs of the digestive system by showing an overhead transparency from an anatomy book and briefly describing what each organ does. Organize the class by birth months and reassemble students in the basic form of the digestive system, using the transparency as a reference. Use beanbags as food particles and start a progression of the food through the system. Start with the mouth group and instruct them to pass the food on to the next organ until the food exits the body. Ask questions of each group about what their job is in the digestion process. Rotate the groups until everyone has played all the organs of the digestive system. In closing, reassemble the students into their regular class formation, and ask questions about the separate organs and their functions. Use the transparency as a guide. Make sure that everyone has answered at least one question.

Materials Needed: overhead transparency of digestive system organs, beanbags

Processing Question: How would your life be different if your digestive system did not work properly?

○ **Integration:** Science

✓ **Assessment:** Students can correctly identify the organs of the digestive system and their functions.

Source: South Carolina State University 2002

Dramatizing the Circulatory System   Grades 4–5

Valued Outcome: Students will be able to describe the function of the circulatory system.

National Health Education Standard: 1

Description of Strategy: Students will dramatize how the heart and blood work together. Sixteen students will be required for this activity. Three students will represent the blood, four the valves, two the ventricles, two the atria, two the venae cavae, one the aorta, and one each for the pulmonary artery and pulmonary vein. Have the students stand in the proper position of a heart. Have the "blood" follow the proper path of blood through the heart's structure.

✓ **Assessment:** Students can accurately portray how the heart and blood work together.

Senses Activity   Grades 4–5

Valued Outcome: Through role-playing the students will have a better understanding of what a person without a sense or senses experiences.

National Health Education Standard: 1

Description of Strategy: Select two or three role-players by picking numbers. Describe a setting in which one of the players does not have one or two of the five senses. Give brief instructions on the situation (such as a blind person crossing a road) being reenacted in the skit. At the end of each skit, take five to ten minutes to discuss questions such as: What happened? Why did it turn out the way it did? Did it turn out the way you thought it would?

Processing Question: What important roles do the senses play in our lives?

✓ **Assessment:** Students can state how each of the five senses play important roles in daily human life.

Excretory System   Grades 4–5

Valued Outcome: Students will identify the major organs of the excretory system.

National Health Education Standard: 1

Description of Strategy: Introduce the organs of the excretory system by showing an overhead transparency from an anatomy book and briefly describing what each one does. Divide the class into groups by shirt color, and have the students form the excretory system by using the different groups as different organs. Use tightly sealed bottles of colored water to represent different liquids. During this time the teacher may ask questions of the different groups pertaining to their organ's operation or contribution to the system. Rotate the groups until everyone has played all the organs of the excretory system. In closing, reassemble the students into their regular class formation, and ask questions about the separate organs and their functions. Use the transparency as a guide. Make sure that everyone has answered at least one question.

Materials Needed: overhead transparency of excretory system, different colors of water in small sealed bottles

Processing Question: How do organs of the excretory system break down fluids into components that our body can consume and discard the rest in the form of waste?

○ **Integration:** Science

✓ **Assessment:** Students can correctly identify the organs of the excretory system and their functions.

Source: South Carolina State University 2002

The Nervous System   Grades 4–5

Valued Outcome: Students will be able to describe the function of the nervous system.

National Health Education Standard: 1

Description of Strategy: Tell students that they are going to act like the parts of the nervous system. Form the class into a circle, with each student standing an arm's length apart. Have them cup their hands in front of them to form a "mailbox." Drop a message in one student's hands and have that student pass the message along to the student to his or her right, and so on.

Explain that the students are acting as the sensory nerve pathways. Stop the message by tapping a student on the head. This student represents the brain. The "brain" then passes the message to the next student on his or her right, and so on. Explain that the students are acting as motor nerve pathways. Stop the message again by tapping a student on the head. This student represents an effector (muscle or gland). The student then reads the message, which gives a command such as to touch your toes or stand on one leg. Everyone follows the directions. Send additional messages, indicating that the class is functioning like the nerve pathways and brain of the nervous system.

Materials Needed: bits of paper for the nerve messages

Processing Question: What role does the nervous system play in helping our bodies function?

○ **Integration:** Science

✓ **Assessment:** Students can correctly identify the parts of the nervous system and their functions.

Inside-Out   Grades 4–5

Valued Outcome: Students will be able to illustrate, through creative writing, the functions of different body systems.

National Health Education Standard: 1

Description of Strategy: Divide the class into groups of five, and ask each group to write a fantasy play about a girl or boy who is able to travel through a human body, meeting different body systems along the way. You should serve as a resource, but avoid giving too much direction, thus stifling creativity. Have the students perform their plays, with one acting as the traveler and the others representing body systems or specific organs.

Materials Needed: paper, pencils

Processing Question: How are the body systems positioned in the body?

○ **Integration:** Writing, Science

✓ **Assessment:** Students' plays accurately describe the function of several different organs and body systems.

Dramatizations: Personal Health

Immunization   Grades 3–5

Valued Outcome: Students will be able to explain the importance of immunizations and will advocate getting needed immunizations.

National Health Education Standards: 1, 8

Description of Strategy: Read and discuss the story *The Berenstain Bears Go to the Doctor* by Stan and Jan Berenstain. This book describes Sister and Brother Bears' well-patient visit to the doctor. The reason for using this book is to describe what each student may have experienced when he or she went to the doctor for a well-patient visit and to explain what an immunization shot is. After reading the story, ask questions such as "Have you ever gone to the doctor when you were not sick?" Explain that this is called a well-patient visit. Also ask, "What did the doctor do when you went for a well-patient visit?" Possible responses include that the doctor listened to the student's heart and breathing; looked at eyes, ears, and throat; weighed or measured the student; gave a shot; or did blood work. Ask students why the doctor would give a shot to someone who wasn't sick. Explain that these types of shots are called "immunizations" and they help protect people from illnesses. Point out that people used to die of different illnesses, but now doctors immunize children so that they can never get these illnesses. Also mention that sometimes it takes more than one shot to protect against an illness. Have students role-play doctor visits. Provide them with doctor kits and let them role-play well-patient visits. Be sure they include immunizations as part of the visit. Explain that the exams they role-play will be done over clothing and that nobody should remove any clothing.

Materials Needed: *The Berenstain Bears Go to the Doctor* (Berenstain and Berenstain 1981a), toy doctor kits for students, a picture of a syringe or a child getting a shot

Processing Questions:

1. What immunizations have you had?
2. What does the word *immunization* mean?

○**Integration:** Reading, Science

✓ **Assessment:** Students can describe what an immunization is and how it works and can explain why immunizations are necessary.

Source: Health Strategies, Inc. 2002a

Tanning Booths   Grades 4–5

Valued Outcome: Students will be able to explain the hazards of tanning booths.

National Health Education Standard: 8

Description of Strategy: Instruct the students to work in small groups and write a script about tanning booths. One group could role-play a conversation between a potential customer and a tanning parlor attendant about the safety precautions practiced by the salon. Another group could enact a situation in which a customer fails to follow proper precautions in the tanning booth. A third group could role-play a person who seeks counsel from a dermatologist after several visits to the tanning booth.

Materials Needed: pencils and paper

Processing Questions:

1. What are the dangers to the skin and other body systems from exposure to tanning booths?
2. What are the proper precautions to follow when using tanning booths?

✓ **Assessment:** Students can list five hazards of tanning booths.

Wearing Braces   Grades 4–5

Valued Outcome: Students will be able to verbalize the benefits of wearing dental braces.

National Health Education Standard: 8

Description of Strategy: Have a student role-play the part of a parent who is trying to convince his or her child (another student) of the benefits of wearing dental braces. Another dramatization regarding braces could involve one student role-playing a child who wears braces to school for the first time and another student reacting to the braces with ridicule.

Processing Questions:

1. What are the benefits of wearing braces?
2. How can a person be prepared to handle ridicule from friends when he or she is wearing braces?

✓ **Assessment:** Students can list five benefits of wearing braces.

Discussion and Report Techniques: Body Systems

The Five Senses   Grades K–2

Valued Outcome: Students become familiar with the five senses.

National Health Education Standard: 1

Description of Strategy: Introduce the five senses by reading to the class one of the many excellent books available on the topic. Introduce each sense by pointing to the body part that accompanies it. Point to one body part at a time and, as a group, have the students say the sense that is related to that body part. Teach the word *sense*. Display large posters of the senses throughout the room while teaching this unit. Tell the students that this week, while learning about our senses, they will put together a book of senses to put in their portfolio and take home to their parents at the end of the week.

Materials Needed: book about the five senses, large posters of the senses

Processing Questions:

1. Which sense is involved in smelling a flower?
2. Which sense is involved in picking up a coin?
3. Which sense helps us watch the clouds?
4. Which sense helps us hear music?
5. Which sense helps us enjoy food?

✔ **Assessment:** Students can name the five senses and the body parts associated with each.

Source: Ezell 1992, 81

How Does the Heart Work?   Grades K–2

Valued Outcome: Students will understand the concept of circulation: Blood is pumped through tubes (blood vessels) through the body and back to the heart, and the heart beats faster when you exercise.

National Health Education Standard: 1

Description of Strategy: On the board or on chart paper, draw a picture of a train that has an engine and at least two cars. Draw tracks under the train, extending in both directions. Ask students to identify the picture and describe what a train does. Explain that a train's job is to transport. It picks up things at one place, carries them along a route, and delivers them to another place. Write the word *blood* on one train car. Ask the students, "How is the circulatory system like a railroad?" Tell them to imagine that the train is the blood. Encourage students to extend the analogy. The tracks are the blood vessels; the stations along the route are the heart, lungs, and body. The circulatory system carries and delivers blood to all parts of the body following a particular route, just as the train carries and delivers goods to stations along its route. Display a poster of heart anatomy (available from the American Heart Association). Explain that the blood follows a certain route each time it returns to the heart. Point to and name the four chambers of the heart as you describe the route that the blood travels: right atrium, right ventricle, lungs, left atrium, left ventricle, rest of body. Encourage students to say the names with you.

Then give students a handout that has a picture of the heart on it (see Worksheet 10.1 on page 482). Have them use the poster to help trace the route that the blood travels as it passes through the heart and label the parts of the heart. Ask students why oxygen is important. Ask them what carries oxygen all around the body. Also, ask them what happens to the heart if it needs more oxygen. Show the students how to place a stethoscope to listen to their own hearts. Then ask them to work with a partner to listen to each other's hearts. Have partners take turns using the stethoscope, counting the number of beats in one minute.

Have them listen to their own hearts, count the beats in one minute, and write the number down.

Next, have the students jump up and down for one minute. Have them listen to their own hearts, count the number of heartbeats in one minute, and write down the number.

Materials Needed: board or chart paper, drawing utensil, large picture of the heart anatomy, handout with a picture of the heart for each student, stethoscopes, clock or a watch with a timer

Processing Questions:

1. Why is oxygen important?
2. What happened to your heart rate when you exercised?
3. What happened to your heart rate when you ate or after walking?

○ **Integration:** Science, Math

✔ **Assessment:** Students demonstrate comprehension of the basic concepts of circulation.

Source: American Heart Association 1996, 39

Sense of Touch   Grades K–3

Valued Outcome: Students will identify different ways and reasons we use our sense of touch and describe how things feel using their sense of touch.

National Health Education Standard: 1

Description of Strategy: Introduce the sense of touch by walking around the room with a rock and having the students touch it and describe what they feel. Explain to the students that they are using one of their five senses, the sense of touch. Tell them that we use our skin and hands to touch objects. Read the book *Touching and Feeling* by Henry Pluckrose. This book tells about the different textures of things, how we sometimes use our sense of touch to send messages to others, and how blind people and puppies use their sense of touch to see. This book also gives descriptive words for things we touch.

Pass out an assortment of objects (such as cotton balls, sandpaper, apples, oranges, bananas, and marshmallows). Explain that you will choose students one at a time to describe what the object in front of them feels like when they touch it. Encourage them to use the descriptive words from the book. Collect the objects from the students. Tell them that the sense of touch is important to our daily lives. Explain that it is important for them to let someone know if they cannot feel something they touch because something may be wrong.

Materials Needed: *Touching and Feeling* (Pluckrose 1998), objects that have different textures, an example of Braille text

Processing Questions:

1. How do we use our sense of touch in daily life?
2. What are some words you might use to describe things we touch?

○ **Integration:** Reading

✓ **Assessment:** Students can describe five ways we use our sense of touch.

Learning about the Five Senses   Grades 2–3

Valued Outcome: Students will be able to identify situations that use the five senses.

National Health Education Standard: 1

Description of Strategy: In a group activity with the students sitting close together, discuss briefly the five senses: sound, sight, smell, taste, and touch. Students will go back to their seats and have a matching quiz. The quiz would be set up as follows.

Word Bank

sound   sight   smell   taste   touch

Fill in the Blank

1. When you look at a bird, you are using your sense of _____.
2. When you bite into a sour lemon, you are using your sense of _____.
3. When you feel the roughness of a tree, you are using your sense of _____.
4. When you listen to the beat of a drum, you are using your sense of _____.
5. When you identify the scent of a candle, you are using your sense of _____.

Materials Needed: matching quiz and pencils for each student

Processing Questions:

1. How many senses do humans have?
2. Can you use all of your senses at once?

✓ **Assessment:** Students can correctly fill in the matching quiz.

Identifying Leaves (Sight)   Grades 3–5

Valued Outcome: Students will be able to describe what their eyes are used for and how different life would be without sight.

National Health Education Standard: 1

Description of Strategy: The class will go outside, and each student will pick three different types of leaves off trees or bushes and bring them inside. When all the students get back in the classroom, have them spread out their leaves across their desks. Each student will then be blindfolded and will be asked to feel the leaves and try to find some differences between them. After a few minutes, the students will take off their blindfolds and, without looking at the leaves, write down the differences between the leaves. They will then look at each individual leaf and visually compare the differences between leaves. Students need to record on a piece of paper all of their comparisons and then present their observations to the rest of the class. After each student's presentation, ask him or her which experiment was easier to do: the one using their eyes or the one blindfolded? Record the answer of each student on a piece of paper.

Materials Needed: blindfold for each child, various leaves, pencils and paper

Processing Question: Why are our eyes important?

○ **Integration:** Science

✓ **Assessment:** Students can describe several ways their lives would be different without sight.

Source: Mace-Matluck and Hernandez 1993

Review of the Senses   Grades 3–5

Valued Outcomes: Students will be able to explain what the senses do and how they work together.

National Health Education Standard: 1

Description of Strategy: Name some things that you enjoy. Have the students give examples of what they enjoy. Show the class pictures that illustrate the senses and have students recall what senses are stimulated and how they work together. Divide the class into five groups. Give each group a piece of construction paper and assign each one a sense. Have the students draw or cut out pictures from magazines and then glue them on to the construction paper. Tell them to write captions about the pictures. Then have each group explain the senses related to each picture and state one way to care for and protect that sense.

Materials Needed: pictures illustrating the senses, magazines, five pieces of construction paper, markers, scissors, glue

Processing Questions:

1. How does each sense work?
2. How should you care for each of the senses?
3. How can you protect each sense?

○ **Integration:** Art

✓ **Assessment:** Students can accurately state the function of each of the senses and give several ideas of how the senses can be protected and cared for.

My Five Senses   Grades 3–5

Valued Outcome: Students will be able to describe how often they use their senses every day.

National Health Education Standard: 1

Description of Strategy: Begin by going outside to take a walk. Ask students to pick a partner to talk to about their experiences on the trip. (This will help them remember more details from their trip.) Walk for twenty minutes. After the walk, have the students brainstorm about their experiences with their partner on a piece of paper. Have students form into groups of four. Give each group seven minutes to brainstorm their ideas, then have each group describe one of their experiences to the rest of the class. Then have the students get back with their partners and identify the following from their original list: three experiences for sight, three for hearing, three for touch, three for smell, and three for taste. Provide magazines and scissors, and ask students to cut examples of people using their five senses from magazines or newspapers.

Materials Needed: pencils and paper, magazines, scissors

Processing Questions: Can you name something you do every day that uses each of the five senses?

✓ **Assessment:** Students can identify three experiences from their walk relevant to each of the five senses.

Source: Mace-Matluck and Hernandez 1993

Tracing Body Systems Grades 3–5

Valued Outcome: Students will identify, describe, and diagram parts of various body systems.

National Health Education Standard: 1

Description of Strategy: Students are divided into groups of four to five. Assign each group a body system (skeletal, digestive, respiratory, muscular, circulatory, and so on). Each group receives a six- to eight-foot piece of bulletin board paper. One student lies down on the paper while the other group members trace the outline of his or her body. Once the body is traced, the students work cooperatively to diagram their assigned body system. Groups may choose to draw directly on the paper or cut and paste parts individually. You can make this project as detailed as you wish. You may have the group write a report and/or have the students make a presentation explaining functions of individual and/or specific parts of the organ system to the rest of the class.

Materials Needed: six- to eight-foot pieces of bulletin board paper, scissors, markers, crayons, glue, white and colored paper, resource materials with diagrams for each system

Processing Question: Why is it important to know how the body's systems work together?

✓ **Assessment:** Students can demonstrate their understanding of the function of the assigned body system using correct terminology.

Effects of Smoking on the Lungs Grades 3–5

Valued Outcome: Students will discuss the negative effects of smoking cigarettes, especially the effects smoking has on the lungs.

National Health Education Standards: 1, 7

Description of Strategy: Discuss with students the effects of cigarette smoke on human lungs. Have students find statistics of smoking related to the human body. Show the students pictures of human lungs damaged by cigarette smoke and pictures of healthy human lungs of nonsmokers. Have the students work in small groups and make a list of positive and negative effects of smoking. Students then will discuss and compare their lists with the rest of the class.

Materials Needed: paper, pencils, resource material and statistics on smoking, pictures comparing lungs of a smoker and a nonsmoker

Processing Questions:

1. What is the job of our lungs?
2. What are the effects of smoking cigarettes?
3. What will happen to a person who smokes over a long period of time?

✓ **Assessment:** Students can list five negative effects on the body from smoking cigarettes.

Which Organ Am I? Grades 4–5

Valued Outcome: Students will be able to identify the different organs of the body.

National Health Education Standard: 1

Description of Strategy: Make large cards with the names of one organ printed on each. Distribute cards to several students and have them stand in front of the class wearing or holding their card. Have each student describe the job of his or her organ in the body. This activity could also be used for body systems rather than organs.

Materials Needed: large cards with names of one organ on each

Processing Question: What are the specific jobs of each body organ?

✓ **Assessment:** Students can correctly identify the organs of the body and describe their functions.

Tracing the Blood Flow Grades 4–5

Valued Outcomes: Students will be able to describe the path of blood through the heart, the parts of the heart, and how to care for the circulatory system.

National Health Education Standard: 1

Description of Strategy: Instruct the students on the path of blood through the heart. Provide them with a diagram of the heart, such as Worksheet 10.1 on page 482, to help them understand the pathway of the blood in the heart. On this worksheet, have students trace the pathway of blood and match the parts of the heart with the correct labels. Have students shade blue the sections of the heart that transport blood carrying carbon dioxide (deoxygenated blood) and shade red the sections of the heart that carry blood with a fresh supply of oxygen (oxygenated blood).

Materials Needed: Worksheet 10.1, red and blue pencils

Processing Questions:

1. What is the main job of the circulatory system?
2. What are the main components of the blood?
3. What are the main structures of the circulatory system?

✓ **Assessment:** Students can correctly complete the worksheet.

Muscular System Debate   Grades 4–5

Valued Outcome: Students will identify the importance of voluntary and involuntary muscles and be able to give examples of each kind of muscle.

National Health Education Standard: 1

Description of Strategy: Divide the class into two groups for a debate. One group will argue that voluntary muscles are the most important to the human body, and the other group will contend the involuntary muscles are most important. Each group should have several minutes to prepare arguments and should be able to support its argument with specific examples of a muscle and its function. After the debate, provide time for discussion.

Processing Question: How does the importance of voluntary muscles compare with involuntary muscles?

✓ **Assessment:** Students can give examples of involuntary and voluntary muscles and describe the functions of each type.

Voluntary Health Organization Panel   Grades 4–5

Valued Outcome: Students will identify organizational purposes and duties of such voluntary health organizations as the American Heart Association, the National Kidney Foundation, and the American Lung Association.

National Health Education Standard: 8

Description of Strategy: Invite representatives from several voluntary health organizations that deal with a specific organ or body system, such as the American Heart Association, National Kidney Association, and American Lung Association, to address the class. Their presentations should be geared to the age of the students and should include facts about each organization's founding, purpose, and projects. Use a panel discussion format.

Processing Question: How do voluntary health organizations help promote our health?

✓ **Assessment:** Students can accurately describe the function and role of the various health organizations.

Virtual Body   Grades 4–6

Valued Outcome: Students will be able to discuss each of the body systems' functions and to use various activities to demonstrate the different functions.

National Health Education Standard: 1

Description of Strategy: Assign groups of students an organ system, and have students explore the website for The Virtual Body (www.medtropolis.com/Vbody.asp). Based on what they learn, they will complete one group activity and make a presentation to the class. Each student in the group must have an equal part to do. For example, students could make clay models of a body system and explain what it does. They could also play a game like Jeopardy. If four students are in a group, then three group members could be the contestants and the other group member could be the host. When presentations are finished, have two different groups get together and test each other on what they learned about the other group's body system.

Materials Needed: computers with Internet access, list of materials as compiled by students

Processing Questions:

1. What is the purpose of the respiratory system?
2. What two organs are located in the digestive system?

✓ **Assessment:** Students can verbally demonstrate familiarity with the functions of the different body systems, using appropriate vocabulary and examples.

Source: MEDtropolis 2002

Discussion and Report Techniques: Personal Health

Presentation by Health Professionals   Grades K–5

Valued Outcome: Students will be able to identify the duties of various health professionals.

National Health Education Standard: 3

Description of Strategy: Invite various health professionals (such as a dentist, orthodontist, optometrist, ophthalmologist, or audiologist) to address the class, describe their occupation, and inform students about sound personal health practices.

Processing Question: How do health professionals help promote our health?

✓ **Assessment:** Students can accurately describe the roles of the various health professionals and their impact on personal health promotion.

Sleeping and Relaxing   Grades 3–5

Valued Outcome: Students will be able to describe how sleep and relaxing affects their personal health.

National Health Education Standard: 7

Description of Strategy: Describe what happens to the body during sleep—activity decreases, the muscles relax, and the heartbeat slows down. To illustrate this, have students count their own heartbeat. Then have them lie down and relax for ten minutes in complete silence. After ten minutes have passed, have the students count their heartbeat again. Discuss the difference between the two heart rates and how important rest and sleep are for the body. Explain that sleep restores energy that keeps their bodies healthy and helps control muscles. Explain how those who go without sleep can lose energy, be quick tempered, easily distracted, and make many mistakes. Finally, have students write a paragraph on how sleep affects their health.

Materials Needed: clock, pencils and paper for each student

Processing Questions:

1. Why is sleep necessary?
2. Describe what happens to the body if deprived of sleep.
3. What happens to the body during sleep?

✓ **Assessment:** Students can list five ways that sleep benefits their personal health.

Fitness for Life   Grades 3–5

Valued Outcome: Students will be able to explain the importance of a wellness lifestyle and will also be able to name some things they can do to develop this type of lifestyle.

National Health Education Standards: 7, 8

Description of Strategy: Talk to the students about how a healthy lifestyle will improve their lives. Give examples of how their diet affects their health and examples of how their exercise habits affect their health. Supply students with various craft materials. Have each student cut out a heart shape from red or pink poster board, write his or her name on it, and use yarn to tie the heart shape from

the center of the top wire on a wire clothes hanger. Have each student cut out a long rectangle that will hang directly from the bottom wire of the hanger. On this piece have students write "My Wellness Lifestyle." Students will cut shapes from remaining poster board. On each shape they will write what they can do to develop their wellness lifestyle (e.g., walking, eating fruits). Each student will share his or her mobile with the rest of the group and tell what options he or she used. When all students have shared, hang the mobiles in the classroom as a reminder of the things they can do to improve their health.

Materials Needed: wire clothes hangers, colored yarn, colored poster board (at least seven different colors, including red or pink), markers, scissors, hole punch

Processing Question: What behaviors can you incorporate into your lifestyle to improve your health?

○ **Integration:** Art

✓ **Assessment:** Students can demonstrate an appreciation of the benefits of a wellness lifestyle and can describe at least five effective ways to promote it.

Screening Procedures   Grades 4–5

Valued Outcome: Students will list and describe screening procedures used in school systems.

National Health Education Standard: 3

Description of Strategy: Prepare an outline of the various health screening procedures that are commonly used in school systems. Include screening measures that may not be available in your school but are used widely. Ask each student to choose one health screening procedure and write a report about it. Collect the reports and collate them into a health screening procedure booklet that can be used as a resource.

Materials Needed: outlines of health screening procedures to hand out to students

Processing Questions:

1. What health screening procedures are used in your school?
2. What occurs during each health screening procedure?

✓ **Assessment:** In their written reports, students demonstrate an understanding of the screening procedure, how to access it, and its importance in promoting health.

Experiments and Demonstrations: Body Systems

Properties of Skin   Grades K–3

Valued Outcome: Students will examine the skin of the foot and its properties.

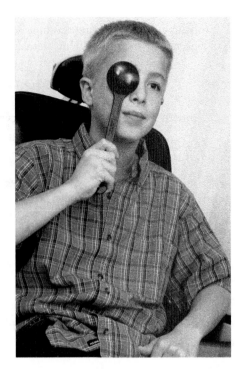

Periodic health screening will aid a child's ability to learn.

National Health Education Standard: 1

Description of Strategy: Ask students to take off both shoes and one sock so that one foot is bare and one is covered with a sock. Have them feel the difference between their skin and the sock covering the other foot. Let them notice that one foot feels cooler than the other does. Ask them to pull on the skin covering their foot and feel if some places are more sensitive than others.

Have each student trace his or her foot on a white sheet of paper and mark with a red marker which places are more sensitive. On the back of the paper, have each student write why they think one foot is cooler than the other.

Materials Needed: red markers, white paper, pencils

Processing Question: Why is it important to keep the hands and feet covered in cold weather?

✔ **Assessment:** Students can explain the benefits of covering their feet during cold weather.

Seeing Is Important   Grades K–5

Valued Outcome: Students will be able to analyze the importance of sight and experience blindness.

National Health Education Standard: 1

Description of Strategy: Explain the structure of the eye using a visual aid (model, poster, etc.). Pass out individual mirrors and have the students look at their eyes. Have students draw the color of their eyes. Have each student place the frames from a pair of glasses on their eyes and look at himself or herself in the mirror.

Discuss taking care of your eyes. How did it feel to wear glasses? Discuss eye exams. Discuss what it is like to be blind. Place the students in groups of two, in which one student wears a blindfold while the other student leads him or her around the classroom.

Materials Needed: an eye visual (model, poster, etc.), mirrors, paper, crayons or markers, eyeglass frames, blindfolds

Processing Question: If you were blind, how would your life be different?

✔ **Assessment:** Students can describe the importance of sight in their lives and can name several ways their lives would be different without sight.

Follow Your Nose   Grades K–5

Valued Outcome: Students will be able to describe the importance of smell.

National Health Education Standard: 1

Description of Strategy: Place three film containers on a table. Put a cotton ball that has a different scent in each container. Have the students smell each container. Students guess what each smell is by selecting the correct picture (e.g., lemon, cinnamon, or peppermint).

Materials Needed: film containers; cotton balls; scented extracts such as lemon, cinnamon, or peppermint; pictures of items the extracts are derived from

Processing Question: How does the nose help us smell?

✔ **Assessment:** Students can describe the sense of smell and its importance.

Body Drawings   Grades 3–5

Valued Outcome: Students will trace the outline of their bodies on a large sheet of paper and label the internal body systems. Students will weigh and measure their bodies.

National Health Education Standard: 1

Description of Strategy: Have the students work in pairs, and have the first student trace around the second student's body while the second student is lying down on a large sheet of paper. Then switch and repeat the process. Each student may then draw and label the internal body systems. On the reverse side, have the students list at least two reasons why each body system is important to general health. You may also wish to weigh and measure the students, and let them use the body drawings to keep up with these measurements throughout the school year. Tack the completed body drawings on the wall, interspersing body parts side of some with the written side of others.

Materials Needed: butcher paper, markers, scale, measuring tapes, pencils

Processing Questions:

1. How is body weight determined?
2. How tall is each individual?
3. What is the relative significance of each body system?

✔ **Assessment:** Students demonstrate awareness of their weight and height. Students can correctly list two ways each body system contributes to their health.

Bone Transformation   Grades 4–5

Valued Outcome: Students will familiarize themselves with the bones and how they function.

National Health Education Standard: 1

Description of Strategy: To begin this activity, discuss the shapes of the bones and the purpose of those shapes, using model bones. Hand out a copy of a drawing of a bone to each student, and have students cut it out and place it in any position on a piece of paper. Working in groups of three or four, have the students discuss and list many different and unusual things bones could become. Each student illustrates a bone development or bone growth on his or her own piece of paper. When the students are done with their transformations, have them discuss and share them with the class.

Materials Needed: model bones, copies of a drawing of a bone for each student, pencils, crayons, drawing paper

Processing Questions:

1. Why do bones have to be certain shapes to perform their functions?
2. Why is the shape of the bone important?

✔ **Assessment:** Students demonstrate an understanding of how bones function in the human body.

Brain Viewing   Grades 4–5

Valued Outcome: Students will compare the parts of an animal brain to that of a human brain.

National Health Education Standard: 1

Description of Strategy: Obtain the brain of a sheep or cow. Have students compare the parts of the animal brain to those of a human brain, using a model of the human brain for the comparison. Contact a local farmer or a butcher to obtain the brain of a sheep and/or a cow.

Materials Needed: sheep or cow brain, model of human brain

Processing Question: Compare the animal's brain to the human brain with regard to size and shape.

◯ **Integration:** Science

✔ **Assessment:** Students can make accurate comparisons between the brain of a human and the brain of an animal.

Nerve Messages   Grades 4–5

Valued Outcome: Students will demonstrate how nerve impulses work.

National Health Education Standard: 1

Description of Strategy: Have students rub their finger across coarse sandpaper, then explain how the nerves in the fingers send messages to the brain and the limbs.

Materials Needed: sandpaper

Processing Question: How does the nerve send messages to the brain and then to the limbs?

◯ **Integration:** Science

✔ **Assessment:** Students can describe how nerve impulses work using appropriate vocabulary.

Joint Experiment   Grades 4–5

Valued Outcome: Students will be able to differentiate between the types of joints in the skeletal system.

National Health Education Standard: 1

Description of Strategy: This will introduce joints into the lesson. There will be six stations that will be completed in order. Each station has a simple experiment and questions.

Station 1: Hinge joints—Have the students open and close the classroom door or a closet door. They must watch the hinges closely. Have them name a part of their body that moves like a hinge.

Station 2: Ball-and-socket joints—Have the students hold a tennis ball against the concave bottom rim of a cup (or even the top rim as long as the cup has a smaller diameter than the ball). Rotate the cup over the ball's surface. Have them name a part of their body that works like a ball-and-socket joint.

Station 3: Gliding joints—There will be a zipper at this station (at least twelve to eighteen inches long). Have the students bend the zipper and move it in curving patterns. (Do not unzip the zipper.) A gliding joint works with several bones bending together. Have them name a gliding joint area.

Station 4: Pivot joints—A globe will be at this station. Instruct the students to spin the globe. A pivot joint rotates around an axis. Can the students think of an area of their body that pivots?

Station 5: Fixed joints—This station will have two pieces of paper glued together. These papers do not move or slide. There are bones in our body that do not move; they are fixed in one place. Have the students name one.

Station 6: No joints—Have the students walk without bending their legs. Have them write their names without bending their fingers. What other things would be hard to do without joints?

Materials Needed: access to a hinged door, cup, tennis ball, zipper, globe, paper glued together

Processing Question: What would happen to our bodies if we didn't have joints?

○ **Integration:** Science

✓ **Assessment:** Students can differentiate between the five different joint types and give examples of body parts that use each of these joints.

Source: Calvert County Public Schools 2002

Ears Help Us Hear   Grades 4–5

Valued Outcome: Students will be able to explain the importance of hearing.

National Health Education Standard: 1

Description of Strategy: Explain the structure of the ear using a visual (model, poster, etc.) of the ear. Take the students outside and listen to the sounds. Record the sounds heard outside, and brainstorm other sounds. Shake two tin cans, one with only one or two marbles in it and one with several marbles in it. Have students listen and identify which can has more marbles and why. Have students complete a short essay on their favorite sound.

Materials Needed: an ear visual (model, poster, etc.), audio recording device, marbles, two tin cans

Processing Question: Explain the importance of hearing in your everyday life.

○ **Integration:** Science, Writing

✓ **Assessment:** Students' essays demonstrate their understanding of the importance of hearing in their everyday lives.

Experiments and Demonstrations: Personal Health

Covering Sneezes and Coughs   Grades K–1

Valued Outcome: Students will identify the importance of covering their mouths during sneezes and coughs and will demonstrate how to avoid spreading germs when they cough or sneeze.

National Health Education Standards: 7, 8

Description of Strategy: Discuss germs. Explain that certain germs in our body may make us sick. Tell students that germs are too tiny to see, but they can be spread from one person to another. Discuss how to care for people with illness and the importance of preventing illness from spreading. Some discussion points should be that medicine helps to fight off germs so people feel better and that it is important to try not to let the germs go to anyone else's body.

Discuss the ways germs spread. Ask students to brainstorm some ways that germs can get from one body to another. Possible responses include breathing on someone, coughing on someone, sneezing on someone, or touching someone after they have touched something with germs on it. Demonstrate how germs may travel. Put warm water in a spray bottle set to very fine mist. Stand back from the class and spray the air above students to show how far a sneeze or cough can reach. Ask students to raise their hands if they felt any water. Tell students that germs may go this far when someone sneezes or coughs.

Some discussion points should be to instruct the students to feel the area around them. Ask the students if the water only landed on them. The answer should be no. Ask the students if their hands got wet. Ask what would happen if, instead of water in a spray bottle, that was a real sneeze or cough. Possible answers include "we would get covered in germs" or "the area around us would get covered in germs." Another point of discussion should include how students can keep their sneezes and coughs from reaching other people. Discuss ways to avoid spreading germs. Discuss the steps to take if you have to sneeze or cough. Have students practice these steps. First, get a tissue; second, cover your mouth or nose; third, cough or sneeze; and finally, throw the tissue away. Teach the students this rhyme and have them act out each step as they say it: "May I have a tissue, please, to cover my mouth and nose? I need to cough or sneeze, and then, away it goes!"

Materials Needed: facial tissues, spray bottle filled with warm water

Processing Questions:

1. What should you do to avoid spreading germs when you cough or sneeze? Why is this important?
2. What are some ways to spread germs other than coughing or sneezing?
3. Why is it important to wash our hands after using the restroom?

✓ **Assessment:** Students can accurately describe how to avoid spreading germs when they cough or sneeze and explain why this is important.

Source: Health Strategies Inc. 2002b

Germs   Grades K–2

Valued Outcome: The students will be able to explain that germs are smaller than the eye can see but are still destructive.

National Health Education Standards: 7, 8

Description of Strategy: Ask the students, "What is a germ? Why is it important to wash your hands?" Divide the class into three groups. Have each student put a small amount of hand lotion on his or her hands and rub them together. Have each student sprinkle a small amount of glitter into their hands while holding them over a bucket. Tell them to spread the glitter over their hands. Let the students know that the glitter represents the germs. Have the first group try to rub the glitter off with a dry towel. Have the second group wash the glitter off with cold water only, and have the last group wash their hands with warm, soapy water. Then have everyone wash his or her hands in warm soapy water. Explain to the students that if they wash their hands every hour, they can prevent illnesses and bacterial infections.

Materials Needed: glitter, paper towels, hand lotion, bucket, hand soap, access to sinks or to tubs of warm, soapy water and cold water

Processing Questions:

1. What was the best method for getting the germs (glitter) off?
2. Why is it important to properly wash your hands?

○ **Integration:** Science

✓ **Assessment:** Students can accurately describe the best hand-washing procedures and their importance to health.

Source: A to Z Teacher Stuff 2002a

Four Kinds of Teeth   Grades K-2

Valued Outcome: Students will be able to name the four kinds of teeth (incisors, cuspids, bicuspids, and molars) and describe the purpose of each type.

National Health Education Standard: 1

Description of Strategy: Create worksheets for each of the four types of teeth and label them. Hand out one set of worksheets and four pieces of paper to each student. Explain that there are different types of teeth, each one with a name and a job to do. Have students hold up the incisors worksheet. Explain that the incisors are located in front of the mouth and have sharp, chisel-shaped crowns that cut food. Have them cut a sheet of paper with scissors, simulating what their incisors do to food. Next, have students hold up the cuspids worksheet and explain that there is one cuspid next to each incisor. Cuspids are pointed to help tear food and are sometimes called canine teeth; have the students tear the paper. Next, have students hold up the bicuspids worksheet and explain that there is one bicuspid (or premolar) located next to each cuspid. Bicuspids crush and tear food; have the students act like

they are crushing and tearing the paper. Have the students hold up the molars worksheet. Explain that molars grind food; have the students act out the molars' job by grinding and smashing the paper.

Materials Needed: four tooth cutouts per child, four pieces of paper and one pair of scissors for each child

Processing Questions:

1. What role do the cuspids play in eating?
2. What role do the bicuspids play in eating?

○ **Integration:** Science

✓ **Assessment:** Students can accurately name and describe the functions of the four types of teeth.

Source: Sevaly 1997, 83–98

Fingerprints   Grades K–5

Valued Outcome: Students will compare fingerprints and recognize the different configurations of each.

National Health Education Standard: 1

Description of Strategy: Provide students with white paper and a stamp pad. Have them press their fingertips on the stamp pad and then on the paper. Ask students to label the resulting fingerprints with their names. Then let them compare each other's prints to see that no two patterns are exactly the same. Discuss the anatomy of the skin ridges that form fingerprints (and footprints).

Materials Needed: stamp pad, white paper

Processing Questions:

1. Why do we have ridges on the fingertips?
2. Why do we each have unique fingerprints?

✓ **Assessment:** Students demonstrate an understanding that fingerprints are unique and can accurately describe the anatomical details of the skin ridges that form prints.

Daily Water Intake   Grades K–5

Valued Outcome: Students will be able to describe how much water they should drink each day (one quart).

National Health Education Standard: 7

Description of Strategy: Make the following statements about water and the ways it helps your body:

- Water in blood helps blood flow through the body, carrying nutrients and oxygen.
- Water helps cool our bodies when we sweat.
- Water helps our bodies remove wastes.
- Our bodies need two or more liters of water each day to replace water that they use.

Place the students in pairs. Each pair needs either a 4-ounce glass, an 8-ounce bottle of water, a 32-ounce pitcher of water, or a 16-ounce thermos. Each group also needs a liter-sized container filled with water. Have the groups measure out how many of their containers equal one liter of water. Have students record their answers on a worksheet. Have four groups work together to complete the worksheet. Display a picture of bottled water, watermelon, fruit juice, celery, lettuce, and a tomato. Ask students which foods are sources of water (all of them are). Have students cut out pictures of foods that are sources of water. Have each student make a collage.

Materials Needed: one liter of water for every two students, worksheet; 4-ounce water glasses, 8-ounce bottles, 32-ounce pitchers, and 16-ounce thermos for each group of eight students; picture of bottled water, watermelon, fruit juice, celery, lettuce, and a tomato; magazines, scissors, and construction paper for collages

Processing Questions:

1. What is the value of drinking water instead of other drinks?
2. How do you know if you are drinking enough water each day?

○ **Integration:** Science, Math

✓ **Assessment:** Students can accurately describe how water is important for personal health, identify sources of water in foods, and state how much water they should drink each day.

Source: Health Strategies, Inc. 2002c

Dental Hygiene   Grades 2–3

Valued Outcome: Students will be able to describe what is good and bad for their teeth.

National Health Education Standard: 7

Description of Strategy: Ask the students about their first visit to the dentist and how they felt about it. Ask if they felt scared and nervous. Talk about what they think is good and bad for their teeth, and ask them what they think will happen if they do not brush their teeth, and how they can keep their teeth in good shape. Read the book *Berenstain Bears Visit the Dentist* by Stan Berenstain and Jan Berenstain and talk about Brother and Sister Bears' visit. What happened to them? What did the dentist say about their report on their teeth?

Explain to the students that they will be doing an experiment. Tell them that a hard-boiled egg represents their teeth. Soda in a cup represents all the bad things for their teeth. Have each student drop his or her "tooth" into the soda. Ask them what they think will happen if the tooth is left in the soda overnight. Have the students write a sentence or two about the first time they went to the dentist.

Have them illustrate their sentences so they can hang the drawings around the room. Distribute toothbrushes and toothpaste to each student.

Materials Needed: *Berenstain Bears Visit the Dentist* (Berenstain and Berenstain 1981b), one hard-boiled egg for each student, toothbrushes for each student, toothpaste, a cup for each student, paper and pencils, dark soda

Processing Questions:

1. Is it normal to be scared and nervous on the first visit to the dentist?
2. What will happen if you do not brush your teeth?

○ **Integration:** Reading, Science, Art

✓ **Assessment:** Students can describe the importance of brushing their teeth and visiting the dentist.

Source: A to Z Teacher Stuff 2002b

Pupil Dilation and Constriction   Grades 3–5

Valued Outcome: Students will describe how light influences the dilation and constriction of the pupil of the eye.

National Health Education Standard: 1

Description of Strategy: Pair students and have them face one another so they can see their partner's eyes. Tell them to look at their partner's pupils for a few seconds and observe their pupil size. Then, at your signal, ask all students to close their eyes and not reopen them until you tell them. Explain that on your signal, they are to open their eyes and look quickly at their partner's pupils. Give the signal after about 45 seconds, and have the students note the constriction of the pupils on being exposed to light.

Processing Question: What is the purpose of the dilation of the pupil?

○ **Integration:** Science

✓ **Assessment:** Students can accurately describe how pupils respond to changes in light and why.

Sound Localization   Grades 3–5

Valued Outcome: Students will understand that having two ears, one on each side of the head, helps us perceive sound direction more accurately than if we only had one ear.

National Health Education Standard: 1

Description of Strategy: Pair students. One student is blindfolded and sits in a chair. The other student, who acts as the tester, stands nearby and taps a pencil against a glass. The blindfolded student points to the direction he or she believes the sound is coming from. Have the tester move to several locations throughout the room, sometimes holding the glass high above the floor and sometimes holding it low. Repeat this with several other students to note differences. Also do the experiment with several blindfolded students who have one ear plugged to note differences in sound localization ability.

Materials Needed: blindfolds, glass jars or drinking glasses, pencils

Processing Question: How does sound enhance the quality of our lives?

○ **Integration:** Science

✓ **Assessment:** Students demonstrate their understanding of how having two ears helps us to better perceive sound direction.

Shadow Play   Grades 3–5

Valued Outcome: Students will demonstrate the difference between proper and improper posture.

National Health Education Standard: 7

Description of Strategy: The purpose is to gain an understanding of various postural defects and practice posture improvement. The materials you will need are a shadow screen (a bedsheet may be used), lights, and equipment for holding up the sheet. This is an excellent way for students to compare and dramatize good and bad posture. Act as the narrator and discuss various aspects of maintaining good posture while standing, sitting, walking, and reading. As you discuss each posture, one student standing behind the screen will demonstrate poor posture while another demonstrates proper posture. The roles of the shadow casters can be changed so that all students participate.

Materials Needed: shadow screen (bedsheet), lights, equipment to hang shadow screen (clothespins, wire, etc.)

Processing Questions:

1. What part does posture play in overall personal health?
2. How does poor posture affect the function of internal organs?

✓ **Assessment:** Students can accurately demonstrate proper posture while standing and sitting.

Health Habits   Grades 3–5

Valued Outcome: Students will identify four simple health habits, explain the need to stay healthy, and demonstrate simple health habits.

National Health Education Standards: 7, 8

Description of Strategy: Demonstrate the proper care of teeth, skin, hair, and nails. For the care of teeth, show students how to properly brush and floss. For the skin, show

students how to use soap and water to wash the hands. For the hair, show students how to brush or comb the hair. For the nails, demonstrate how to use a nailbrush to scrub underneath the nails and how to use fingernail clippers. After demonstrating each technique to the class, introduce the idea of a health fair to students and allow them to suggest what they need to plan for one. Have the students set up the health fair in the classroom. Possible suggestions include labeling and setting up four separate areas, each for care of teeth, skin, hair, and nails (have parents help out with the health fair and see what the children have learned about how they can take care of themselves). Tell the students that in order to prevent the spread of communicable diseases they should not share their toothbrushes, combs, or brushes. Students should go to each station and properly demonstrate the particular technique for that station.

Materials Needed:

- **Teeth station**—cups (paper or plastic), water, toothpaste, a mirror, and a basin. Bring extra *new* toothbrushes so that each student can have his or her own to practice the activity.
- **Skin station**—a basin of water, mild soap, and paper towels.
- **Hair station**—a mirror. Students who have their own comb or brush could use this area. Make sure to have a pack of *new* combs to pass out to the students who forgot to bring their own.
- **Nails station**—have a basin of water, soap, nail cutter, and nailbrush.

Processing Questions:

1. What do we do to take care of our bodies?
2. What health habits can prevent the spread of communicable diseases?

✓ **Assessment:** Students can correctly demonstrate good health habits at each station and verbally express an appreciation of the importance of healthy habits.

Source: Bajah and IICBA Organization 2002

Aerobic and Anaerobic Activities   Grades 3–5

Valued Outcome: Students will be able to distinguish between aerobic and anaerobic activities so that they can participate in those activities that would benefit their endurance.

National Health Education Standards: 1, 7

Description of Strategy: Review the meaning of *aerobic* (something you can do for a long time), *anaerobic* (something that makes you out of breath), and *couch potato* (nonintellectual, sitting activities). Give each student a picture of a sport or activity (indicate on the picture whether it is aerobic, anaerobic, or couch potato), and a three-column handout labeled with each category. Designate three places around the room with signs that say "aerobic," "anaerobic," and "couch potato." Have each student get up and act out the activity; the other students guess the activity by raising their hands and allowing the demonstrator to call on them. After the students guess the activity, say "Go," and have the students stand under the sign that they think best represents the type of activity. Have the demonstrator say what kind of activity it is, and give each student who is in the correct place a sticker to put on his or her handout under the correct heading. Many of the activities could be aerobic or anaerobic based on the intensity of the activity. Explain this to the students. If a student can explain why he or she chose aerobic over anaerobic (or vice versa), let him or her also have a sticker.

Materials Needed: pictures of activities (one for each student in your room); large signs with the words *aerobic,* *anaerobic*, and *couch potato*; stickers; three-column handout with anaerobic, aerobic, and couch potato headings for each student

Processing Questions:

1. Can you distinguish between activity types?
2. Which activities are better for your health?

✔ **Assessment:** Students demonstrate their understanding of the differences between aerobic, anaerobic, and "couch potato" activities by standing under the correct signs during the activity.

Demonstration of Correct Brushing
Grades 3–5

Valued Outcome: Students will demonstrate, in front of the class, the importance of brushing their teeth.

National Health Education Standards: 7, 8

Description of Strategy: Define plaque. Use a mouth model and "invisible" (clear plastic) plaque tiles to demonstrate how plaque builds up after eating without brushing and flossing. Tell the students that plaque is caused by germs that can damage teeth by making holes called cavities. Use the mouth model, toothbrush, floss, and plaque tiles to demonstrate that brushing and flossing will rid teeth of plaque. Instruct the students to take turns brushing and flossing the mouth model. Have the students explain how brushing removes plaque from teeth.

Have students chew red "plaque" tablets that show where plaque is on teeth and, looking in a classroom mirror, observe where the darkest red stains are on their teeth. Pass out a toothbrush and a trial-size toothpaste that students can take home for practice.

Materials Needed: large model of set of teeth, large toothbrush, dental floss or colored yarn, toothbrushes and toothpaste for each child, plaque tiles (clear plastic), red "plaque" tablets

Processing Questions:

1. What is the correct way to brush your teeth?
2. Why is it necessary to brush regularly and correctly?

✔ **Assessment:** Students can demonstrate the correct brushing and flossing procedures and can verbally communicate the importance of proper dental care.

Sources: Merritt 2002; Smoak 2002

Teeth Problems
Grades 4–5

Valued Outcome: Students will demonstrate proper dental hygiene.

National Health Education Standard: 7

Description of Strategy: Discuss with students the various problems (such as cavities, root canals, loss of enamel, false teeth, and so on) that could occur from not taking care of their teeth. Discuss and list on the board or on an overhead transparency the proper steps for taking care of their teeth:

- Brush teeth after every meal.
- Use dental floss before brushing teeth.
- Rinse mouth with mouthwash.
- Take regular trips to the dentist.
- Limit the amount of sugar you consume.

Have each student copy these steps as a reminder of the proper dental hygiene procedures. Distribute toothpaste and a toothbrush to each student. Invite a dentist or dental hygienist to demonstrate the proper techniques for brushing teeth.

Materials Needed: board or overhead projector, markers, paper, pencil, toothpaste, and a toothbrush for each student

Processing Question: What are the proper steps for good dental hygiene?

✔ **Assessment:** Students can list five steps to take for proper dental hygiene.

Teeth and Digestion
Grades 4–5

Valued Outcome: Students will learn about the roles that teeth, saliva, and digestive enzymes play in digestion.

National Health Education Standard: 1

Description of Strategy: Give students a saltine. Have them chew it without swallowing and note what happens. Explain that teeth grind food. At the same time, saliva and digestive enzymes in the mouth act on the food. Students should note how the taste of the cracker sweetens as this happens. The chewed cracker is being changed to a moist bolus so that it can be swallowed easily.

Materials Needed: saltine crackers

Processing Question: What significant part do the teeth play in digestion?

✓ **Assessment:** Students can describe the roles the teeth, saliva, and digestive enzymes play in digestion.

Sleep Needs   Grades 4–5

Valued Outcome: Students will identify different needs for sleep with regard to age groups.

National Health Education Standard: 1

Description of Strategy: To demonstrate the varying needs for sleep at different ages, have students interview several people of different ages (such as siblings, peers, parents, grandparents). Instruct students to write down the names and ages in chronological order by age. Have them report on the different needs for sleep for people of different ages.

Materials Needed: paper, pencils

Processing Questions:

1. How much sleep does the student need?
2. Why do sleep needs vary at different stages of life?

✓ **Assessment:** Students will accurately determine the correct amount of sleep they need at each age level.

Puzzles and Games: Body Systems

The Sound Matching Game   Grades K–5

Valued Outcome: The class will play a game to help them understand that many different sounds can sometimes sound a lot alike.

National Health Education Standard: 1

Description of Strategy: Fill two film containers with rice, two with beans, two with water, and so on for all the materials listed under Materials Needed. Place them on a table so that pairs are not next to each other. Explain how we use our ears. Then have the students shake the containers and listen carefully to the sound. Ask them to match up pairs that sound the same. Once the children have played the game, they can peek inside the containers to see if their answers are correct.

Materials Needed: twenty camera film containers (or similar sized opaque containers), rice, beans, water, popcorn, dry cereal, sand, gravel, crumbled dried leaves, marbles, paper clips

Processing Question: What is the most important function of our ears?

✓ **Assessment:** Students express an appreciation of the sense of hearing.

I See   Grades 3–5

Valued Outcome: Students will be able to describe the sense of sight and explain how to protect the eyes from injury.

National Health Education Standards: 1, 7

Description of Strategy: Begin with a game of "I See." The class moves to music. When the music stops, the students freeze and stare straight ahead. Point at something and ask a student to describe what he or she sees without actually naming it. Have the other students guess what the object is (give them three guesses). Repeat this a few times; try asking them to describe a color. Gather the students; discuss why we have eyes and ways they keep us safe—for example, seeing oncoming traffic. Make a chart of ways to protect the eyes from injury. Include the fact that the eyes have eyelashes, eyelids, and tears for protection.

Materials Needed: music, music player, chart paper, markers

Processing Question: How many ways do our eyes and our sense of sight help us in everyday life?

✓ **Assessment:** Students can explain how sight contributes to our well-being and name three ways to protect the eyes from injury.

Blood Jeopardy   Grades 3–5

Valued Outcome: Students will play a game by matching parts of the blood with statements about the circulatory system.

National Health Education Standard: 1

Description of Strategy: Using an overhead projector and transparencies, write short statements about various parts of the blood and/or circulatory system. Divide the class into teams and have them guess the part of the blood to which the statement applies. Various numbers of points can be awarded according to the difficulty of the statement.

Materials Needed: overhead projector, transparencies, overhead markers

Processing Question: What are the various functions of the blood?

✓ **Assessment:** Students can correctly complete the matching activity.

Body Parts Puzzle   Grades 4–5

Valued Outcome: Students will correctly put together a puzzle of organs of the different body systems.

National Health Education Standard: 1

Description of Strategy: Divide the class into groups. Provide each group with a sealed package containing body parts made of construction paper and a large piece of paper that has the outline of the human body on it. At your signal, the groups open their packets and place the organs where they should be in the body. Record the amount of time it takes each group to complete its puzzle. With the same groups, repeat this activity a few days later and record the time again. Have students compare their timed results to see if they improved.

Materials Needed: construction paper cut into shapes of organs of different body systems, butcher paper with outline of human body, timer or clock, paper and pencil for teacher

Processing Question: What are some examples of how the body systems work together to keep us healthy?

○ **Integration:** Science

✓ **Assessment:** Students can work together to correctly complete the puzzle.

Body Organs Game   Grades 4–5

Valued Outcome: Students will be able to describe the organs of the body and their functions.

National Health Education Standard: 1

Description of Strategy: Have students study the organs in a human body and focus on their functions. Then conduct a game similar to a spelling bee. Have the students stand. Each student is given the name of a body organ and asked to tell the function, or vice versa. If the answer is wrong, the student sits. The game ends when one person is left standing.

Processing Question: What are the major body organs and their functions?

✓ **Assessment:** Students can correctly describe the functions of body organs.

Memory Game   Grades 4–5

Valued Outcome: Students will repeat a sequence of movements to test their memory skills.

National Health Education Standard: 1

Description of Strategy: This game allows the students to see how the brain can store and use information. Divide the class into teams. Read several body actions, such as "touch your nose," "touch your toes," and "clap your hands." Each team takes turns to see how many actions can be followed in the sequence you read before members of the team become disorganized.

Materials Needed: list of sequences of body actions

Processing Question: How does the brain store information?

✓ **Assessment:** Students demonstrate their understanding of the limitations of memory.

Bean Bag Toss   Grades 4–5

Valued Outcome: Students will identify endocrine glands and their hormones while tossing a bean bag through holes in a cardboard box.

National Health Education Standard: 1

Description of Strategy: Cut several holes in the bottom of a large cardboard box. Label each hole with the name of a different endocrine gland and secure the box in front of a wall. Each student has three chances at tossing a bean bag through the holes. Score one point for getting the bag into the hole and two points if the student can name one function of the gland or one of the hormones it secretes. Each function or hormone may be identified only one time. Tally scores and announce the winners. Repeat this game periodically; make sure to change the order so that students who were first during the previous game have to go last, and vice versa.

Materials Needed: cardboard box, bean bags, scissors, marker

Processing Questions:

1. What is the function of each gland in the endocrine system?
2. What is the function of each of the hormones secreted by these glands?

✓ **Assessment:** Students can correctly identify the functions of several endocrine glands or their hormones.

Puzzles and Games: Personal Health

Take Time For Personal Health   Grades 4–5

Valued Outcome: Students will list different roles, functions, and health practices associated with various components of personal health.

National Health Education Standards: 1, 7

Description of Strategy: Divide the class into groups, and assign each group a different component of personal health, such as care of the hair, skin, teeth, eyes, or ears, and the need for exercise, sleep, and relaxation. Allow the groups two minutes to list as many roles, functions, or health practices associated with that component as they can. Read each list for accuracy and determine which group won the round by having the most accurate statements. Play several more rounds; explain that each time the listings must be different. See not only which group can list the most per round, but also which group is able to list the most at the end of the game.

Processing Questions:

1. What are the roles and functions of the hair, skin, teeth, eyes, and ears?
2. What are the personal health habits needed for each of these organs in order for the body to work efficiently?

✓ **Assessment:** Students can list at least three positive health practices for each component of personal health.

Other Ideas: Body Systems

Body Builders   Grades K–3

Valued Outcome: Students will construct craft-stick figures, simulating bones, muscle, and skin.

National Health Education Standard: 1

Description of Strategy: Have each student make a character with "bones," "muscles," and "skin." Craft sticks provide the frame; yarn wrapped around sticks represents muscles; and cloth scraps serve as skin. Additional features can be added to give each model some unique characteristics.

Materials Needed: craft sticks, yarn, cloth scraps

Processing Question: How do the bones, muscles, and skin work together to make the body more efficient?

○ **Integration:** Art

✓ **Assessment:** Students demonstrate an understanding of how bones, muscles, and skin are structured on the human body.

Other Ideas: Personal Health

Dressing for the Weather   Grades K–2

Valued Outcome: Students will understand that dressing appropriately for the weather can prevent illness.

National Health Education Standard: 7

Description of Strategy: Make an extra-large boy paper doll and an extra-large girl paper doll along with an accompanying and varied wardrobe for all kinds of weather. Let the students take turns each day dressing the dolls appropriately for the day's weather or for different seasons.

Materials Needed: paper dolls, doll clothes

Processing Question: How can we dress appropriately for weather in order to prevent illness and/or discomfort?

✓ **Assessment:** Students will describe the correct way to dress in cold weather and explain how this can help prevent illness.

11 Sexuality Education

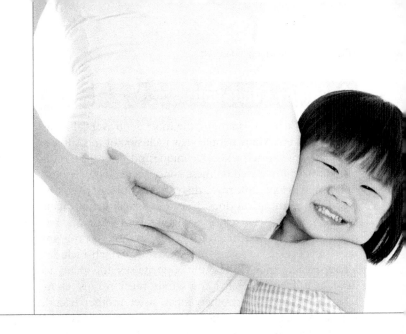

Valued Outcomes

After completion of this chapter, you should be able to:

- Identify the goals of a sexuality education program.
- Discuss the social aspects of sexuality and family living.
- Discuss marriage, parenthood, and divorce.
- Trace the psychological development of sexuality.
- Describe the anatomy and physiology of the male and female reproductive systems.
- Explain the problems of family abuse and violence.

Reflections

After reading this chapter, reflect upon the type of training you believe an elementary education teacher would need to have in preparation for teaching sexuality education. Be specific in the type of content to be covered in the training. Do you think some type of certification is needed? What (if any) qualities does a teacher need to teach sexuality education? What should the emphasis be focused on at the elementary level?

A comprehensive sexuality education program respects the diversity of values and beliefs represented in the community and will complement and augment the sexuality education received from students' families.

—Sexuality Information and Education Council of the United States (2002)

NATIONAL HEALTH EDUCATION STANDARDS

1. Students will comprehend concepts related to health promotion and disease prevention to enhance health.

2. Students will analyze the influence of family, peers, culture, media, technology, and other factors on health behaviors.

Sexuality Education

Sexuality education is among the most controversial areas facing teachers. Many people view inclusion of this subject as an attempt to teach sexual technique and lower the morals of today's youth. Based on these concepts, sexuality education would involve little more than teaching the act of coitus. **Sexuality education** does deal with sexuality, but this is not the same thing as sex. Sexuality involves one's total being and identity. An effective sexuality education program seeks to develop an individual's sexuality, which includes an appreciation for self and the opposite sex, the ability to develop fulfilling personal and family relationships, comfort with sexual roles (mother, father, sister, brother, friend, wife, or husband), recognition of bodily functions as related to reproduction, understanding how emotions play a part in sexual behavior, maturing attitudes toward the function of sex, the responsibility of being a member of a family, and, overall, a healthy attitude toward life.

The Sexuality Information and Education Council of the United States (SIECUS) says that "sexuality education is a lifelong process of acquiring information and forming attitudes, beliefs, and values. It encompasses sexual development, sexual and reproductive health, interpersonal relationships, affection, intimacy, body image, and gender rroles" (SIECUS 2011). The council goes on to state that comprehensive school-based sexuality education that is appropriate to students' age, developmental level, and cultural background should be an important part of the education program at every age. The program should respect the many values and beliefs represented in a community and complement/augment the sexuality education received in the home.

The primary responsibility for teaching facts, attitudes, and values about sexuality should remain with the parents. However, there is frequently a gap between the education children receive about family life in their homes and their level of questioning, need, and interest. School is not the only source of information outside the home. Churches and other organizations can contribute significantly in this area. The school is an increasingly important contributor to education about family life. Before a family life curriculum can be taught, parental approval must be obtained. Most communities will support such a program if the school administration and community understand what is to be taught. This is the most important first step, which cannot be ignored if sexuality education is to be successful.

The appreciation for self must start early in life and be built on each year if children are to feel comfortable with their sexuality through the preadolescent, adolescent, and adult years. As should be emphasized in all aspects of health education, children must recognize that they will eventually have to accept the responsibility of their sexuality.

If society is not willing to promote comprehensive sexuality education, then that component of a student's total being will be shortchanged. Personal and social problems such as unwanted pregnancies, sexually transmitted infec-

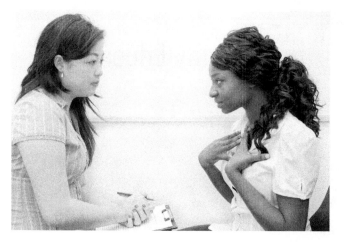

It is important that a positive self-image be developed if children are to grow to adulthood with the ability to respect others.

tions (STIs), sexual unresponsiveness, and divorce will continue to plague society. A worthwhile educational effort in sexuality and family life must include social, psychological, moral, and biological components. In this chapter, these areas of concern are examined while providing the necessary overview of content for teaching sexuality education.

Implications for Sexuality Education

Few subjects in society evoke more discussion and controversy than sexuality education courses taught in our schools. It is amazing that one of the most significant aspects of our being is such a taboo topic. Humans are sexual from the moment they are born until well into old age. The adage that we are sexual beings from womb to tomb is certainly true. Although humans have learned a great deal about sexuality that can be taught in the educational process, we often seek to repress and hide sex information and avoid discussing sexuality with our children. Many people believe that it is better to ignore unwanted pregnancies, the increasing rate of STIs, and the many misconceptions of the nation's youth.

There are basically two philosophical positions concerning sexuality education in our society. One group promotes the concept of abstinence-only education, and the second group advocates comprehensive sexuality education. Both positions stem not only from the desire to promote specific sexual ideologies and social visions, but also from each group's perception that the opposition represents a crucial component in an encroaching political movement. What is at stake is each group's visions of morality, family, and gender (Nelson 1996, 16).

Parents greatly influence the views their children hold concerning sexuality. Parents provide the young child with a basic orientation by the verbal and nonverbal messages they send concerning nudity, masturbation, sex values, and so on. If the message is that sex is shocking, dirty, or disgusting, this is transmitted to the child. These types of messages are likely to interfere with enjoyable healthy sexuality in the adult years. It is important to note that when children learn about sex and sexuality from their parents, the information is more likely to be accurate and positive than that learned from peers. Children are more likely to view sex as "dirty" or something to be ashamed of if learned from peers. Research indicates that adolescents who report good communication with parents are more likely to use contraception than adolescents who report poor communication, and adolescents who receive sex education from their parents are more likely to behave in ways consistent with their knowledge.

Sexuality education must include an open learning atmosphere, improved materials, and improved training of educators. In addition, the curricular planning process, the implementation of the curriculum, training of the teachers, and multimedia materials should all be open to parents and the community for inspection and evaluation.

Abstinence-Only Sexuality Education

The dilemma facing educators and schools is the teaching of abstinence versus responsibility. In question is whether schools should approach sexuality education from the perspective that all sexual problems can be avoided if students remain sexually abstinent or if a more pragmatic approach should be followed, acknowledging that young people are going to be sexually active and that issues associated with such activity need to be discussed so sexual responsibility can be advocated. This latter approach fits well with the wellness approach and self-responsibility. However, since the early 1980s, a variety of abstinence education programs have been adopted by many states. In these curricula, students are taught that chastity is the only answer and that premarital sex can only lead to disease, pregnancy, and emotional turmoil. Opponents of this approach point out that such views can cause extreme reactions toward sex. In addition, issues such as preventing pregnancy, HIV, and other STIs are not discussed in abstinence programs. Omitting such information from sexuality education is actually dangerous to the welfare of students. Most educators favor a middle position on teaching sexuality education: Abstinence is encouraged, but with the realization that students may have premarital intercourse and that they do need to be informed and responsible for protecting themselves from unwanted pregnancies and possible infection with HIV or some other STI.

The federal government does not dictate sexuality education or its content in schools; four federal statutes preclude the federal government from doing so. Those four statutes are the Department of Education Organization Act, Section 103a; the Elementary and Secondary Education Act, Section 14512; Goals 2000, 314 (b); and the General Education Provisions Act, Section 438 (SIECUS 2006). With these statutes and keeping in mind that the federal government does not have a policy concerning sexuality education, a number of federal programs have been instituted that provide funding for strict abstinence until marriage education. Beginning in 1996 and continuing today, through funds available from the Maternal and Child Health Bureau, states can apply for grants for teaching sexuality education. However, if applications are funded, each state receiving funds must agree to the following stipulations. The sexuality program:

1. must have as its exclusive purpose teaching the social, psychological, and health gains to be realized by abstaining from sexual activity;
2. teaches abstinence from sexual activity outside marriage as the expected standard for all school-age children;
3. teaches that abstinence from sexual activity is the only certain way to avoid out-of-wedlock pregnancy, sexually transmitted infections, and other associated health problems;
4. teaches that a mutually faithful, monogamous relationship in the context of marriage is the expected standard of human sexual activity;
5. teaches that sexual activity outside of the context of marriage is likely to have harmful psychological and physical effects;
6. teaches that bearing children out of wedlock is likely to have harmful consequences for the child, the child's parents, and society;
7. teaches young people how to reject sexual advances and how alcohol and drug use increase vulnerability to sexual advances; and
8. teaches the importance of attaining self-sufficiency before engaging in sexual activity. (SIECUS 2006)

In 2009, President Barack Obama signed legislation that represented the first-ever cuts to abstinence-only-until-marriage programs. This legislation also included elements that begin to undo some of the sexual and reproductive health program restrictions that were instituted under the previous administration. Specifically, additional monies were provided for family planning resources and to combat the HIV/AIDS epidemic, as well as providing seed funds to create a National AIDS Strategy. Currently, federal monies are not available for teaching sexuality education programs other than abstinence. At the present time, states must still agree to the eight guidelines listed above if they are to receive funds.

Where Do Children Learn About Sexuality?

In 1999, the Henry J. Kaiser Family Foundation conducted a study that determined 59 percent of adolescents ten to twelve years old and 45 percent of adolescents thirteen to fifteen years old indicated that they personally learned the "most" concerning sexuality from their parents. The same study found that 44 percent of parents of ten- to twelve-year-olds and 70 percent of thirteen- to fifteen-year-olds said they had talked with their children concerning relationships and becoming sexually active.

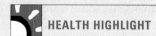

HEALTH HIGHLIGHT | **State Mandates: General Requirements for Sex and HIV Education**

State	Sex Education* Mandated	HIV Education Mandated	When Provided, Sex or HIV Education Must:				Parental Role		
			Be Medically Accurate	Be Age Appropriate	Be Culturally Appropriate and Unbiased	Cannot Promote Religion	Notice	Consent	Opt-Out
Alabama		X		X					X
Arizona				X			HIV	Sex	HIV
Arkansas									
California		X	X	X	X	X	X		X
Colorado		X	X	X	X		X		X
Connecticut		X							X
Delaware	X	X							
Dist. of Columbia	X	X		X			X		X
Florida			X	X					
Georgia	X	X					X		X
Hawaii			X	X					
Idaho									X
Illinois		X		X					X
Indiana		X							
Iowa	X	X	X	X	X		X		X
Kentucky	X	X							
Louisiana				X		X	X		X
Maine	X	X	X	X					X
Maryland	X	X							X
Massachusetts							X		X
Michigan		X	X†	X			X		X
Minnesota	X	X							X
Mississippi‡				X			X		X
Missouri		X		X			X		X
Montana	X	X							
Nevada	X	X		X			X	X	
New Hampshire		X							X
New Jersey	X	X	X	X	X		X		X
New Mexico	X	X							X
New York			X		HIV				HIV
North Carolina	X	X	X	X					
North Dakota	X								
Ohio	X	X							X
Oklahoma		X					X		X

HEALTH HIGHLIGHT **State Mandates (*continued*)**

State	Sex Education* Mandated	HIV Education Mandated	When Provided, Sex or HIV Education Must:				Parental Role		
			Be Medically Accurate	Be Age Appropriate	Be Culturally Appropriate and Unbiased	Cannot Promote Religion	Notice	Consent	Opt-Out
Oregon	X	X	X	X	X		X		X
Pennsylvania		X		HIV			X		HIV
Rhode Island	X	X	X	X	X				X
South Carolina	X	X		X			X		X
Tennessee	X	X		HIV					X
Texas				X			X		X
Utah^Ω	X	X	X		X		X	X	X
Vermont	X	X		X					X
Virginia				X			X		X
Washington		X	X	X	X		X		X
West Virginia	X	X					X		X
Wisconsin		X	X	X	X		X		X
TOTAL	**21+DC**	**33+DC**	**13**	**27+DC**	**9**	**2**	**22+DC**	**3**	**35+DC**

* Sex education typically includes discussion of STIs.

† Sex education "shall not be medically inaccurate."

‡ Localities may omit state-required topics, but may not include material that "contradicts the required components."

Ω State also prohibits teachers from responding to students' spontaneous questions in ways that conflict with the law's requirements.

Source: Guttmacher Institute, Sex and HIV Education, *State Policies in Brief*, (as of September 2011), New York: Guttmacher Institute, 2011. www.guttmacher.org/statecenter/spibs/spib_SE.pdf, accessed September 2011.

Children also learn about sexuality from sources outside the home such as friends, teachers, neighbors, television, music, books, advertisements, and toys. They learn from institutions such as churches, synagogues, and other places of worship as well as from community agencies and schools. To help illustrate this concept, another study conducted by the Kaiser Foundation found that teenagers identified the sources from which they had learned "a lot" about pregnancy and birth control. Forty percent indicated teachers, school nurses, or classes at school; 36 percent named parents; and 27 percent named friends other than boyfriends or girlfriends (Henry J. Kaiser Foundation 2002).

School-Based Sexuality Education

Sexuality education taught by trained teachers can add significantly to children's ongoing learning. The content should be developmentally appropriate and should include topics on issues such as self-esteem, family relationships, values, communication techniques, dating, and decision-making skills. It is imperative that communities plan sexuality programs to respect the diversity of values in the classroom and community.

The primary goal of any sexuality education effort is to promote adult sexual health. It seeks to assist young people in understanding a positive view of sexuality and provide information that can help them protect their health and make sound decisions.

In 1990, SIECUS brought together a group of professionals representing a cross section of foundations, associations, government agencies, and the medical profession to formulate a framework to promote and facilitate the development of comprehensive sexuality education programs. This task force was to develop curricula, textbooks, and programs, as well as evaluate existing programs. It produced the document *Guidelines for Comprehensive Sexuality Education: Grades K–12 (Guidelines)* that outlines the steps needed in establishing comprehensive sexuality education programs. In 2004, the *Guidelines* were updated to reflect more recent societal and technological changes.

According to the *Guidelines*, a comprehensive sexuality education program has four goals:

1. **To provide accurate information about human sexuality**—Topics include growth and development, human reproduction, anatomy, physiology, masturbation, family life, pregnancy, childbirth, parenthood, sexual response, sexual orientation, contraception, abortion, sexual abuse, HIV/AIDS, and other sexually transmitted infections.

2. **To provide an opportunity for young people to develop and understand their values, attitudes, and beliefs about sexuality**—Teachers should help them understand their family's values, develop their own values, increase self-esteem, develop insights concerning relationships with families and individuals of both genders, and understand their obligations and responsibilities to their families and others.

3. **To help young people develop relationships and interpersonal skills**—Education should help young people develop communication and decision-making skills, assertiveness, peer refusal skills, and the ability to engage in satisfying relationships. This includes helping to develop the capacity for caring, supportive, noncoercive, and mutually pleasurable intimate and sexual relationships.

4. **To help young people exercise responsibility regarding sexual relationships**—Topics include abstinence, pressure to become prematurely involved in sexual intercourse, the use of contraception and other sexual health measures, prevention of STIs, and sexual abuse (SIECUS 2004).

▪ Guidelines for Comprehensive Sexuality Education

The *Guidelines for Comprehensive Sexuality Education Grades: Kindergarten–12ᵗʰ Grade* are organized into six key concepts. In addition, they contain a total of 36 topics and 778 developmental messages at four levels of development:

- **Level 1: Middle Childhood**—Ages five through eight; early elementary school
- **Level 2: Preadolescence**—Ages nine through twelve; upper elementary school
- **Level 3: Early Adolescence**—Ages twelve through fifteen; middle school/junior high
- **Level 4: Adolescence**—Ages fifteen through eighteen; high school

The *Guidelines* are value-based, and the task force has attempted to develop specific values found in most communities in a pluralistic society. However, every community should review these values to make sure they are consistent with community norms and diversity. The values expressed in the *Guidelines* include (SIECUS 2004):

- Sexuality is a natural and healthy part of living.
- All people are sexual.
- Sexuality includes physical, ethical, social, spiritual, psychological, and emotional dimensions.
- Every person has self-worth.
- Young people should view themselves as unique and worthwhile individuals within the context of their cultural heritage.
- Individuals express their sexuality in varied ways.
- Parents should be the primary sexuality educators of their children.
- Families provide their children's first education about sexuality.
- Families share their values about sexuality with their children.
- In a pluralistic society, people should respect and accept the diversity of values and beliefs about sexuality that exist in a community.
- Sexual relationships should never be coercive or exploitative.
- All children should be cared for and loved.
- All sexual decisions have effects and consequences.
- All persons have the right and the obligation to make responsible sexual choices.
- Individuals, families, and society benefit when children are able to discuss sexuality with their parents and/or trusted adults.
- Young people develop their values about sexuality as part of becoming adults.
- Young people explore their sexuality as a natural process of achieving sexual maturity.
- Premature involvement in sexual behavior poses risks.
- Abstaining from sexual intercourse is the most effective method of preventing pregnancy and STI/HIV.
- Young people who are involved in sexual relationships need access to information about health care services.

HEALTH HIGHLIGHT | **Key Concepts in a Comprehensive Sexuality Education Program**

1. ***Human Development***
   Reproductive anatomy and physiology
   Reproduction
   Puberty
   Body image
   Gender identity and orientation
2. ***Relationships***
   Families
   Friendship
   Love
   Dating
   Marriage and lifetime commitments
   Parenting
3. ***Personal Skills***
   Values
   Decision making
   Communication

   Assertiveness
   Negotiation
   Looking for help
4. ***Sexual Behavior***
   Sexuality throughout life
   Masturbation
   Shared sexual behavior
   Abstinence
   Human sexual response
   Fantasy
   Sexual dysfunction
5. ***Sexual Health***
   Contraception
   Abortion
   STDs and HIV infection
   Sexual abuse
   Reproductive health
6. ***Society and Culture***

   Sexuality and society
   Decision making
   Communication
   Assertiveness
   Negotiation
   Finding help
   Gender roles
   Sexuality and the law
   Sexuality and religion
   Diversity
   Sexuality and the arts
   Sexuality and the media

   Source: SIECUS 2004

Any community or school considering the development or evaluation of an existing sexuality education program should consider the *Guidelines* and the topics provided by the task force. The group responsible for such development should represent a cross section of the community, and the curriculum developed must meet the needs and approval of that community. The complete *Guidelines* are available from SIECUS at www.siecus.org.

Teaching Sexuality Education

Like all teaching, sexuality education requires teachers to use effective communication skills; empathize with their students; understand the needs, interests, and characteristics of the various age levels; and believe in the need to develop students' critical thinking skills. Effective sexuality educators must be comfortable with their own sexuality and be able to overcome any embarrassment or self-consciousness they may feel. Another aspect of being an effective sexuality educator is use of appropriate terminology. Kilander pointed out more than 40 years ago that using acceptable terminology helps children learn to respect their bodies, helps prevent negative connotations for body parts and functions, provides a common vocabulary for children, and makes children more comfortable when asking questions (Kilander 1968).

The acceptance of any program must involve the community in the planning process. People are more comfortable if they have opportunities to give input and to view the content, materials, and activities associated with the curriculum. Successful sexuality programs have a high degree of parental involvement, administrative efforts at teacher training, a cooperative relationship between a school and a family planning agency, and strong support from the school board (Scales 1984). However, the value system taught to each child should come from the family. The attitudes the students reflect are still the responsibility of the family to instill. The school can impact the student by providing knowledge, decision-making training, and opportunities for examining sexuality issues in a nonthreatening environment. At their best, sexuality education programs in the school can strive to help students recognize and have insight into their own values. These values should be drawn from the family and the institutions most important in their lives, such as the church or synagogue. What is important to remember concerning sexuality education is that, even though opponents have received a lot of attention, most Americans support such education in the schools. As teachers we must take a stand for sexuality education and strive to make sure what students receive in the classroom is balanced and accurate.

TEACHING TIP

Introduce the student to a decision making model such as POWER and the use of refusal skills (see Chapter 4) prior to teaching relationships, personal skills, and sexual behavior components of sexuality education.

Dear Parent/Guardian:

Our school is developing a program in family living, including sexuality education, following the guidelines recommended by the Steuben County Board of Education. Selected teachers have been trained in the program. The philosophy of the program stresses

- the awareness and importance of family, religious, and moral values in making personal decisions
- understanding the need for consideration, love, respect, and responsibility in family life
- recognition of responsibilities to the school, the community, and society

We recognize that you, as parents, have the major responsibility for the formation of desirable attitudes toward family living and sexuality education. The role of the school is to support your efforts. We have the professional resources to create a comprehensive, sequential, and up-to-date program that will assist your child in developing these important life attitudes. The course contents, books, and multimedia materials for this program have been carefully screened. Every effort is being made to meet the varied needs and interests of our children.

We invite you to join us in developing our school program. Our first parent workshop has been scheduled for _____ (date) at _____ (time) in room _____. You are invited to review our course of study and the instructional materials. You are also welcome at any time to discuss this program with me.

Your interest and cooperation, as evidenced by the return of the tear-off form below, is very valuable to us. The response form also allows you the option of having your child excused from the program.

Sincerely,

Principal

_____

Please return to _____ (school name) on or before _____ (date).
_____ I would like to have my child excused from the Sexuality Education program.
_____ I can attend the parent workshop.
_____ I cannot attend the parent workshop.
I would like an appointment to speak with _____ my child's teacher _____ the principal.

Parent/Guardian Signature: _____ Date: _____

As Susan Spalt (1996) has suggested, every school professional should repeat the Serenity Prayer of Alcoholics Anonymous: "God grant me the serenity to accept the things I cannot change, courage to change the things I can, and wisdom to know the difference."

Any teachers who teach in the sexuality education program at any level need to train in that area. Teachers also need to be objective concerning controversial issues and have the ability to appreciate the views of others. Of course, a sense of humor helps, as well as being comfortable with one's own sexuality. Finally, they need a broad base of knowledge concerning the biological, psychological, and social aspects of human sexuality (Byer and Shainberg 1994, 422). What seems to be most important as schools examine the issues of teaching sexuality education is keeping in mind what will best serve the needs of the student. Following are guidelines essential for offering quality sexuality education programs (SIECUS 2006).

1. Sexuality education should be offered as part of an overall comprehensive health education program.

2. Teachers must be trained for sexuality education, receiving training in human sexuality including the philosophy and strategies of sexuality education.
3. The community must be involved in the development and implementation of sexuality education programs.
4. Curricula and materials should reflect cultural diversity and reflect all elements of society.
5. Young people must be given an opportunity to explore their own and society's attitudes/values and to develop or strengthen social skills.

Social Aspects and Values of Family Living

Various cultural, historical, legal, religious, and other institutional factors influence families and the sexuality roles within the family. It is important to remember that many forms of the family can be found. With this in mind, some typical characteristics of the family will be examined.

▪ Types of Families

The family fulfills a most important role in providing stability for the individual and society. The term *family* is used to describe two or more people living together who are related by blood, marriage, or adoption (Eshleman 2003). A nuclear family might be composed of a husband and wife, a brother and sister, one parent and a child or children, or both parents and one or more children. An extended family consists of a number of nuclear family groupings, often with blood ties. Extended family members can include uncles, aunts, grandparents, or cousins.

People who marry will be part of at least two different nuclear families, one in which they are born and one they start after selecting a marriage partner. The nuclear family to which we are born is the first and most basic provider of socialization. The extended family also has an influence on our socialization.

▪ The Changing Nature of the American Family

American youth in past generations generally grew up in one city or town, married someone from the surrounding area, and lived in the immediate locality. Chances were that members of the extended family, such as aunts, uncles, and grandparents, lived in the area also. In today's society, the nuclear family may be intact, but chances are that the extended family is not. For example, parents and grandparents may live in widely separate locations. As a result, grandparents may visit only on holidays or other special occasions. Thus, the interaction between these family members is not as frequent as it was in the past. The mobility of today's society and frequent job changes or transfers have served to separate the nuclear family from the extended family.

The advent of two-career households has brought about several changes as well. Families tend to have fewer children, and the care of the children may be left to daycare centers or other individuals who are not family members. Consequently, children may come in contact with caretakers of various ages who influence the social/psychological and value system development of the child.

In 2002, 19.3 million adults were divorced, representing 9.9 percent of the population. Almost 28 percent of all children under eighteen (19.8 million) lived with one parent; 84.5 percent of these children lived with their mother (Single Parent Central 2002).

Divorce may also change children's perspectives and the roles and responsibilities they have to handle. Estimates indicate that 50 percent of all children under the age of eighteen will spend some time in a female-parent-only situation. Several researchers have found that the divorce rate in North American society is strongly correlated with

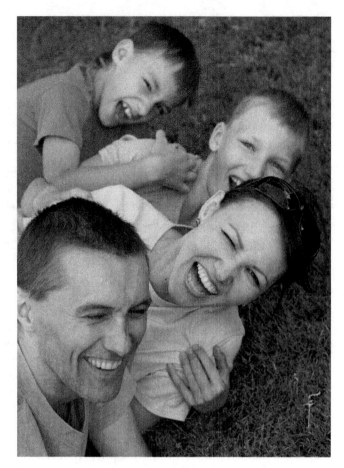

The family serves an important role by providing stability in the individual and society.

a significant increase in sexual problems, juvenile delinquency, and emotional and psychological maladjustment (Haas and Haas 2003, 320).

In the past, the value system an individual initially accepted was a combination of beliefs fostered by social engagement with the church, family, and school. Now, young people can witness a whole spectrum of values in a relatively short period of time by passive viewing, listening, or reading through television, video games, computers, and other media.

Individuals become socially, morally, and psychologically influenced by all the factors just described. Understanding the world is perhaps more difficult than ever because of these transitions and because of a barrage of mixed signals. No wonder, then, that many young people are confused about their roles in, and the expectations of, society.

The family has changed. However, it seems that people will always need others to whom they are bonded through closeness, sharing, and love. Such factors as the dual-career family, in which both the father and the mother share child-rearing and household responsibilities, have required adjustments to the family model of the past. And divorce, separation, and death have made

HEALTH HIGHLIGHT | **How Do You Know It Is Love?**

Strong, DeVault, and Sayad (1999) have suggested several factors that indicate some common experiences of an individual in love:

- Valuing the partner's presence
- Being able to communicate concerning intimate things
- Giving emotional support to the partner
- Sharing oneself and one's possessions with the partner
- Being able to understand each other

- Being able to count on the partner in time of need
- Holding the partner in high regard
- Feeling happiness with the partner
- Tolerating the partner's idiosyncrasies, routines, or forgetfulness
- Physically expressing love by hugging, kissing, making love
- Giving material evidence such as gifts, flowers, small favors, sharing tasks
- Expressing nonverbal feelings such as feeling happy, more content,

more secure when the person is present
- Giving nonmaterial evidence such as emotional and moral support in times of need and respecting the opinion of the partner
- Offering self-disclosure such as revealing intimate facts about oneself
- Verbally expressing affection such as saying "I love you"

Source: Strong, Devault, and Sayad 1999

single-parent families common. Because the stigma of divorce is not as great as it once was and more opportunities exist for women to work, couples who in the past stayed together, often unhappily, now have the option of divorcing. An interesting aspect of divorce is that the fastest growing type of single-parent family is the male-headed household. Another outgrowth of divorce is the blended family, which brings together children from previous marriages. When divorced parents remarry, blending the children may well be the largest problem they need to overcome.

Another interesting change in family structure is the return of adults to the home of their parents because of divorce and/or lack of job opportunities. These adults are referred to as *boomerang children*, because they left the household once but now return to live with their parents. Situations in which children return to the parents' home can cause adjustment problems for everyone. Issues of financial responsibility, privacy, and household responsibilities are all important.

Another issue for the family is the growing elderly population. As people live longer, caregiving for the elderly often falls to the family. In two-career families, this can create financial, as well as career-related, challenges.

Even with the problems and issues facing families today, couples continue to marry, remarry, and have children. Whatever problems are faced by the family, the desire to give love, share love, and be a part of the family unit will continue to perpetuate the family.

Concepts of Love and Family

Children can discuss what they like in friends and begin to realize that choosing the person with whom they want to spend their life is a very important decision. Some

concepts to discuss in relation to family life are love and intimacy, courtship and marriage, parenthood, single parenthood, and divorce.

Love and Intimacy

From the socialization process, we learn that we are supposed to form relationships and "fall in love." Attempting to define love is a difficult task. Without caring, what is thought to be love instead may be strong desire. E. Fromm (1989, 17) wrote that caring and respect for another is central to love and that people can achieve a meaningful type of love only after they are secure in their own identity. Fromm goes on to define mature love as "union under the condition of preserving one's integrity, one's individuality." Fromm suggests that a lover must feel, "I want the loved person to grow and unfold for his own sake and in his own ways, and not for the purpose of serving me" (Fromm 89).

The English language is limited in that only one word is available to describe a wide variety of feelings and relationships called love. The ancient Greeks had several terms to describe more precisely the different kinds of love. *Eros* referred to passionate or erotic love. *Storge* meant affection such as the feelings parents have for their children. *Philia* indicated the type of love in friendships, and *agape* referred to a kind of love associated with the traditional Christian view of being undemanding, patient, kind, and always supportive. In our society, love has been defined in terms of romantic, rational,

Creativity in the Classroom

When discussing love and intimacy have the student find a poem or reading from literature that they feel presents their conceptualization of love.

and mature love. Romantic love is an intense emotional experience that can totally captivate our existence. Rational love is based on acceptance of a partner's imperfections as well as affections and is more likely to lead to fulfilling, long-lasting relationships. Mature love is maintained through communication and separateness of the partners. It involves respect, admiration, and the desire to help each other. Lovers who exhibit maturity are best friends who are committed to each other and their relationship. J. Gevinger-Woititz (1993) states that there are three key ingredients of love. They are:

1. **Intimacy**—The emotional component involving feelings of closeness.
2. **Passion**—The component that reflects romantic and sexual attraction to another individual.
3. **Decision/commitment**—The cognitive component that an individual makes about being in love and committing to the relationship.

According to this model the greater the levels of intimacy, passion, and commitment, the more likely a person is involved in a positive love relationship. As relationships progress, the passionate feelings tend to become less intense and are replaced with a deep, caring, enduring type of love that is capable of sustaining a long-term commitment. This is not to say that passionate love should be allowed to leave relationships. In fact, couples should strive to maintain romance in their relationship. This requires a great deal of effort in learning how to communicate effectively, considering the spouses' feelings, striving to meet one another's needs, and the continuing commitment to the spouse.

To be intimate means to be vulnerable. It means risking rejection or suffocation of one's self. However, compatible partners replace those risks with trust and satisfaction. Essentially, individuals must remain responsible for themselves yet help each other with their goals, problems, and desires. Enjoying, sharing, and caring should be the outcomes of living with someone with whom love and intimacy are shared.

▪ Dating, Courtship, and Marriage

People marry for both personal and societal reasons. There is no single reason why people marry. Some people marry because they do not want to be alone. They want someone to share confidences, and they want to give and receive affection. A happy marriage can offer intimacy, support, and stimulation for personal growth. Some people marry for economic reasons; they may wish to pool their incomes, or one spouse may provide financial security to the other while he or she runs the home and cares for the children. Most people marry because they enjoy a person and can depend on that person in times of need. Marriage theoretically provides someone with whom to share both joy and sorrow.

Marriage serves many functions for individuals, including establishment of a family, companionship, economic strength, emotional security, a sexual outlet, and children. The greater the success in meeting these needs, the greater the likelihood the marriage will remain intact. Because each year more than two million marriages take place in the United States, it seems safe to say that marriages exist to fulfill basic needs associated with the husband–wife relationship. For these individual needs to be met, each partner must be committed to the marriage, develop effective communication skills, and accept the responsibility to nurture and enhance the marriage.

▪ Parenthood

When children enter a family, couples must assume new roles. The wife must become a mother and the husband a father. The exclusive attention of the partners toward each other, as well as the time demands and interests of the couple, must change. Parenthood is a difficult task, yet couples are expected to fulfill this role with little or no formal training. Parenthood is a lifetime commitment. Individuals can quit their jobs or divorce their mate, but there is no honorable way to withdraw from the role of father or mother. Many groups are now providing parenthood education programs that promote parenting skills. These courses attempt to teach ways to facilitate communication between parents and children, improve methods of discipline, and develop appropriate behavior for parents and children.

Advantages and Disadvantages of Parenthood. The obvious advantage of parenthood is the opportunity to love and nurture another human being. The psychological pleasure derived from being part of a loving family and helping to direct its development can bring a couple closer together, with the long-term benefit of pride in having done so. Besides the extreme economic cost of having and raising children, parenthood usually requires an adjustment in the career of at least one of the partners. Further, a child takes away from the emotional sharing time of the couple. Much time is spent in guiding and showing affection to the child. Some personal activities must be changed or eliminated, and there is a constant need to transport the children to and from various activities and functions as they become older.

Single Parenthood. Parenthood is difficult when two partners share the nurturing and love that children require. It can become even more difficult if only one parent is present. Through death, desertion, or divorce, single-parent situations often arise. Some individuals cope quite successfully with single parenthood, whereas others struggle with the many roles and situations they face in raising their children.

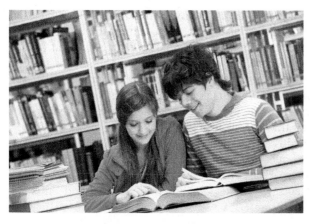

Dating helps in the processes of socialization, personality development, and learning to get along with others.

A single parent may experience a variety of problems. It may be difficult to meet the emotional needs of the child. There are a variety of ways to express love for a child. Telling a child he or she is loved and demonstrating that love with quality time serve to express love; however, the demands of working and maintaining a home may be so overwhelming that a child's emotional needs may not be met adequately. It also may be hard for the single parent to provide proper supervision for the child. Making arrangements for the child's care and supervision is difficult and costly and may take a large share of the budget. In addition, because women tend to make less money than men, households headed by women can experience financial difficulties. Finally, the single parent may experience unfulfilled emotional and sexual needs. Unmet emotional needs can develop because of the lack of time to seek a relationship. Because most single parents wish to hide their sexual involvement from their child, finding a time and place can present problems. Nevertheless, being a single parent does not have to be a disaster. It is important that single parents have sufficient financial, material, and emotional support to meet their own and their child's demands.

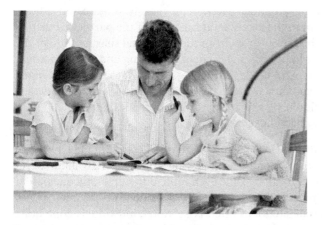

One of the greatest joys of parenthood is the opportunity to love and nurture another human being.

▪ Divorce

The most frequent method for dissolving a marriage is through divorce. Divorce is usually viewed as a failure of the family system, as well as a great personal crisis. However, it is also a way to end physical abuse and emotional tension. Personal factors most often given as reasons for divorce include financial problems, physical abuse, mental abuse, drinking, in-law problems, lack of love, adultery, and sexual incompatibility. Six social factors that seem to have contributed to increased divorce rates are (Byer and Shainberg 2001):

1. **Changing family functions**—Outside sources may now fulfill functions that were once considered primary family responsibilities. These may include medical, religious, and recreational aspects of family life.
2. **Casual marriages**—Hasty and youthful marriages complicated by pregnancy are often unstable.
3. **Jobs for women**—With greater job and career opportunities available to a large number of women, which allows greater economic freedom, a great barrier to divorce is removed.
4. **Decline in moral and religious sanctions**—Although not all churches openly state it, most have taken a more liberal attitude toward divorce. Also, society does not attach the stigma to divorce that it once did.
5. **The philosophy of happiness**—If happiness does not materialize to the degree anticipated, divorce or separation is accepted as a way of dealing with the feeling.
6. **More liberal divorce laws**—The liberalization of divorce laws, including no-fault divorces, has made it easier to terminate a marriage.

The emotional impact of a divorce is most difficult. Anyone who has experienced a divorce will usually describe it as a painful, devastating experience. Problems with finances, personal adjustment, and children can create an extremely stressful situation. Children whose parents are divorcing may develop deep feelings of guilt, fear, anger, loneliness, and/or sadness. Many times children feel that they must take sides in the conflict, which only serves to enhance their feelings of guilt. Because of the emotional conflict between the marriage partners, they may fail to recognize the worry the children feel concerning their own welfare. It is important to remember that despite the family fighting, the children will continue to love both parents. Children need sensitive parents and understanding teachers during and after a divorce. Many children will require counseling, which places an even greater burden on the teacher and school system.

Blended Families

Indications are that about 80 percent of individuals who divorce will remarry. Many times children from previous marriages find themselves in a stepfamily or blended family situation. The transition and adjustment for both the parents and the children may be difficult. Dealing with sibling jealousy, new rules, and striving for affection can put stress on the blended family.

Psychological Aspects of Sexuality and Family Living

Individuals have a wide variety of options for displaying their psychological and physiological traits. Also, in today's society there is greater flexibility in sex roles. This section deals with those psychological aspects of human sexuality and family life that help determine how people feel and react as individuals.

Gender Development

From birth, social expectations largely guide gender development. Parents consciously and unconsciously manipulate their children's gender development from infancy based on the sole criterion of sex. From dress and toys to behavior, the child learns to accept the parameters of being either a girl or a boy. By age two, children know what sex they are and understand some of their society's expectations for that sex. By the time children have reached school age, task orientation and emotional responses are based almost solely on what has been learned about gender. In some cases this process may be beneficial; in other cases it may be detrimental to the potential of both boys and girls.

The key to gender development is the creation of gender equality. Gender is socially constructed from the exercise of cultural conditioning. Making the sexes appear to be opposite and of unequal value requires the suppression of natural similarities by the use of social power. Social power can take the form of pushing boys toward what society considers the more masculine occupations, while girls are expected to follow those occupational paths that women have traditionally followed. An example of stereotypical gender roles is expecting women to become teachers or nurses. In reality, males and females are more like each other than they are different. Both can be reasonable, emotional, aggressive, or passive. Contemporary gender roles are evolving from traditional gender roles in which one sex is subordinate to the other to more equal roles in which both sexes are treated equally and to androgynous roles in which both sexes display the instrumental and expressive traits associated with one sex or the other.

Both males and females have a right to expand their individual potential and not be held to traditional roles and stereotypes. Traditional behavioral roles are learned in the same ways as gender identity. The emphasis should be on the humanness of people, not on their gender. Through such an emphasis, factors that inhibit the complete development of the individual can be discarded. Sharing household duties, child-rearing, and economic responsibilities can all contribute to the personal development of both partners. Males need not always be expected to be aggressive, nor females always passive.

Overcoming traditional gender roles is not easy because they are established early in life and are constantly reinforced throughout the years. Self-evaluation and a sense of adequacy are linked to gender role performances as defined by parents and peers in childhood.

It is important for teachers not to perpetuate artificial gender differences in the classroom. Imperative to this is recognition by teachers that boys and girls do not have innate abilities or disabilities in areas (academic, social, emotional, etc.) because of their gender.

Developing Sexuality

All aspects of human sexuality develop over a long period of time, from early childhood through the adult years. The groundwork for sexual values begins to develop in infancy, as children learn trust, initiative, and love. As they grow older, children try to achieve self-confidence in their interactions with parents, adults, and peers. Development of self-confidence is crucial to the development of the child's sexuality. If children grow up feeling at ease with themselves, they are more likely to appreciate themselves and members of the opposite sex.

Anything that affects a child's developing identity will eventually affect his or her sexuality as well. If the child learns to be defensive, unforgiving, or mistrusting in daily life, these attitudes will carry over into the sexual component of that individual's personality. Consequently, it is imperative that children learn to give and receive love and have a positive self-image if they are to be at ease with their sexuality later in life.

Sexual Orientation. Some children in the classroom may not identify with a heterosexual orientation, that is, sexual attraction to members of the opposite sex. They may instead be sexually attracted to members of the same sex, a homosexual orientation.

Reasons for sexual preference are not well understood. Some research suggests that it may have a biological basis in the size of certain brain structures (Allen and Gorski 2002). Other research suggests genetic, environmental, or hormonal factors may influence sexual orientation. There is probably no single reason or theory that accounts for all differences in sexual preference.

Teachers need to understand that a person's sexual orientation is not a matter of choice. An individual has no more choice about being homosexual than heterosexual. Teacher sensitivity is most important when interacting with gay and lesbian students because these students can become socially isolated, withdraw from activities and friends, have trouble concentrating, and develop low self-esteem (American Academy of Child and Adolescent Psychology 2011). Problems generally begin in early adolescence. Some of the problems encountered by gay/lesbian adolescents may include:

- feeling different from peers
- feeling guilty about their sexual orientation
- worrying about the response from their families and loved ones
- being teased and ridiculed by their peers
- worrying about HIV infection and other STIs
- fearing discrimination when joining clubs, playing sports, seeking admission to college, and finding employment
- being rejected and harassed by others

Biological Components of Sex Education

It is essential for all teachers to have a basic knowledge of the reproductive system and how it works. Obviously all the material presented in this section will not be presented in the elementary classroom, but teachers need the information for their own understanding of the reproductive system.

The Male Reproductive System

The male reproductive system, shown in Figure 11.1, is not as hormonally complex as that of the female because men do not have sexual cycles. The major male sexual endocrine glands are the two *testes*, or **testicles,** which are contained and protected in a saclike structure called the **scrotum.** At puberty, the testes (singular *testis*) begin producing mature **sperm,** the male reproductive cells. Attached to the top of each testis is the **epididymis.** This structure consists of tightly coiled tubes through which the sperm pass to the *vas deferens* (also called the *ductus deferens* or *spermatic ducts*). The two vas deferens serve as storage areas for the

mature sperm and are the means by which sperm move to the urethra. The two vas deferens eventually merge into one structure called the *ejaculatory duct*. This tube connects with the **urethra.** The urethra is a tube that runs the length of the **penis** and is used to transport both urine and semen (described below). The penis is the male organ for sexual intercourse and consists of spongy vascular material called erectile tissue, which swells when blood fills the vascular spaces in response to psychological and/or physical stimulation. The head of the penis is called the *glans penis*. This area contains many nerve endings and is very sensitive to sexual stimulation.

The **seminal vesicles,** the **prostate gland,** and the two **bulbourethral glands (Cowper's glands)** manufacture substances important to the sperm and ejaculate. The seminal vesicles produce a simple sugar, fructose, that adds volume to the ejaculatory fluid, called semen, and activates the movement of the sperm. The prostate gland provides a highly alkaline milky fluid that helps neutralize the highly acidic vagina and facilitates the movement of sperm. The pea-sized bulbourethral glands also produce an alkaline fluid that lubricates and neutralizes the acidity of urine in the urethra. The bulbourethral glands secrete this substance prior to ejaculation of sperm. The combined fluid produced by the seminal vesicles, prostate, and bulbourethral glands, along with the sperm it contains, is **semen.**

It should be noted that the testes constantly manufacture mature sperm from puberty through old age. On release of interstitial cell-stimulating hormone (ICSH) into the bloodstream from the anterior lobe of the pituitary gland, the testes also secrete testosterone. Although it plays many diverse roles, testosterone is needed to trigger the male adolescent growth spurt, which is accompanied by

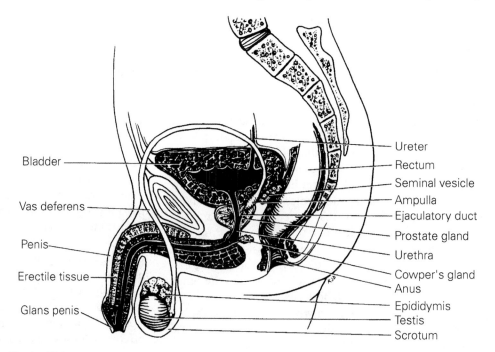

Figure 11.1
The Male Reproductive System

the development of secondary sex characteristics, including appearance of facial and genital hair, deepening voice, oilier skin, and increased muscle size and mass.

The Female Reproductive System

The female reproductive system, shown in Figure 11.2, is composed of the external genitalia and the internal organs consisting of the vagina, uterus, uterine tubes (fallopian tubes or oviducts), and ovaries. The external genitalia are the *labia majora* (the outer lips, or folds) and the *labia minora* (the inner lips, or folds). The **clitoris** is a small structure at the top of the labia minora that facilitates sexual stimulation. The **vagina** is an elastic canal extending from just behind the cervix to the opening of the external genitalia. It serves as the organ for sexual intercourse and

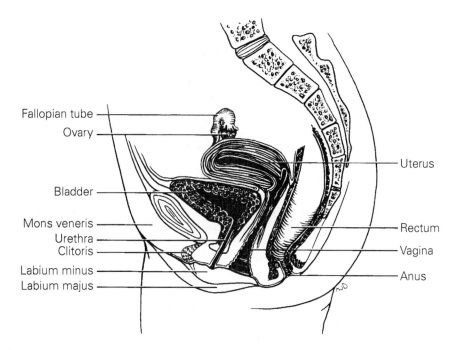

Figure 11.2
The Female Reproductive System

as the birth canal. The **uterus** (or womb) is a pear-shaped organ where the fetus develops. The uterus has three layers: the *perimetrium* (outer layer), the *myometrium* (muscular middle layer), and *endometrium* (inner layer). The endometrium is sloughed off during menstruation. Two armlike projections called the *uterine tubes* branch from the top of the uterus. These tubes are three to five inches long and have *fimbria* (small fingerlike projections) at the far ends next to the ovaries. Through these tubes the eggs, or ova, pass. If fertilization takes place, it occurs in the upper third of one of the uterine tubes. Two **ovaries** produce ova and secrete hormones that bring about the development of the female secondary sex characteristics, such as the rounding of the female figure, breast development, and pubic hair.

Each ovary contains 200,000 to 400,000 saclike structures called follicles that store immature egg cells. At the onset of puberty several follicles are activated in the ovary each month by follicle-stimulating hormone (FSH) being released into the bloodstream from the anterior lobe of the pituitary gland. Only one follicle will evolve into a mature ovum and simultaneously secrete estrogen. Estrogen signals the uterus to prepare for a potential pregnancy by filling its lining with blood and nutrients for nourishment of the embryo. As the maturing follicle and its ovum move to the surface of the ovary, with the follicle

continuing to secrete estrogen, luteinizing hormone (LH) is released into the bloodstream from the anterior lobe of the pituitary. The production of LH causes the follicle to rupture and release the mature ovum into the uterine tubes. This process, known as ovulation, usually occurs midway into the monthly reproductive cycle of twenty-eight days. This cycle is shown in Figure 11.3.

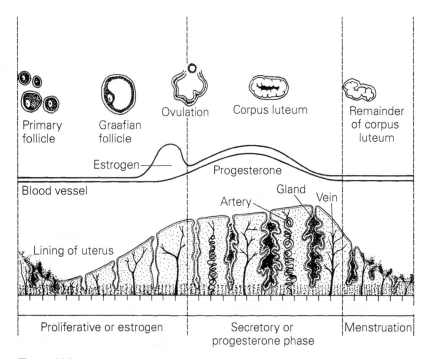

Figure 11.3
The Female Monthly Reproductive Cycle

During ovulation, estrogen is at its highest level and causes cessation of additional secretions of FSH. At the same time, LH continues to be secreted and produces closure of the ruptured follicle. The empty follicle, now called the *corpus luteum*, and the mature ovum begin to produce another hormone, in addition to now-declining levels of estrogen, called *progesterone*. Progesterone further prepares the uterus for implantation of a fertilized egg and continues to maintain the uterus during pregnancy.

From the moment that conception occurs, the woman's body begins to change. Through pregnancy a weight gain of seventeen to twenty-four pounds is normal and looked on as desirable because this helps ensure adequate development of the fetus. The average fetus weighs approximately seven pounds at birth. Table 11.1 lists the development of the fetus through each trimester.

If the mature ovum is not fertilized within twenty-four to forty-eight hours after ovulation, it disintegrates, thus diminishing the amount of estrogen and progesterone in the bloodstream. Around the twenty-fourth day of the cycle, the corpus luteum also stops secreting progesterone and estrogen. As a result, several days later the uterus expels its blood-rich lining through the vagina in a process referred to as menstruation (Figure 11.3). Following menstruation, the reproductive cycle begins again in preparation for possible fertilization and pregnancy. Menstruation begins with puberty. The onset of menstruation is called menarche.

Conception

Conception occurs when a single sperm fertilizes an egg to produce a zygote. Conception usually occurs in the upper third of the uterine tube and must take place in the first or second day following ovulation. To facilitate conception, the sperm go through a series of biochemical changes known as *capacitation*, which enables penetration of the egg (Kelly 2006, 281). When a sperm

> **TEACHING TIP**
>
> Use overheads, anatomical charts, or plastic models when teaching the functions and structures of the female and male reproductive systems. The visuals help to promote understanding as well as providing another learning cue for the student.

Table 11.1   Development During Pregnancy
First-trimester development
• A small mass of cells is implanted in the uterus.   • The mass of cells becomes the embryo until seventh/eighth week.   • Development into a fetus begins after seventh/eighth week.   • Major organ systems are present and recognizable.   • During the fourth to eighth weeks, the eyes, ears, arms, hands, fingers, legs, feet, and toes develop.   • By the seventh week, the liver, lungs, pancreas, kidneys, and intestines have formed.   • By the end of the first trimester, the fetus weighs two-thirds of an ounce and is about 4 inches in length.   • From this time on, development consists of enlargement and differentiation of the existing structures.
Second-trimester development
• By the end of the fourteenth week, movement can be detected.   • By the eighteenth week, a fetal heartbeat can be detected.   • By the twentieth week, the fetus will open its eyes.   • Around the twenty-fourth week, the fetus is sensitive to light and can hear sounds. It will also have periods of sleep and wakefulness.
Third-trimester development
• Fat deposits form under the skin.   • During the seventh month, the fetus turns in the uterus to a head-down position.   • By the end of the eighth month, the fetus weighs an average of 5 pounds, 4 ounces.   • At birth, the average infant weighs approximately 7.5 pounds and is 20 inches long.

enters an egg, the membrane thickens to prevent further penetration by sperm.

▪ Genetics

The human body is made up of trillions of cells that perform various specialized functions. Each cell contains a *nucleus*, which contains genes that provide the hereditary information in smaller rod-shaped bodies called *chromosomes*. Twenty-two pairs of auto-somal (non-sex-determining) chromosomes account for individual facial features, hair color, height, body build, and a myriad of other characteristics. Gender is determined by the twenty-third, or sex-determining, chromosomal pair. One member of the pair is an X chromosome inherited from the mother's ovum. The other (inherited from the father's sperm) can be either an X or Y chromosome. If a Y chromosome is present, the offspring is male; if no Y is present, the offspring is female.

Mitosis is ordinary cell division. This process results in two new cells that each contain the full complement of forty-six chromosomes. *Meiosis* is the cell division by which sperm and ovum are formed. These cells are called *gametes* and contain only twenty-three chromosomes. When a male gamete (sperm) unites with a female gamete (ovum), the twenty-three pairs unite to form the complete set required to produce a new individual from the zygote.

▪ The Embryonic Period

Immediately after conception, the zygote begins to divide to form other cells. It travels down the uterine tube and within ten days attaches to the uterine wall. From the time it attaches to the wall until the eighth week, it is called an embryo. The embryo divides into three layers of cells from which the various body organs and systems develop. The innermost layer, the *endoderm*, becomes the digestive and respiratory systems; the next layer, the *mesoderm*, forms the skeletal, muscular, circulatory, and reproductive systems; and the *ectoderm*, or outermost layer, becomes the nervous system and skin. The head develops first, and the lower body develops last. After eight weeks, the embryo is called the fetus. (For simplicity, both the embryo and fetus will be described as the embryo in the following two paragraphs.)

The *amnion* is a thin protective membrane that is filled with a fluid called the *amniotic fluid*. This fluid serves as insulation and protection for the embryo against shocks and blows to the mother's abdomen. The fluid also permits changes in position as growth and movement occur. The *umbilical cord* connects the placenta and the developing embryo.

The *placenta* is the organ through which nutrients, vitamins, antibodies, and other substances (such as drugs, alcohol, and diseases) are moved inward. Waste products, such as nitrogen compounds and carbon dioxide, are carried outward to diffuse across the placenta to the mother's blood, which carries them to the mother's kidneys and lungs for disposal (in urine and exhaled gas). This is accomplished even though there is no mixing of the embryo's and mother's blood. The placenta is expelled shortly following the birth of the child and is referred to as the *afterbirth*.

▪ Multiple Births

Several factors contribute to multiple births. Heredity, the increased use of fertility drugs, age of the mother, and social factors seem significant (Haas and Haas 2003). Some families are genetically more likely to have multiple births than others are. Women in their thirties and forties are more likely to have multiple births than are women in their twenties.

Identical twins develop from a single fertilized ovum that divides to form two individuals. Such twins are always the same sex and look alike. *Fraternal twins* develop from two different ova fertilized at the same time. However, fraternal twins may not be of the same sex and look no more alike than any other siblings born to the same parents.

Triplets usually involve two fertilized ova, one of which separates and then develops into twins. *Quadruplets* usually involve two fertilized ova that then divide and develop into two pairs of identical twins.

▪ Childbirth

The process of childbirth occurs in three stages and is referred to as labor (Figure 11.4). This process begins when the amniotic sac that has protected the fetus ruptures and the amniotic fluid flows from the vagina. Labor pains occur at regular intervals, usually fifteen to twenty minutes apart, with the cervix dilating three to four inches to permit passage of the fetus through the vagina. This first stage of labor may last twelve to sixteen hours (or even longer) for the first birth but usually is shorter in subsequent births.

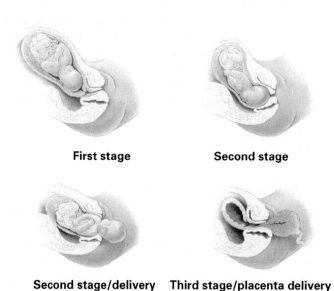

First stage   **Second stage**

Second stage/delivery   **Third stage/placenta delivery**

Figure 11.4
The Three Stages of Birth

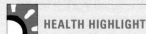

Psychological Signs

1. Fear of being alone with a specific person
2. Sleep disturbances, such as nightmares, fear of going to bed, and fear of sleeping alone
3. Irritability or short temper
4. Clinging to parent or parents
5. Unexplained fears
6. Changes in behavior and schoolwork or in relating to friends or siblings
7. Behaving like a younger child (regression)
8. Sexual sophistication or knowledge greater than age group
9. Running away from home or fear of going home

Physical Signs (Caused by Sexual Acts)

1. Difficulty in walking or sitting
2. Pain or itching in genital areas
3. Torn, stained, or bloody underwear
4. Bruises or bleeding in external genitals, vagina, or anal areas
5. Sexually transmitted diseases
6. Pregnancy

Source: From *Human Sexuality*, Second Edition, by Nancy W. Denney and David Quadagno, © 1992. Used by permission.

The second stage begins when the cervix has fully dilated and the baby's head enters the vagina. It ends with the birth of the baby. Contractions are quite severe and last from a minute to a minute and a half, with a two- to three-minute interval between contractions. The contractions serve to move the baby down the birth canal. Just before the head of the child appears, it rotates to the side to pass the pelvic bone. The neck and shoulders emerge, and the rest of the body follows rather quickly.

The third and final stage lasts only a few minutes and consists of the delivery of the placenta. The placenta separates from the wall of the uterus and is expelled as afterbirth. It is examined to determine that all of the organ has been delivered.

Occasionally, complications arise during labor. For example, some conditions may require a *caesarean section* (or *c-section*). When this procedure is used, an incision is made through the abdominal wall and another in the uterus, and the baby is removed. The reason for a caesarean section is usually a contracted pelvis, through which the baby is unable to pass into the vagina. Other reasons are that the baby is in a breech (buttock or leg presenting first) position; the placenta has prematurely separated from the uterus, causing a loss of oxygen; a vaginal infection is present; or the mother is incapacitated because of injury or trauma. To help identify potential complications, a fetal monitor may be used during the birth process. Recently, caesarean sections have been used by healthy women to deal with the unpredictability of the onset of labor.

Unwanted Pregnancies

The abortion issue is far from settled. Many states have circumvented the 1973 Supreme Court ruling that allowed abortions by establishing laws that make abortions difficult to obtain. The U.S. Congress has placed restrictions on federally funded abortions by prohibiting Medicaid funds from being used to pay for the procedure except when the mother's life is in danger. The issues associated with abortion continue to be hotly debated.

If the decision is made to not terminate an unwanted pregnancy, there are other options. The woman may choose to keep her child or place the infant for adoption. In general, the younger the woman is, the more difficult her decision. Parenting is a demanding job, and if the woman is single, the difficulty is even greater. Many times she must rely on her parents or other relatives to aid in caring for the child. Unfortunately, too often the maturity necessary to be a good parent is lacking. The woman is faced with the difficulty of supplying a safe place for the child to grow and develop, providing adequate nutrition, developing sufficient economic resources, and having a secure, supportive environment. The options open to a single, young parent may be severely lacking from a social, educational, and economic perspective. Even if marriage occurs, the chance of a teenage marriage surviving is much less than if marriage occurs later in life.

Adoption is also a difficult decision, but many couples want to provide the love, closeness, and resources a child needs. Being an adoptive parent is no different from being a natural parent. The same love, rewards, and frustrations are experienced by both parents and children.

Problems of Child Abuse and Violence

Child abuse consists of any act of commission or omission that endangers or impairs a child's physical or emotional health and development (Childhelp USA 2011). The major forms of child abuse are:

- **Physical abuse**—any nonaccidental injury to a child. This includes hitting, kicking, slapping, shaking, burning, pinching, hair-pulling, biting, choking, throwing, shoving, whipping, and paddling.
- **Emotional abuse**—any attitude or behavior that interferes with a child's mental health or social development. This includes yelling, screaming, name-calling, shaming, negative comparisons to others, and telling a child he or she is "bad," "no good," "worthless," or a "mistake."

HEALTH HIGHLIGHT | **Information for Teachers on Abuse**

1. Child sexual abuse (molestation) involves the misuse of power by an adult or older child to engage a younger child in sexual activities to gratify the perpetrator's (offender's) needs.

2. Both touching and nontouching offenses are included in the category of sexual abuse. Examples of nontouching behaviors include showing children pornography or having children pose for pornographic pictures. Touching offenses include fondling and penetration.

3. Although the actual behavior involved in child sexual abuse varies, the following characteristics are common:
   a. It usually starts at an early age, before children are aware of the inappropriate nature of the acts.
   b. The adult takes advantage of the child's need for approval, trust, and lack of knowledge.
   c. The behavior is surrounded with secrecy.
   d. The adult uses authority to threaten, bribe, or trick the child into complying.
   e. The child feels responsible for the abuse.

4. The child's reaction to the situation depends on his or her perception of the offense and the reactions of those important to him or her, rather than the legally defined severity of the offense.

5. Current information suggests that at least 1 in 4 girls and 1 in 7 boys are physically molested by the age of eighteen. In 80 to 90 percent of the reported cases, the perpetrator is someone who is known to the child; in over 50 percent of the cases, the offender is a family member.

6. Most often, the perpetrator is someone the child knows well. The child may be emotionally tied to the individual and may even love him or her. Therefore, it should be emphasized that abuse can happen with someone we know or love; do not overemphasize danger from strangers.

7. Some children are aware of the inappropriateness of abusive behavior but are still unable to terminate it. Others are unable to recognize or respond appropriately to abusive or potentially abusive behaviors.

8. The educator should be sensitive to the manner in which material is presented and to the reactions of the students. Disclosure is often vague or indirect.

9. Define the subject according to the child's age. For young ones, explain that, although most adults are good and caring, some do not make good decisions about touching children. They may try to touch children on private parts of the body for no good reason. A broader range of offenses and behaviors can be included when defining molestation to older children. Describe examples of touching and nontouching behaviors to make sure they understand the entire concept.

10. It is equally important for children to understand the characteristics of healthy interpersonal and familial relationships. Indicate that most adults do care and want to help children. Describe examples of positive interpersonal relationships as well as negative ones in teaching the material.

11. Lessons for younger children need to stress developing the self-confidence and self-esteem needed to resist the attention and gifts often "earned" through participating in the abuse. Older children should begin to recognize characteristics of cooperative and exploitative relationships and relate these to their daily activities.

12. Touches can be categorized according to one's personal reaction to the touch. Good touches make one feel warm, secure, or happy; bad touches make one feel angry, hurt, or ashamed. Those touches that confuse are often sexual touches or touches that are delivered in a contradictory manner that perplexes the child. Teachers can refer to resource materials, the local school district, or the state department of education for additional information.

13. Lessons should include opportunities to role-play and use the skills taught. For examples of assertiveness and decision-making activities, refer to the various resource materials available through state departments of education and local school districts.

Source: Administration for Children and Families

- **Sexual abuse**—any sexual act between an adult and child. This includes fondling, penetration, intercourse, exploitation, pornography, exhibitionism, child prostitution, group sex, oral sex, or forced observation of sexual acts.

- **Physical neglect**—failure to provide for a child's needs in the form of supervision, housing, food, clothing, medical care, and hygiene.

- **Emotional neglect**—failure to provide affection and support necessary for the development of emotional, social, physical, and intellectual well-being.

Child abuse is a particularly difficult problem to combat because the abuse usually occurs in the home and because there is often a public reluctance to intervene or report what is thought to be a private matter.

Data reported in 2007 tracked over 3 million reports of child abuse (some reports did include multiple children). Out of these reports, 899,000 children were found to be victims of abuse or neglect. Sixty percent of these children were found to be neglected, 17.4 percent were physically abused, 7.6 percent were sexually abused, and 4.2 percent were emotionally abused. Data indicate that rates of victimization decline as the age of the child increases. As reported in 2006 data, the rate for victimization was 12.1 per 1,000 children except for sexual abuse. The rate for sexual abuse was 1.7 victims per 1,000 female children compared to 0.4 victims per 1,000 male children. The perpetrators of these acts of child abuse or neglect were reported as 60 percent female and 40 percent male. A perpetrator is most often a parent or other caretaker, such as a relative, babysitter, or foster parent, who has maltreated a child. Almost 80 percent of victims were abused by a parent or parents. The mother acting alone was responsible for 58 percent of neglect victims and 32 percent of physical abuse. The father acting alone was responsible for 29 percent of child neglect cases and 22 percent of abuse cases. There were approximately 1,530 child fatalities in the year 2006. Youngest children were the most vulnerable. Children younger than one year old accounted for 44 percent of child fatalities, and 85 percent of fatalities were children younger than six years of age (U.S. Department of Health & Human Services 2008).

Aside from the obvious physical effects, a child's psychological development can be seriously handicapped by abusive treatment. Many abused children are emotionally affected for the rest of their lives. A child who is abused in the home is one who loses the chance to be a child. Unable to understand why they are being punished, these children come to believe that they deserve such treatment because they are "bad." They see the world as cold and hostile and have little faith in themselves or in their ability to succeed in life. They learn that using force is an acceptable way to deal with others and, tragically, often become child abusers themselves.

Parents most often become physically or emotionally abusive because of their own history of abuse, failure to understand the needs of their children, or as a response to unmanaged stress. They typically do not have the self-confidence, ingenuity, and ability to cope with crises within the family. Crisis presents a greater danger for them than for someone with better coping skills. Even a minor occurrence may be enough to lead to loss of self-control and an abusive attack on an innocent child. In many instances, abusing adults reverse roles with their children, requiring the child to love and care for them without providing the emotional support the child needs.

With sexual abuse, abusers may actually convince themselves that they are doing a child a favor by showing him or her the "facts of life" in a more loving way than an outsider would do (Office of the Attorney General 1985). In 90 percent of child sexual abuse cases, the offenders are male and are often described as being unassertive, withdrawn, and emotionless. Other characteristics include a history of either physical or sexual abuse, alcohol or drug abuse, little satisfaction with sexual relationships with adults, lack of control over their emotions, and occasionally mental illness (Prevent Child Abuse America 2011). There is hope for reeducation of the adult if the matter can be brought to the attention of the proper authorities. Successful therapy seems directly related to the perpetrator's willingness to change.

Every state has laws that make it mandatory for teachers to report suspected abuse. Not every bruise should be considered abuse, but if a pattern of injury is observed, teachers should report this concern. Proper authorities include the state's department of family and child services or a local health agency.

Chapter In Review

Summary

- No area in health education is more controversial than that of sexuality education.
- The majority of teachers and parents support sexuality education.
- Some individuals oppose sexuality education.
- Schools can assist students in developing critical thinking skills, communication skills, self-esteem, and a solid knowledge base.
- The family should provide the value base on which students make their decisions.
- Sexuality education at the elementary level consists of many components, including biological aspects, self-esteem, relationships, personal skills, social mores, and sexual health.
- The family is the basic unit of society. The family is an institution in transition, leading to variations of family units such as single-parent and blended families.
- Factors that may contribute to the divorce rate include changing family functions, casual marriages, increased job availability for women, decline in moral and religious sanctions, the philosophy of happiness, and more liberal divorce laws.
- Human sexuality develops over an extended length of time, ranging from early childhood to the adult years.
- The various structures of the male and female reproductive system are designed to enable human reproduction.
- Unwanted pregnancies are a continuing issue; the options available for consideration are keeping the child, planning for adoption, or terminating the pregnancy. For all three options, there are consequences that must be faced by the individuals involved.
- Estimates are that about 3 million children are maltreated by their parents and other adults each year.
- Every state has laws that require teachers to report suspected abuse.

Discussion Questions

1. What are some reasons for opposition to sexuality education?
2. What are some of the groups that oppose sexuality education, and what are their grounds for opposition?

3. Discuss the anatomy and physiology of female and male reproductive systems.

4. What important functions does the family fill?

5. What factors should the classroom teacher be aware of when there are children of divorce in the classroom?

6. What are the shortcomings of inflexible gender roles?

7. Differentiate among and explain the different types of abuse.

8. What are the key concepts that a comprehensive family life and sexuality education program should contain?

Critical Thinking Questions

1. Does sexuality education promote premature sexual activity? On what rationale do you base your opinion?

2. Does sexuality education belong in the home, school, or both?

3. From what sources did you discover your sexual information? What effect has that had upon your perception of sexuality?

4. In today's world, is it realistic to expect to marry once and have it last a lifetime?

5. To what extent should a couple stay married for the sake of the children involved?

Access more material online at www.pearsonhighered.com/anspaugh. At this companion website for *Teaching Today's Health,* you'll find chapter quizzes, web links, flashcards, a glossary, additional Worksheets, and more to help you succeed.

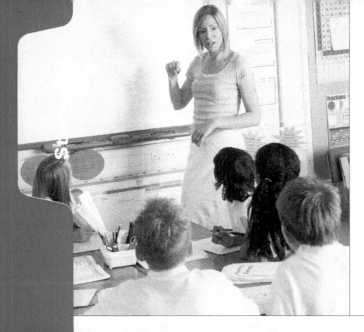

Strategies for Teaching Sexuality Education

12

Sexuality education should assist young people in understanding a postive view of sexuality, provide them with information and skills for taking care of their sexual health, and help them make sound decisions now and in the future.

—*Guidelines for Comprehensive Sexuality Education Fact Sheet (SIECUS 2004)*

Valued Outcomes

After completion of this chapter, you should be able to:

- Provide learning opportunities for a variety of topics related to sexuality education.
- Discuss the different types of families.
- Help students identify why each member of a family is important and what roles each member has.
- Present the interpersonal skills necessary for strengthening individual and family relationships.
- Help students identify why a positive self-image is necessary.
- Help students identify why the understanding of self is a foundation for succe's transition to adulthood.
- Discuss children's rights; no one should be mistreated, taken advantage of, or abused by another person.
- Discuss the physical, social, and emotional growth of the male/female.
- Discuss procreation.
- Discuss menstruation and the process that healthy females experience.
- Help students develop wholesome attitudes toward sexuality.
- Help students understand how sexual values and decisions are often individual decisions.

Reflections

Review the quote at the beginning of this chapter. What topic taught at the elementary and middle school levels would be most difficult for you to deal with in the classroom? Discuss what information you would need to have as a teacher to be successful in teaching the topic(s). What sensitive areas for students and parents would you be most concerned about when teaching the content?

Building Self-Esteem and Responsible Decision Making

Traditionally, providing sexuality education has been the responsibility primarily of the family. Organized religion and other social institutions have also played a significant role. For a variety of reasons, these sources are no longer completely adequate. The schools, by supplementing—not replacing—traditional sources, can provide well-designed and tested sexuality education programs that can benefit all concerned—children, parents, and society in general.

The classroom is a nonthreatening atmosphere where reliable and accurate information can be presented about sex and family matters. But sexuality education is more than just factual information. An effective program must be based on the development of self-esteem and responsible decision making. If children learn to feel good about themselves, they are less likely to be open to exploitation, and less likely to need to exploit others in sexual and family functioning. Sexuality education strives to teach equality and respect between the sexes and an appreciation for self and others.

The suggestions in this chapter will help you work toward these goals. These learning opportunities will assist students in obtaining factual knowledge, developing their value systems, and growing psychologically as individuals.

Shown to the right of each activity title in this chapter is the suggested grade level(s) for which the activity might be appropriate. Through modification, many of the suggested activities could be used at various grade levels. This modification could include the changing of questions that might be more age appropriate for the activity than those provided.

Information Assessment Strategies

Finding Answers through Technology
Grades 4-8

Valued Outcome: Students will be able to access information to answer their questions concerning sexuality.

National Health Education Standards: 1, 2

Description of Strategy: The sexuality education website www.sexetc.org is a reliable website that offers answers and discussion of sex and sexuality issues. The website, run by Rutgers University, can be accessed via a web browser or through mobile devices. The available information includes a Sex in the States section, FAQs, and definitions for over 400 sex terms. The information is offered in order to help people understand and make use of the most accurate information possible regarding sex and sexuality. When discussing sexuality issues and concerns, the students (with the help of the teacher) should formulate thoughtful questions and then research them on the reliable website. Additionally, important terms can be researched on the website so students have an accurate understanding of what some terms really mean rather than relying on peers for the information.

Materials Needed: computer with Internet access or mobile device with online access

Processing Questions:

1. What are the important facts found regarding the question(s) under consideration?
2. What questions do you have in regard to the answers found at the website?
3. What questions do you have in regard to the terms researched?

✓ **Assessment:** Have the class write their reactions to the answers they found. Are they what the student thought the answers should/would be? The students can develop a vocabulary list and be assessed by their ability to define the terms.

Rights and Responsibilities
Grades 4–6

Valued Outcome: Students will be able to identify the factors that help families live in happy environments.

National Health Education Standards: 2, 8

Description of Strategy: Have the class prepare two-column lists of their rights and responsibilities as family members. Under the rights column, they may list such things as being provided with food and shelter, having free time to play or watch television, being allowed to express their opinions on certain family matters, and spending their allowances as they wish. Under the responsibilities column, students may list such things as keeping their rooms clean, taking out the trash, helping with housework, caring for a younger sibling, being honest in family matters, and accepting parental decisions. After the lists have been prepared, discuss the significance of the items listed. Ask questions such as the processing questions below.

Materials Needed: pencils or pens and paper

Processing Questions:

1. Do you think your rights and responsibilities are equally balanced?
2. How have your rights and responsibilities changed as you have gotten older?
3. Do boys in a family have certain rights and responsibilities that girls do not have?
4. Do girls in a family have certain rights and responsibilities that boys do not have?
5. How much input should children have about their rights and responsibilities?
6. If you made all the rules in your home, what changes might you consider? Why?

7. What do your rights and responsibilities suggest to you about your own level of maturity?
8. How would you feel if you had no responsibilities?

✓ **Assessment:** Students can give at least three examples of how their rights and responsibilities contribute to a functional family.

Attitude Inventory— How Do I Feel? Grades 4–6

Valued Outcome: Students will identify feelings concerning family, friends, and themselves.

National Health Education Standard: 2

Description of Strategy: Prepare individual sheets like the one shown here, and ask the students to offer their opinion about each statement. Follow with a general class discussion, and then ask students to write a paragraph about three things they learned from their responses.

Materials Needed: attitude inventory sheet for each student, pencils

Processing Questions:

1. Were there questions that were difficult to answer?
2. Why were the answers to some of the questions difficult?
3. What three things did you learn from your responses?

○ **Integration:** Writing

✓ **Assessment:** In their written reflection, students demonstrate an understanding of the influence that family, peers, media, and other factors have on their attitudes about relationships.

Getting to Know Me Grades 4–5

Valued Outcome: Students will be able to list their unique characteristics.

National Health Education Standard: 4

Description of Strategy: Prepare sheets or cards with the following statements or categories on them. Pass out a sheet to each student to complete, then collect and shuffle all the responses. Either as a class or in small-group activity, see if students can identify each other by the responses. Have the students consider what this suggests about the unique individuality of each person.

Something that I do well: _____

Music that I like: _____

Three words that describe me: _____

If I could have a dream come true, it would be: _____

How Do I Feel?

	Agree	Disagree	Not Sure
1. Each child is an important member of his or her family.	____	____	____
2. Families do a lot of fun things together.	____	____	____
3. Mothers should hug and kiss their children more than fathers should.	____	____	____
4. Children who have no brothers or sisters are unhappy.	____	____	____
5. Mothers and fathers should not hug and kiss each other in front of their children.	____	____	____
6. The more I learn about myself, the better I like myself.	____	____	____
7. Children who don't help with the housework should not get an allowance.	____	____	____
8. The best way to learn about sex is to ask friends.	____	____	____
9. I'd be too embarrassed to ask my parents about sex.	____	____	____
10. Sometimes I dread becoming a teenager.	____	____	____
11. I have trouble telling friends how I really feel.	____	____	____
12. My friends often pressure me to do things I don't want to do.	____	____	____
13. When a friend does something wrong, I usually tell the person how I feel.	____	____	____
14. Children should be allowed to set some of the family rules.	____	____	____
15. Adults are free to do what they want most of the time.	____	____	____

☆ TEACHING IN ACTION | **Daily Lesson Plan**

Lesson Title: Information Please

Date: February 12, 2012   **Time:** 10:00 A.M.   **Grade:** Five   **Teacher:** Faris

I. National Health Education Standards

Health Education Standard 3: Students will demonstrate the ability to access valid information and products and services to enhance health.

II. National Health Education Standards Performance Indicator

3.5.1 identify characteristics of valid health information, products, and services.

III. Valued Outcomes

- Students will be able to identify sources of information concerning sexuality questions.
- Students will be able to identify the characteristics of accurate information concerning sexuality questions.
- Students will be aware that one lone source cannot supply all the needed information for every sexuality question.

IV. Description of Strategy

1. Prepare a worksheet that lists the following possible sources of information on sexuality: movies and television shows, health teachers, ministers/priests/rabbis, friends, the Internet, parents, library books, physicians, newspapers, magazines, and school textbooks.
2. On the worksheet, have the students rank the items in the list, starting with "1" for the most likely source for them to get information and "11" for the least likely source of information.
3. Discuss the rankings with the class and have students point out the pros and cons of each source. Give students helpful hints on deciphering what is accurate sexuality information.
4. Discuss the sources of information that are trying to sell a product or have a hidden message (this could be true of many types of health information, not just sexuality information).
5. Avoid encouraging students to eliminate any one source of information. Remind them that it is always best to seek multiple sources of information to get the most complete information.

V. Materials Needed

- worksheet for ranking sources

VI. Formative Evaluation

Benchmarks
- Level 1: Student was able to identify some sources of information concerning sexuality questions.
- Level 2: Student was able to identify all sources of information concerning sexuality questions.
- Level 3: Student was able to identify all sources of information concerning sexuality questions and list the pros and cons associated with each.
- Level 4: Student was able to identify all sources of information concerning sexuality questions and list the pros and cons associated with each. Student was able to describe the best way to get accurate and complete information on sexuality questions.

VII. Points of Emphasis

1. Explain that some sources of information concerning sexuality are better to use than others.
2. Emphasize the importance of using multiple sources of information.
3. Explain how having the right information concerning sexuality leads to better decision-making skills and confidence.

Teacher Evaluation
1. Keep the lesson as taught?   yes _____   no _____
2. What I need to improve _____
3. Next time make sure _____
4. Strengths of lesson Strategies _____

TEACHING IN ACTION | **Daily Lesson Plan**

Lesson Title: Love, Love, Love

Date: February 5, 2012   **Time:** 9:00 A.M.   **Grade:** Six   **Teacher:** Land

I. National Health Education Standards

Health Education Standard 2: Students will analyze the influence of family, peers, culture, media, technology, and other factors on health behaviors.

II. National Health Education Standards Performance Indicator

2.8.2 describe the influence of culture on health beliefs, practices, and behaviors.

III. Valued Outcomes

- Students will be able to identify different types of love toward various members of society.
- Students will able to list nonsexual ways to express love toward others.
- Students will be able to describe how culture influences perceptions of love.

IV. Description of Strategy

1. Have the class talk about and give examples of all the different people whom they love. This could include parents, siblings, grandparents, friends, or classmates, just to name a few.
2. Then describe to the students the different kinds of love (romantic, familial, religious, platonic, etc.) and various types of families (for example, nuclear or extended) that give and receive these different kinds of love.
3. Have students write down appropriate ways to express love to family members or friends verbally, by the tone of their voices, by body language, and by actions toward each other.
4. Discuss with students ways to express love, and discuss how culture influences our attitudes toward love. Ask students: "What are some symbols of love that we see through television, movies, magazines, etc., and are these symbols accurate portrayals of love?"

V. Materials Needed

- Pen/pencil
- Paper

VI. Formative Evaluation

Benchmarks

- Level 1: Student was able to identify several types of love in their family.
- Level 2: Student was able to identify all types of love in their family and describe the differences.
- Level 3: Student was able to identify all types of love in their family and describe the differences. Student was able to list a few appropriate ways to express love to different family members, friends, etc.
- Level 4: Student was able to identify all types of love in the family and describe the differences. Student was able to list appropriate ways to express love to different family members, friends, etc., and discuss how culture influences our perception of love.

VII. Points of Emphasis

1. Explain how the different types of love are appropriate for different members of society (family members, friends, significant others, etc.).
2. Remind students that love can be expressed verbally and nonverbally.
3. Explain how the influence of culture sometimes defines our views and expectations of love.

Teacher Evaluation

1. Keep the lesson as taught?   yes _____ no _____

2. What I need to improve _____

3. Next time make sure _____

4. Strengths of lesson _____

What I like to do in my spare time: _____

I'm looking forward to: _____

One thing I like about myself: _____

Who am I? _____

Materials Needed: one prepared paper or card for each student, pencils

Processing Questions:

1. Were there any questions that were difficult to answer?
2. What were you proud of in your answers?
3. What would you like to change about your answers?
4. Did anything surprise you about your answers?

✓ **Assessment:** Students can name specific positive attributes about themselves.

How My Decisions Affect Others   Grades 5–6

Valued Outcome: Students will list how they think their decisions to perform various tasks affect their family.

National Health Education Standards: 5, 8

Description of Strategy: Use the following list as an example. Students should consider different situations they may face and think about how the decisions they make affect their family. Have students record their responses and then discuss them as a class.

If I Decided to...	I Think My Family Would Feel...
say no to a drug a friend offered me	_____
not clean my room after being told to do so	_____
try to do my best in math	_____
do my homework for a week without being reminded	_____

Materials Needed: list of situations for each student

Processing Questions:

1. Do your actions affect the people around you?
2. Can you do things that will make life easier for your family?

✓ **Assessment:** Students demonstrate awareness of how their decisions affect those around them.

That's My Opinion   Grades 6–8

Valued Outcome: Students will develop insight into what boys and girls look for and expect from individuals of the opposite sex.

National Health Education Standard: 2

Description of Strategy: This activity is designed to help boys and girls understand the many misconceptions about qualities desired by the opposite sex. Divide the class into groups of males and females and assign a recorder and spokesperson for each group. Have each group respond to the questions "I like girls (boys) who..." and "I dislike girls (boys) who..." The recorder keeps a record of all responses and the spokesperson reads the responses aloud (the teacher may wish to screen the responses first).

Materials Needed: pencils and paper

Processing Questions:

1. What did the boys seem to like about the girls? What did they dislike?
2. What did the girls seem to like about the boys? What did they dislike?
3. Why do you think there were differences between the two lists for both the likes and dislikes?
4. What do you think we can learn from the likes and dislikes of boys and girls?

✓ **Assessment:** Students can identify qualities valued by the opposite sex.

Me and My Self-Confidence   Grades 7–8

Valued Outcome: Students will recognize that many people are very successful even though they may not look perfect.

National Health Education Standards: 2, 4

Description of Strategy: Discuss characteristics that can cause people to feel self-conscious, such as being overweight or underweight, being very short or very tall, having a large nose, or having skin problems. Note that some of these characteristics are either temporary or ones that can be changed while others are permanent or difficult to change. All characteristics can actually become an asset. Discuss famous individuals noted for unique or unusual physical features. These might include Barbra Streisand and her nose or Dudley Moore and his height. Emphasize that each of these individuals relied on developed talent rather than inherited physical characteristics to achieve success and that self-confidence was often the key to success.

Processing Questions:

1. Can you name some people you really admire who may have an unusual physical characteristic?
2. What physical characteristics do you have that you feel are less than perfect?
3. What characteristics and talents do you have that make you proud?

✓ **Assessment:** Students demonstrate awareness of how they perceive themselves.

HEALTH HIGHLIGHT | **What's Happening?**

Martin Heesacker, in *Portraits of Adjustment*, has stated, "Long-term studies indicate that many of the behavioral, psychological, and academic problems shown by children following divorce are traceable to conflict in the dysfunctional family prior to the divorce." Some of the research findings indicate that girls tend to act out less than boys do; that eleven-year-old boys whose parents had divorced within the last year had 19 percent more behavioral and academic problems than eleven-year-old boys living in an intact family did; and divorces tended to generate their own problems, whether in reducing economic well-being or in further disrupting relations among parents and children.

Source: Heesacker 1994, 254

Legal Rights　　　　　　　　　　Grades 7–8

Valued Outcome: Students will learn what sexual abuse is and what options they have if they are abused.

National Health Education Standards: 3, 7

Description of Strategy: Unfortunately, many children in this country are sexually abused. Such abuse may come from other family members or from trusted adults or friends. Often, children are completely unaware of their legal and moral rights in such instances. After becoming informed on legal recourse available in your area, present an objective lecture on the subject to your class. It is very important that you preface your discussion by emphasizing that the child has no reason to feel guilty or ashamed for being a victim of sexual exploitation of any kind. Further, point out that there are authorities who can protect against that person ever hurting them (reprisal) again. Suggest sources that children can turn to for help if such exploitation is occurring. A good first choice is the school psychologist, counselor, or physician.

Processing Questions:

1. Is it ever a child's fault if he or she is sexually abused?
2. If you are being treated in a way that makes you think you are being abused, what should you do?
3. Who are some people you could tell if you are being abused?

✓ **Assessment:** Students can define sexual abuse and name several resources available to them and their peers in case of abuse.

Decision Stories

Present decision stories such as the following, using the procedures outlined in Chapter 4, pages 60–62. The content of the stories that you present should be appropriate for the developmental levels of your students. The examples here range from stories suitable for the early elementary grades to the upper grades, but remember that appropriateness must be determined in the social context of your own group.

For each of the decision stories, write a list on the board of ideas generated by the class for how each situation should be dealt with. Ask the students to discuss the merits of the methods suggested.

✓ **Assessment for Decision Stories:** Students can identify health-enhancing behaviors and exhibit positive decision-making skills.

Am I Stuck with Me?　　　　　　　Grades K–3

Kevin is overweight and not very good at sports. He is often chosen last in team sports and games; although this bothers him, he tries to make a joke of it. In fact, he makes a great many jokes because he wants the other kids to like him. And they do. They think Kevin is a lot of fun. But Kevin doesn't just want to be the class clown. He wants the other kids in class to respect him for who he is. He would like the girls in class to think more highly of him too.

Focus Questions:

1. What might Kevin do to feel better about himself?
2. Are there some things that he should not change? Why or why not?

National Health Education Standards: 5, 8

The Crush　　　　　　　　　　　Grades 4–6

Jackie couldn't seem to stop thinking about the boy who lived down the street. He was a lot older than she was, and he thought she was "just a kid." Jackie went out of her way to be around him. She hoped that he would invite her out on a date, even though she wasn't really old enough to start dating. Then one day Jackie saw him with another girl—one closer to his own age. She felt terrible. How could he do this to her?

Focus Question: What should Jackie do next?

National Health Education Standards: 2, 5

John's World

Grades 4–6

John's parents were divorced last year. John is living with his mother, but he sees his father regularly. One weekend, while John is staying with his father, he finds out that his father is going to get married again. "John," his father says. "This is Janet. I know that you're going to like each other." But John doesn't like his father's fiancée. He is still feeling bad about the divorce. Now this! Will this woman become his stepmother? What will happen to his real mother? What kind of a family will this be? John is confused, very angry, and deeply unhappy.

Focus Questions:

1. Should John pretend he likes this woman, or should he treat her badly so she will know how he feels?
2. What could John say to his father about this situation?

National Health Education Standards: 2, 4

Stories or Facts

Grades 4–6

One day after school, some of the girls are talking about how babies are made. Susan is listening with interest. Some of the things she hears are new to her. She has learned a little bit about sexuality education from her parents and in school, but she is still not sure about all the details. Now she is more confused than ever. She wishes that she knew which of these things were really true.

Focus Questions:

1. What can Susan do to get accurate information?
2. Who should she try to talk with?
3. Should she rely on her friends for information?

National Health Education Standards: 2, 3

Being Friendly

Grades 4–8

Sharon was playing in her backyard one day when Mr. Smith, the man next door, asked her if she would like to come over and have some ice cream. Mr. Smith had always been nice, so Sharon accepted his invitation. Once inside his house, Sharon learned that Mrs. Smith was not there. Mr. Smith started putting his arms around Sharon and brushing up against her. That made Sharon feel uncomfortable. Sharon wanted to leave, but Mr. Smith was very anxious to have her stay.

Focus Questions:

1. Is Mr. Smith acting appropriately?
2. What should Sharon do in this situation?
3. Should she worry about hurting Mr. Smith's feelings?
4. How should Sharon react if the person touching her is her stepfather or another relative?

National Health Education Standards: 4, 5, 7

Fooling Around

Grades 6–8

Bob and his friend George are spending the afternoon together in George's home. It is raining, so they have to stay inside. George's parents are not at home. The two boys start to talk about sex. Then George suggests that the two of them "fool around" together and play with each other's bodies. Afterward, Bob feels that maybe he did something wrong. He feels guilty and frightened. The next day, he feels even worse. He is afraid to tell his parents what happened.

Focus Question: What should Bob do?

National Health Education Standards: 2, 5

The Party

Grades 6–8

Tina's friend Marie is having a party and has invited Tina. At the party, Tina knows only a few of the other guests. Everyone seems to be having a good time. There is music, and the boys and girls are dancing. Later, Tina notices that some of the couples are kissing and making out. A boy named Carl comes over to her. "Would you like to dance with me?" he asks. She is not sure. She doesn't really know Carl. What if he tries something? What could she do? She feels flattered that Carl is paying attention to her, but she is also unsure of herself in situations like this.

Focus Questions:

1. What should Tina do?
2. What are some possible reasons she feels uncomfortable?
3. What decisions does Tina have to make now and in the future?

National Health Education Standard: 4

Dramatizations

The Answer Is No

Grades 4–6

Valued Outcome: Students will gain experience in having to tell others they may not do something they want to do. Students will then report how it feels to be in the position of saying no.

National Health Education Standard: 4

Description of Strategy: Have the students work in pairs of their own choosing. Explain that one student will play the part of a parent, and the other will play the part of that parent's child. The child will ask permission from the parent to go to a party where both boys and girls will be present. The student acting the part of the child will explain about the party—who will be there, where it will be, and so on. After listening, the student acting as parent refuses permission. The son or daughter argues for permission but is still refused. Let several pairs of students act out the situation in front of the class, but do not require anyone to do so who does not wish to participate. Discuss how the different pairs of students handle the same situation. Then, without forewarning the class that you will do so, have selected pairs of students switch roles and repeat the activity. Use discretion in choosing which pairs of students to use for this second part of the activity. Be prepared to discuss how the parents might feel when they have to say no.

Processing Questions:

1. What differences do you note in individual roles when these roles are reversed?
2. What did you learn from this activity?
3. How do you think parents feel when they have to say no?
4. What are some potential reasons for saying no?
5. Why might saying yes be good or bad?

✔ **Assessment:** Students can name several reasons why it can be best for parents to refuse permission.

Superkid
Grades 5–6

Valued Outcome: Students will verbally list ways that life is difficult for everyone, no matter what talents or gifts they have.

National Health Education Standards: 1, 2

Description of Strategy: Have the students work in pairs. One student plays the part of Superkid and the other will be his or her press agent. Each pair decides what abilities each Superkid will have. These abilities might include flying, speaking any language, singing or playing a musical instrument so well that the person is a superstar, possessing great athletic talent, and so on. First, the student playing the press agent introduces the Superkid and describes his or her abilities in the most glowing terms. Then, Superkid acknowledges his or her popular acclaim but notes to the class that life is not perfect even for a Superkid. Have the student explain why being a Superkid isn't as completely wonderful as the press agent has said. If the person is described as an athlete, for example, he or she might explain the anxieties about getting injured on the field, the pressure of competition, and so forth.

Processing Questions:

1. Does anyone have all their problems taken care of?
2. Is it possible that extreme talents sometimes can create more problems?
3. If you had one incredible ability, what would you like it to be?
4. What talents do you have that make you super in some way?

✔ **Assessment:** Students demonstrate their understanding that everyone has problems.

How Would You Handle It?
Grades 6–8

Valued Outcome: Students will act out commonly faced situations.

National Health Education Standards: 1, 2, 4

Description of Strategy: Divide the class into pairs; make sure that close friends are not paired. (There will be no role switching in this activity.) Have each pair act out situations such as the following:

- asking for and getting a date
- asking for and being refused a date
- introducing a friend to one's parent (a third child should play the part of the friend)
- telling a divorced parent that you don't care for the person the parent is dating
- introducing yourself to a member of the opposite sex to whom you feel attracted
- being polite to someone you don't like
- handling rejection when socially rebuffed

Processing Questions:

1. Which of the preceding situations do you find the most difficult?
2. What is most important when attempting to convey a message to someone?
3. How many ways can you think of to handle each of the situations?

✔ **Assessment:** Students demonstrate their ability to use interpersonal communication skills to enhance health and relationships.

Understanding Others
Grades 7–8

Valued Outcome: Students will imitate personal characteristics that they do not have.

National Health Education Standards: 1, 2

Description of Strategy: Not everyone is alike; some people are bossy, and others are shy. Assign different roles to various children, such as Noisy Ned, Bossy Betty, Shy Sam, Iceberg Irene, Chatterbox Chester, Silent Sylvia, Blustery Ben, Whirlwind Wanda, Studious Stu, Laughing Larry, Somber Sarah, and Flighty Frank. Make sure that the children assigned to each role do not have the characteristics of the role they are to play. One by one, have each child act out the part for a few minutes.

Processing Questions:

1. How can you deal with these different personality types?
2. What do you find appealing about the characteristics of each personality type?

3. Why might others be put off by some of these characteristics?
4. Why is it good that all people are not alike?

✓ **Assessment:** Students demonstrate an understanding of differences in personality traits and the positive and negative effects the traits have on others.

Discussion and Report Techniques

Being My Own Perfect Friend   Grades 1–6

Valued Outcome: Students will be able to assess the qualities they desire in themselves and others who are friends.

National Health Education Standards: 2, 7

Description of Strategy: Ask the students to make a list of five qualities they would like in a perfect friend. Have them describe each of these qualities in a sentence, such as "My perfect friend gives me good advice when I am not feeling happy" or "My perfect friend accepts me for who I am." Ask students to share their ideas in class, and prepare a master list on the board, poster board, or overhead projector.

Materials Needed: index cards or sheets of paper, pencils, board, posterboard, or overhead projector and markers or pens

Processing Questions:

1. How can each of you be your own perfect friend?
2. If you cross out "my perfect friend" in your sentences and substitute the word "I," what do you notice about the sentence?
3. How can each of us be more of a "perfect friend" to ourselves instead of sometimes being our own "worst enemy"?
4. What are the implications for ourselves and our friends?

✓ **Assessment:** Students can name several qualities that make someone an excellent friend, and can use those examples to explain how each person can be an excellent friend to him- or herself.

Solving Problems   Grades 4–6

Valued Outcome: Students will develop possible choices for solving problems they may encounter.

National Health Education Standard: 5

Description of Strategy: Divide the class into an even number of groups of four or five each. One student in each group will be a recorder. Have each group write three problems that require a decision. Emphasize that these problems should be typical ones that their age group faces and should be about relationships or risky behavior. When finished, pair the groups and have them exchange problems. Each group then writes possible solutions for the new problems. The recorders can report the results to the class.

Materials Needed: pencils and paper

Processing Questions:

1. Did any groups list the same problems?
2. Is it always easy to make positive decisions?
3. Does it sometimes help to get other opinions about what to do?

✓ **Assessment:** Students demonstrate the ability to use decision-making skills to enhance health or reduce risk.

Opportunities for All   Grades 4–6

Valued Outcome: Students will recognize and name professions that were once male- or female-dominated but in which both genders now have increasing opportunity to participate.

National Health Education Standard: 1

Description of Strategy: In years past, many occupations were considered as appropriate only for males or females. Today, this social attitude is changing, as are our conceptions of gender roles and gender stereotyping in general. After discussing this point with the class, divide the class into small groups to talk about and research individual instances of changing professions for the sexes. Have some groups look into changing occupational opportunities and others look at changing social or familial roles. For example, many police officers in cities and towns throughout the nation are now women, and some men now stay home and care for the children. Ask each group to compile a report on how changes in their area of research have resulted in greater opportunity for both men and women.

Processing Questions:

1. Do you think it is appropriate for females to engage in all professions? Why or why not?
2. Do you think it is appropriate for males to engage in all professions? Why or why not?
3. What profession do you think you would like to be a part of when you grow up?

○ **Integration:** Social Studies

✓ **Assessment:** Students can name at least five professions that were once dominated by a particular gender and discuss reasons for the change in gender roles.

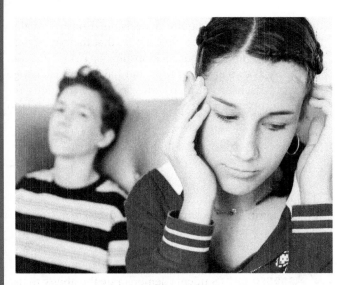

In developing relationships, adolescents need to rely on their values and learn to communicate effectively.

Dictionary with a Difference   Grades 4–6

Valued Outcome: Students will develop a page about themselves in a "human dictionary."

National Health Education Standard: 4

Description of Strategy: Have students make a "dictionary" about themselves to be exhibited in the classroom. Each child has a page that is his or her dictionary entry. Included should be a picture, below which is the last name, first name, the phonetic respelling, and birth date. There should be a line telling the age and grade, a line listing identifying characteristics, a line for interests, and a qualitative statement (for example, I am good at basketball, baseball, and swimming).

Materials Needed: photos of students, paper, pencils or pens

Processing Questions:

1. What is something really special about yourself?
2. How are you different from the way you were last year?

○ **Integration:** Writing

✓ **Assessment:** Students can identify positive characteristics in themselves.

Growing Up   Grades 6–8

Valued Outcome: Students will complete sentences describing how they will respond to various situations associated with growing up.

National Health Education Standards: 5, 7

Description of Strategy: The passage to adulthood can be an especially awkward and confusing time as young people struggle with new signals from their bodies and the maturing young men and women around them. Many will experience emotional changes, mood swings, feelings of uncertainty, and increased feelings of independence and sexuality. A positive and confident attitude can help them handle these changes better.

As students grow, fewer adults will be making decisions for them, but the pressure to be part of the peer group will increase. They will need to rely on their own values to help make the choices most appropriate for developing a positive and healthy life. Have your students complete the following statements.

- I want to drive my friend's car, but I don't have my license. I'm going to _____.
- I know my girlfriend has cramps because she has her period. I'm going to _____.
- My parents can use my help around the house more often. I think I'll _____.
- I haven't developed physically as fast as my friends. This makes me feel _____.
- I have acne on my face. I will _____.
- My parents are going away next weekend. I'm going to _____.
- Some of my friends like to talk about sex. This makes me feel uncomfortable. I should _____.

Materials Needed: list of statements for each student

Processing Questions:

1. Why are some of the statements more difficult to deal with than others?
2. Is a person's maturity indicated by what he or she says? does?
3. Are there certain pressures to say or do certain things? Give examples.
4. Can you identify some decisions based upon these statements that might (or might not) indicate good decision making?

✓ **Assessment:** Students' responses demonstrate their ability to make good decisions to enhance health and relationships.

Individual Reports   Grades 7–8

Valued Outcome: Students will learn more about human development.

National Health Education Standards: 1, 3

Description of Strategy: As appropriate for the developmental level of your particular students, assign individual report topics on aspects of physical and emotional growth. Have the students use a health textbook and other approved informational sources to research particular areas, such as the growth spurt that occurs in adolescence, puberty, menarche, first social encounters with the opposite sex, and dating behavior in the early teen years. On a separate sheet of paper, have students list questions for which they did not find answers during their research. Consult with each student on an individual basis to assist in finding appropriate solutions to these questions. In doing this activity, rely on the advisory committee to your sexuality education program for appropriate responses to individual student questions or dilemmas.

Materials Needed: paper, pencils or pens, reference materials

Processing Questions:

1. What kinds of questions do you have for which you did not find answers?
2. What did you learn that you did not know before about human development?

○ **Integration:** Writing

✓ **Assessment:** Students demonstrate the ability to access valid sources of information about human development.

Experiments and Demonstrations

Guppies
Grades K–3

Valued Outcome: Students will become familiar with the concept of reproduction and birth and their variation among different species.

National Health Education Standard: 1

Description of Strategy: After discussing the concept that all living things can reproduce, let students observe the birth process in live-bearing fish. Obtain some young female guppies and young male guppies. Raise them in separate aquariums. Point out to the class the physical differences between the females and the males. Note that the female guppy is larger and somewhat drab in coloration in contrast to the smaller, brightly colored male. Explain that in many animal species there are obvious differences between males and females, as there are with human beings. When the fish are mature, place one or more males in the tank with the females. In a few weeks, one or more of the females will become pregnant. This will soon be obvious. With luck, birth may take place while class is in session. Have the children observe the birth process. Also point out differences in the birth process for different species; for example, many fish and all birds are egg layers. (As soon as the female guppies give birth, separate the adults from the young, as guppies are cannibalistic.)

Materials Needed: functioning aquarium apparatus, guppies, fish food

Processing Questions:

1. What are some examples of species where their babies are not born alive? How are they born?
2. Were you born alive?

○ **Integration:** Science

✓ **Assessment:** Students demonstrate an understanding that birth is a natural part of the life cycle of living things.

Puzzles and Games

Word Search for the Reproductive System
Grades 4–6

Valued Outcome: Through a word search puzzle, the students will become more familiar with words associated with reproduction.

National Health Education Standard: 1

Description of Strategy: Create a word search and have the students find and circle each of the words listed. The words may read in any direction—up, down, across, or diagonally.

Materials Needed: word search worksheet and pencils for each student

Processing Questions:

1. Can you define all the words in the word search list?
2. Can you use the words in a sentence?

✓ **Assessment:** Students can correctly define the vocabulary words or use them in a sentence.

Reproductive System Crossword Puzzle
Grades 6–8

Valued Outcome: Students will increase their vocabulary about reproduction.

National Health Education Standard: 1

Description of Strategy: Prepare a crossword puzzle worksheet.

Materials Needed: crossword puzzle worksheet and pencils for each student

Processing Questions:

1. Can you define all the words in the crossword puzzle?
2. Can you use each word in a sentence?

✓ **Assessment:** Students can correctly define the vocabulary words or use them in a sentence.

Scrambled Sentences   Grades 7–8

Valued Outcome: Students will review the reproductive system by unscrambling sentences.

National Health Education Standard: 1

Description of Strategy: Create a worksheet using the following scrambled sentences about the human reproductive systems. Have the students unscramble the sentences.

canal acts birth as the vagina a _____
(*The vagina acts as a birth canal.*)
ova the hormones and ovaries produce _____
(*The ovaries produce ova and hormones.*)
tubes occurs in fertilization the uterine _____
(*Fertilization occurs in the uterine tubes.*)
begins females in at menstruation puberty _____
(*Menstruation begins in females at puberty.*)
in the fetus uterus the develops _____
(*The fetus develops in the uterus.*)
are cells the male sperm reproductive called _____
(*The male reproductive cells are called sperm.*)
testes produced in the cells sperm are _____
(*Sperm cells are produced in the testes.*)
fluids other and semen of made is up sperm _____
(*Semen is made up of sperm and other fluids.*)
puberty begin at sperm produced to be _____
(*Sperm begin to be produced at puberty.*)
at testosterone the triggers spurt male puberty growth _____
(*Testosterone triggers the male growth spurt at puberty.*)

Materials Needed: worksheet for each student generated from scrambled sentences above

Processing Questions:

1. Are there any terms you did not understand?
2. Can you take each unscrambled sentence and describe the process that is occurring within each situation?

✔ **Assessment:** Students can correctly unscramble the sentences and further describe the processes in their own words.

Matching Parts and Functions   Grades 7–8

Valued Outcome: Students will review information on the reproductive system by labeling the parts in a team competition.

National Health Education Standard: 1

Description of Strategy: Draw a large diagram of the female reproductive system on the board. Draw leader lines from each of the parts, and allow room for labeling. Prepare a similar diagram for the male reproductive system. (Refer to Figures 11.1 and 11.2 on pages 194 and 195.) Divide the class into two teams. Point to a part on either diagram and ask the first player from Team A to identify it. If the student knows the answer, he or she should come to the board and label the part. If the student does not know the correct answer, the first player from Team B gets a chance. Score one point for each correct answer. After a part has been correctly labeled, ask the next player to explain one function of that part. If the student knows the correct answer, she or he should come to the board and write the function next to the name of the part.

Materials Needed: board and markers or overhead projector and pens

Processing Questions:

1. What were the most significant things we learned?
2. What were some of the most difficult questions to answer?

✔ **Assessment:** Students can name the anatomical features of the male and female reproductive systems and can accurately describe their functions.

True or False   Grades 7–8

Valued Outcome: Students will review information about human sexuality through team competition.

National Health Education Standard: 1

Description of Strategy: Divide the class into two teams and ask each player to decide whether a statement that you make is true or false. Score one point for each correct answer. Then write each of the true statements on the board. Review the true statements at the end of the game. Sample statements might include the following:

- Girls should not swim during menstruation. (false)
- A wet dream is a sign that a boy is reaching puberty. (true)
- Fertilization leading to pregnancy occurs when a sperm unites with an egg. (true)
- The beginning of menstruation means that a girl can now become pregnant. (true)

Materials Needed: board and markers, prepared list of statements

Processing Questions:

1. What were the most difficult questions to deal with? Why?
2. Were there questions you wanted to know more about?

✔ **Assessment:** Students can accurately assess the truth of statements relating to human sexuality.

Other Ideas

Family Activities
Collage
Grades K–3

Valued Outcome: Students will make a collage of activities they engage in with their families.

National Health Education Standard: 2

Description of Strategy: Have each student search through magazines to find pictures of family activities. These activities can include watching television together, going on trips or outings, working around the house, talking with one another, and so forth. Explain to the students that the pictures they choose need to represent a family activity. Thus, a picture of a television set by itself can represent watching television together, an airplane can represent a trip to relatives in another part of the country, and so on. Have each student prepare a colorful collage and then explain to the class the meaning of each component.

Materials Needed: poster board, magazines, scissors, glue

Processing Questions:

1. What activities do you do most often with your family?
2. What family activities are your favorite?

○ **Integration:** Art

✔ **Assessment:** Students can describe several family activities they participate in.

Growing Up
Grades K–4

Valued Outcome: Students will increase understanding of the growth process.

National Health Education Standard: 1

Description of Strategy: Have each student trace his or her hand on a sheet of paper. Ask the students to take their tracings home, and have one or both parents trace their hands over the child's tracing.

Materials Needed: paper, pens

Processing Questions:

1. Is your parent's hand larger than yours? Why?
2. How do body parts grow?
3. Will your whole body be larger when you are grown?

✔ **Assessment:** Students demonstrate an understanding of the concept of growth.

Families Are Different
Grades 4–6

Valued Outcome: Students will realize that any family structure can provide a loving and healthy environment for personal growth, even if that family structure is not "typical."

National Health Education Standard: 2

Description of Strategy: Invite adults of your acquaintance to come to class to discuss the different types of families in which they grew up. Include individuals from a wide variety of familial backgrounds, including traditional American nuclear families, extended family situations, single-parent families, and so forth. This is not an easy activity to do, but it can be a most valuable one. Your guests should not gloss over any difficulties they had growing up in their particular situation, but children should not get the impression that singular events are typical of any situation.

Materials Needed: guest speakers who can effectively address identified issues

Processing Questions:

1. Are all families the same?
2. Can you be a normal person if you do not live with your mother and/or father?
3. Is growing up easy for anyone?

○ **Integration:** Social Studies

✔ **Assessment:** Students can describe several ways that family structures differ and can identify misleading stereotypes in the media about the "typical" family.

Inherited Traits
Grades 4–6

Valued Outcome: Students will realize that some personal characteristics are inherited.

National Health Education Standard: 1

Description of Strategy: The human genetic code contains information about thousands of inherited traits. These include hair, eye, and skin color; shape of ears and nose; and general physique. Emphasize to your class that even individual rates of growth are to a large extent genetically controlled, which explains why some children grow more quickly than others. To demonstrate that some genetic traits are less obvious than others, ask the class to roll their tongues. Some students will be able to roll their tongues, but others will be unable to do so. This ability is a genetic trait.

Processing Questions:

1. What are some other characteristics that you have that are unique?
2. Does having a certain genetic trait make you better or worse than anyone else?

○ **Integration:** Science

✓ **Assessment:** Students can identify several traits in themselves that they inherited from their parents.

My Family Tree   Grades 4–6

Valued Outcome: Students will develop a family tree and discuss characteristics they might have inherited from other family members.

National Health Education Standards: 1, 2

Description of Strategy: Distribute copies of Worksheet 12.1 on page 483. Have each student prepare his or her family tree (younger children may need the assistance of their parents to fill in the names). After the diagrams are completed, discuss the family trees. This may be an area where sensitivity will be needed since some students may be adopted or have stepparents. If you have adopted students in class, have them add roots to the tree representing their birth parents. If approached carefully, this activity may provide an opportunity to discuss what adoption is, why people adopt, and which traits any of the adopted children in the class perceive they have that are similar to those of their adoptive parents.

Materials Needed: photocopies of Worksheet 12.1 for each student

Processing Questions:

1. What physical features do you have in common with siblings, parents, grandparents, stepparents, and so on?
2. Do you have any interest(s) similar to those of your ancestors?
3. Which relative do you think you most resemble?

✓ **Assessment:** Students can identify several characteristics they may have inherited from family members.

Caught in the Act   Grades 4–6

Valued Outcome: Students will observe and record classmates' behaviors.

National Health Education Standard: 8

Description of Strategy: What positive behaviors do you see your classmates use? Are they responsible, cooperative, or courteous? Provide Worksheet 12.2 (page 484) to your students. Students should observe their fellow classmates and try to catch their classmates in the act of good behaviors.

Materials Needed: worksheet 12.2 for each student

Processing Questions:

1. Why is it important for us to be responsible, cooperative, and courteous?

2. How do you feel when someone is not responsible, cooperative, and courteous?
3. How does it make you feel when you are responsible, cooperative, and courteous?

✓ **Assessment:** Students can describe how responsibility, cooperation, and courtesy benefit the community and promote positive interpersonal relationships.

Responsibility   Grades 4–6

Valued Outcome: Students will list the responsibilities of different family members.

National Health Education Standard: 7

Description of Strategy: Give each student a copy of the chart on Worksheet 12.3 (page 485). Have the students write their name and their family members' names in the top row. Have them put an X in each column that includes a responsibility each person has in the home. Add other responsibilities if desired.

Materials Needed: Worksheet 12.3 chart for each student, pencil or pen

Processing Questions:

1. What are the consequences of people not completing their responsibilities?
2. Do you always fulfill your responsibilities?
3. Do you have to be reminded to do your jobs around the house?

✓ **Assessment:** Students can explain how each individual's fulfillment of his or her responsibilities supports the family.

Helping Others   Grades 4–6

Valued Outcome: Students will develop a list of ways that they can help their friends and family.

National Health Education Standard: 8

Description of Strategy: Provide each student with a copy of Worksheet 12.4 (page 486). Using this worksheet, have students compile a list of things they can do to help out family and friends. These acts of kindness need not be big chores or sacrifices. They can be little things that may make a difference in the day of the people they love.

Materials Needed: Worksheet 12.4 and a pencil for each student

Processing Questions:

1. Was it difficult to think of ways to help any of the people on the list? Why?
2. Do you feel you have helped the people on the list as much as you should?

3. How does helping others make you feel?

✓ **Assessment:** Students can identify five actions they can and would like to take that would help support their friends and family members.

The Menstrual Cycle   Grades 5–6

Valued Outcome: Students will learn the different phases of the menstrual cycle.

National Health Education Standard: 1

Description of Strategy: About every twenty-eight days, a new menstrual cycle begins in the female body. The cycle begins with the shedding of the lining of the uterus. This is called menstruation and takes about four or five days. For the next several days, the lining (or endometrium) is very thin, and an egg cell in an ovary begins to ripen. The lining starts to thicken, and, by the fourteenth day, a ripened egg is released into a uterine tube. This is called ovulation. The endometrium continues to thicken as the egg moves toward the uterus. If the egg is not fertilized, it disintegrates and menstruation takes place, which signals the beginning of a new cycle. Have students use Worksheet 12.5 on page 487 to indicate each step of the cycle.

Materials Needed: Photocopy of Worksheet 12.5 for each student

Processing Questions:

1. What is menstruation?
2. Why is menstruation called a twenty-eight-day cycle?

✓ **Assessment:** Students can accurately describe the different phases of the menstrual cycle.

Why Are They Like That?   Grades 5–6

Valued Outcome: Students will have an opportunity to ask questions about the behavior of the opposite sex.

National Health Education Standards: 1, 2

Description of Strategy: Certain aspects of the behavior of boys is often a puzzle to girls and vice versa. Have each student write one question about some aspect of the "typical" behavior of the opposite sex that is puzzling or perhaps annoying. The questions should be unsigned. Collect all the questions and read aloud those that seem most germane to a discussion of behavior among boys and girls at your class's grade level. Have volunteers attempt to explain the point of view of the opposite sex that might shed light on a particular aspect of behavior. For example, at a certain age girls may be more interested in boys than boys are interested in girls as a result of maturational differences. Therefore, girls may be attracted to older boys, thus giving boys their

own age the feeling that they are not seen as sexual peers. Act as moderator in the discussion, and provide factual information as necessary.

Materials Needed: slips of paper, pencils or pens

Processing Questions:

1. Did you learn anything new about the opposite sex?
2. Do you think the behavior of the opposite sex makes any more sense than it did before?
3. Do males and females think the same way?

✓ **Assessment:** Students can describe several reasons that members of the opposite sex are perceived to behave a certain way. Students can name several real differences between male and female behavior.

Why Not?   Grades 6–8

Valued Outcome: Increase student awareness of possible consequences of some kinds of sexual behavior.

National Health Education Standards: 1, 7

Description of Strategy: After discussion and approval of this activity by all members of the family life advisory committee (or through the approval process at your school), invite various representatives of sex education groups in your community to lecture to the class on the ramifications of certain sexual decisions that each individual must make, such as the decision to have intercourse outside of marriage. Make it clear before the activity that you as the teacher are not advocating any behavior that goes against general community norms.

Materials Needed: guest speakers who are screened carefully before talking to the group

Processing Questions:

1. Is it wise to make sexual decisions based on how you feel at a certain time?
2. What are some reasons for delaying some kinds of sexual behavior?

✓ **Assessment:** Students can name several possible negative consequences of sexual activity and can describe how delaying sexual activity can be a healthy decision.

Family Rules   Grades 7–8

Valued Outcome: Students will list various rules they are supposed to follow every day.

National Health Education Standard: 7

Description of Strategy: Create a worksheet of the following chart and give a copy to each student. Discuss with the students the different kinds of rules they may be expected to follow every day. Two rules are given. Have the students discuss rules and then complete their own daily lists, placing an X in the columns of the days they successfully followed each rule.

	M	T	W	Th	F	Sa	S
Get up on time							
Brush my teeth							

Materials Needed: worksheet for each student

Processing Questions:

1. Are some rules more difficult to follow? Why?
2. Why are there rules to follow?
3. What would happen if there were no rules? Would you really like that?

✓ **Assessment:** Students are able to identify the benefits of having each rule in place.

Advice Column
Grades 7–8

Valued Outcome: Students will ask questions about family and human sexuality.

National Health Education Standard: 1

Description of Strategy: With your assistance and supervision, have the class put together a newspaper advice column. First, have each student write a letter to the column asking for some advice about a sexuality or family life matter. Students may ask for simple factual information, such as "What is masturbation?" or for advice on handling a personal problem, such as "How can I ask someone for a date?" Collect all the letters, which should be unsigned or signed with a pseudonym such as "Puzzled" or "Wondering," and group the letters into categories. Restate a typical example of each category, writing the paraphrased statement on the board or overhead projector. Then have each student write an advice column to answer the question. Again using your discretion, collate the different suggestions offered and discuss them with the class. Properly handled, this activity can offer you important insights into the sexual development of students in your class. As "managing editor" of the advice column, however, you must make sure that topics covered stay within guidelines set up for your school's sexuality education program.

Materials Needed: paper, pencils or pens, board and markers or overhead projector and pens

Processing Questions:

1. What did you learn that you did not know before?
2. What do you think is the most important part of relationships with others?
3. Did you find out what you most wanted to know?

✓ **Assessment:** Students demonstrate appropriate awareness of concepts of human sexuality.

13 Substance Use and Abuse

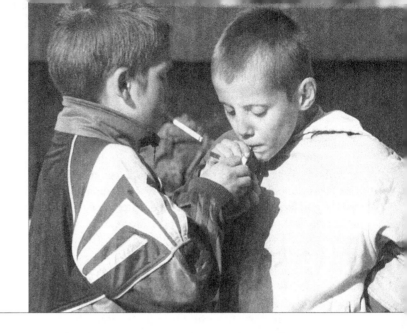

Valued Outcomes

After completion of this chapter, you should be able to:

- Define substance use, misuse, and abuse.

- Identify reasons that people abuse substances.

- Describe the various effects of different drugs on the body.

- Describe how tobacco advertising influences youths to use tobacco products.

- List recommendations for schools to reduce alcohol, tobacco, and other drug abuse problems among their students.

- Give examples of the signs and symptoms of substance use and abuse.

- Describe the most effective drug abuse education and prevention programs.

Reflections

As you read through the chapter, note the patterns of use of the various drugs and the reasons some youths abuse drugs. As you consider these facts, think of how you could develop an effective substance abuse prevention program for your community.

Adolescents and other young adults who use drugs and alcohol often take risks that endanger their health and the health of others.

—National Institute on Drug Abuse (2011)

NATIONAL HEALTH EDUCATION STANDARDS

1. Students will comprehend concepts related to health promotion and disease prevention to enhance health.

2. Students will analyze the influence of family, peers, culture, media, technology, and other factors on health behaviors.

3. Students will demonstrate the ability to access valid information and products and services to enhance health.

4. Students will demonstrate the ability to use interpersonal communication skills to enhance health and avoid or reduce health risks.

5. Students will demonstrate the ability to use decision-making skills to enhance health.

7. Students will demonstrate the ability to practice health-enhancing behaviors and avoid or reduce risks.

Substance Abuse

Substance abuse (drug abuse) is a potential problem among virtually all students. Risk factors are those factors that contribute to, or increase the risk of, developing substance use and abuse problems. To prevent substance use and abuse, risk factors should be identified and ways to reduce the impact of risk factors should be developed. Effective substance abuse prevention education focuses on decreasing the risk factors while also increasing protective factors (those factors that help prevent substance use and abuse).

In this chapter, we examine those substances that are commonly abused or misused. Some of them have little or no therapeutic value but can be purchased by adults for their personal use. Over-the-counter (OTC) drugs, such as cough medicines, can have beneficial effects when used carefully. Because many people wrongly consider these drugs to be essentially harmless, however, misuse and abuse are common. Prescription drugs, such as tranquilizers, are more closely controlled, but these substances are also widely abused. Finally, we look at illegal substances, such as marijuana, heroin, hallucinogens, club drugs, and cocaine.

■ Reasons for Substance Abuse in Youths

Individuals misuse or abuse drugs for a variety of reasons. Young people are especially likely to do so for the following reasons:

- **Curiosity**—Humans intrinsically desire to experience the unknown; this desire is especially pronounced during the ages of strong peer influence, when many of a youngster's friends are experimenting with drugs.
- **Low self-esteem**—Many individuals have poor opinions of themselves. By using drugs, these people attempt to avoid coming to grips with their feelings of inadequacy. Drugs thus serve as a coping mechanism.
- **Peer pressure**—Particularly during adolescence, individuals have a strong need to belong. If peers are abusing drugs, there is strong pressure on the part of all members of a group to do likewise.
- **Adult modeling**—Young people want to feel grown up, and they view taking drugs as a form of adult behavior to be emulated. Smoking tobacco or marijuana, drinking alcohol, or taking pills may all result from adult modeling.
- **Mood alteration**—Some people take drugs simply to change their psychological state. The mellow feeling or the excitement produced is the motivation for this behavior.
- **Boredom**—Many young people, especially during the teenage years, are unsure about their place in society.

The activities of childhood no longer interest them, but they are not yet able to engage in adult activities. As a result, they feel bored with life.

- **Alienation**—Some individuals feel that they have little or no power to control their own destiny. They may also feel unwanted and unloved. Often, such people have few friends and view themselves as social misfits. Drugs provide an outlet for the expression of feelings of alienation.

The National Survey on Drug Use and Health provides insights regarding trends in youth substance abuse. The Health Highlight box on page 224 has excerpts from the 2009 survey.

■ Possible Symptoms of Substance Abuse in Youth

Drug use is a preventable behavior, and drug addiction is a treatable disease. As with many other diseases, the sooner it is detected and addressed, the sooner a sick person can begin to get well. How can a teacher tell if a student is abusing drugs? This is a difficult question when behavioral signs and symptoms are used as a basis for suspicion. It can be difficult to separate the typical adolescent behavior from drug-induced behavior.

No one factor determines who will use drugs and who will not, but several indicators can alert adults that a young person might be involved in substance abuse:

- sudden decline in school achievement
- smoking cigarettes
- a change in the child's friends or peers
- parents' loss of trust in the child
- a change in the child's personality
- withdrawal from extracurricular activities that were previously important to the child
- missing classes, missing school, or habitually late to school
- negative change in appearance and/or personal hygiene
- lack of communication with parents and/or other adults, such as secretiveness, unexplained phone calls, and hostility to questions
- going out every night
- unexplained disappearance of family funds or family and personal possessions
- increased aggressiveness toward others, such as fighting and hostility
- heavy use of OTC preparations to reduce eye reddening

It is important to note that just because a student exhibits some of the behaviors listed above that doesn't mean that child is abusing drugs.

Effects of Drugs on the Body

A **drug** is any substance that has mind-altering properties or in other ways interacts with and modifies the structure and function of the body. Drugs include OTC and prescription medicines, caffeinated beverages, alcohol, tobacco, illegal substances, herbs, and volatile chemicals such as airplane glue, correction fluid, and paint.

Drug use generally implies that the drug is being used legally, the user is following the directions on the label or directions from the health care provider, and the drug is being used for a legitimate, medical reason.

Drug misuse includes the unintentional or inappropriate use of prescribed or nonprescribed medicine that results in the impaired physical, mental, emotional, or social well-being of the user. Sometimes drug misuse is not intentional, such as not complying with prescription medication instructions.

Drug abuse generally refers to chronic, excessive use of a drug. Drug abuse may also refer to a person's intent. If a person drinks to excess for the purpose of getting drunk, that could be considered abuse. If a person uses an illegal drug for any reason, that is considered abuse. This includes anyone under the age of twenty-one drinking alcohol, if their state considers this action illegal (underage drinking). See Table 13.1 for a list of commonly abused drugs and some of the associated health risks.

Table 13.1	Commonly Abused Drugs*	
	Substances (with Common Names)	**Selected Acute Effects and Health Risks****
Tobacco	• **Nicotine:** cigarettes, cigars, bidis, smokeless tobacco	Chronic lung disease; cardiovascular disease; stroke; various cancers; adverse pregnancy outcomes
Alcohol	• **Ethyl alcohol:** liquor, beer, wine	Lowered inhibitions, slurred speech, nausea, loss of coordination, visual distortions, impaired memory, sexual dysfunction, loss of consciousness, increased risk of injuries and violence, fetal damage (in pregnant women), depression, liver and heart disease, fatal overdose
Cannabinoids	• **Marijuana** (dope, ganja, grass, bud, Mary Jane, pot, reefer, green, weed) • **Hashish** (boom, gangster, hash)	Slowed reaction time; distorted sensory perception; impaired balance and coordination; increased heart rate and appetite; impaired learning and memory; anxiety; panic attacks
Opioids	• **Heroin** (smack, dope, junk, skunk, China white) • **Opium** (big O, block)	Euphoria; drowsiness; impaired coordination; dizziness; confusion; nausea; sedation; slowed or arrested breathing; hepatitis; HIV; fatal overdose
Stimulants	• **Cocaine** (blow, bump, coke, crack, rock, snow) • **Amphetamine** (bennies, speed, uppers) • **Methamphetamine** (meth, ice, crank)	Increased heart rate, blood pressure, body temperature, and metabolism; feelings of exhilaration; increased energy, mental alertness; tremors; irritability; anxiety; panic; paranoia; violent behavior; psychosis, weight loss, insomnia; cardiac or cardiovascular complications; stroke; seizures
Club Drugs	• **MDMA** (Ecstasy, X, E) • **Flunitrazepam** (Rohypnol, forget-me pill, roofies)*** • **Gamma-hydroxybutyrate** (GHB)***	*Ecstasy*: Mild hallucinogenic effects; increased tactile sensitivity; lowered inhibition; anxiety; chills; sweating; teeth clenching; muscle cramping; depression; impaired memory; hyperthermia *Rohypnol*: sedation; muscle relaxation; confusion; memory loss; dizziness; impaired coordination *GHB*: drowsiness; nausea; headache; disorientation; loss of coordination; memory loss/unconsciousness; seizures; coma
Dissociative Drugs	• **Ketamine** (Special K) • **PCP and analogs** (angel dust) • **Dextromethorphan** (DXM, Dex, Robotripping)	Feelings of being separate from one's body and environment; impaired motor function; anxiety; tremors; numbness; memory loss; nausea *Also, for ketamine*: analgesia; delirium; respiratory depression and arrest; death *Also, for PCP and analogs*: psychosis; violence; slurred speech; hallucinations *Also, for DXM*: euphoria; confusion; dizziness; distorted visual perceptions

(continued)

Table 13.1	Commonly Abused Drugs (*continued*)	
	Substances (with Common Names)	**Selected Acute Effects and Health Risks****
Inhalants	• **Solvents:** paint thinners, gasoline, glues • **Gases:** butane, propane, aerosol propellants, nitrous oxide • **Nitrites:** isoamyl, isobutyl, cyclohexyl	Stimulation; loss of inhibition; headache; nausea or vomiting; slurred speech; loss of motor coordination; wheezing/cramps; muscle weakness; depression; memory impairment; damage to cardiovascular and nervous systems; unconsciousness; sudden death
Hallucinogens	• **LSD** (acid, blotter, cubes, yellow sunshine) • **Mescaline** (buttons, cactus, peyote) • **Psilocybin** (magic mushrooms, shrooms)	Altered states of perception and feeling; hallucinations; nausea *Also, LSD and mescaline*: increased body temperature, heart rate, blood pressure; loss of appetite; sweating; sleeplessness; numbness, dizziness, weakness, tremors; impulsive behavior; rapid shifts in emotion *Also, for LSD*: flashbacks, Hallucinogen Persisting Perception Disorder *Also for psilocybin*—nervousness; paranoia; panic
Anabolic steroids	• **Anadrol, Oxandrin, Equipoise** (roids, juice, gym candy, pumpers)	Hypertension; blood clotting and cholesterol changes; liver cysts; hostility and aggression; acne *In adolescents*: premature stoppage of growth *In males*: prostate cancer, reduced sperm production, shrunken testicles, breast enlargement *In females*: menstrual irregularities, development of beard and other masculine characteristics

* Commonly abused drugs not in this table include: Salvia divinorum, prescription medications (CNS depressants, stimulants, opioid pain relievers), other depressants (barbiturates, benzodiazepines)

** Some of the health risks are directly related to the route of drug administration. For example, injection drug use can increase the risk of infection through needle contamination with staphylococci, HIV, hepatitis, and other organisms. See full table available at www.nida.nih.gov/drugpages/drugsofabuse.html for routes of administration.

*** Associated with sexual assaults.

Source: National Institute on Drug Abuse. 2011. *Commonly Abused Drugs*. (Full text of table available at www.nida.nih.gov/drugpages/drugsofabuse.html)

▪ Route of Administration

Drugs can be taken orally in the form of pills, capsules, or liquids. They may be injected intravenously (directly into the bloodstream through a vein), intramuscularly (into a muscle), or subcutaneously (under the skin). Certain substances may be inhaled. Others may be administered topically, that is, by the external application of the substance to the skin or mucous membranes.

The amount of time required for a drug to take effect largely depends on the technique employed to administer it. The method of administration yielding the strongest and most rapid effect is intravenous (IV) injection. This procedure is considered the most dangerous because the risk of infection, vein collapse, or overdose is extremely high. Overdose is a significant problem with IV injection because chemicals enter the circulatory system rapidly, bypassing the body's first line of defense. Smaller amounts of a drug are needed intravenously than for any other form of application.

Intramuscular injection works most rapidly in the deltoid muscle and least rapidly in the buttocks because the blood supply in the buttocks is poor. Subcutaneous injection can be extremely irritating to the tissue. Topical administration is usually short-acting and may damage the skin or mucous membranes because the chemical being administered often serves as an irritant.

Even oral ingestion creates problems. This technique requires the drug to enter the bloodstream by passing through the stomach, where it may be destroyed or altered to an inactive form. Then the substance must be lipid (fat) soluble in order to cross cell membranes and reach its target. Lipid-soluble products tend to be retained by the body and show cumulative effects; if water soluble, the substance is rapidly excreted by the body. Substances absorbed in the digestive tract then go to the liver before being absorbed into general circulation. The function of the liver is to break down chemicals for excretion, so at least some of the substance may be inactivated there. Ultimately, oral ingestion creates difficulty in controlling the actual dosage absorbed by the body.

▪ Distribution

Drugs are carried to body parts through the bloodstream. Some drugs are absorbed and then excreted quickly. Aspirin is an example of a drug that is excreted within a few hours. Other drugs are cumulative and are excreted very slowly. It may take several days to build up the level of the drug in the body to produce the desired therapeutic effect. Once drug levels are built up, only maintenance doses are needed to maintain the drug's level. Certain heart medications are of this type.

▪ Dosage

Dosage is the amount of a drug that is administered. The dosage determines the effect of the substance on the body, or the dose-response relationship. The larger the amount taken, the greater the probability of several different effects. The *threshold dose* is the minimum amount required to produce a therapeutic effect. The dose in which maximum effect is obtained is called the *maximum dose*. The *effective dose* is the dose needed to produce a desired effect. A *lethal dose* is the amount of drug that will produce death. The ratio between the effective dose and the lethal dose is the *therapeutic index*. This is obtained by dividing the amount of a lethal dose by the amount required for an effective dose. The higher the index, the lower the chance of a given dosage being lethal.

Another important concept concerning dosage is the potency, or the difference in effective doses between drugs that are used for the same purpose. For example, substance A may require twice the dosage to achieve the same effect as substance B. Therefore, substance B is a more potent drug. The time required for the substance to produce an effect after the body receives it is called the *time response*. As a general rule, the more quickly an effect appears, the shorter its effectiveness.

The presence of more than one drug can produce what is called *synergism*, in which the combined action of the drugs is greater than the sum of the effects of any one of the drugs taken alone. For example, some drugs *potentiate*, or increase the effect of, another drug. The effect of one substance may be enhanced because of specific enzymes, formation of more potent metabolites, or for unknown reasons. Pesticides, traces of hormones in meat and poultry, traces of metals in fish, nitrites, nitrates, herbs, and a wide range of chemicals used as food additives have been shown to interact with and potentiate some drugs. The classic example of synergism causing a dangerous potentiation is that a safe dose of alcohol, when mixed with a safe dose of a barbiturate, can become lethal by depressing respiration. Conversely, a drug that acts as an *antagonist* blocks or interferes with the function of another drug when used in combination with it, or it may inhibit a normal biological compound, such as a hormone.

▪ Expectations of the User

The mood of the user and the setting in which the drug is taken may also affect the reaction to the drug. If the person expects the substance will help a problem or produce a particular effect, then the probability of that effect actually occurring increases. The effect may occur even when the substance administered is only a placebo, or inert substance. The *placebo effect* is quite common. Friends, soft lights, and music may help create an environmental setting for particular drug effects.

Placebos are substances that produce an apparent cure or perceived health improvement based on the expectations of the user. Many patients report improvements after taking simple sugar pills that they believed were powerful drugs. Clinicians and scientists accept the placebo effect as a central phenomenon in medicine and ascribe the phenomenon to the body's self-protective effort for healing (National Library of Medicine 2005. Self-Healing, Patents, and Placebos. www.nlm.nih.gov/hmd/emotions/self.html).

▪ Frequency of Use

When some drugs are used frequently, larger dosages are required to maintain the effect. This is called *tolerance*. There are several forms of tolerance discussed here. *Disposition tolerance* concerns the rate at which the body disposes of a drug. Certain drugs tend to increase the rate of action of enzymes in the liver and, consequently, the deactivating of the drug. For example, alcohol and barbiturates cause the liver to increase production of metabolic enzymes that deactivate certain drugs. Alcohol and barbiturates are examples of drugs that cause the liver to produce the metabolic enzymes. Another important point is that these enzymes are not very discriminating; therefore, tolerance to one substance may lead to tolerance of other drugs that are pharmacologically similar. This effect is called *cross-tolerance*. Usually a heavy drinker will exhibit tolerance to barbiturates, tranquilizers, and anesthetics.

Evidence indicates that a considerable degree of central nervous system tolerance to certain drugs may develop independent of changes in the rate of absorption, metabolism, or excretion. This is called *pharmacodynamic tolerance* and occurs when the nervous tissue or other target tissues adapt to the substance so that the effect of the same concentration of a chemical decreases. In the case of *reverse tolerance*, users will have the same response to a lower dose of a drug that they had with initial higher doses. Reverse tolerance is believed to be primarily a learning process and does not result from a physiological response. However, it is possible for some drugs, such as marijuana, to be stored in the fat cells and released later as the fat cells are broken down. The fact that drug products remain in the body for extended periods of time may account for some of the reverse tolerance effect (Ray and Ksir 2002, 417). Usually, tolerance to a substance that requires increasing amounts of a chemical to maintain normal body functioning will lead to a physical dependence.

Some drugs, such as aspirin, cause neither physical tolerance nor dependence. *Psychological dependence* implies a pattern of compulsive drug use characterized by a continued craving for a drug and the need to use the drug for effects other than pain relief. If the person stops taking a drug after a period of time, the person might experience anxiety as a withdrawal symptom.

Substance dependence, either physiological or psychological, appears to be synonymous with substance abuse. The model of addiction-producing drugs is based on the

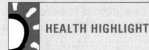

Perceived Harm in Drug Use among Youths: A Focus on Alcohol, Cigarettes, and Marijuana

The 2009 National Survey on Drug Use and Health (NSDUH) showed overall decreases in the years 2002–2009 in the percentages of youths who used alcohol, cigarettes, and marijuana (compared by (1) lifetime use, (2) use in the past year, and (3) use in the past month), although yearly numbers at times show increases in usage. Data shows that the perception that substances might cause them harm remains an important factor influencing whether or not youths will use these substances. Historically, declining levels of perceived risk have been associated with subsequent increases in rates of use, and this still seems to hold true.

Alcohol and Cigarettes: In the years 2002–2008, data shows a nearly

20 percent decline in youths using alcohol in the past month. However, between 2008 and 2009, there were no significant changes in the rates of current alcohol use. A similar result was seen for use of cigarettes in the past month. It was found that rates of current youth smoking declined by about 30 percent between 2002 and 2008, then remained unchanged in 2009. Although the rates of use of alcohol and cigarettes were unchanged between 2008 and 2009, there was a decline during this time period in youths' perceived risk of harm in having four or five drinks of alcohol nearly every day or smoking one or more packs of cigarettes per day.

Marijuana: Rates of marijuana use for the past month in studies declined in the years 2002–2006, were similar in 2006–2008, and increased between 2008 and 2009. In 2007, 54.7 percent of youths aged twelve to seventeen, reported that they thought there was a great risk of harm in smoking marijuana once or twice a week; this number declined during the following two years, to 49.3 percent in 2009.

Source: Substance Abuse and Mental Health Services Administration. (2010). *Results from the 2009 National Survey on Drug Use and Health: Volume I, Summary of National Findings.* (Additional information available at www.oas.samhsa.gov/NSDUH/2k9NSDUH/2k9ResultsP.pdf.)

---

opiates, which require the development of tolerance, along with physical and psychological dependence. Opiates, alcohol, and barbiturates are examples that fit the traditional addiction model.

Over-the-Counter Drugs

Over-the-counter medicine is also known as OTC or non-prescription medicine. All these terms are interchangeable and refer to medicine that you can buy without a prescription. The U.S. Food and Drug Administration (FDA) states that these medications are safe and effective when you follow the directions on the label and as directed by your doctor (FDA, Consumer Education: Over-the-Counter Medicine, April 2008. www.fda.gov/cder/consumerinfo/otc_text.htm).

Most OTC drugs are somewhat effective in relieving the symptoms of the mild illnesses and disorders for which they were developed, as long as they are used according to directions. However, despite regulation by the Federal Trade Commission and other government agencies, advertising claims for many OTC products are often misleadingly optimistic. As a result, when the product fails to produce instant relief, some individuals may be tempted to exceed the recommended dosage in hopes of additional or faster aid. This sort of misuse can create health hazards. Additional health hazards are created when those with a predilection to addictive behavior, such as alcoholics, become dependent on and thus abuse such OTCs as cough syrup.

Individuals should also recognize that there is some risk involved in using any medication, including aspirin, even when the directions are carefully followed. First, there is a possibility of allergic reaction. In rare cases, such reactions can be fatal. The Dietary Supplement and Nonprescription Drug Consumer Protection Act of 2006 requires the FDA to establish systems for collecting data about serious adverse reactions that people experience while using certain nonprescription drugs and dietary supplements (GovTrack.us 2006). Second, relief provided by an OTC drug may mask symptoms of another illness or underlying disorder. For this reason, self-medication should only be attempted when the problem is minor and obvious, as in the case of a mild cold.

Another risk in using OTC drugs comes from *synergism.* As mentioned earlier, if two or more drugs or medications are taken at the same time, one substance can cause an increase or decrease in the potency of another. This synergistic reaction can have harmful and even fatal results.

As with any drugs, OTC drugs can have a stronger effect on children than on adults. For example, children's aspirin, formerly thought to be safe, has been identified as a cause of a severe reaction that can lead to death under certain conditions. Epidemiological research has shown an association between the development of Reye's syndrome and the use of aspirin (a salicylate compound) for treating the symptoms of influenza-like illnesses such as chicken pox and colds. The U.S. Surgeon General, the FDA, the Centers for Disease Control and Prevention (CDC), and the American Academy of Pediatrics recommend that aspirin and combination products containing aspirin not be given to children under eighteen years of age during episodes of fever-causing illnesses (National Reye's Syndrome Foundation 2008).

Depressants

Drugs that slow down, inhibit, or depress the nervous system are classified as depressants. The most commonly used depressant drug is alcohol. There are dozens of other depressants, most of which are prescription drugs. Whether obtained legally or illegally, however, depressants are among the most common of misused and abused drugs.

Depressants can have a calming effect, and strong depressants can produce sleep. The use of depressants has an extremely high risk of both physical and psychological addiction. Prolonged use builds up a tolerance, which may eventually lead to a coma and death. The withdrawal process from depressants can be life threatening and should be carried out under medical supervision. Because of the high risk of addiction and tolerance, many doctors are reluctant to prescribe these drugs as sleep aids.

Depressant drugs have four main effects on the body. As *sedatives*, they can produce relaxation. As *tranquilizers*, they can reduce anxiety and act as muscle relaxants. As *hypnotics*, they can promote sleep. As *anesthetics*, they can create a loss of sensation. Various depressant drugs differ in their potencies, but in sufficient amounts they can all produce these four effects.

The sedative-hypnotics include barbiturates and tranquilizers. Examples of barbiturates by trade name include Amytal, Nembutal, and Seconal. Commonly prescribed tranquilizers include Valium, Librium, and Miltown. Both of these types of drugs are usually taken orally, although some can be given intravenously as a general anesthetic.

▪ Alcohol

Ethyl alcohol is the active ingredient in beer, wine, and distilled beverages, such as whiskey. Ethyl alcohol is not as toxic as are some other forms of alcohol, such as isopropyl alcohol, which is used as rubbing alcohol. In this discussion, we use the term *alcohol* to refer to ethyl alcohol. Alcohol is a colorless, flammable liquid formed by the fermentation of fruits, juices, or cereal grains. Alcoholic beverages contain varying amounts of alcohol, depending on the type of beverage. Beer usually contains from 5 to 7 percent alcohol. Wines may vary from 11 to 20 percent. Distilled beverages have the highest alcohol content. This content is measured by the proof of the beverage, which is a number that is twice the alcohol content. For example, a 100-proof whiskey contains 50 percent alcohol, whereas a 90-proof whiskey contains 45 percent.

The use of alcohol by youths remains a problem, despite declining levels of use and increased awareness of the inherent dangers. The U.S. Department of Health and Human Services reports that approximately 10 percent of nine- to ten-year-olds report that they have started drinking and that nearly one-third of youths begin drinking before age thirteen. They have also noted that by age fifteen, approximately 50 percent of boys and girls have had a whole drink of alcohol, and by age 21, approximately 90 percent have done so (U.S. Department of Health and Human Services 2011). Further, alcohol use among young people appears to stimulate a progression to other drug use.

The use of alcohol and tobacco among youth is correlated with other health problems, including adolescent suicide, homicide, school dropout, delinquency, early sexual activity, sexually transmitted infections (STIs), unwanted pregnancy, and motor vehicle crashes. Alcohol-related traffic crashes are the leading cause of death and spinal cord injury for young Americans. Young adults are unlikely to develop alcohol problems if the age of first use is delayed beyond childhood and adolescence.

Effects of Alcohol. Alcohol is a central nervous system depressant. In small doses, the substance has a mellowing or tranquilizing effect. The individual may feel relaxed and free from tension. As a result, behavior may become less inhibited, leading to the misconception held by some that alcohol is a stimulant. Actually, what appears to be stimulated, or at least animated, behavior results from the anesthetic, depressant effect that alcohol has on the cerebral cortex area of the brain.

The effects of alcohol on the body correspond with the amount of alcohol in the system. The amount of alcohol can be measured by the percentage of the blood that is composed of alcohol. In large amounts, alcohol impairs brain activity, muscular control, coordination, memory, reaction time, and judgment. Heavy intake over a short period can bring about a dulling of the senses. Continued heavy drinking can result in coma and death.

Consumption of alcohol over a long period can result in damage to the brain and liver. The brain may be damaged to the extent that memory, judgment, and learning deteriorate. Cirrhosis of the liver is a potentially fatal condition caused by alcohol damage. Cirrhosis of the liver does occur in nonalcoholic drinkers, but this is rare.

Even moderate amounts of alcohol consumed by pregnant women can have adverse effects on the fetus. Alcohol can have a deleterious effect on the developing fetus, resulting in a condition known as *fetal alcohol syndrome* (FAS). A child born with FAS may suffer permanent impairment. Characteristics of the condition include low birth weight, smaller head circumference, abnormal formation of the nose, small fingernails, smaller stature, poor joint movement, ear abnormalities, and mental retardation.

In moderation, alcohol does not seem to harm the adult body permanently. However, an adult who decides to partake of alcoholic beverages should exercise care. Alcohol should be consumed slowly, with adequate food in the stomach. Individuals should also recognize that tolerance to alcohol is cumulative. More of the substance may be required to produce the pleasant, mellow effect associated with its use. Drinking without recognizing the potential dangers of alcohol can lead to tragedy.

Why Do Youths Begin Abusing Alcohol?

Decisions to drink are influenced by an array of interacting individual and environmental factors. Two main reasons are reported: to see what it is like and to be sociable. Youths drinking is usually group behavior with rituals of sharing and turn-taking, free from adult control. Teens also report drinking to feel good, to feel grown-up, to relax, to get away from problems, and to relieve boredom.

Parents and other family members play a crucial role in the development of their children's drinking patterns and establishment of future habits, and peers play an important role in present lifestyle issues and activities. For teens who go on to develop problems with alcohol abuse, risk factors such as genetic predisposition or conduct disorder may be evident. However, no one factor can play a role without being influenced by other factors. Psychosocial, biomedical, and psychological problems are associated with the consumption of alcohol in adolescents—a population experiencing rapid change due to physical, psychological, social, and cognitive development. Accident statistics are a prime indicator of this.

Alcohol drinking is also associated with sexual risk-taking, which creates risk for teenage pregnancy, STIs, and HIV/AIDS. Although a direct causal relationship between the two has not been empirically shown and may not be generally applicable to all adolescents, alcohol is perceived by adolescents and some adults as a sexual disinhibitor.

Alcohol and other drug abuse may also contribute to the higher rates of low birth weight and mortality among infants born to adolescent mothers. Alcohol use is associated with psychiatric conditions such as depression, conduct problems, and antisocial behavior. Prolonged use can result in psychological problems such as escapism, poor self-image, and alienation. Alcohol can affect mood, judgment, and self-control, resulting in such outcomes as suicidal behavior.

Finally, alcohol dependence in itself can be a consequence of alcohol abuse, a health problem affecting both mental and physical health. Youth represents a risky population of alcohol users and abusers, one in which the consequences of use tend to be more severe than with adults. Prevention, intervention, and treatment are required to effectively reduce present and future harm.

Drinking and Accidents.

Alcohol remains the primary cause of automobile accidents among drivers. Alcohol is involved in 50 percent or more of all fatal traffic accidents. Without question, drinking and driving don't mix. Two of the many groups who are keeping the drunk-driving issue alive by increasing awareness of the problem are MADD (Mothers Against Drunk Driving) and SADD (Students Against Drunk Driving). MADD also serves to mobilize the public to help individuals modify their drinking habits and protests the judicial system when an individual with a history of drunk driving is allowed to continue to drive. MADD has been successful in reducing the legal blood-alcohol concentration in various states and has initiated several effective programs to limit drinking and driving.

The purposes of SADD include helping students save their own lives and the lives of others, educating students on the problem of drinking and driving, developing peer counseling among students about alcohol use, and increasing public awareness and prevention of alcohol abuse. An important feature of the SADD program is the "Contract for Life," a teenager–parent contract in which the teenager agrees to call the parent for advice and/or transportation at any time from any place if the teenager or his or her driver has had too much to drink. The parent in return agrees to transport the teenager and also agrees to seek sober transportation for him- or herself in a similar situation.

Alcoholism and Alcohol-Related Problems.

Perhaps the area of greatest concern among substance abuse professionals is alcoholism among young people. According to the National Council on Alcoholism, alcoholism is the number one drug problem among the nation's youth. Forty percent of children have tasted alcohol by age ten. The average age for a first drink is just under thirteen. Nearly 30 percent of teenagers have experienced negative results from abuse of alcohol. These range from auto accidents to arrests, to detrimental effects on schoolwork, and others mentioned earlier in this chapter. Ironically, 42 percent of fourth-graders failed to recognize alcohol as a drug. Only 72 percent of children in the upper grades realize it is a drug and, therefore, dangerous.

Definitions of the term *alcoholism* vary from source to source. In general, the disease alcoholism can be described as when a person is unable to choose whether he or she will drink and is unable to stop drinking. Alcoholics use the substance in such a way that their personal, social, and occupational behavior is interfered with or totally disrupted. The problem is common among people from all walks of life, including the clergy, homemakers, politicians, factory workers, musicians, police officers, and retired people. Both rich and poor, young and old, are susceptible. As many as 10 million Americans have a serious drinking problem.

The disease model of alcoholism has received support from many medical practitioners and has been endorsed by the American Medical Association and other professional groups. The National Institutes of Health's National Institute on Alcohol Abuse and Alcoholism (2011) notes that research shows that the risk for developing alcoholism runs in families; researchers are working to discover the specific genes that put people at risk. The genes a person inherits partially explain predisposition, but lifestyle is a factor. Particular friends, stressors, and how readily available alcohol is also are factors that may increase a person's risk for alcoholism. It is important to note that alcoholism is not a foregone conclusion, no matter the predetermined risks. A child of an alcoholic parent will not automatically be an alcoholic, and some people develop alcoholism if nobody in their family has a drinking problem. Knowing risk can help a person take steps to avoid developing problems with alcohol (NIH 2011). Bliss (2009) notes that the disease model of alcoholism may rely too much on biological factors at the expense of other lifestyle factors. The spiritual and holistic conceptualizations of alcoholism are gaining some popularity.

Ethnicity as well as heredity may also play a role in alcoholism. Many Asians, for example, have a genetic variant of aldehyde dehydrogenase that is slower than the allele found in non-Asians. This is typically blamed for the accumulation of acetaldehyde that is associated with the marked facial flushing and increased heart rate that many Asians experience when drinking alcoholic beverages.

Regardless of how important the heredity factor is, social and psychological factors also influence the development of alcoholism. Because alcohol is generally accepted in our society, many individuals feel free to use it. Too often, however, use leads to misuse, and alcoholism is the result. The drug becomes a crutch for dealing with everyday problems until the individual can no longer get along without it.

Alcohol-related problems are all too common in our society. Aside from the thousands of traffic deaths and injuries that occur each year because of alcohol abuse, alcohol is also related to the high divorce rate, job absenteeism, crimes of violence, suicide, and social disorder. Alcoholics and their families can receive help from many sources, including such nonprofit groups as Alcoholics Anonymous (AA). AA is a support group of fellow alcoholics designed to help each other remain sober. There are also many commercial alcoholic treatment programs. These can be expensive, but many insurance companies now pay for such treatment. Al-Anon, Alateen, and Alatot are groups specifically established to assist the families of alcoholics. Al-Anon is a group for spouses, relatives, and friends of alcoholics. Alateen and Alatot are groups that are designed for children of alcoholics. These groups are designed to help friends and relatives understand the alcoholic and thereby better cope with the alcoholic's lifestyle. These groups also help the family members understand the roles they play as codependents—that is, the behavior of family members that sometimes enables the alcoholic to continue his or her lifestyle. For example, if a spouse calls her alcoholic husband's employer and tells the employer that her husband will not be at work because he is sick, this action enables the alcoholic to continue his behavior.

Prevention of Alcohol Abuse. The key to dealing with adolescent alcohol and other substance use is prevention, which should begin in early childhood and continue throughout adolescence. Prevention programs can be school-, family-, or community-based. The information-only and "scare tactic" approaches of the past are now considered ineffective. The mass media approach, although information-oriented, is useful in increasing public awareness and putting an issue on the social agenda. Current programs tend to be more psychosocial in approach, addressing social, cognitive, biological, attitudinal, and developmental factors aimed at building skills within a supportive group context.

School-based programs have the advantage of being able to use age-specific strategies in a learning environment. Highly structured programs are appropriate for younger ages. Community approaches depend on a coordinated effort on behalf of the public and private agencies and other groups within the community. Possible community strategies include recreational alternatives for youth and community.

Barbiturates

Barbiturates have historically represented one of the nation's biggest drug abuse problems. Generally known as downers, barbiturates are often taken as a way of escaping from the problems of daily living. The Drug Enforcement Administration states that although many people have used barbiturates therapeutically without harm, concern about the addiction potential of barbiturates and the increasing number of fatalities associated with them led to the development of alternative medications, such as benzodiazepines (which, although rarely fatal, share many of the undesirable side-effects of barbiturates).

The effects of barbiturates depend on the dosage ingested. In small doses, a person feels drowsy, uninhibited, and intoxicated. In moderate amounts, depressants produce a state of intoxication that is remarkably similar to alcohol intoxication. In high doses, the user staggers as if drunk, develops slurred speech, and is confused. At higher doses, the person is unconscious (coma), and death from cardiac or respiratory arrest is very possible (Barry 2002, 3). Some people use depressants in order to obtain a "high" or to counteract the effects of stimulant drugs. The margin of safety between a safe and a lethal dose is very narrow; therefore, barbiturates are considered dangerous and are less likely to be prescribed than safer alternatives.

Withdrawal symptoms associated with the discontinued use of barbiturates indicate a strong physical dependence of the body on the drug. There is a similarity among the withdrawal symptoms seen with most drugs classified as depressants, like barbiturates. Withdrawal symptoms may include insomnia and anxiety, tremors and weakness, and in its most severe form, seizures and delirium. Withdrawal from barbiturates can be life threatening, and therefore should be supervised by a physician (U.S. Department of Justice 2005).

Tranquilizers

Tranquilizers are classified as major and minor. The major tranquilizers, such as Thorazine, are used to treat psychosis. Minor tranquilizers, such as Valium and Librium, are prescribed for stress and anxiety and are also useful as muscle

HEALTH HIGHLIGHT | **FDA Approves New Formulation for OxyContin**

OxyContin, an extended-release narcotic used for management of pain, has been popular in the illicit drug marketplace. In 2008, about half a million people used the drug nonmedically for the first time. The active ingredient in OxyContin is twice as potent as morphine, and rapid growth in prescriptions of the drug led to higher distribution and so increased availability for abuse. In 2010, the U.S. Food and Drug Administration approved a new formulation of the controlled-release drug intended to help discourage misuse and abuse of the medication. Through crushing pills, people intent on abusing the previous formulation have been able to release high levels of oxycodone all at once; this can result in a fatal overdose.

This reformulation of OxyContin is intended to prevent the drug from being crushed to release more medication. The hope is that this may result in less risk of abuse and/or overdose.

Source: U.S. Food and Drug Administration. 2010. FDA Approves New Formulation for OxyContin. (More information available at www.fda.gov.)

relaxants. However, partly because they are so widely prescribed, such tranquilizers are often abused. Physical and psychological dependency can result. Symptoms of physical dependency include drowsiness and slurred speech. Psychological dependency may be characterized by increased irritability and irrational fear. As is the case with barbiturates, withdrawal from tranquilizers can be highly traumatic and should be monitored by a physician.

Cross-Tolerance and the Depressant Drugs

Tolerance to depressant drugs can be developed fairly quickly. Higher and higher doses of the drug must be taken to produce the desired relaxing effect. As mentioned earlier, tolerance to one kind of depressant drug also produces tolerance to other types of depressant substances that are not even being taken. The danger of cross-tolerance may not be as obvious to drug abusers as it should be. Once tolerance to one depressant drug has developed, the individual may decide to switch to another depressant in hopes of achieving the same desired effect. However, because of cross-tolerance, the outcome is not as hoped. A higher dose may then be taken. If the new drug is more potent, a fatal overdose may result.

Narcotics

Narcotic drugs are produced for the most part from opium and its derivatives, although some are synthesized substances. Such drugs act on the central nervous system and gastrointestinal tract. They are excellent painkillers, but they can be highly addictive, both physically and psychologically. Opium, morphine, codeine, and heroin are derived from the opium poppy. Morphine is a potent painkiller used primarily to relieve severe pain such as that caused by acute sickle-cell crisis and heart attack. Codeine is often used in conjunction with acetaminophen to relieve moderate pain; codeine is also effective in suppressing the cough reflex.

Heroin

Heroin is not used for medical purposes and is one of the most dangerous drugs abused. The drug can be smoked, swallowed, injected under the skin, or injected directly into a vein. The latter method is used most often by heroin addicts because the drug reaches the brain most quickly this way. The desired effect is a sudden rush of euphoria, followed by a dreamy state of complete relaxation. This period may last up to several hours, depending on a variety of factors, including the strength of the dosage.

Although considered physiologically "clean" in the sense that it does not damage organs, heroin is extremely addictive, and a user soon may live for no other reason than to inject more heroin. Tolerance also quickly develops, leading to a need for higher and higher or more frequent doses of the drug. The result is too often a fatal overdose, which results in death from cardiorespiratory failure.

Withdrawal from heroin is agonizing. It is characterized by chills, fever, diarrhea, and vomiting. However, painful as it is, heroin withdrawal is seldom life threatening. Still, most heroin addicts, even when they would like to quit, find it almost impossible to do so because of the craving they have developed for the drug.

The dangers from heroin use are manifold. Aside from weight loss, lethargy, sexual inadequacy, and the constant problems of withdrawal that require regular doses of the drug, injection of heroin can lead to other health problems, including hepatitis and HIV/AIDS because of dirty needles and anemia caused by disregard for proper nutrition. "Street heroin" is always sold in an adulterated state (such as being mixed with baking soda or milk sugar) so that the actual percentage of heroin is small. Toxic adulterants in heroin sold on the street can also kill.

After the Harrison Act of 1914, there was a decline in the number of addicts using opiates, including heroin. In the early years after World War II, heroin use slowly increased in the lower class, partially because it was inexpensive. During the 1950s and 1960s, heroin use spread rapidly. Because of laws, eradication programs in Turkey and Mexico, and diminished supplies, heroin use in the United States fell slightly in the 1970s and 1980s. The National Survey on Drug Use and Health (NSDUH) reports that in 2009, there were 180,000 persons aged twelve or older who had used heroin for the first time within the past twelve months. The number of heroin initiates was significantly higher than the 100,000 average annual number of heroin initiates during 2002 to 2008 (National Institute on Drug Abuse 2010).

Stimulants

Stimulants are drugs that stimulate, or speed up, the nervous system. Physiologically, the stimulant drugs increase heart rate, blood pressure, and amount of circulating blood sugar. They also constrict the blood vessels and dilate bronchial tubes and the pupils of the eyes. Some can produce a temporary euphoria.

▪ Caffeine

The most common stimulant is caffeine, which is contained in coffee, tea, cola drinks, and even chocolate. Caffeine is a mild stimulant that is often abused. Moreover, it is a drug and should be recognized as one that can lead to health problems.

Caffeine is absorbed quickly into the bloodstream and reaches a peak blood level in about thirty to sixty minutes. It increases mental alertness and provides a feeling of energy. However, high doses of caffeine can overstimulate and cause nervousness and increased heart rate. Caffeine can also cause sleeplessness, excitement, and irritability. In some cases, high doses of caffeine can induce convulsions.

Coffee or cola drinking, let alone chocolate eating, cannot be considered drug abuse by most commonly accepted standards. But some individuals seek out caffeine for its own sake, in OTC products and in illegal substances to produce a caffeine "high." Because it is not considered a dangerous drug, the opportunities for caffeine abuse are often overlooked by the authorities.

▪ Amphetamines

Amphetamines, or "uppers," represent a more serious stimulant drug abuse problem than caffeine. These drugs have limited legitimate and useful medical applications, but because of their wide availability, they are often abused.

Amphetamines can be helpful if taken correctly, or they can be detrimental to a person's health if taken incorrectly or illegally. Amphetamines are used in many medical treatments. Ritalin is a prescription drug that aids in attention deficit hyperactivity disorder (ADHD), and Sudafed is an OTC drug that is a powerful nasal decongestant. Adderall, an amphetamine that was once used to treat exogenous obesity, has been outlawed in some states because of abuse. Adderall has also been used to treat cases of ADHD and narcolepsy. Many states in the United States restrict the use of Adderall as an anorectic agent (i.e., for the treatment of anorexia); the long-term effects of Adderall are not known.

Vyvanse is another drug used to treat ADHD, but there are significant side effects, including slowing the growth of children, seizures, and eyesight changes or blurred vision (FDA 2010).

The FDA has approved short-term use of amphetamines for weight-loss programs but has warned against their potential for abuse. The U.S. medical associations have asked all physicians to be more careful about prescribing amphetamines. Only 1 percent of amphetamine prescriptions are now written for weight loss, compared with 8 percent in 1970. In fact, amphetamine use is currently recommended only for narcolepsy and some cases of hyperactivity in children.

Methamphetamine (Meth). A potent and commonly abused form of amphetamine is methamphetamine, or meth, a white, odorless, and bitter-tasting powder. Methamphetamine, also called speed, is an illegal, highly addictive drug that is cheaper and has longer-lasting effects than cocaine does. Methamphetamine is a relatively easy and inexpensive stimulant to make, so the Comprehensive Methamphetamine Control Act was passed in 1996 to discourage its illicit manufacture.

More facts about methamphetamine (from the Substance Abuse and Mental Health Services Administration 2010):

- Methamphetamine's ability to release dopamine rapidly in reward regions of the brain produces an intense euphoria, or "rush." Repeated abuse can lead to addiction.

- In 2008–2009, about 41 percent of past year methamphetamine users aged twelve or older reported they obtained the meth they used most recently from a friend or relative for free; about 29 percent bought it from a friend or relative.

- Methamphetamine can be prescribed by a doctor, but the medical uses are limited.

- Most of the meth abused in the United States comes from superlabs, but it can be made in small, illegal laboratories, where production endangers the surrounding people and environment.

- Transmission of HIV and hepatitis B and C can be consequences of meth abuse as a result of decisions made during periods of impaired judgment and inhibition while under the influence.

- There are no medications approved to treat meth addiction.

▪ Cocaine

Known on the street as "snow" or "coke," cocaine is an illegal drug that continues to rise in popularity. Currently, cocaine trafficking and consumption represent one of the most significant drug problems in the United States. The groups most vulnerable to cocaine use include adolescents and young adults who demonstrate higher than average levels of tobacco, alcohol, and especially marijuana use.

The risk of becoming a cocaine user does not decrease after the teen years. Initiation to cocaine use occurs anytime from adolescence to adulthood.

According to the National Institute on Drug Abuse 2009 Monitoring the Future survey, among eighth-, tenth-, and twelfth-graders there were continuing declines reported in the use of powder cocaine. Significant declines in use were measured from 2008 to 2009 among twelfth-graders across all three survey categories: lifetime use decreased from 7.2 percent to 6.0 percent; past-year use dropped from 4.4 percent to 3.4 percent; and past-month use dropped from 1.9 percent to 1.3 percent. Their perceived risk of harm associated with powder cocaine use increased significantly during the same period.

Cocaine is legal and useful for limited medical purposes. Because of its vasoconstrictive and anesthetic properties, cocaine is used as a local ingredient in Brompton's cocktail, a preparation for treating severe pain in individuals who have a terminal illness.

Cocaine is taken to produce a feeling of intense euphoria and boundless energy. As this fades, depression—sometimes severe—follows, along with the strong desire for another dose, or "hit." Although physical dependence is not strong with cocaine, psychological dependence is common and can be very potent. Paranoid thinking, hallucinations, and psychosis can occur with heavy, extended use. Withdrawal symptoms from cocaine are limited to mild depression and anxiety with limited use.

Cocaine is most often found in the form of a white powder that can be snorted (absorbed into the bloodstream through the nasal tissues) or dissolved in water and then injected (with a needle, directly into the bloodstream). Crack is a name given to the processed rock crystal form of cocaine, which, when heated, produces vapors that are smoked; the smoke absorbs rapidly into the bloodstream through the lungs. The intensity and duration of cocaine's effects—which include from 5 to 30 minutes of increased energy, reduced fatigue, and mental alertness—vary depending on intake of the drug through snorting, injection, or smoking. The high wears off fairly quickly, so the drug must be taken again to sustain it. (National Institute on Drug Abuse 2010).

A process used for purifying or refining cocaine is called *freebasing*. This method produces a more potent form of cocaine that has an accelerated and intense high. The drug is heated to a high temperature and mixed with other substances, some highly volatile, resulting in explosion on occasion. The final mixture is then smoked in a water pipe.

Cocaine's action on the body most directly affects the cardiovascular system. Heart rate increases and small blood vessels constrict, thus raising blood pressure. This sudden increase in cardiac activity, coupled with vasoconstriction, leads to an elevated risk of cardiac ischemia, resulting in heart attack or rhythm disturbances. These risks can occur when using small amounts, either by sniffing, snorting, smoking, or IV use. The absence of an underlying heart condition *does not* make an individual immune from cardiac consequences.

The most effective treatment of cocaine dependence is behavioral intervention; the personalized combination of treatment, social support, and other services helps to optimize outcomes for the patient. There are no FDA-approved medications for treating cocaine addiction, although research is ongoing (NIDA 2010).

▪ Tobacco

Tobacco has been used for hundreds of years. It can be sniffed in the form of snuff, chewed (placed between the gum and lips), or smoked. Smoking is the most popular use of tobacco. Cigarettes became popular in the early 1900s; previously, tobacco was usually chewed or smoked in a pipe.

Tobacco use is the single most preventable cause of disease, disability, and death in the United States (CDC 2011). It is estimated that each year 443,000 people die as a result of smoking or secondhand smoke exposure; another 8.6 million have a serious illness caused by smoking. More than 80 percent of the approximately 46.6 million U.S. adult cigarette smokers began smoking before they were eighteen. Adolescent smokeless tobacco users are more likely than nonusers to smoke cigarettes as adults. Rates of smoking in adolescents decreased before remaining stable since 2003, but an increasing number of U.S. high school students have reported using smokeless tobacco products in recent years (CDC 2011).

The Centers for Disease Control and Prevention (2009) advocate that "evidence-based, statewide tobacco control programs that are comprehensive, sustained, and accountable have been shown to reduce smoking rates, tobacco-related deaths, and diseases caused by smoking." The younger a person is when he or she starts to smoke, the more likely he or she is to become a long-term smoker and to develop smoking-related diseases. Preventing adolescents from taking up smoking is far more cost-effective than treating the addiction and resulting diseases later in life.

According to a study by the U.S. Department of Health and Human Services (DHHS), children in this country can easily buy cigarettes, in violation of the law. However, DHHS also found that where state and local officials take their responsibilities seriously and devise enforcement tools that are workable and effective, these laws can be successfully enforced. Preventing the use of tobacco products will do more to enhance the length and quality of life in the United States than any other step that could be taken.

Effects of Tobacco Smoking. According to the U.S. Surgeon General, cigarette smoking is the primary avoidable cause of death in our society and the most important health issue of our time. More deaths are caused each year by tobacco use than by human immunodeficiency virus (HIV), illegal drug use, alcohol use, motor vehicle injuries, suicides, and murders combined. Cigarette smoking causes about one out of every five deaths each year. (This estimate includes deaths from secondhand smoke exposure.) On average, adults who smoke cigarettes die

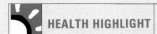

| HEALTH HIGHLIGHT | **Young People and Smoking** |

According to the Centers for Disease Control and Prevention, the following is the updated information regarding youth and smoking:

- Each day in the United States, approximately 4,000 adolescents aged twelve through seventeen years try their first cigarette.
- Each year cigarette smoking accounts for approximately one of every five deaths, or about 438,000 people. Cigarette smoking results in 5.5 million years of potential life lost in the United States annually.
- Although the percentage of high school students who smoke has declined in recent years, rates remain high: 19 percent of high school students report current cigarette use (smoked cigarettes on at least one day during the thirty days before the survey).

- Forty-six percent of high school students have tried cigarette smoking, even one or two puffs.
- Eleven percent of high school students have smoked a whole cigarette before age thirteen.
- Nearly 9 percent of high school students (15 percent of male and 2 percent of female students) used smokeless tobacco (e.g., chewing tobacco, snuff, or dip) on at least one day during the thirty days before the survey.
- Fourteen percent of high school students smoked cigars, cigarillos, or little cigars on at least one day during the thirty days before the survey.
- All states have laws making it illegal to sell cigarettes to anyone under the age of eighteen, yet 14 percent of students under the age of eighteen who

currently smoke cigarettes reported that they usually obtained their own cigarettes by buying them in a store or gas station during the thirty days before the survey.
- Cigarette companies spent more than $15.2 billion in 2003 to promote their products.
- Children and teenagers constitute the majority of all new smokers, and the industry's advertising and promotion campaigns often have special appeal to these young people.
- Eighty-three percent of young smokers (ages twelve through seventeen) choose the three most heavily advertised brands.

Source: Centers for Disease Control and Prevention. 2010. *Tobacco Use by Young People: Tobacco Use and the Health of Young People.* (Available at www.cdc.gov/HealthyYouth /tobacco/facts.htm.)

four years earlier than nonsmokers do. Based on current cigarette smoking patterns, an estimated 25 million Americans who are alive today will die prematurely from smoking-related illnesses.

The primary drug in tobacco is nicotine. A typical filter cigarette contains between 1 and 2 mg of nicotine, with about 90 percent of this amount being absorbed when inhaled. Nicotine acts as a stimulant on the heart and nervous system, causing an increased heartbeat and elevated blood pressure and constricted blood vessels that leads to decreased skin temperature. Blood loses some of its ability to carry oxygen because of the carbon monoxide in tobacco smoke, which is more readily picked up by hemoglobin.

Cigarette smoke also contains chemicals known collectively as *tars*. These substances have been identified as carcinogens, or cancer-causing agents. Smoking is a major cause of lung cancer and may contribute to other forms of malignancies as well. Smokers not only run an increased risk of developing cancer, they also have much higher rates of coronary heart disease. Emphysema, a breathing disorder that results from deterioration of lung tissue, is also associated with cigarette smoking, as are many other respiratory diseases.

The relationship between a mother's smoking and harmful effects on a developing fetus has been established. According to the National Institute on Drug Abuse (2009), in the United States, it is estimated that about 16 percent of pregnant women smoke during their pregnancies. Carbon

monoxide and nicotine exposure as a fetus can contribute to fetal growth retardation, decreased birthweight, later learning and behavioral problems, and an increased risk of obesity in children (NIDA 2009). As reported by the Office of the Surgeon General, there is link between prenatal exposure to nicotine and adolescents' use of tobacco. Daughters of women who smoked cigarettes while they were pregnant are four times more likely to start and continue smoking during adolescence than daughters of women who did not smoke during pregnancy (Office of the Surgeon General 2006). Smoking during pregnancy may also be associated with spontaneous abortions and sudden infant death syndrome (SIDS) (NIDA 2009).

Although cigarette smokers run the highest risk of developing health problems, use of tobacco in other forms can also lead to serious problems. For example, pipe smoking is related to cancer of the lip; both pipe and cigar smokers run a higher risk of developing cancer of the mouth, larynx, and esophagus. Snuff dippers, or people who use smokeless tobacco, have a higher incidence of oral cancer than do nonusers.

Secondhand and Sidestream Smoke. Although an individual may choose not to smoke, being in an enclosed area with smoking forces him or her to smoke involuntarily. Sidestream smoke is the smoke that comes from a burning cigarette. Secondhand smoke is exhaled from the smoker. This smoke has much higher concentrations of some irritating and hazardous substances than mainstream, or inhaled, smoke does. Carbon monoxide is especially significant with secondhand smoke. With several people smoking in an enclosed area, the Environmental Protection Agency's safe limit recommendation for carbon monoxide can be exceeded. Most standard air-filtration systems do not remove carbon monoxide gas from the air. Only dilution with fresh air can lower carbon monoxide levels.

Nicotine from sidestream smoke generally settles out of the air, with only small amounts being absorbed from heavily polluted air. Other carcinogens are absorbed in small amounts, but the carcinogenic effect is not known. Other substances from sidestream smoke probably are not hazardous, just irritating to nonsmokers. People who have cardiovascular disease or pulmonary disease can be adversely affected.

Secondhand smoke causes an estimated 3,000 lung cancer deaths, and more than 35,000 coronary heart disease deaths occur each year among adult nonsmokers in the United States. Each year, secondhand smoke is associated with an estimated 8,000–26,000 new asthma cases in children. Exposure to secondhand smoke causes an estimated 150,000–300,000 new cases each year of bronchitis and pneumonia in children aged less than eighteen months, 7,500–15,000 of which will require hospitalization.

A report from the CDC (2008) found that 46 percent of Americans show biologic exposure to the deadly toxins found in cigarette smoke. Recent studies indicate that 21 million children (or 35 percent of children) are exposed to secondhand smoke on a regular basis (CDC 2008).

Why People Smoke. People begin smoking for some of the same reasons that apply to drinking. Adult modeling and peer pressure are certainly factors. The appeal produced by cigarette advertising also plays a part. Some people abuse tobacco to be more alert, and others use it to relax. (The mood of the smoker plays a role in the perception of the abuser.) Many smokers find smoking extremely pleasurable. Some claim that cigarettes curb anxiety, sadness, and boredom. Some smoke because of habit, with various cues (immediately after a meal, with coffee, or being around other smokers) triggering the habit of tobacco abuse. The nicotine present in tobacco products has been shown to be addictive. Nicotine stimulates the adrenal glands, resulting in a discharge of epinephrine (adrenaline); this stimulation causes an increase in blood pressure, respiration, and heart rate. Nicotine also increases dopamine levels in the reward circuits of the brain, offering pleasurable feelings for many tobacco users. Long-term brain changes from continued nicotine exposure can result in addiction (National Institute on Drug Abuse 2009).

A very forceful motivation for smoking is advertising. Cigarette manufacturers spend approximately $4 billion each year promoting cigarettes and the acceptance of smoking. Cigarette advertising reveals very few facts about cigarettes, but rather appeals to individual needs, a memory of good feeling, the universal need for companionship,

and a desire for escape and adventure. Cigarette ads also are designed to reduce one's anxieties about growing old, being alone, and losing one's health and sex drive. Free samples may encourage initiation of tobacco use among children and adolescents, especially when distributed at youth-oriented events, such as concerts. Cigarette sponsorship of sporting events allows cigarette brand names to be shown or mentioned on television (even though cigarette commercials are prohibited in the broadcast media), and cigarette sponsorship of televised sporting events is reported to increase cigarette brand recognition among children.

The impact of such advertising on potential smokers (primarily young people) is substantial. Studies reviewed by the National Cancer Institute indicate that tobacco advertising and promotional activities are important catalysts in the smoking initiation process (National Cancer Institute 2011). Many in the public health community believe that 1) tobacco companies purposely market to youths because they know that few people initiate smoking in adulthood, and 2) the tobacco industry's advertising and marketing strategies are effective and are responsible for increasing the rate at which young people start smoking. It has been shown that changes in advertising methods are associated with variations in the rates at which youths begin smoking (Cummings *et al.* 1995; Gilpin and Pierce 1997).

Tobacco companies increasingly market to girls and women, who account for about 20 percent of the smokers in the world (CDC 2010). In examining why women begin smoking (an act of rebellion, social acceptance, and other reasons), advertisers are able to effectively market to this target group.

A study by the CDC shows that antismoking strategies are needed in childhood to counteract the effects of advertising. Findings from the CDC's Youth Risk Behavior Surveillance System indicate that students who smoke their first cigarette at less than twelve years of age are more likely to become regular and heavy smokers than students who begin smoking at a later age. Students who participate in sports activities smoke less than students who do not participate in sports.

Recently, there has been less emphasis placed on tobacco prevention education in schools and/or programs that deal with tobacco or drug prevention that are isolated from other components of the coordinated school health program. There need to be more tobacco use prevention efforts in the schools and communities, and in order to be effective, these efforts need to be an integral part of an overall health behavior change program within a coordinated school health program. Eventually, these programs should reinforce tobacco use prevention among youth and promote tobacco nonuse as a norm within U.S. culture.

Reducing the Hazards of Smoking. The best way to avoid the hazards of smoking is simply not to smoke. This means not beginning in the first place or giving up the habit if smoking has already begun. People who smoke should also recognize the possible harmful effects of secondhand smoke on others. Inhaling smoke produced by a smoker can aggravate respiratory conditions and may even be the cause of such conditions in a nonsmoker. Those who refuse to stop smoking can lower the risk they run by choosing a brand of cigarettes with low tar and nicotine, by smoking fewer cigarettes, by taking fewer puffs and not inhaling deeply, and by not smoking the cigarette all the way down to the end.

Smokeless Tobacco. Chew, snuff, and other forms of oral tobacco have chemicals known to cause cancer and other adverse health effects, contrary to claims made that it is a safe alternative to smoking tobacco. These products can cause bad breath and stained teeth; gum disease; destruction of the bone sockets around the teeth; tooth loss; leukoplakia (white sores in the mouth that can be precancerous); cancer of the mouth, tongue, throat, esophagus, stomach, and pancreas; and increased risk of heart disease, heart attacks, and stroke (American Cancer Society 2010).

Marijuana

Marijuana is a prepared mixture of the crushed leaves, flowers, small branches, stems, and seed of the hemp plant, *Cannabis sativa*. Hashish is a more potent resin derived from this plant. Depending on various factors, including the amount of drug taken, the type of drug, the setting, and the mood of the user, cannabis intoxication may resemble the effects of alcohol, a sedative, a stimulant, or a hallucinogen. Marijuana in low to moderate doses causes a sedative effect. However, at higher doses, marijuana produces effects quite similar to hallucinogens. Like powerful hallucinogens, there is little cross-tolerance for marijuana and, for example, lysergic acid diethylamide (LSD). In average doses, it acts much like alcohol.

After alcohol and nicotine, marijuana is the third most popular recreational drug in the United States—in other words, it is the dominant illicit drug. Under the Controlled Substances Act (CSA), Congress listed marijuana in Schedule I. Schedule I substances have a very high potential for abuse, and no accepted medical use in the United States. According to the 2009 Monitoring the Future survey, the rates of lifetime marijuana use among young people hasn't significantly changed in the years 1995 to 2009 as reported by 8th grade students (19.9% decreased to 15.7%), 10th grade students (34.1% decreased to 32.3%), and 12th grade students (41.7% nominally increased to 42%).

Although marijuana tolerance can develop, the frequent user may actually require less of the drug to gain the effects of the drug over time. Physical dependence seems to be rare. There is a danger of psychological dependence, however.

▪ Effects of Marijuana Use

Short-term or long-term marijuana use can have the following effects:

- **Effects on the brain**—THC, the active ingredient in marijuana, connects to specific nerve cell sites in the brain called cannabinoid receptors and influences the activity of those cells. There are many of these cannabinoid receptors in the parts of the brain that influence pleasure, memory, thought, concentration, sensory and time perception, and coordinated movement. Short-term use of marijuana can produce effects such as problems with memory and learning, distorted perception, difficulty in thinking and problem solving, loss of coordination, and increased heart rate.

- **Effects on the heart**—The user's risk of heart attack more than quadruples in the first hour after smoking marijuana.

- **Effects on the lungs**—Smoking marijuana produces many of the same respiratory problems as smoking tobacco, including persistent cough and phlegm production, more frequent acute chest illness, a heightened risk of lung infection, and a greater tendency to obstructed airways. Smoking marijuana increases the likelihood of developing cancer of the head or neck. The more marijuana smoked, the greater the increased risk of cancer. Marijuana smoke contains 50 to 70 percent more carcinogenic hydrocarbons than does tobacco smoke.

- **Effects on learning and social behavior**—Marijuana use can lead to depression, anxiety, and personality disturbances. Marijuana detrimentally affects a person's ability to learn and remember information. Someone who smokes marijuana every day may be functioning at a reduced intellectual level all of the time. Workers who smoke marijuana do not work as effectively as their nonsmoking peers do.

- **Effects on pregnancy**—Babies exposed to marijuana during pregnancy display altered responses to visual stimuli, increased tremulousness, and a high-pitched cry, which may indicate neurological problems in development. Marijuana-exposed children have been observed to have more behavioral problems in infancy and preschool years than unexposed children have, and they demonstrate poorer performance on tasks of visual perception, language comprehension, sustained attention, and memory. In school, marijuana-exposed children are more likely to exhibit deficits in decision-making skills, memory, and the ability to remain attentive (NIDA 2010).

▪ Medical Marijuana

The FDA has not approved the use of botanical marijuana for medicinal purposes. However, various states allow its use to treat all or some of the following:

- **Glaucoma**—Marijuana smoking is used to reduce the fluid pressure of the eye in a glaucoma patient.

- **Chemotherapy-caused nausea and vomiting**—As far back as 1982, the National Academy of Sciences stated that medication containing tetrahydrocannabind (THC), the active ingredient in marijuana, was the only kind of medicine that was effective in reducing the severe nausea caused by certain drugs used to treat cancer. It has been demonstrated in research studies that THC is more quickly absorbed from marijuana smoke than from *oral* preparations.

- **Appetite stimulant**—There may well be a stimulating influence on food intake in advanced cancer patients who use marijuana in conjunction with chemotherapy.

- **Antiasthmatic effect**—Short-term smoking has produced a bronchodilation effect in patients with bronchial asthma.

- **Seizures, spasticity, and other nervous system disorders**—The National Institute on Drug Abuse has been reporting since 1980 that marijuana is useful in treating some epilepsy disorders (NIDA 1980).

- **Muscle-relaxant action**—Limited studies suggest that marijuana is effective in relieving muscle spasms common in patients who have multiple sclerosis.

Some prescription drugs have effects similar to marijuana. One of these is the drug Marinol, available in the form of a pill (but other delivery methods are being studied). Synthetic THC is the active ingredient, found to relieve the nausea and vomiting associated with chemotherapy for cancer patients and to assist with loss of appetite with AIDS patients (U.S. Drug Enforcement Agency 2011).

Research on the antinausea and antivomiting effects of smoking marijuana may not be consistent because of varying potency, which is dependent on the source of the marijuana.

Should marijuana be an accepted drug?

Marijuana is an unstable substance that has a poor shelf life. It may contain more than 1,000 chemicals, of which only about 400 are currently known. It contains dozens of things that may not be useful in treating a specific problem. At best, marijuana is a controversial drug. Although it may not be as harmful as some researchers report, it certainly is not harmless. Any use of THC for medical purposes does not stand as an endorsement for the recreational aspects of the drug.

Inhalants

Substances that are inhaled to produce altered states are called *inhalants*. These substances are classified as volatile solvents and aerosols. Common inhaled chemicals are fingernail polish remover, lacquer thinners, glue, gasoline, and correction fluid. Inhalation is a rapid means of ingesting substances, equivalent to IV injection in the time required to reach the brain. Altered consciousness can be achieved within one to two minutes of inhaling a large concentration and five to ten minutes with low doses.

Inhalants can also be ingested through the mouth. This method is called *huffing*.

Although they differ in makeup, nearly all abused inhalants produce short-term effects similar to anesthetics, which act to slow down the body's functions. When inhaled in sufficient concentrations, inhalants can cause intoxication, usually lasting only a few minutes. However, sometimes users extend this effect for several hours by breathing in inhalants repeatedly. Repeated inhalations make them feel less inhibited and less in control. If use continues, users can lose consciousness. Sniffing highly concentrated amounts of the chemicals in solvents or aerosol sprays can directly induce heart failure and death within minutes of a session of repeated inhalations. This is most common in cases of abuse of butane, propane, and chemicals in aerosols. High concentrations of inhalants also can cause death from suffocation by displacing oxygen in the lungs and then in the central nervous system so that breathing ceases (NIDA 2008).

Designer Drugs

Designer drugs are substances created in a laboratory by using chemistry to change the properties of another drug (e.g. cocaine, morphine). The resulting "designer" drugs typically have a new, different effect on the brain or behavior (National Institute on Drug Abuse 2011). Compounds are altered to give the appearance of the original drug, and, to some extent, the effects, but the drugs contain only legal substances. They are often called *look-alikes*. The most familiar designer drugs have been amphetamine look-alikes that contained caffeine, ephedrine, and phenylpropanolamine hydrochloride—the same ingredients as in many OTC diet and cold compounds. Designer cocaine may consist of powdered sugar and a topical anesthetic such as benzocaine. The user experiences sinus numbing, but the cocaine rush is absent. Naive users may be fooled, but experienced coke users quickly recognize the imposter.

In addition to differing in chemical makeup, some designer drugs are more dangerous than the drugs they imitate. They may contain very dangerous drugs that can be lethal in very small amounts, so when the user injects his or her usual dose, it may be fatal. Other effects such as brain damage and paralysis have occurred. Designer drugs are banned in the United States by a bill passed in 1986.

Club Drugs

According to the U. S. Department of Health and Human Services, Substance Abuse and Mental Health Services Administration (SAMHSA), the term *club drugs* refers to a wide variety of drugs often used at all-night dance parties ("raves"), nightclubs, and concerts. Club drugs can impair senses, memory, judgment, and coordination. Some common effects of club drugs include loss of muscle and motor control, blurred vision, and seizures. Club drugs such as methylenedioxymethamphetamine (MDMA or ecstasy) are stimulants that increase the heart rate and blood pressure and can lead to heart or kidney failure. Research studies have shown that regular use of ecstasy produces long-lasting, perhaps permanent, damage to the brain's ability to think and store memories.

Other club drugs, such as gamma-hydroxybutyrate (GHB), are depressants that can cause drowsiness, unconsciousness, or breathing problems. GHB and another drug, rohypnol, can cause a kind of amnesia; users may not remember what they said or did while under the effects of the drug. These drugs are sedatives and are often referred to as date rape drugs because victims become unconscious or immobilized. Most club drugs are odorless and tasteless. Some are made in a powder or liquid form that makes the drug easier to slip into a drink without a person's knowledge.

Because club drugs are illegal and often produced in makeshift laboratories, it is impossible to know exactly what chemicals were used to produce them. How strong or dangerous a club drug is varies. Higher doses of club drugs can cause severe breathing problems, coma, or even death.

Sometimes it is difficult to tell if someone is using these drugs, but there are warning signs, such as:

- problems remembering things recently said or done
- loss of coordination, dizziness, and fainting
- depression
- confusion
- sleep problems
- chills or sweating
- slurred speech

It is illegal to buy or sell club drugs, and club drugs can be addictive. It is also a crime to use any controlled substance to aid in sexual assault. Mixing club drugs together or with alcohol is extremely dangerous. The effects of one drug can magnify the effects and risks of another.

Hallucinogens

Hallucinogens are substances that occur naturally or are produced synthetically and that distort the user's perception of reality. Such drugs cause sensory illusions that make it difficult to distinguish fact from fantasy. Perhaps the most widely known hallucinogen is lysergic acid diethylamide (LSD), which was first synthesized in 1938. Although still occasionally used in medical research, the drug has no commonly used therapeutic applications. Even a tiny amount is enough to cause hallucinations, which manifest themselves in intensified colors, individualized sound perceptions, and bizarre visions that may be pleasant or extremely frightening. In mentally unstable individuals, LSD can produce psychotic reactions. There is also a danger of so-called flashbacks in which an individual

will suddenly have hallucinations weeks after having last ingested the drug. LSD does not cause physical dependency or seem to result in brain damage or birth defects, as once supposed. However, a "bad trip," or unpleasant experience while under the influence of the drug, can have long-lasting psychological effects.

Other hallucinogens are either derived from peyote, a kind of cactus that grows in Mexico and the American Southwest, or made synthetically. Most have effects similar to those produced by LSD, but some are particularly dangerous because of unpredictable side effects. One of the more common of these illegal drugs is phencyclidine hydrochloride (PCP), known as "angel dust." Originally synthesized as an animal tranquilizer, PCP is a relatively easy chemical to manufacture illegally. The drug is usually mixed with tobacco or marijuana and ingested by smoking.

PCP produces perceptual distortions, feelings of depersonalization, and changes in body image. Apathy, sweating, and auditory hallucinations may also result. High doses produce a stupor and overdose coma that can last for several weeks. This period can be followed by weeks of a confused mental state. In some individuals PCP also has been reported to precipitate extremely violent behavior, including murder.

Drug Education

Evaluation research on drug education prevention programs done over the last thirty years indicates that these programs have not been effective. In fact, the findings state that these programs essentially had no effect on the drug problem. Although studies of more recently developed programs are more optimistic, the findings still do not provide strong evidence of highly effective programs. The goals of these programs have been to affect three basic areas: knowledge, attitudes, and behavior. The programs have had some success in increasing knowledge and, to a lesser extent, changing attitudes toward drugs; however, increases in knowledge and changed attitudes do not mean much if the actual drug behavior is not affected. In fact, those programs that only increase knowledge tend to reduce anxiety and fear of drugs and may actually increase the likelihood of drug use. For example, one approach in the past was to provide students with complete information about all the possibilities of drug abuse, from the names of every street drug, to how the drugs are usually ingested, to detailed descriptions of possible effects of the drugs, and to possible consequences of an overdose. Given the inquiring nature of children, such an approach could well amount to a primer on how to take drugs, not how to avoid them.

The only effective approach to drug education is one in which children come to see that drug abuse constitutes unnecessary and self-abusive consequences. Teachers must provide realistic alternatives. Too often, the real appeal of such drugs as marijuana or alcohol is dismissed by asking children to take up a sport or go bike riding or learn to play a musical instrument. Such suggestions are fine as far as they go, but they often fail to take into account the personal problems that may tempt children into drug abuse.

Education programs that address social influence show the most promise in reducing or delaying onset of drug use. Psychological approaches in which social influences and skills are stressed are more effective than other approaches. The most effective programs in influencing both attitudes and behavior are peer programs that included either refusal skills—with more direct emphasis on behavior—or social and life skills, or both.

TEACHING TIP

There are a lot of wrong ways to teach drug abuse prevention. Scare tactics don't work. It's also best to avoid placing too much emphasis on the drugs themselves and how they are used. Rather than preventing abuse, this method sometimes encourages it! Instead, focus on the person rather than the drug. Teach resiliency skills like assertiveness, decision-making skills, and self-esteem.

In order for drug abuse prevention to be effective with youths, it is important that the message be reiterated early and reinforced consistently by authority figures such as parents, teachers, coaches, and mentors (Office of National Drug Control Policy 2011). A number of programs, taught as part of an overall Coordinated School Health Program, have been shown to be effective in improving outcomes for students. The National Institute on Drug Abuse (2011) has found that programs including the Caring School Community Program, Guiding Good Choices, Life Skills Training Program, Lions-Quest Skills for Adolescence, Project ALERT, and Project STAR contain strategies that have proven effective. These programs focus on preventing the onset of drug use through strategies such as using a sense of community; teaching personal responsibility, communication, and decision making; increasing knowledge about consequences; strengthening family involvement; and focusing on social influences.

A drug abuse education program is not an easy undertaking. For every strategy that has been proposed, there have been critics with good and plausible arguments as to why that strategy is the worst one possible. There are even those, including many parents, who feel that the best approach is no approach at all. This is the concept that if adults don't mention drugs, then the problem doesn't really exist. This view seems out of touch with reality, and yet it is understandable considering how so many drug education programs have led to unfortunate results.

The use of scare tactics in any health education program, including drug abuse education programs, is counterproductive. Children soon learn to recognize the difference between fact and possible fiction. Attempts to equate the dangers of marijuana with those of heroin, suggestions that any drug can kill or permanently impair an individual, and other dire warnings, no matter how true, are often disregarded as propaganda.

Teachers must never lie about the dangers of drugs or play down the problems that children are facing that may make drugs seem to be an appealing way to cope. Effective drug education walks a fine line, one that requires teachers' sensitivity to the environment in which children must live and function. It is always important to point out that, no matter what the circumstances, each individual has a choice and must make a choice about substance use or abuse. Drug education must be a part of a comprehensive mental health education program. Only when children realize that drugs are not the answer to a problem, but part of the problem, can instruction be considered successful.

Chapter In Review

Summary

- A drug is any substance that alters bodily functions.

- Drugs can be misused or abused.

- Reasons for substance abuse include low self-esteem, mood alteration, curiosity, peer pressure, boredom, alienation, and adult modeling.

- Drugs act on the body by stimulating or depressing cellular activity.

- Even when drugs are prescribed for medical purposes, there is a possibility that abuse can result.

- Over-the-counter drugs are usually safe when taken as directed, but ingestion of any drug, no matter how mild, can cause health hazards.

- Advertisements for OTC drugs can often lead people to believe that the drugs are safer and more effective than they actually are.

- Alcohol is one of the most commonly used and abused drugs.

- Alcohol can easily lead to psychological and physical dependency.

- The disease of alcoholism can and does occur in youth.

- Alcoholics and their families can receive help from many sources, such as AA.

- Barbiturates are depressants, and amphetamines are stimulants. If abused, these drugs can cause serious health problems or death.

- The narcotics class of drugs includes opium, morphine, and heroin.

- Heroin is extremely addictive and can lead to psychological breakdowns and irrational acts.
- With any street drug, the user can never be sure of just what chemicals are contained in the dose sold.
- Caffeine is the most commonly used stimulant.
- Amphetamines can be helpful if taken correctly, but methamphetamine is a commonly abused and highly addictive drug that can cause numerous health problems.
- A stimulant drug that is currently one of the most dangerous we have in our society is cocaine, known as "snow," "coke," or "crack."
- Crack is cheap and readily available and is smoked and absorbed into the bloodstream in less than ten seconds.
- Smoking tobacco is a serious health problem.
- Smokers often become psychologically and physically dependent on tobacco.
- Tobacco companies' advertising and promotional activities have led many children to start smoking and to use smokeless tobacco.
- Smoking is a difficult habit to break, but failure to do so can lead to a variety of serious diseases, including cancer and emphysema.
- Sidestream and secondhand smoke can cause similar problems to nonsmokers who live and/or work with smokers.
- Smokeless tobacco can lead to similar problems as smoking tobacco.
- Marijuana, for various reasons, is in a classification by itself.
- Ongoing research is determining the possible medicinal effects of marijuana.
- Most abused inhalants produce short-term effects similar to anesthetics. Death can result.
- Designer drugs are created in a laboratory to change the properties of another drug. They are banned in the U.S.
- Club drugs include MDMA, GHB, and rohypnol, the latter two of which are considered date rape drugs.
- Hallucinogenic drugs include LSD and PCP.
- Although not physically addictive, hallucinogens can lead to psychological breakdowns and irrational acts.
- Substance education is a difficult topic, one in which there are no easy answers regarding the correct course of action.
- Factual information must be provided, and yet substance education must not be allowed to become a primer on how to take drugs.
- Effective drug abuse education programs are needed to change not only knowledge and attitudes, but behavior as well.
- Community mores and lifestyles must be considered so that information and advice given are realistic and practical.
- The best course is to build self-esteem in students so that drugs are not seen as a viable alternative for coping with personal problems.

Discussion Questions

1. What is the definition of a *drug*? Give examples of substances that qualify as drugs under this definition.
2. List six common reasons for substance abuse, especially as these reasons apply to young people.
3. What factors contribute to the misuse and abuse of OTC drugs?
4. Describe the effects of alcohol on the body at various blood-alcohol concentration levels.
5. List six factors that contribute to the habit of smoking tobacco.
6. Discuss the adverse effects of smokeless tobacco.
7. Discuss cocaine and the various forms of the drug.
8. Why is marijuana considered to be a harmful substance? How can it effectively be used medicinally?
9. What approach to substance education is the most effective, and why?
10. What are the characteristics of a good substance abuse prevention program in the schools?

Critical Thinking Questions

1. There appears to be a thin line between use, abuse, and misuse. Do you think an underage person (e.g., someone who is under twenty-one and drinking alcohol) can use alcohol responsibly? Explain your answer relative to the law prohibiting the use of alcohol by those under the age of twenty-one.
2. There are a variety of reasons why some people begin to abuse drugs, and they appear to be unique for each individual. Can you synthesize the factors into the most common reasons for beginning abuse of substances?
3. Explain why some people continue to abuse substances even when they know about the harmful effects of the drugs on their body.
4. Explain your side of the debate regarding whether or not marijuana should be legalized.
5. How do you feel that the tobacco settlement monies should be used by the states?

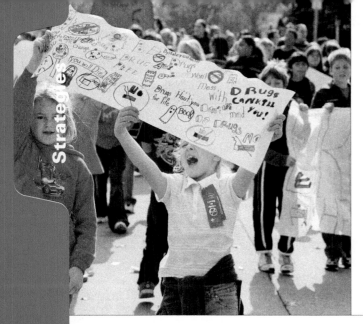

Strategies for Teaching about Substance Use and Abuse

 14

It is important for teachers to realize that there are almost as many reasons for drifting into substance abuse as there are different kinds of drugs.

NATIONAL HEALTH EDUCATION STANDARDS

1. Students will comprehend concepts related to health promotion and disease prevention to enhance health.

2. Students will analyze the influence of family, peers, culture, media, technology, and other factors on health behaviors.

3. Students will demonstrate the ability to access valid information and products and services to enhance health.

4. Students will demonstrate the ability to use interpersonal communication skills to enhance health and avoid or reduce health risks.

5. Students will demonstrate the ability to use decision-making skills to enhance health.

7. Students will demonstrate the ability to practice health-enhancing behaviors and avoid or reduce risks.

8. Students will demonstrate the ability to advocate for personal, family, and community health.

Valued Outcomes

After completion of this chapter, you should be able to convey the following to your students:

- Dealing effectively with personal problems is important in preventing substance abuse.
- Poor self-image increases the potential for substance abuse.
- Drugs should be taken only when a doctor prescribes them and only in the amount prescribed.
- People use and abuse drugs for physical, emotional, and social reasons.
- Certain drugs can be legally purchased only with a doctor's prescription.
- Some drugs, called over-the-counter drugs, can be purchased without a doctor's prescription.
- Smoking is dangerous to health.
- Tobacco smoke can be harmful to those who do not smoke, as well as to smokers themselves.
- Alcohol is a drug.
- Misuse of alcohol can cause physical, emotional, and social problems.
- Alcoholism is a disease.
- Alcoholism can lead to many health problems.
- Barbiturates can cause both physical and psychological dependency.
- Cocaine and crack are very dangerous drugs and should not be used under any circumstances.
- Amphetamines, like barbiturates, can be dangerous if abused.
- Illegal drugs, including narcotics and hallucinogens, can have unpredictable and serious health consequences.

Reflections

Consider the possibility that you have a student who is abusing an illegal drug, and he or she has confided in you. What are the realistic steps that you would take as a teacher in this situation? What other pieces of information would you need? Consider the personal, ethical, and legal ramifications. Which of the strategies in this chapter would be useful to help teach students to take responsibility for their actions?

The Challenge of Substance Abuse Education

Elementary school children need to be provided with learning experiences that will help them develop attitudes and values that build self-esteem and respect for the body so that drug taking is not seen as a way of coping with life. They must be taught to accept responsibility for their own behavior so that they will know how to deal with the problem of drugs in society.

The challenge of drug education is not to make every child a drug expert, nor to frighten children with scare tactics. Instead, it is to help children recognize that there is no need for them to misuse or abuse any drug, regardless of what reason they may have for being tempted to do so.

It is important for teachers to realize that there are almost as many reasons for drifting into substance abuse as there are different kinds of drugs. A youngster may wish to start smoking for an entirely different reason from the reason a youngster might begin amphetamine abuse. The temptation to take a particular drug may not stem from any self-destructive impulse, although sometimes it does. The problem is that the resultant behavior is always self-destructive, in varying degrees, regardless of the motivation. If children recognize this fact, and if they are on their way to building a strong self-image, then substance abuse is far less likely to occur in later years.

Shown to the right of each activity is the suggested grade level(s) for which the activity might be appropriate. However, many of the suggested activities could be modified for use at various grade levels.

Information Assessment Activities

Where Do You Stand? Grades K–5

Valued Outcome: Students will be able to clarify their values regarding substance abuse.

National Health Education Standards: 2, 4

Description of Strategy: Draw a chalk line on the floor. Explain to your students that the line is a continuum on how they feel about various decisions. One end of the line represents complete disagreement with a position, and the other end represents complete agreement. Or the line could represent degrees of willingness or unwillingness.

Then ask for volunteers to demonstrate where they stand on a variety of questions that you put forward. Try to keep the questions nonthreatening and nonincriminating. Questions that you might ask include: Where do you stand on smoking cigarettes? Where do you stand on drinking alcohol? How willing would you be to tell a friend who takes drugs that you do not approve of that behavior? How dangerous do you think it is to take a drug that you don't know anything about?

Materials Needed: chalk

Processing Question: Which of the questions were hardest for you to answer? Why do you think that is?

✔ **Assessment:** Students demonstrate awareness of their own values regarding substance abuse.

Sentence Completion Grades 3–5

Valued Outcome: Students will be able to complete statements with their own values-related answers.

National Health Education Standards: 4, 7, 8

Description of Strategy: Ask the students to complete statements such as the following with values-related answers:

For me, smoking is . . .

If I saw another student using drugs, I would . . .

Some people start drinking alcohol because . . .

Drugs are . . .

To me, substance abuse means . . .

The best reason for not taking any drugs is . . .

One thing I don't believe about drugs is . . .

If I made the laws about drugs, I would . . .

I was surprised to learn that drugs . . .

People who take drugs . . .

Materials Needed: handout for each student, pencils

Processing Question: What factors in your background influence your values regarding substance abuse?

✔ **Assessment:** Students' responses demonstrate awareness of their own values regarding substance abuse as well as a personal interest in practicing health-enhancing behaviors.

Smoking and the Law Grades 4–5

Valued Outcome: Students will gain awareness of tobacco regulation and clarify their own values about smoking.

National Health Education Standards: 1, 2

Description of Strategy: After you have discussed the definition of a drug, point out that tobacco qualifies under the definition. Note that although smoking is known to be hazardous to health, tobacco products can be purchased legally by adults. Ask students to consider the implications of this fact. Point out that each individual must make a decision about smoking. Then have the students consider the following question: Should laws be passed that prevent people from smoking in certain public places?

Processing Questions:

1. Should cigarettes be made illegal? Why or why not?
2. What legal rights should smokers have?
3. What legal rights should nonsmokers have?
4. What are some reasons to be considered in making such laws?
5. How do you feel about laws regulating smoking?

○ **Integration:** Social Studies

✓ **Assessment:** Students demonstrate awareness of the influence of government regulation and community pressure on smoking behavior and clarify their own values regarding smoking.

Smoking and You
Grades 4–5

Valued Outcome: Students will be able to list reasons why a person might decide not to start smoking.

National Health Education Standards: 2, 4, 5

Description of Strategy: Have each student prepare a list with two columns. In the first column, ask the students to write reasons why they think a person might want to start smoking. In the second column, have them list reasons why a person might decide not to start smoking. Talk over the various reasons that the students list in a general discussion. Which reasons in each column are rational ones? Which are irrational ones?

Processing Question: What are the emotional and social reasons a person might start smoking?

✓ **Assessment:** Students will be able to list five reasons why a person might decide not to start smoking.

Drug Abuse Prevention Newspaper
Grades 4–5

Valued Outcome: Students will be able to utilize their Internet skills to research information about specific drugs and complete a student-oriented "Drug Abuse Prevention" newspaper.

National Health Education Standards: 2, 3

Description of Strategy: Set up the students in groups of three or four. Each group of students will research information about a specific category of drugs (e.g., marijuana laws; youth and smoking; SADD). It may be helpful to assign a topic to students. The students will access appropriate Internet sites (.gov sources are recommended) to find reliable information about a topic related to their assigned category. They will then write a brief (100-word) article using their information in a newspaper article format; students should be sure to organize the research so they can keep their information and source documentation on file. Then, they will format the information and upload it onto the class webpage (intranet).

Materials Needed: access to Internet, word processing or layout program, school intranet

Processing Questions:

1. How can the media/newspaper articles affect drug use/abuse behaviors?
2. Were you surprised by information you found when researching your topic?
3. How is writing an article about a topic different from reading what other people have written about it?

○ **Integration:** Language Arts

✓ **Assessment:** The students will be evaluated on their ability to write the articles, list supporting sources, and successfully upload the articles in newspaper format on the school intranet server.

Living without Drugs
Grades 4–5

Valued Outcome: Students will be able to describe alternative ways to alleviate various health problems.

National Health Education Standards: 1, 2, 7

Description of Strategy: Have the students bring in advertisements for health-related products from magazines and newspapers. Look especially for ads that deal with stress ailments, such as headaches, backaches, insomnia, and diarrhea. After comparing and discussing the ads, have the students brainstorm alternative ways to deal with these problems. Alternatives to medication may include taking time to talk to a friend or loved one, listening to soft music, eating properly, exercising, drinking plenty of water, or doing something special.

Materials Needed: newspapers and magazines

Processing Question: Why is our society so drug dependent?

✓ **Assessment:** Students can list several health-enhancing alternatives to relying on drugs to resolve or prevent health problems.

Living with Drugs
Grades 4–5

Valued Outcome: Students will be able to explain the connection between societal problems and substance abuse.

National Health Education Standard: 1

Description of Strategy: Have the students collect and bring in magazine articles and newspaper clippings about accidents, domestic problems, violence, suicide, and crime. Discuss the clippings and the role drug or alcohol use may have played. Have the class members consider

TEACHING IN ACTION | **Daily Lesson Plan**

Lesson Title: Caffeine: The Common Drug

Date: February 20, 2012   **Time:** 11:00 A.M.   **Grade:** One   **Teacher:** Rashid

I. National Health Education Standards

Health Education Standard 7: Students will demonstrate the ability to practice health-enhancing behaviors and avoid or reduce health risks.

II. National Health Education Standards Performance Indicator

7.2.1 demonstrate healthy practices and behaviors to maintain or improve personal health.

III. Valued Outcomes

- Students will identify products that contain various amounts of caffeine.
- Students will describe the dangers of consuming too much caffeine.
- Students will make educated choices for alternatives to caffeine.

IV. Description of Strategy

1. Discuss with students what caffeine does to the body including common undesirable side-effects (rapid heartbeat, sleep inhibitions, headaches, etc.).
2. Display food and beverage items that contain various amounts of caffeine and some that do not have caffeine. Include soft drinks, milk, juice, coffee, tea, chocolate, and water.
3. Ask students to identify the items that have caffeine and the items that are uncaffeinated. Afterwards arrange the foods in order of the amount of caffeine they have. This will show students that some caffeinated items do not have as much caffeine as other items do.
4. Explain the importance of consuming caffeinated products in moderation. Also, explain the importance of calcium, and describe the negative effect that caffeine and carbonation have on calcium absorption. Show students some foods that provide calcium.
5. Encourage students to select uncaffeinated foods, such as milk, juice, or water, instead of soft drinks.

V. Materials Needed

- caffeinated and uncaffeinated food items
- table

VI. Formative Evaluation

Benchmarks

- Level 1: Student was able to identify products containing caffeine.
- Level 2: Student was able to identify products containing caffeine and list reasons why consuming too much caffeine is not healthy.
- Level 3: Student was able to identify products containing caffeine. Student was able to list reasons why consuming too much caffeine is not healthy and to list alternative foods.
- Level 4: Student was able to identify products containing caffeine. Student was able to list reasons why consuming too much caffeine is not healthy and to list alternative foods. Student was able to describe the benefits of calcium and explain the interaction between calcium and caffeine and soft drinks.

VII. Points of Emphasis

1. Explain what happens in the body when too much caffeine is consumed.
2. Explain the importance of making good decisions regarding food/beverage choices.
3. Explain that caffeine in moderation is not dangerous.

Teacher Evaluation

1. Keep the lesson as taught?   yes _____   no _____

2. What I need to improve _____

3. Next time make sure _____

4. Strengths of lesson _____

TEACHING IN ACTION | **Daily Lesson Plan**

Lesson Title: Stimulants

Date: February 20, 2012   **Time:** 1:00 P.M.   **Grade:** Seven   **Teacher:** Conway

I. National Health Education Standards

Health Education Standard 8: Students will demonstrate the ability to advocate for personal, family, and community health.

II. National Health Education Standards Performance Indicator

8.8.1 state a health-enhancing position on a topic and support it with accurate information.

III. Valued Outcomes

- Students will understand how tobacco, alcohol, and other drug use affects crime rates and the economy.
- Students will identify government programs that help fight stimulant abuse.
- Students will identify several positions on the government's role in fighting stimulant abuse.

IV. Description of Strategy

1. Explain that drug use costs the United States billions of dollars every year.
2. Explain that a portion of the taxes that their parents pay supports government institutions (military, police, prisons, and hospitals) that are actively involved in preventing drug use. Make the connection between drug use and crime in the community.
3. Identify how drug use is fought in the United States (police enforcement, prosecution, prison terms, etc.).
4. Have students discuss how they feel about their families having to pay for fighting drug use. Ask students to describe other ways that this money could be used.
5. Have students write a report about a stimulant and its effect on the economy or crime rates. Instruct students to use a media source (newspaper or magazine article, television news report) for their report. This will help them make connections between stimulant abuse and crime/economic issues.

V. Materials Needed

- none

VI. Formative Evaluation

Benchmarks

- Level 1: Student was able to identify government programs that fight stimulant abuse.
- Level 2: Student was able to identify government programs that fight stimulant abuse and can list a few ways stimulant use affects crime rates and the economy.
- Level 3: Student was able to identify government programs that fight stimulant abuse and can list many ways stimulant use affects crime rates and the economy.
- Level 4: Student was able to identify government programs that fight stimulant abuse and can list many ways stimulant use affects crime rates and the economy. Student was able to argue several positions on the government's role in fighting these problems.

VII. Points of Emphasis

1. Explain the correlation between stimulant abuse and crime rates.
2. Explain how the cost of fighting stimulant abuse affects students and their families.
3. Explain how money spent on anti-drug programs could be spent on other things or saved.

Teacher Evaluation

1. Keep the lesson as taught?   yes _____   no _____

2. What I need to improve _____

3. Next time make sure _____

4. Strengths of lesson _____

reasons why these things might have occurred and what kinds of actions can be taken to avoid them in their own lives (alternatives to destructive behavior).

Materials Needed: newspapers and magazines

Processing Question: Why is there such a positive correlation between substance abuse and violence/crime?

○ **Integration:** Social Studies

✔ **Assessment:** Students demonstrate awareness of the link between substance abuse and social ills.

Drug Rating Scale   Grades 4–5

Valued Outcome: Students will express their opinions about drugs.

National Health Education Standards: 1, 4

Description of Strategy: Have the students complete the following rating scale on their beliefs about drugs. Then have a classroom discussion about why they feel the way they do.

1. strongly agree   2. agree   3. don't know/neutral
4. disagree   5. strongly disagree

__ It is okay to smoke marijuana every once in a while.
__ Crack cocaine is the worst drug a person can take.
__ Nicotine in cigarettes is a drug.
__ Smoking cigarettes is not good for your health.
__ Tripping on acid only affects you once, and then you never feel the effects of the drug again.
__ The best thing I can do when asked to take drugs by someone is to say no and walk away.
__ Drinking alcohol is not the same as taking a drug.
__ Alcohol won't hurt you.
__ I can smoke now and then quit when I get older, and it won't hurt me.
__ The only kind of people who take drugs are bad students who are always getting in trouble.

Materials Needed: handout for each student, pencils

Processing Questions:

1. Why should we say no to drugs?
2. What happens when people take drugs?
3. If a person takes drugs, will it affect him or her for the rest of his or her life?

✔ **Assessment:** Students demonstrate an awareness of the harmful effects of substance use and abuse.

Decision Stories

Present decision stories such as the following, using the procedures outlined in Chapter 4, pages 60–62.

For each of the decision stories, write a list on the board of ideas generated by the class for how each situation should be dealt with. Ask the students to discuss the merits of the methods suggested.

Assessment for Decision Stories: Students can identify health-enhancing behaviors and exhibit positive decision-making skills.

Drugs in the Neighborhood   Grades 3–5

Darlene knows that some of the older kids in her neighborhood are using and selling drugs. They don't seem to care that Darlene sees what they are doing. "It's none of your business," one of them told her. But Darlene is not so sure. A couple of her friends bought some of these drugs and have started using them. Darlene doesn't know what will happen in the neighborhood next.

Focus Question: What can Darlene do about the drug problem in her neighborhood?

National Health Education Standards: 2, 5, 8

Mom Drinks Too Much   Grades 3–5

Often, when David arrives home from school in the afternoon, his mother is sitting in the living room with a glass or a bottle beside her. Sometimes she is very loving, and other times she seems very angry at him. Sometimes she is asleep on the couch, and he has trouble waking her up. Sometimes mom can't fix supper for David and his younger sister. David knows that his mom uses alcohol more than she should. She is frequently depressed and upset. David is afraid of how his mom will act when he comes in every day, and he is afraid that she will get hurt. He also worries about who is taking care of his sister when he is not there. David constantly worries about what will happen to his family if his mom does not stop drinking.

Focus Question:

1. What actions should David take?
2. Who does he need to talk to about his problems?
3. Who might be able to help David, his sister, and his mom?

National Health Education Standards: 2, 3, 5

Want a Smoke?   Grades 4–5

Mark always walks home from school with a group of friends. One day, two of his friends light up cigarettes. Mark is surprised because he didn't know that they had started smoking. "Want a smoke?" his friend Jim asks. His other friend George says, "Try one." Mark can see that Jim and George are trying to look grown up. He wants to look grown up, too. The other two boys in the group are not smoking. Mark wonders what he should do.

Focus Question: What should Mark say to his friends?

National Health Education Standards: 2, 5

Sleepover
Grades 4–5

Leah had been looking forward to tonight. It is her tenth birthday, and she is having a sleepover party in her backyard. Her parents were letting Leah and her two friends, Casey and her sister, Allison, sleep in her tent. The girls had eaten sandwiches and were about to play cards when Casey pulled out a pack of cigarettes from her coat pocket. "Hey, let's have a cigarette," she says. Casey and Allison both take out a cigarette. Casey offers the pack to Leah. "No, I don't want to," she says. "What's the matter, big baby? Are you scared?" asks Casey. "We didn't know we were sleeping over with such a baby. Maybe we'd better go home." Leah had been having lots of fun, but she did not know that her friends smoked.

Focus Question: What should Leah do?

National Health Education Standards: 2, 5

Problems at Home
Grades 7–8

Michael's problems at home are getting worse, and he feels he has nowhere to turn. He is very lonely and frightened about what is happening in his life. His parents are always fighting. They don't seem to have any time for him anymore. He wants so much to have someone show him love and concern. He also wishes that he could just leave his problems behind him.

Focus Question:

1. What are some methods of coping that Michael might try?
2. What might be the consequences of each of these methods?

National Health Education Standards: 3, 7

Dramatizations

I'm No Dummy
Grades K–2

Valued Outcome: Students will be able to demonstrate refusal skills.

National Health Education Standard: 4

Description of Strategy: Have the students make and use hand puppets to act out skits about drug use and abuse. One puppet, for example, might be offered drugs by other puppets. "I'm no dummy," the first puppet replies and then gives reasons for refusing.

Materials Needed: paper lunch bags or cloth for making puppets, markers

Processing Question: What is the best way to refuse the offer of drugs?

✔ **Assessment:** Students will demonstrate their ability to effectively use interpersonal communication skills to refuse offers of drugs.

Drug Abuse Prevention Decision Story Presentation
Grades 3–5

Valued Outcome: The students will be able to use information from a health-related Decision Story to produce and deliver a presentation to their classmates.

National Health Education Standards: 2, 3

Description of Strategy: After you have covered a decision story with the class, instruct students to use Microsoft PowerPoint or a similar presentation program to develop each aspect of the decision story and the decision they reached. They could do this individually or in assigned groups. Each slide should be illustrated by an appropriate picture related to that aspect of the decision story. The final presentations can be narrated live or recorded beforehand. The presentation could also be uploaded to a school intranet site.

Materials Needed: access to a computer and presentation software; access to Internet or software program with pictures

Processing Questions:

1. How can technology be used to deliver health education messages to students?
2. In thinking through each step of the decision to prepare the presentation, did the final decision change based on further reflection?

✔ **Assessment:** The students will be evaluated on setting up the PowerPoint presentation and delivery of the PowerPoint presentation to the class.

Peers Helping Other Peers
Grades 3–5

Valued Outcome: Students will be able to persuade a peer to prevent drug abuse.

National Health Education Standards: 4, 8

Description of Strategy: Have the students role-play a drug-related incident. Pick four students who are willing to participate in the role-playing. Without the class hearing, explain to the four students that they are at the mall and see a couple of friends. They watch their friends walk around to the back of the mall. Deciding they want to see what their friends are up to, they follow them. Little did they know that their two friends were doing drugs. Once approached, they started acting really funny. The good students are to tell their friends the effects of the drugs on their body and to help them understand that what they are doing is wrong. Explain to the students they are to use their prior knowledge from the unit on substance abuse to persuade the students to quit. After this is accomplished, ask the rest of the class to tell the four students what they did wrong or what they did right. Follow this with discussion on what they could have done to prevent the drug use.

Processing Questions:

1. What can you do as a student to keep your friends off drugs?
2. What would you do if approached with a harmful substance?
3. What can you do for the community to cut down substance abuse?

✓ **Assessment:** Students demonstrate their ability to use interpersonal communication skills to advocate healthy choices about drugs.

Drug Court   Grades 3–5

Valued Outcome: Students will gain awareness of legal penalties that are enforced for drug-related offenses.

National Health Education Standard: 1

Description of Strategy: Have the students role-play various drug-related court cases. In this court, the class acts collectively as judge and jury. Various students come before the court acting the part of the arresting officer. They explain to the court that they have arrested an individual on a drug charge and then describe the offense. In each case, the defendant has already pleaded guilty to the charge. It is up to the court to decide what sentence or decision to make. The class must come up with a consensus on each offense. Follow each decision with a general discussion. Also note to the students what penalty might have been given in an actual court.

Processing Questions:

1. Why is it illegal to use/abuse certain drugs?
2. What penalties are given to those who illegally use/abuse drugs?

○ **Integration:** Social Studies

✓ **Assessment:** Students demonstrate awareness of the social and legal consequences of drug abuse.

What Would Happen If...?   Grades 3–5

Valued Outcome: Students will be able to simulate various activities while pretending to be under the influence of certain kinds of drugs.

National Health Education Standard: 1

Description of Strategy: After discussing the effects that various kinds of drugs can have on the body and brain, have students role-play situations in which a person attempts an activity while under the influence of a certain kind of drug. For example, what would happen if an airline pilot tried to land a plane while under the influence of alcohol? What would happen if a surgeon tried to operate while under the influence of a hallucinogen? Have one student play the affected person. Another student, at the last minute, steps in and saves the day. After the activity, emphasize to the class that sometimes no one can keep a tragedy from happening. Bring this point home by discussing drunk-driving statistics or other examples from the news.

Processing Questions:

1. What effects do drugs have on the body?
2. How can the effects of drugs affect one's job performance?

✓ **Assessment:** Students demonstrate understanding that drug use impairs function and the risks the drug user imposes on others.

Dangers of Huffing   Grades 4–5

Valued Outcome: Students will discuss the difficulties of peer pressure and ways of overcoming and reversing peer pressure. Students will be able to name some of the dangers of inhaling chemicals.

National Health Education Standards: 1, 2, 4, 5

Description of Strategy: Divide the class into small groups of four or five students each. Give the groups pretend bottles of glue. Have a couple of students play the role of the persuader and the other students in the group play the role of the reluctant ones. Have the students discuss how it felt to be pressured and the possible effects of inhaling chemical products. Then have the students brainstorm ways to handle these situations and ways they might actually reverse peer pressure by preventing the other members of the group from participating.

Materials Needed: pretend bottles of glue

Processing Questions:

1. What are the dangers of inhaling chemicals?
2. What are some ways you could avoid situations like these?

✓ **Assessment:** Students can name a danger of inhaling chemicals and demonstrate their ability to use decision-making skills and interpersonal communication skills to overcome negative peer pressure and make healthful choices about inhaling chemicals.

Past, Present, and Future Drug Users and Abusers
Grades 4–5

Valued Outcome: Students will be able to explain and discuss the effects, consequences, and solutions of substance use and abuse.

National Health Education Standards: 1, 2

Description of Strategy: Have four or five students role-play the effects and consequences of substance use and abuse. The selected students should have background knowledge on their substance and its effects and consequences. Provide appropriate information for the various drugs to ensure that students disseminate the correct information. Have the other students ask questions about the selected students' "experiences" with substance use and abuse. As a class, have students discuss different outcomes and solutions that would prevent future use and abuse of substances.

Materials Needed: note cards with appropriate information

Processing Questions:

1. What are some of the effects and consequences of substance use/abuse?
2. What are some reasons people use and abuse substances?

✓ **Assessment:** Students can suggest at least five strategies that would prevent future abuse of substances.

Public Service Messages
Grades 4–6

Valued Outcome: Students will be able to devise a one-minute message on substance education.

National Health Education Standards: 1, 8

Description of Strategy: Divide the class into small groups. Have each group prepare a one-minute public service message for television broadcast about substance eduction. Encourage imagination. Some students may wish to write and sing a song bearing their message. Others may wish to act out a skit. Still others may opt for a panel format. Have each group give its presentations, and have the class discuss each one. You may wish to have the students vote for the most effective presentation.

Materials Needed: optional videotaping equipment to aid discussion

Processing Questions:

1. How can anti-drug messages best be given to the public?
2. What should these messages include?

✓ **Assessment:** Students' presentations demonstrate their understanding of substance abuse issues and their ability to advocate for community health.

Discussion and Report Techniques

Presentation by Health Professionals
Grades K–5

Valued Outcome: Students will learn numerous facts about substance use and abuse from a health professional.

National Health Education Standards: 1, 3

Description of Strategy: With permission from your school administration, invite an official from a substance abuse program to speak to your class about substance use and abuse. Talk with your guest alone before the presentation and emphasize that no scare tactics should be used. The presentation should be factual and objective. Allow time for a question-and-answer session afterward.

Processing Questions:

1. What types of treatment are given in substance abuse programs?
2. How effective are these programs?

○ **Integration:** Social Studies

✓ **Assessment:** Students' questions demonstrate their understanding of the presentation topic.

Dealing with Problems
Grades K–5

Valued Outcome: Students will be able to identify personal problems and then share solutions with each other in class.

National Health Education Standards: 4, 5

Description of Strategy: Divide the class into small groups and have them complete these four sentences:

1. I have a problem…
2. This is what happened…
3. My feelings were (or are)…
4. I need your help to…

Have each group discuss or role-play for the rest of the class a real problem for them personally. Then let the group present their ideas for positive solutions and get the class response.

Materials Needed: pencils and paper

Processing Question: If you find effective solutions to problems, can that keep you from using/abusing drugs?

✓ **Assessment:** Students demonstrate the ability to use decision-making skills and interpersonal communication skills to make healthful choices and avoid drug use.

Who Influences Your Decisions?
Grades K–5

Valued Outcome: Students will learn about decision making and whom they can talk to when making difficult decisions.

National Health Education Standards: 2, 3, 5

Description of Strategy: Talk with students about how all people make decisions every day. Some decisions affect our lives more drastically than others do. There are easy decisions to make—such as which shoes to wear to school—and there are much more difficult decisions—such as what to do if a friend wants to copy your test answers. It is important to know where to go for advice or help when making important decisions. Have students brainstorm a list of people, places, and institutions that are important to consider when making a decision. This list might include family, television, friends, church, and teachers. Have each student decide who or what he or she considers to have the greatest influence on his or her own life. Then have students create collages about the many different influences that affect their thinking and decisions every day.

Materials Needed: paper, magazines, scissors, markers, crayons, glue

Processing Questions:

1. What is the most effective way to make a wise decision?
2. How can effective decision making help prevent a substance abuse problem?

✓ **Assessment:** Students can name several available resources (including people) that can help them make difficult decisions.

The Question Box   Grades 3–5

Valued Outcome: Students will be able to identify personal problems and practice problem-solving skills.

National Health Education Standards: 4, 5

Description of Strategy: Have each student write on an index card a personal problem he or she is concerned about. Students may fill out as many cards as they like, but they are to write only one question per card. No names or other means of identification should be included. Have the students place their cards in a large ballot box. Allow them to place additional questions in the box for a week. After class, open the box and screen out any cards that inadvertently reveal any problems that would lead to identification of the student involved. Compile a numbered list of concerns from the remaining cards, hand out copies of the list, and randomly assign each student a number from the list. Each student should explain to the class how he or she would deal with the problem. Allow other students who have different opinions to add comments.

Materials Needed: index cards, pencils, ballot box, handout for each student of compiled list of concerns

Processing Question: What type of problems in relationships or school could lead to a substance abuse problem?

✓ **Assessment:** Students demonstrate the ability to use effective decision-making skills to resolve personal problems in a healthy way.

Smoking   Grades 3–5

Valued Outcome: The students will be able to recall the detrimental effects of smoking by writing a short paragraph on the topic.

National Health Education Standard: 1

Description of Strategy: Ask students to sit in a circle and talk about what smoking does to the body. Hold up a smoking advertisement and ask the students what the advertisement tells them about smoking. For example, does it make you look cool? Have the students respond as a group. Then have students draw pictures of how they think healthy lungs look compared to the lungs of a smoker. Tell students to write a short paragraph about other detriments of smoking.

Materials Needed: smoking/cigarette advertisement, pencils and paper

Processing Question: How do advertisements try to influence young people to smoke?

○ **Integration:** Writing

✓ **Assessment:** Students' written responses include at least five detrimental effects of smoking.

Resiliency Skills Blog   Grades 4-5

Valued Outcome: Students will analyze the influence of family, peers, culture, media, technology, and other factors on health behaviors. Students will be able to set up, make entries into, and implement a blog on the Internet.

National Health Education Standard: 2

Description of Strategy: After studying a unit on resiliency skills, introduce students to the concept of "blogging." Instruct them to set up a blog on the school's or district's intranet to blog about their thoughts on assertiveness, decision making, and self-esteem. The students can have one class blog or their own individual blogs. Students should brainstorm about ways to "Say No," to avoid situations where they might be pressured to use drugs, and how to make wise decisions. They can blog about real-life situations they have experienced or might experience. If students have individual blogs, when students visit each other's blogs they can brainstorm with them, provide feedback, and offer suggestions.

Materials Needed: computers, blog template and instructions, school intranet (This would be much more secure than an Internet blog, where the entries would be visible to others outside the school network.)

Processing Question:

1. How can resiliency skills be used to prevent or delay drug use?
2. Is the brainstorming process different in social media composed to in person?
3. What might be the drawbacks to having a public blog?

○ **Integration:** Language Arts

✓ **Assessment:** The students will be graded on their ability to set up, make entries in, and publish their blog on the school intranet network.

Saying No to Drugs   Grades 3–5

Valued Outcome: Students will demonstrate drug awareness.

National Health Education Standard: 7

Description of Strategy: Discuss with the students what drugs are. Explain to them that drugs can hurt them badly, and it is not good to use them. Tell the students that it is all right to say no to using drugs and that people who want them to try drugs are not their friends. Allow the students to talk about drug abuse. Advise them on the right and wrong thing to do. Tell them about famous people who have died from drug abuse. Following the discussion, give each student a piece of drawing paper and some crayons or markers. Give them suggestions for drawing campaign signs against using drugs (e.g., "Just Say No"). Have them make the signs as colorful and noticeable as possible. Hang the signs throughout the school as a reminder to the rest of the students that drug abuse is not welcome.

Materials Needed: crayons or markers, paper

Processing Questions:

1. What should you do if someone offers you drugs?
2. What is drug abuse?
3. Are drugs good for your body?

○ **Integration:** Art

✓ **Assessment:** Student projects demonstrate their awareness of the negative consequences of substance abuse.

Effects of Drug Use   Grades 3–5

Valued Outcome: Students will become aware of the effects of drugs on the body.

National Health Education Standard: 1

Description of Strategy: To begin this activity, define the word *drug*. Explain how some drugs can be helpful and others harmful. Then, discuss how some drugs that are helpful can be harmful if used wrongly. Divide the students into groups of four. Give each group an index card with a drug use situation on it. Have each group discuss a particular situation and decide if the drug being used is helpful or harmful and why. Then, write *harmful* and *helpful* on the board. Have each group share the situation they discussed and say whether the drug is helpful or harmful. Write the situation down. To close this activity, summarize why it is important to know how and what drugs are used for. Also discuss a few helpful things that drugs do and a few harmful things they do.

Materials Needed: index cards, board, markers

Processing Questions:

1. Why is it important to know about the effects of drugs?
2. How can people abuse helpful drugs and make them harmful?

✓ **Assessment:** Students demonstrate an awareness of positive and negative effects of drug use and can differentiate between appropriate and inappropriate use of drugs.

Smoking Marijuana   Grades 4–5

Valued Outcome: Students will learn about physical effects and legal consequences of smoking marijuana.

National Health Education Standard: 1

Description of Strategy: Invite a juvenile court representative to class to speak about the legal consequences of using drugs. The activity before the lesson will include discussion of students' experiences with jail or criminal activity. The follow-up activity will consist of asking the speaker a series of questions. Each student should be handcuffed for a few seconds.

Materials Needed: handcuffs (provided by juvenile court representative)

Processing Questions:

1. Why is it important not to smoke marijuana?
2. What did the juvenile court representative cite as a legal consequence of using marijuana?

○ **Integration:** Social Studies

✓ **Assessment:** Students can describe the physical effects and legal consequences of smoking marijuana.

Preventing Drinking and Driving   Grades 4–5

Valued Outcome: Students will learn about using decision-making steps to make healthful decisions about alcohol use.

National Health Education Standards: 4, 5, 8

Description of Strategy: Provide students with this scenario: Your older sister arrives to pick you up from the movies but has had too much to drink, and you know it. You both have to get home soon, and your sister is determined to get behind the wheel. What can you do to prevent this from happening? Have the students individually jot down their ideas, then break them up into small groups to compare notes, and have each group pick and present one of their preventive measures to the rest of the groups.

Materials Needed: pencils and paper

Processing Question: What would you do to prevent someone from drinking and driving?

✔ **Assessment:** Students demonstrate their ability to apply decision-making skills and strategies to make and promote healthy decisions about alcohol use.

Source: U.S. Department of Education 2001

Dangers of Smoking   Grades 4–5

Valued Outcome: Students will be able to explain and discuss the dangers of smoking.

National Health Education Standard: 1

Description of Strategy: Give the students information about the dangers of cigarette smoking. Working individually, have the students create slogans or posters for a class anti-smoking campaign. Ask the principal to judge the students' work and present small prizes for originality and creativity.

Materials Needed: construction paper, markers, crayons, colored pencils, scissors, glue

Processing Questions:

1. Why do you think people smoke?
2. Why do you think it is so hard for people to quit smoking?

○ **Integration:** Art

✔ **Assessment:** Students demonstrate an understanding of the dangers of smoking.

Source: American Lung Association 2002, 2003

The Space Colony   Grades 4–5

Valued Outcome: Students will be able to originate a drug policy and drug laws for a new planetary settlement.

National Health Education Standards: 5, 8

Description of Strategy: Tell the class that they are about to travel to a new planet by spaceship. On this planet there are no governments or laws. As a group, the class must decide on the drug policy and drug laws for the new planetary settlement. The class, acting as a committee,

must decide what drugs, if any, are to be taken to the new planet and how such drugs will be distributed or made available. Have the class keep in mind that drugs include useful medications, but that such medications can be abused. Laws relating to the misuse of drugs on the new planet must also be discussed. After thorough discussion, have the class come to a consensus about a drug policy on the new planet. Write their conclusions on the board. Then have each student prepare an individual report, including any dissenting opinions. Students must support their opinions.

Materials Needed: markers, board

Processing Questions:

1. Why are drug laws needed?
2. Are current laws effective in preventing substance abuse? Why or why not?

○ **Integration:** Social Studies, Writing

✔ **Assessment:** Student reports demonstrate their ability to use decision-making skills to make healthful choices and to advocate for community health.

Individual Reports   Grades 4–5

Valued Outcome: Students will be able to initiate research and prepare a report on a drug-related problem.

National Health Education Standards: 1, 3

Description of Strategy: Ask students to research a drug-related problem and prepare individual reports on what they find. Topics can include smoking and health, alcohol abuse and accidents, drugs and the law, and dangers of substance abuse.

Processing Questions:

1. What is the relationship between smoking and health?
2. What are the dangers of substance abuse?

○ **Integration:** Writing

✔ **Assessment:** Student research reports demonstrate their understanding of their topic and their ability to access valid health information.

Defending Yourself from Pressure   Grades 4–6

Valued Outcome: Students will see that the media does not always portray life accurately, especially regarding substance abuse, and will learn techniques that can help them resist false advertising.

National Health Education Standards: 2, 7

Description of Strategy: Explain the effects alcohol, smoking, and illegal substances may have on the body.

Ask for examples in which drugs have had an ill effect on someone. Then have the class discuss why people become involved in such things. Lead the class in discussing peer pressure, what is considered "cool," and the effects of the media. Have the class discuss how the media influences our way of thinking and how they can defend themselves from such pressures. At the end of the discussion, have the students make a substance abuse collage from magazine advertisements. Have them develop a theme such as "just say no to false advertisement" for their collage. Students should be able to explain their slogans and collage clippings and tell how the pictures apply to the slogan. Grade them on (1) doing the project and doing it well, (2) originality, (3) time and effort put into it, and (4) explanation of collage. When the collages are done, display them around the school (such as in the cafeteria) to remind other students of false advertising.

Materials Needed: poster board, magazines for clippings, construction paper or markers, glue, scissors

Processing Questions:

1. How does the media misrepresent information?
2. What are some ways you can resist false advertising?

○ **Integration:** Social Studies, Art

✓ **Assessment:** Students demonstrate an understanding of how the media can influence health behavior and can describe techniques to recognize and resist false advertising.

Just Saying No Is Our Final Answer! Grades 5–6

Valued Outcome: The student will be able to use his or her prior knowledge of substance abuse/use to organize a drug-free school environment.

National Health Education Standard: 8

Description of Strategy: Divide the class into small groups. Assign each group different roles in making their school a drug-free school. For example, have the class decide on different strategies that would get the drug-free message out to the students and to the community. Different strategies might include posters, videos, or special programs with different activities informing the students of the harmful effects of substance abuse. Have each group give at least a one- to two-minute presentation of the strategy that they would use to make their school a drug-free environment. After the presentations, discuss with the class the positive and negative aspects of each presentation.

Processing Questions:

1. What are other ways to promote a drug-free school environment?
2. What can you do as a student to promote a drug-free community?

✓ **Assessment:** Students' presentations demonstrate their ability to advocate for community health.

Researching Substance Abuse Grades 5–8

Valued Outcome: Students will learn more about different drugs and know the effects that drugs have on the human body.

National Health Education Standards: 1, 3

Description of Strategy: Discuss different types of drugs with the students. Allow the students to share anything (within reason) they know about the different drugs and the effects they have on the human body. Tell the students that they will be writing a research paper on drugs and the effect they have on the body. Make materials such as encyclopedias, written information on drugs or drug abuse, and Internet access, if possible, accessible to the students throughout the entire time they are working on the project. Have the students pick a drug or type of drug, and describe it and the effects it has on the human body. First, have them research their topic; this can be started on the first day of the assignment. Make sure they document their information. The second step is a rough draft. Finally, have students correct the rough draft and turn in the final copy. Have each student make an oral presentation of his or her research paper.

Materials Needed: paper and pencils, research materials such as encyclopedias, drug abuse manuals, computer(s) with Internet access

Processing Question: What are the types of drugs?

○ **Integration:** Writing

✓ **Assessment:** Student reports demonstrate their understanding of their topic and their ability to access valid health information.

Debating Drug Abuse Grades 5–8

Valued Outcome: Students will be able to explain the pros and cons of taking drugs.

National Health Education Standards: 2, 4, 8

Description of Strategy: Divide the class into two groups. Half the class should be on one side of the room (Side A), and the other half should be facing them (Side B). Tell the students on Side A that they are against taking drugs and cannot stand to be around those who do. Tell Side B that they all take drugs, and they think drugs should be legal. These two sides are both given this question: "Should drugs be legalized?" Give the students the rest of the class period to do research. On the next day, hold a debate between Side A and Side B. Side A should detail the facts of the effects of drugs, and Side B should give excuses about those facts and excuses that people taking drugs would make. Then discuss the harm that drugs do cause with the exceptions of the drugs that are legal for medicinal purposes only.

Processing Questions:

1. Should all drugs be legalized?
2. Is it dangerous to take illegal drugs without a prescription?

✔ **Assessment:** Students can articulate the negative effects of drug abuse and can differentiate between appropriate and inappropriate uses of drugs. Students demonstrate the ability to recognize the influence of media, peers, culture, and government on people's behavior regarding drug use.

Experiments and Demonstrations

Smoking Machine   Grades K–5

Valued Outcome: Students will become aware of what cigarette smoking does to the body.

National Health Education Standard: 1

Description of Strategy: The purpose of this demonstration is to show the effect of cigarette tars on the human body by way of analogy. Check with school and state policies regarding experiments in the classroom before engaging in this demonstration. If there are no policies prohibiting the experiment, send a letter home to the parents or guardians that informs them in advance of this demonstration. Be sure to perform this experiment in a well-ventilated room and place the apparatus where students will not inhale the smoke.

You will need a large glass bottle, a two-hole rubber stopper, glass delivery tubes, a cigarette holder, cigarettes, and a small hand pump. Most of this equipment can be found in a school chemistry lab or can be obtained from a scientific supply house. Set up the apparatus as shown in Figure 14.1.

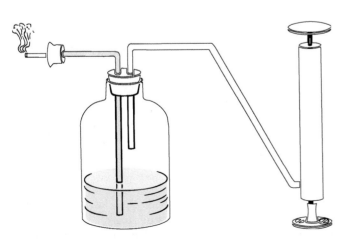

Figure 14.1
Smoking Machine Apparatus

Fill the bottle halfway with water. Place a cigarette in the holder and light it. Operate the pump to draw smoke from the cigarette into the bottle and water. Continue to pump until the cigarette is burned completely. Burn additional cigarettes as necessary until tars can be seen in the water. Have the students examine the water and note the distinct smell. Tars may also collect in the glass tubing. Ask students how this demonstration illustrates what happens when a person smokes a cigarette.

Materials Needed: water, a large glass bottle, a two-hole rubber stopper, glass delivery tubes, a cigarette holder, cigarettes, a small hand pump

Processing Questions:

1. What happens to cigarette smoke when it enters the body?
2. What are the short-term and long-term health effects of cigarette smoking?

○ **Integration:** Science

✔ **Assessment:** Students demonstrate their awareness of the harmful physical effects of smoking on the body.

Goldfish Demonstration   Grades K–5

Valued Outcome: Students will learn about the toxic qualities contained in cigarette smoke.

National Health Education Standard: 1

Description of Strategy: Check with school and state policies regarding experiments in the classroom before engaging in this demonstration. If there are no policies prohibiting the experiment, send a letter home to the parent or guardian that informs them in advance of this demonstration. Be sure to perform this experiment in a well-ventilated room.

Before you begin, explain to the class that there are hundreds of chemical substances in cigarette smoke including nicotine, cyanide, formaldehyde, lead, arsenic, and carbon monoxide, which are all poisons. Set up a smoking machine apparatus like the one shown in Figure 14.1. This time, first add two or three goldfish to the water in the bottle. Then process three or more cigarettes by using the pump. The fish will begin to lose their equilibrium as they are affected by the chemicals in the cigarette smoke. *As soon as this begins to happen,* remove the fish by pouring the water into a net. Place the fish into a bowl of clean water. *Do not pour the contaminated water into the clean water as you do this, or the fish will die from continued exposure to the contaminants.*

Materials Needed: water, a large glass bottle, a two-hole rubber stopper, glass delivery tubes, a cigarette holder, cigarettes, a small hand pump, two or three goldfish, fish net

Processing Questions:

1. What are some of the chemicals in cigarette smoke?
2. How does the body react to these chemicals when they enter the body?

◯ **Integration:** Science

✓ **Assessment:** Students demonstrate their awareness of the harmful physical effects of smoking on the body.

Breathalyzer Demonstration   Grades K–5

Valued Outcome: Students will learn the dangers of drinking and driving.

National Health Education Standard: 1

Description of Strategy: Invite a local police officer to demonstrate how a Breathalyzer works. This device is used to test the amount of alcohol in a person's bloodstream. Have the officer explain the dangers of drinking and driving. The officer should note that even a small amount of alcohol has a deleterious effect on driving ability.

Processing Questions:

1. What are the effects of alcohol on the body?
2. Why do police officers have to test drivers' blood-alcohol concentration?

✓ **Assessment:** Students can describe the effects of alcohol on body function and give reasons why alcohol should not be consumed before driving.

Saying No!   Grades 3–5

Valued Outcome: Students will recognize the power in asserting themselves when confronted with possible substance abuse.

National Health Education Standards: 4, 7

Description of Strategy: This lesson in assertiveness is accompanied by a physical demonstration of how assertiveness strengthens itself with repetition. Students are encouraged to develop an arsenal of assertive responses about why they won't indulge in a harmful substance. The more they practice their responses, the more powerful their will becomes. Sample responses might include "No! That is harmful, and I won't become involved with it." Or "I've seen (heard) what can happen by using that. It's not for me." Or "I respect my body too much to do that to it." Assertive behavior includes more than just a set of words. Encourage students to be firm and quick with their rejections of the substance. Help students realize that anyone who would tempt them to harm themselves in such a way is definitely not a friend, no matter how long the student may have known them.

To illustrate the importance of willpower, hold one dowel out in front of you with both hands (thumbs extended toward the middle of the rod). Explain to the class that the dowel represents willpower and the ability to say "No!" to using harmful substances such as cigarettes, drugs, or alcohol. Tell the students if they are tempted by someone to try such a harmful substance for the first time (slowly and firmly place pressure on the center of the dowel by pulling the ends in toward you), their will is being tested just as the strength of the dowel is being tested. Ask the students, if a person has never said "No!" to this substance before, do they think that person's will could withstand the temptation? (Allow students to offer responses. Their answers may vary.) Continue the even pressure until the dowel breaks in the middle. Explain to the students that since some people never learn to say "No!" their will could break easily the first time. Now take four dowels and stack two on top of the other two. Secure the grouping of dowels at either end with rubber bands. Hold them out in front of you as you did earlier. Explain that these four dowels represent someone who has said "No!" several times before. Ask the students if they think it will be easier or harder for their will to be broken. (Allow for student responses.) Again, with the thumbs extended toward the middle of the bundle of four dowels, attempt to pull back on the ends (holding the dowels away from students). More than likely, it will be rather difficult to break this bundle. Explain to the class that putting the four dowels together is as if someone had been able to say "No!" four times to the offer of a dangerous substance.

Materials Needed: five wooden dowels, each approximately eighteen inches long

Processing Questions:

1. What are some good responses when confronted with drugs?
2. What is likely to happen to someone who has never said no before?
3. Is it easier to say no after you have said it once before?

✓ **Assessment:** Students will be able to offer at least three assertive responses when confronted with drugs.

Impaired   Grades 4–5

Valued Outcome: Students will be able to describe how drug and alcohol use diminishes the ability to perform tasks that require manual dexterity.

National Health Education Standard: 1

Description of Strategy: Divide the class into teams of equal size (five or six students per team). Explain that each person must thread a nut all the way onto a bolt and off again; when each student has finished, he or she passes the bolt and nut to the next teammate and repeats the process until the entire team has completed the task. Time this process and record each team's time. Repeat this process with students wearing gloves or mittens and again record each team's times. Repeat the process with students wearing the sunglasses smeared with Vaseline or hand lotion and record the time again.

Materials Needed: for each team: one pair of gloves or mittens, one bolt and corresponding nut, one pair of sunglasses that have been covered with Vaseline or lotion, a stopwatch, paper

Processing Questions:

1. How is the use of the gloves and the sunglasses comparable to the way drugs and alcohol can impair you?
2. Compare the time each team took to complete the three different tasks. How can this relate to the impact of drugs and alcohol on reaction time?
3. Can you list some daily tasks (even some jobs) that would be influenced by alcohol and other drug use?

✓ **Assessment:** Students can describe how drug and alcohol use impairs manual dexterity and can give examples of how daily tasks would be negatively influenced by drug and alcohol use.

Source: Wolfanger 2001

Sobriety Testing Stations   Grades 4–5

Valued Outcome: Students will be able to identify each of the different sobriety tests and how they are used to detect the amount of alcohol consumed by a person. Students will also understand the physical effects of drinking alcohol.

National Health Education Standard: 1

Description of Strategy: Before class, set up the four stations described below. At each station, have directions written out on index cards. At the beginning of the class, show a fifteen-minute video about the consequences of DUIs (driving under the influence) and DWIs (driving while intoxicated) and the different field sobriety tests used to determine alcohol consumption. After the video, pair students up and have them visit each station and do the activities described.

- **Station 1: Breathalyzers**—The first station will have two Breathalyzers. Have students try using the Breathalyzers.
- **Station 2: Vision Impairment**—This station has two pairs of "fogged" sunglasses (use Vaseline or lotion on the lenses) to show the students how vision is affected after consuming alcohol. While wearing the sunglasses, have students walk up to the board and write down a sentence that is read to them from the index card at that station.

- **Station 3: Visual Tracking**—This station has five small pen lights. Use the lights to dilate the pupils of the eyes. Have students:

  1. Shine the light into their partner's eyes with his or her permission, and watch how the person's pupils change shape. If the person had been drinking, his or her pupils would stay dilated.
  2. Move the light around in several directions and have their partner follow it with the eyes only (not moving his or her head). If the person had been drinking, he or she would not be able to smoothly follow the path of the light or of any object.

- **Station 4: Walking a Line**—Attach a three-inch-by-ten-feet piece of tape to the floor. Have one partner put palms together and, while standing, raise the hands straight up above the head. While looking directly up, and with the help of the other partner, have the student spin around five or six times until disoriented. Immediately, have the person who was spinning try to walk in a straight line along the tape.

Then, assemble students into five groups. Have each group write down and perform a skit that relates to the things they did in the four stations or to what they learned from the stations and the fifteen-minute video. These skits will be used to check for understanding.

Materials Needed: index card of instructions for each station, two Breathalyzers, two pairs of fogged sunglasses, five small pen lights, video about consequences of DUIs and DWIs and the field sobriety tests that are used to determine how much alcohol a person has consumed, roll of wide masking tape, additional blank index cards (Note: Your local police department or sheriff's office may also lend you some Breathalyzer tests for educational purposes and may have officers who present alcohol awareness programs with additional specialized equipment.)

Processing Question: What did you learn from the stations about the physical effects of alcohol?

✓ **Assessment:** Students' skits demonstrate their understanding of how sobriety tests work and can describe the physical effects of drinking alcohol.

Smoking Aerobics   Grades 4–5

Valued Outcome: Students will be able to show how smoking tobacco affects a person's everyday physical activity.

National Health Education Standard: 1

Description of Strategy: Have each student check his or her heart rate using a stethoscope or by placing their fingers along the side of their necks. Do a ten-minute aerobic routine with the students to raise their heart rates.

After exercising, have them check their heart rate again and compare it with their first reading. Then have them do the following:

- Write any two facts you know about smoking.
- Write down your two favorite physical activities.

Now give each student a straw. While they are breathing through the straw, lead students through the same aerobic routine as before. The straws represent the restricted air passages through which a smoker breathes when doing physical activity. At the end of the exercise, have the students check their heart rates again to see if there is a difference compared to the first heart rate taken. Then have students do the following and discuss their answers as a class.

- Write two words expressing feelings you experienced when doing aerobics while breathing through the straw.
- How can smoking affect the two favorite physical activities that you wrote down?

Materials Needed: stethoscopes, straws

Processing Question: How can smoking affect your fitness?

○ **Integration:** Physical Education

✓ **Assessment:** Students can articulate how smoking has a negative effect on their ability to perform physical activities and can explain how smoking can make a person less physically fit.

Source: PE Central 2000c

How to Say No to Smoking   Grades 5–8

Valued Outcome: Students will describe the dangers of smoking and learn assertive techniques for saying no to smoking.

National Health Education Standards: 1, 4, 7

Description of Strategy: Describe assertiveness, how to say no, and nonverbal behavior that accompanies saying no assertively. Provide a sponge to represent the lung and dark poster paint to apply to a sponge to represent the effects of tar and nicotine on the lungs and have students describe what they see. Discuss how to make the decision to want to say "no" by making a list of pros and cons. After discussing how harmful smoking is and how to not give in to peer pressure, reinforce it by having the students role-play. For example, one student could be offering a friend a cigarette while another student would decide what to say to him or her.

Materials Needed: sponge, dark poster paint

Processing Questions:

1. What does cigarette smoking do to your lungs?
2. What would you say to a peer who offers you a cigarette to smoke?

✓ **Assessment:** Students can clearly demonstrate refusal skills during the role-play.

Puzzles and Games

Drugs Spell Trouble   Grades 3–5

Valued Outcome: Students will be able to match the names of drugs with clues about those drugs.

National Health Education Standard: 1

Description of Strategy: Give students Worksheet 14.1 on page 488 or create your own puzzle. Have students write the name of the drug that answers each clue given in the letter spaces provided. The completed puzzle spells out vertically a message about substance abuse.

Materials Needed: worksheets for each student, pens or pencils

Processing Question: What clues about drugs can identify those drugs?

✓ **Assessment:** Students can correctly complete the worksheet.

Smoking Crossword Puzzle   Grades 3–5

Valued Outcome: Students will be able to use their knowledge of the detrimental health effects of smoking to complete puzzles.

National Health Education Standard: 1

Description of Strategy: Provide students with a cross-word worksheet. After you have discussed smoking in class, have the students complete the puzzle.

Materials Needed: puzzle worksheet for each student, pens or pencils

Processing Question: What are the detrimental effects of smoking?

✓ **Assessment:** Students can correctly complete the worksheet.

Let's Play Tic-Tac-Toe   Grades 3–5

Valued Outcome: Students will be able to distinguish facts from misconceptions with regard to several substance abuse–related statements.

National Health Education Standard: 1

Description of Strategy: Using Worksheet 14.2 on page 489, tell the students to write "T" in the squares with true statements and write "F" in the squares with false statements. Each square corresponds with the question having the same number. How many students scored tic-tac-toe?

Materials Needed: tic-tac-toe worksheet 14.2 for each student, pens or pencils

Processing Questions:

1. Why are there so many misconceptions about substance abuse?
2. How can we reduce the number of misconceptions in the public about substance abuse?

✔ **Assessment:** Students can correctly complete the worksheet.

Safe Use of Medicines Grades 3–5

Valued Outcome: Students will learn to identify the safe use of several common over-the-counter (OTC) medicines.

National Health Education Standards: 1, 3, 7

Description of Strategy: In advance, make a transparency of the front side of a flattened box or wrapper for several OTC items for use on an overhead projector. Cut a piece of construction paper to cover the transparency. Then cut this paper into four or five interlocking shapes, creating a sort of jigsaw puzzle. Number each piece according to its difficulty, from 1 to however many total pieces are used to cover the image; the most obvious puzzle piece clues would have the higher numbers on them. Place number 1 over the directions for the medication's use. Use a little bit of tape to hold each cover piece to the transparency.

Divide the class into groups. Explain to the class that on the overhead is the image of an OTC medicine with which they may be familiar. It is presently covered by several pieces of a jigsaw puzzle. Each group in rotation will be asked a true-false question about the safe use of OTC medicine. If the group answers the question correctly, the students ask to have a specifically numbered piece of the puzzle removed. They then have ten seconds to see if they can identify the mystery medication. If no one correctly guesses the product, the puzzle piece is replaced on the overhead, and the second team is offered a true-false question with the possibility of removing a puzzle piece and correctly identifying the hidden product. When a correct identification of the hidden product is given, that team obtains a point value equal to the sum of the numbered puzzle pieces left on the transparency. If the puzzle originally had four pieces and only the number 1, number 2, and number 4 pieces were left on the transparency, that team would score 7 points. Continue the game until either all the true-false questions have been covered or all the images have been identified. The highest score wins.

Materials Needed: the outer boxes or wrappers of several well-known OTC medicines—aspirin, nasal spray, acetaminophen, eye drops, and so on; transparency sheets (one for each product); overhead projector; several sheets of construction paper (one for each product); true-false questions; clear tape

Processing Questions:

1. Can an OTC drug be bought without a doctor's prescription?
2. What should you do before taking an OTC drug?

✔ **Assessment:** Students demonstrate their understanding of the safe use of OTC drugs by answering questions correctly.

Other Ideas

My Choice, Your Choice... Consequences! Grades K–2

Valued Outcome: Students will be able to explain to a friend or peer why he or she does not use or abuse substances.

National Health Education Standards: 4, 8

Description of Strategy: Have the students make hand puppets using a sock or paper sack. Decorate faces on the puppets using markers or colored buttons. After the puppets are completed, have the students decide whether or not his or her puppet will have a positive name, such as Sober Joe, or negative name, such as Bobby Booze. Pair students up so that each pair has a positive and negative puppet. Working in pairs, have the students tell why he or she does not use or abuse substances. For example, one puppet—Bobby Booze—may tell Sober Joe how he sneaked into his dad's cabinet and had a sip of alcohol. The other puppet—Sober Joe—should tell Bobby Booze his reasons for not drinking.

Materials Needed: socks or paper bags, buttons (different colors) or other materials to use to decorate the puppets, glue, markers

Processing Questions:

1. What is your best refusal line to the peer pressure to use substances?
2. How can you be a positive influence on your friend(s), if they begin to use/abuse substances?

◯ **Integration:** Art

✔ **Assessment:** Students can articulate several reasons not to abuse drugs. Students demonstrate the ability to be a positive influence on peers.

Dealing with Peer Pressure Grades K–5

Valued Outcome: Students will be able to describe how peer pressure can be a positive and/or negative influence with regard to substance abuse.

National Health Education Standard: 2

Description of Strategy: Divide the class into groups of six to eight. Have each group form a circle and place pieces of candy in the center of each group. Give five members of each group a slip of paper stating that they are to eat the candy and attempt to get anyone not eating it to do so. Give the remaining students in each group a slip of paper stating that they should not eat the candy and should resist all attempts to get them to do so. Let this interaction go on for about five minutes. Then ask the students to take their regular seats. Ask the following questions:

What were you feeling when you were doing this exercise?

What do you think the purpose of this exercise was?

What is peer pressure?

Why is it important to know about peer pressure?

Materials Needed: written instructions for each student, pieces of candy

Processing Questions:

1. What is peer pressure?
2. How can peer pressure be a positive factor in your life?
3. How does negative peer pressure lead to substance abuse?

✓ **Assessment:** Students can define peer pressure and explain how it can be a positive or negative influence on decisions about drugs.

Affirmations
Grades K–5

Valued Outcome: Students will be able to describe how support from friends can prevent substance abuse problems.

National Health Education Standard: 2

Description of Strategy: Have each student come to the front of the class and say, "Sometimes I don't feel so good about myself." Then have the student turn his or her back to the class. Have other students then volunteer to affirm one fine quality about that individual. Every student should get three affirmations from the class. These may refer to being a loyal friend, being kind, being a good student, being fair, being friendly, and so on.

Materials Needed: none

Processing Questions:

1. How can young people offer moral support to their friends through praise?
2. How can such praise prevent substance abuse problems?

✓ **Assessment:** Students can list three ways in which support from friends can prevent substance abuse problems.

Informational Interviews and Presentations
Grades 3-5

Valued Outcome: The students will be able to make and deliver to their classmates an audio/video documentary of an interview.

National Health Education Standard: 3

Description of Strategy: Divide the students into groups of four or five. Each group should either choose or be assigned a topic or person to interview who may have some relation to the topic of drug use. Interviewee ideas could include a school liaison drug officer, a pharmacist, someone who has quite smoking, an older student who has refused to use drugs or alcohol, or another related topic/person. Give students guidelines on the focus of the interviews; specifically, they might ask their opinions about drug use and abuse, the difference between legal and illegal drug use, difficulties faced by people who are trying to quite smoking, or strategies they used to overcome peer pressure. The students should formulate their own questions in preparation for the interviews, guided by your topic suggestions. Each group will need to have access to and learn how to use a video camera and a computer-related recording program. During the next few days in class, the groups will edit their video, and then the groups will deliver their interview presentation to the class.

Materials Needed: video camera (for each group or shared among the class), access to a computer with a recording program (e.g., Garage Band or GoldWave)

Processing Questions:

1. How can technology be used to deliver health education messages to students?
2. How does talking to a person with experience in a topic help inform views and aid in making smart decisions?

○ **Integration:** Social Studies

✓ **Assessment:** The students will be evaluated on each phase of the interview: 1) questions asked; 2) editing the footage; and 3) presentation of the documentary to the class.

Slogans
Grades 3–5

Valued Outcome: Students will be able to develop a list of slogans against drug use.

National Health Education Standards: 2, 4, 8

Description of Strategy: Have the students develop a list of slogans used by tobacco, alcohol, and OTC drug manufacturers. Discuss what the slogans are attempting to convince the consumer to do. Discuss the irrational appeal often used in this advertising approach. Then have

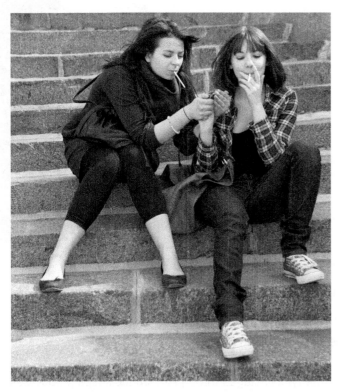

Peer pressure can be a positive or negative influence in a person's life.

the students come up with counterslogans that seek to convince the consumer to do the opposite.

Processing Question: How can anti-drug messages convince the public not to abuse drugs?

✓ **Assessment:** Students demonstrate the ability to recognize marketing tactics used by alcohol, tobacco, and drug companies and generate anti-drug slogans that demonstrate their ability to advocate for healthy behavior and choices.

Drug Collage   Grades 3–5

Valued Outcome: Students will be able to describe the harmful effects of tobacco use.

National Health Education Standard: 1

Description of Strategy: Have the students create a collage showing in detail the effects of tobacco use, and state reasons that they believe people start using tobacco. They can find information by searching magazines they have brought to class and finding tobacco ads. They can also use articles from the newspaper about drug-related incidents that have happened recently that they can cut out and paste to the backboard for their collage.

Materials Needed: magazine advertisements, newspapers that have a youth editorial section, paper, markers, glue

Processing Question: What are some harmful effects that tobacco products bring to a person's health and overall lifestyle?

Integration: Art

✓ **Assessment:** Students demonstrate their understanding of the negative effects of tobacco.

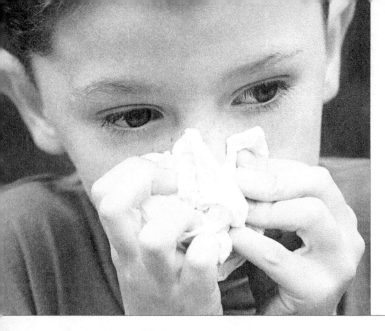

Infectious and Noninfectious Conditions

You can do more for your own health and well-being than any doctor, or any exotic medical service.

—Joseph Califano, former Secretary of Health, Education, and Welfare

Valued Outcomes

After completion of this chapter, you should be able to:

- Describe the disease agents for infectious and noninfectious conditions.
- Describe the typical stages through which a disease progresses.
- Describe how the body is protected from disease.
- Discuss the major childhood communicable diseases.
- Discuss the human immunodeficiency virus.
- Discuss cardiovascular disease and several types of cancer.
- Identify the risk factors associated with the major noninfectious diseases.
- Discuss the recent trends in the diagnosis and treatment of diseases.

Reflections

Helping children understand how diseases are prevented is important to their long-term quality of life. Check your state's requirements for vaccinations and immunizations. Are there risks associated with any of the suggested or required vaccinations? What are your feelings concerning the potential risks?

NATIONAL HEALTH EDUCATION STANDARDS

1. Students will comprehend concepts related to health promotion and disease prevention to enhance health.

3. Students will demonstrate the ability to access valid information and products and services to enhance health.

7. Students will demonstrate the ability to practice health-enhancing behaviors and avoid or reduce risks.

Diseases—Then and Now

Many conditions affect the quality of life. Over the past centuries, the types of diseases that have killed and debilitated humans have changed. At one time infectious diseases were the biggest killers, but now chronic diseases are the leading causes of death. Some say that the infectious diseases may again become our biggest enemy, especially in the form of the acquired immunodeficiency syndrome (AIDS) epidemic, which is caused by the human immunodeficiency virus (HIV).

Communicable Diseases

At various times throughout history, communicable diseases such as the bubonic plague, smallpox, syphilis, and polio have been common throughout the world. Occasionally a disease such as Legionnaires' disease also causes an epidemic. Currently the HIV/AIDS epidemic threatens the welfare of people here and throughout the world. The common cold, influenza, and the persistence of the many childhood diseases also are constant problems (see Table 15.1).

The Stages of Diseases

When a pathogen invades a human host, the body's reaction to the invasion proceeds through several broad phases—incubation, prodromal, clinical, convalescence, and recovery. Figure 15.1 illustrates these typical stages.

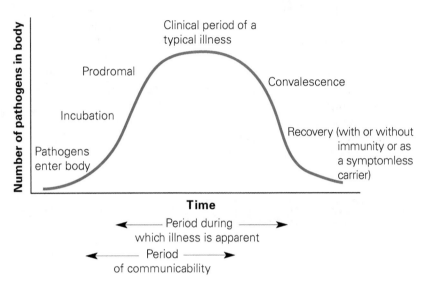

Figure 15.1
Typical Periods of Illness

Table 15.1	**The Pathogens**	
Type	**Characteristics**	**Examples of Disease Caused**
Viruses	The smallest pathogens. Composed of nucleic acid and protein. Made up of DNA or RNA but not both. Known as obligate intracellular parasites because they must live in living host. Penetrate cells and use cells' nucleic acids to replicate viruses. May burst out of cell, destroying it, or the cell degenerates and viruses are released as cell dies.	Warts; hepatitis A, B, C, D, E; measles; polio; mumps; oral and genital herpes
Bacteria	Single-celled microorganisms. Abundant in our environment, but very few are pathogenic to humans. Three common forms: rod shaped or bacilli, round or cocci, and spiral or spirilla. Cause harm by releasing toxins (poisons) and need not invade cells to cause disease.	Tuberculosis, strep throat, tetanus, gonorrhea, Legionnaires' disease
Rickettsias	A genus of small bacteria. Resemble both viruses and bacteria. Like viruses, they are intracellular parasites. Transported by insects and other arthropod vectors.	Rocky Mountain spotted fever, typhus, Q fever
Fungi	Single-celled or multicelled plantlike organisms. Release enzymes that digest cells. Seek a favorable climate for reproduction on food or anywhere there is high humidity, warmth, and oxygen supply.	Candidiasis, ringworm
Protozoa	Single-celled microscopic parasitic animals. Release toxin and enzymes that destroy cells or interfere with their functions.	Trichomoniasis, malaria, amoebic dysentery, African sleeping sickness
Helminths	Multicellular parasitic animals. Vary in size from relatively small (pinworms) to a length of several feet. May lodge in various parts of the body and block the digestive tract, blood, and lymph vessels.	Pinworms, tapeworms, trichinosis

The incubation stage is the time between initial infection and the appearance of symptoms. The incubation period can be as short as a few hours (for the common cold) or as long as a few years (as in the case of HIV). The prodromal stage is the short period in which the body begins to react to the pathogens. Fever, headache, nasal discharge, and irritability are common but the actual characteristics of the disease are not yet apparent, and diagnosis may be difficult. The disease is usually highly communicable during this period. The clinical stage is the time when the disease is at its worst. The characteristics of the disease are readily identified. The convalescence stage is the period in which the host feels better but may or may not feel like returning to normal activities. The recovery stage is the time in which recovery seems complete. However, the disease may still be communicable. The host may relapse, recover with immunity to the disease, recover but not have immunity, or recover from the disease but be a source (carrier) for the disease.

Protection against Diseases

For an infectious disease to invade a human host, some change must take place in either the host or the environment. The mere presence of a pathogen does not necessarily lead to infection; the host must be susceptible to the disease. Factors such as age, sex, stress level, nutrition, and genetic makeup influence susceptibility. For a pathogen to gain entry to a human host, it must overcome several effective barriers. These barriers are summarized in Table 15.2.

▪ The Immune System

If the defenses listed in Table 15.2 do not prevent development of a disease, the host body turns to another powerful line of defense. **Immunity** is the state of being protected against diseases or through the activities of the immune system. When the host is invaded by a pathogen, the immune system swings into action to destroy the infectious agent. Anything that invades the body and causes the immune system to react is called an **antigen** (foreign body). The body develops **antibodies** that destroy or lessen the effects of the invading antigen. Each type of antibody is specific for each type of antigen. For example, antibodies for measles have no effect on the common cold antigens.

The immune system works in several ways to protect against diseases and infections. The first is through **phagocytosis,** which is the ingestion and destruction of pathogens by several different types of white blood cells (Thibodeau and Patton 1993). **Humoral immunity** is the protection provided by antibodies derived from B cells. In **cellular immunity** T cells are activated and attack microbes or abnormal cells such as viral or tumor cells. Figure 15.2 illustrates these three mechanisms.

Table 15.2	The Body's Defenses against Disease
Barrier	**Defense against Pathogens: Viruses, Bacteria, Fungi, Protozoa, Rickettsias, Helminths**
Skin	Skin must break for invader to penetrate
Body Secretions	Sweat and oil glands kill or repel invaders
	Secretions at body entrances such as earwax, tears, and nasal secretions contain enzymes that destroy invaders
Mucous	Trap and engulf invaders
Membranes	Cilia function to sweep invaders toward body openings
	Contain enzymes that destroy or slow pathogen reproduction
Enzymes and Compounds in Blood	Kill invader by causing it to burst, destroying its cell membrane, preventing/slowing reproductive cycle
Immune System	Antigen/antibody response
	White blood cell action
	Attempts to reject unrecognized enemies or develop antibodies against them
Interferon and Natural Substances	When virus invades, protein is produced that protects healthy cells making subsequent infections difficult *Properdin:* large protein that destroys gram-negative bacteria *Polypeptides:* same action as properdin *Lysozyme:* enzyme that kills bacteria; found in saliva, tears, and breast milk

Lymphocytes are the type of white blood cells most responsible for the preceding actions. Two forms of lymphocytes are **T cells** and **B cells.** T cells circulate through lymphatic tissue and the bloodstream, neutralizing antigens. **T helpers** or **T suppressor cells,** respectively, increase or release the response of other lymphocytes. When stimulated by an antigen, B cells produce antibodies that destroy the antigens.

Immunity can be developed through having a disease (**natural immunity**) or through **artificial immunity.** Artificial immunity is acquired by vaccination when killed or attenuated (weakened) organisms or **toxins** (poisons) are injected into the body to stimulate antibody formation. Antibodies for a particular antigen can be injected that will provide short-term protection against a disease. (More information on diseases and recommended immunizations is provided in the Health Highlight on pages 262–263.)

ACTION OF PHAGOCYTES

These white blood cells are attracted to infection sites, where they engulf and digest microorganisms and debris.

Adherence

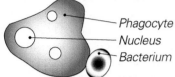

— *Phagocyte*
— *Nucleus*
— *Bacterium*

1 The phagocyte must first contact and recognize a microbe as foreign. This process is assisted by chemicals released during inflammation.

Ingestion

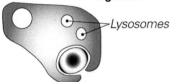

— *Lysosomes*

2 The phagocyte engulfs the microbe in a pouch formed in its membrane. Fluid-filled particles called lysosomes move toward the microbe.

Digestion

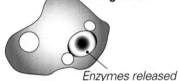

Enzymes released

3 Enzymes within the lysosomes are released into the pouch to help digest the microbe.

HUMORAL IMMUNITY

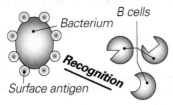

Bacterium   *B cells*
Recognition
Surface antigen

1 A humoral response is started when an antigen (foreign protein)—here on the surface of a bacterium—activates one type of B cell.

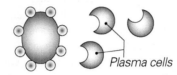

Plasma cells

2 The particular type of B cell multiplies, forming cells called plasma cells, which make antibodies designed specifically to attack the bacterium.

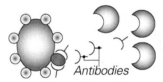

Antibodies

3 After a few days, the antibodies are released and travel to and attach to the antigen. This triggers more reactions, which ultimately destroy the bacterium.

Second exposure

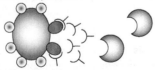

4 Some B cells remain in the body as memory cells; if the bacteria enters the body again, they rapidly produce antibodies to halt the infection.

CELLULAR IMMUNITY

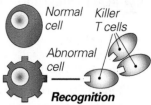

Normal cell   *Killer T cells*
Abnormal cell
Recognition

1 An antigen, here on the surface of an abnormal cell (such as a virus-infected or tumor cell) is identified by, and activates, specific killer (cytotoxic) T cells.

Helper T cell
Killer T cell

2 With the assistance of helper T cells (another type of T cell), the killer T cells begin to multiply.

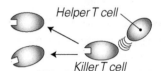

A   *B*

3 The killer T cells travel to, and attach to, the abnormal cells (A), leading to their destruction (B). The T cells survive and may go on to kill more targets.

Second exposure

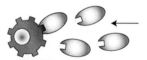

4 Some of the killer T cells remain as memory cells and quickly attack abnormal cells should they reappear (for example, after reinfection with a virus).

Figure 15.2
Actions and Responses of the Immune System

Selected Infectious Diseases

Common childhood diseases include the common cold, chicken pox, rubella (German measles), influenza, rubeola (measles), strep throat, meningitis, tuberculosis, mumps, and pertussis (whooping cough). Of these, the diseases most commonly found in schools are the common cold, influenza, strep throat, and the childhood diseases of chicken pox, mumps, and rubella. To a lesser extent, diseases such as infectious mononucleosis, hepatitis, and human immunodeficiency virus (HIV) are now affecting the classroom. In schools, childhood diseases constitute the greatest problem. Students face days of restricted activity and school absenteeism because of these diseases.

▪ The Common Cold

The cold is the most common of all infectious diseases found in schools. A cold alone is not considered serious, but secondary infections resulting from improper care can be a problem. There are more than 200 different

HEALTH HIGHLIGHT | **Overview of Diseases and Recommended Childhood Immunizations**

Diseases that are generally preventable by following appropriate vaccination schedules (CDC 2011):

Diphtheria: Bacterial disease passed by direct contact with respiratory droplets. Bacteria produce a toxin that can cause weakness, sore throat, low-grade fever, swollen glands in the neck, swelling of the heart muscle, heart failure, coma, paralysis, and death.

Hepatitis A: An infection in the liver caused by a virus spread primarily by the fecal-oral route. Symptoms include fever, tiredness, loss of appetite, nausea, abdominal discomfort, dark urine, and jaundice. Death can result.

Hepatitis B: An infection of the liver caused by a virus spread through contact with blood or other body fluids. Causes a flu-like illness with loss of appetite, nausea, vomiting, rashes, joint pain, and jaundice; infection can result in severe liver diseases, including cancer.

Human Papillomavirus (HPV): A virus most common in people in their teens and early twenties; the major cause of cervical cancer in women and genital warts.

Influenza: A highly contagious viral infection of the nose, throat, and lungs spread through respiratory droplets. Can cause sudden high fever, chills, dry cough, headache, runny nose, sore throat, muscle and joint pain, and extreme fatigue; may lead to hospitalization or death.

Measles: Highly contagious viral disease spread through respiratory droplets. Symptoms usually include a rash, fever, cough, and watery eyes; can also cause pneumonia, seizures, brain damage, or death.

Meningococcal Disease: Caused by bacteria spread through the exchange of nose and throat droplets; a leading cause of bacterial meningitis in children. Symptoms include nausea, vomiting, sensitivity to light, confusion and sleepiness, blood infections, and death. Survivors may lose their arms or legs, become deaf, have nervous system problems, become developmentally disabled, or suffer seizures or strokes.

Mumps: Infectious disease caused by a virus spread in the air by respiratory droplets or through contact with a contaminated object. The virus causes fever, headaches, painful swelling of the salivary glands under the jaw, fever, muscle aches, tiredness, and loss of appetite. Complications can include meningitis, encephalitis, permanent hearing loss, or swelling of the testes, which can lead to sterility in men.

Pertussis (Whooping Cough): Caused by bacteria spread through contact with respiratory droplets. Symptoms include runny nose, sneezing, low-grade fever, and cough; can cause spells of violent coughing and choking. Infected babies can get pneumonia, have seizures, become brain damaged, or die.

Pneumococcal Disease: An infection of the lungs caused by a bacteria spread through contact with respiratory droplets. Sinus and ear infections can result; severe cases can be fatal or result in long-term problems (brain damage, hearing loss and limb loss).

Polio: Caused by a virus spread through contact with the feces of an infected person and through respiratory droplets. Symptoms sudden fever, sore throat, headache, muscle weakness, and pain; infection can result in paralysis and death.

Rubella (German Measles): Caused by a virus spread through coughing and sneezing. Causes a mild illness with fever, swollen glands, and a rash; complications can be very serious in pregnant women.

Tetanus (Lockjaw): Caused by bacteria found in soil that enters the body through a wound. Bacteria produce a toxin that causes spasms and stiffness of all muscles in the body; can lead to "locking" of the jaw (preventing opening of the mouth, swallowing, breathing); death can result.

Varicella (Chickenpox): Very contagious disease caused by the varicella zoster virus spread from a cough, sneeze, or contact with virus particles

---

viruses or rhinoviruses that can cause the common cold. Symptoms usually develop within twenty-four hours after exposure and include teary eyes, obstructed breathing, and a runny nose. When a fever is present, it indicates a secondary infection. Once a cold develops, it typically will run its course in seven to fourteen days.

There is no cure for a cold; antibiotics are of no benefit. Once a cold has developed, bed rest, good nutrition, and plenty of fluids are the best treatment. Over-the-counter cold remedies may help treat the symptoms of the cold but cannot treat the virus itself. A cold is most contagious in the first twenty-four hours.

Aspirin should not be given to children because of the possibility of Reye's syndrome.

▪ Strep Throat

Strep throat is commonly found in the school setting. The causative agent is the streptococcal bacterium. The infection is passed primarily through sneezing, coughing, or the use of soiled objects, such as handkerchiefs, that reach the mouth. Incubation time for strep throat is three to five days. Symptoms may include sore throat, fever, nausea, and vomiting. In some cases, people may develop a rash on the

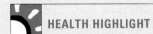

HEALTH HIGHLIGHT (*continued*)

from blisters on the skin. Symptoms include itchy rash with blisters, tiredness, headache, fever; can lead to severe skin infections, pneumonia, and encephalitis.

Recommended immunization schedule for persons aged zero through eighteen years (United States)

The following schedule indicates the recommended ages for routine administration of currently licensed childhood vaccines as of 2011 for children through age eighteen. Any dose not given at the recommended age should be given when indicated and feasible.

Age ▶ Vaccine ▼	Birth	1 month	2 months	4 months	6 months	12 months	15 months	18 months	19–23 months	2–3 years	4–6 years	7–10 years	11–12 years	13–18 years
Hepatitis B	HepB	HepB				HepB							Hep B Series	
Rotavirus			RV	RV	RV[2]									
Diphtheria, Tetanus, Pertussis			DTaP	DTaP	DTaP		DTaP				DTaP		Tdap	Tdap
Haemophilus influenzae type b			Hib	Hib	Hib[4]	Hib								
Pneumococcal			PCV	PCV	PCV	PCV				PPSV		Pneumococcal		
Inactivated Poliovirus			IPV	IPV		IPV					IPV	IPV Series		
Influenza					Influenza (Yearly)									
Measles, Mumps, Rubella						MMR					MMR	MMR Series		
Varicella						Varicella					Varicella	Varicella Series		
Hepatitis A						HepA (2 doses)			HepA Series					
Meningococcal										MCV4		MCV4	MCV4	
Human Papillomavirus													HPV (3 doses) (females)	HPV Series

KEY:

▮ Range of recommended ages for all children

▮ Range of recommended ages for certain high-risk groups

▮ Range of recommended ages for catch-up immunization

Source: Center for Disease Control and Prevention (CDC). Recommended immunization schedule for 2011. (Additional information available at www.cdc.gov/vaccines/recs/schedules/child-schedule.htm)

neck and chest area. Strep throat is treated with antibiotics. Students should be excluded from school until the fever and sore throat are gone for twenty-four to forty-eight hours.

▪ Influenza

Influenza, or flu, is a commonly experienced virus. Three forms of the virus are currently isolated, with a multitude of strains within each variety. Forms of the virus include types A (the most pathenogenic), B, and C. Short-term immunity may be acquired from any particular form, but this does not transfer to a different variety. Today,

fortunately, the flu is not extremely hazardous to normally healthy people. However, deaths can occur in adults over sixty-five, children under five, and people who have chronic diseases.

The symptoms of influenza include aches and pains, nausea, diarrhea, fever, and coldlike ailments. The best treatment for flu is bed rest, ingesting plenty of fluids, eating nutritious foods, and taking medicine, if prescribed. Although obvious symptoms last only a few days, a feeling of weakness may persist for some time, so extra rest may be needed. It is important to take extra care following the flu, so that complications do not develop.

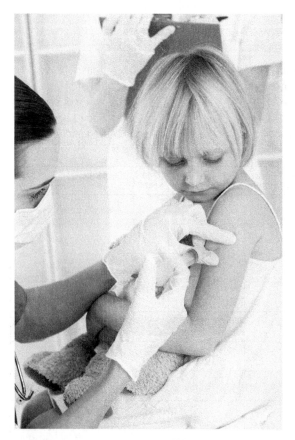

Artificial immunity is acquired by vaccination.

Because influenza is caused by a virus, Reye's syndrome can develop as a secondary disease. Children should not be given aspirin to relieve discomfort as it may contribute to the development of Reye's syndrome. This syndrome can involve the pancreas, heart, kidneys, spleen, and lymph nodes. Symptoms may include an upper respiratory infection, nausea, vomiting, disorientation, coma, and seizures. Although rare, this is a serious and often life-threatening disorder.

Infectious Mononucleosis

Infectious mononucleosis is initiated by the Epstein-Barr virus and is transmitted through saliva, hence its more common name, the kissing disease. In reality, mononucleosis does not seem to be highly contagious. Initial symptoms may include moderate fever, discomfort, lack of appetite, fatigue, headache, and sore throat. Lymph nodes usually become enlarged, as does the spleen about one-third of the time. Occasionally mild liver damage may occur, leading to jaundice for a few days. Diagnosis is made using a blood test. A positive test indicates extremely high levels of mononucleocytes, a type of white blood cell. Treatment consists of possibly prolonged bed rest, sound nutrition, and medicine for secondary problems, as indicated. For two to three months after recovery, the person may feel depressed, lack energy, and feel sleepy during the day. Symptoms may exist up to a year after infection.

Hepatitis

Five types of hepatitis have been isolated: hepatitis A, B, C, D, and E. Hepatitis A is often the result of poor sanitary conditions and is a common infection in the United States, with almost half the adult population carrying antibodies against the virus. Hepatitis A vaccine (Harvix) is highly effective in preventing the illness. If a susceptible person is exposed to hepatitis A, gamma globulin administered within ten days provides protection. Hepatitis A is transmitted through person-to-person, fecal-oral contact, sexual contact with infected persons, and contaminated blood (rare). Persons traveling internationally should receive the hepatitis A vaccine (CDC 2011).

Hepatitis B is currently transmitted primarily by drug addicts sharing contaminated needles and through body secretions such as sweat, breast milk, and semen. Hepatitis B is more serious than hepatitis A, with a higher potential for liver damage. Since 1982, there has been a vaccine that will prevent hepatitis B. The vaccination consists of three injections spaced over a period of several months. Routine vaccination is recommended for anyone under eighteen years of age.

Hepatitis C is caused by the hepatitis C virus, which is found in the blood of an infected person, and the infection is spread by contact with that blood. The sharing of items such as toothbrushes, razors, personal care items, or intravenous syringes can spread this virus. The disease is rarely spread through sexual contact. Further protection consists of getting the A and B vaccinations, not getting a tattoo or body piercing, not having sex with more than one partner, and using latex condoms when having sex (CDC 2011).

Hepatitis D can only be contracted by a person suffering from hepatitis B. The C virus seems to intersect with hepatitis B to create a chronic and more severe form of the disease. Hepatitis D is spread in the same fashion as hepatitis B.

Hepatitis E is similar to hepatitis A but is acute rather than chronic in nature. This type of hepatitis is rare in the United States but has caused large outbreaks in other parts of the world. Direct or indirect contact with an infected person's feces, contamination of food or water supply, raw shellfish, unwashed hands, and cooking utensils may have enough of the virus to cause an outbreak.

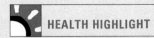

The Occupational Safety and Health Administration (OSHA) has issued regulations concerning job exposure to bloodborne pathogens. Teachers and other school personnel must be aware of the hazards and protect themselves from harm when there is potential contact with body fluids from a child infected with HIV or hepatitis. Obviously the consideration is for more than just casual contact. The beginning point for a teacher's personal safety is to make sure all immunizations are up to date. OSHA standards require that an employer make the hepatitis B vaccination series available to all employees who are exposed to blood or other body fluids on the job. OSHA also requires postexposure evaluation and follow-up to all employees who are exposed.

The Centers for Disease Control and Prevention (CDC) has identified universal precautions for protection or preventing the risk of exposure from any type of bodily substance. These precautions include personal hygiene (washing hands, face, etc.) after potential exposure, wearing personal protective equipment (having a face mask, apron, and rubber gloves), having work practice controls for protocol and procedures for disposing of potentially contaminated materials, and procedures/protocol for cleaning and disinfecting areas of contamination.

It is imperative that every school district have guidelines and protocol for dealing with bloodborne and fluidborne pathogens. The school should provide every teacher with a kit containing the above-listed items. Training should be provided each year on the guidelines/protocol for dealing with blood/fluids in the school setting.

▪ Human Immunodeficiency Virus and Acquired Immunodeficiency Syndrome

HIV can lead to a complex array of diseases resulting in AIDS. The CDC lists a variety of clinical conditions to be used in diagnosing AIDS, along with an HIV-positive seroconversion and a T cell count below 200 (NIAID 2011).

Some of the conditions used in diagnosing AIDS include the following:

Opportunistic Infections (infections that take advantage of a weakened immune system)

- *Pneumocystis carinii* pneumonia (PCP)—a type of lung disease caused by a protozoan fungus, which is usually not harmful to humans
- Tuberculosis—either *Mycobacterium avium-intracellulare* complex (MAI) or *Mycobacterium tuberculosis* (TB); MAI is most common among AIDS patients
- Bacterial pneumonia—caused by several common bacteria
- Toxoplasmosis—disease of the brain and central nervous system

Cancers

- Kaposi's sarcoma—a cancer causing red or purple blotches on the skin
- Lymphomas—cancers of the lymphatic system
- Invasive cervical cancer—more common in women who are HIV-positive

Other Conditions

- Wasting syndrome—involves persistent diarrhea, severe weight loss, and weakness

- AIDS dementia—impairment of mental functions, mood changes, impaired movement as a result of HIV infection of the brain

Other Infections

- Candidiasis (also called *thrush*)—a fungal infection that affects the vagina, mouth, throat, and lungs
- Herpes—a common viral sexually transmitted infection (STI)
- Cytomegalovirus—a virus that, in AIDS patients, can lead to brain infection, infection of the retina, pneumonia, or hepatitis

HIV/AIDS remains a devastating disease. It took eight and one-half years for the first 100,000 cases of HIV/AIDS to be reported. In only two and one-half years, the second 100,000 cases were reported. Since HIV/AIDS was discovered in 1981 in the United States, 617,025 people have died. In 1993, HIV/AIDS became the leading cause of death for Americans between the ages of twenty-five and forty-four. Currently in the United States there are more than one million persons living with HIV/AIDS, and an estimated 42,439 new HIV infections were diagnosed in 2008 (MMWR 2008). The best protection young people have against HIV/AIDS is education and practicing safe sex if they become sexually active. The Health Highlight box "Preventing the Spread of HIV/AIDS and Sources of Information" provides information on preventing the spread of HIV/AIDS and lists sources of information on the nature of HIV treatment and prevention.

Individuals who are infected with HIV may experience a variety of symptoms or may appear to be quite healthy. However, even people with no obvious symptoms can transmit HIV to others. The indicators of possible HIV infection include persistent diarrhea, dry cough, shortness of

HEALTH HIGHLIGHT | **Preventing the Spread of HIV/AIDS and Sources of Information**

Recommendations to reduce the possibility of becoming infected:

- Practice abstinence or mutual monogamy.
- Always use protection (that is, latex condoms and spermicide, such as nonoxynol-9) if having sex with multiple partners or with persons who have multiple partners.
- Do not have unprotected sex with individuals who have HIV/AIDS, those who engage in high-risk behavior, or those who have had a positive test for the AIDS virus.

- Avoid sexual activities that might cut or tear the rectum, vagina, or penis, such as anal intercourse.
- Do not have sex with prostitutes.
- Do not use IV drugs or share needles. Refrain from having sex with IV drug users.

Information on AIDS and HIV

AIDSinfo (800) 448-0440
www.aidsinfo.nih.gov
Information on HIV and AIDS from the National Institutes of Health.

CDC National Prevention Information Network (800) 458-5231
http://cdcnpin.org
Information on education services. Copies of Public Health Service publications available.

CDC-INFO (800) 232-4636
www.cdc.gov/cdc-info
Twenty-four-hour hotline that provides information and referrals for HIV and AIDS.

Local health departments also have valuable information concerning HIV and AIDS.

Source: CDC 2011

---

breath, fatigue, skin rash, swollen lymph glands (neck, armpits, groin), candidiasis, unexplained fever or chills, night sweats (over several weeks), and unexplained weight loss of 10 percent of body weight in less than two months. Women may also experience abnormal Pap smears, persistent vaginal candidiasis (a yeastlike fungal infection characterized by an itchy white discharge), and abdominal cramping as a result of pelvic inflammatory disease (PID). These infections are a result of HIV infection and are caused by immunodeficiency, but they are not yet considered AIDS.

It was previously thought that HIV did little in the body immediately after infection and simply stayed within a few immune system T cells for seven to ten years. It is now known that the real battle starts immediately within the lymph nodes, where day after day, year after year, the body is in mortal combat with the virus before finally exhausting its immune response reserves (Cray and Park 1996, 64).

HIV-1 is the HIV subtype found in the vast majority of infected individuals in the United States. Two tests are currently being used to detect HIV. The enzyme-linked immunoabsorbent assays (ELISA) test is the antibody test initially used. If the ELISA results indicate that the patient has HIV, another test—the Western blot—is administered for confirmation. Since the ELISA is an antibodies test and it may take from two to thirty-six months for antibodies to develop, there is a possibility of a false negative test for HIV antibodies. Usually the Western blot, a more precise antibodies test, shows clearly either HIV-positive or -negative. If there is an inconclusive Western blot test, a person should be retested in six months. Anyone who tests positive for HIV can transmit the virus. Enzyme immunoassays are used to detect the presence of HIV-1 in clinical samples. ELISA tests are used as the primary screening test for HIV-1 infection, and the Western blot tests are used to double-check and confirm positive ELISA results.

Both these variations of agglutination tests use antigen-specific antibodies labeled with specific enzymes to detect the presence of HIV-1 antigens. Additional tests using other techniques may also be performed to detect the presence of HIV and to monitor the status of an HIV-infected patient (Brooks, Butel, and Morse 2001). In addition to the above-mentioned tests, several tests are available that can be used for home or point of service testing, but these tests have not yet been approved by the FDA.

Routes of Transmission. HIV is transmitted primarily through sexual contact. Secondary transmission occurs among intravenous drug users. Screening techniques have reduced the chances of receiving HIV in blood transfusions to approximately one in one million. The heterosexual transmission of HIV has become a significant problem. The CDC has reported that heterosexual transmission makes up 25 percent of new infections. Among females, 80 percent of new infections result from heterosexual contact. Among men, sexual contact between men accounts for the largest percentage of new infections (65 percent). Intravenous drug users and sharing of needles account for 14 percent of new infections in men and 20 percent of new infections in women (CDC 2008). In fact, the potential for an AIDS epidemic through heterosexual transmission of HIV is staggering. Estimates are that one million Americans are already infected with HIV. Considering that the incubation period can be as long as ten years and that the HIV-infected person is unaware of the disease, transmission has the potential to grow exponentially.

In 1986, a second type of HIV virus, HIV-2, was discovered. Studies of HIV-2 are rather limited; while there seem to be many similarities to HIV-1, differences are noted. Both types of HIV have similar means of transmission, and both lead to the opportunistic infections listed

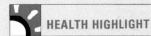

Since most students in this age group are not sexually active or trying drugs, you may decide that the young people you speak with do not need to know the details of how HIV is transmitted through unprotected sexual intercourse and injecting drug use. However, if you think they may be considering or may be doing things that put them at risk of infection, you will need to be sure they know the risk regardless of their age.

Students this age probably have heard about HIV/AIDS and may be scared by it. Much of what they have heard may have been incorrect. To reassure them, make sure they know that they cannot become infected through everyday contact, such as going to school with someone who is infected with HIV.

Students also may have heard myths and prejudicial comments about HIV infection and AIDS. Correct any notions that people can be infected by touching a doorknob or being bitten by a mosquito. Urge students to treat people who are infected with HIV or who have AIDS with compassion and understanding, not cruelty and anger. Correcting myths and prejudices early will help students protect themselves and others from HIV infection and AIDS in the future.

Consider including the following points in a conversation about HIV infection and AIDS with students in the late elementary and middle school levels:

- AIDS is a disease caused by a tiny germ called a virus.
- Many different types of people have HIV/AIDS today—male and female, rich and poor, Caucasian, African American, Hispanic, Asian, and Native American.
- Because a person can be infected with HIV for as long as ten or more years before the signs of AIDS appear, a significant number of young people may have been infected when they were teenagers.
- Correct the many myths concerning AIDS.
- You can become infected with HIV either by having unprotected sexual intercourse with an infected person or by sharing drug needles or syringes with an infected person. Also, women infected with HIV can pass the virus to their babies during pregnancy or during birth. If not treated during pregnancy, there is increased likelihood that the disease will be passed to the baby.
- A person who is infected can infect others in the ways described, even if no symptoms are present. You cannot tell by looking at someone whether he or she is infected.
- People who have HIV/AIDS should be treated with compassion.

Source: CDC 1999

on pages 268–269. However, persons infected with HIV-2 are less infectious early in the course of infection. Most cases of HIV in the United States are HIV-1, whereas HIV-2 is more predominant in West Africa (CDC 2008).

HIV infection is not contracted through contact with food, eating utensils, clothing, furniture, swimming pools, or insects. Such contact as shaking hands, coughing, sneezing, or even living with an HIV-positive person will not result in disease transmission. HIV has been found in tears, saliva, and urine, but transmission through contact with these substances has not been found to be directly implicated (Peterman 1986).

Treatment. At present, no cure is available for HIV/AIDS, and the disease must still be considered fatal. The recommended treatment for HIV is a combination of three or more medications in a regimen called Antiretroviral Therapy (ART). Each ART regimen is tailored to the individual patient. How many drugs and how often the drugs are to be taken are determined by a physician. This combination of drugs is very effective in reducing viral load in an HIV positive person. However, this mode of treatment is not without serious side effects, including diabetes, abnormally high cholesterol and triglyceride levels, shrinking limbs, and bizarre appearance of fat deposits on different parts of the body (United States Department of Health and Human Services 2011).

Today, people infected with HIV have longer and healthier lives, mainly because there are many effective medicines to fight the infection. Most medicines fall into one of the following three categories:

- Reverse transcriptase (RT) inhibitors interfere with a critical step during the HIV life cycle and keep the virus from reproducing.
- Protease inhibitors interfere with a protein that HIV uses to produce infectious viral particles.
- Fusion inhibitors block the virus from entering the body's cells.

While these medicines help people with HIV, they are not perfect. They do not cure HIV/AIDS. People with HIV infection still have the virus in their bodies; even when they are taking medicines, they can transmit HIV to others through unprotected sex and needle sharing (National Institute of Allergy and Infectious Diseases [NIAID] 2011).

Chronic and Noninfectious Diseases

Americans are commonly afflicted by chronic and noninfectious diseases. Diseases of this type are not "caught" but are developed over time, often are progressive in effect, and may be due to genetic predisposition. Under

HEALTH HIGHLIGHT | **Support for Children Who Have HIV Infection in School: Best Practices Guidelines**

I. Preparation of the School Setting

1. An **advisory committee on HIV-related issues** shall be established for the school district and commissioned by the superintendent. Membership shall be composed of health professionals (community physicians, school nurses, and other child and adolescent health workers), parents, teachers, students, persons with HIV infection, attorneys, advocates, and persons representing diversity in the community. At regular meetings, matters shall be discussed concerning HIV that relate to administrative practices, legal and policy questions, educational programs, universal infection control standards, and student welfare. Consultants shall be used as appropriate.

2. The school district shall adopt **policy statements of relevance to students with HIV infection** in collaboration with the advisory committee. These shall conform with state and federal laws and regulations, and draw on state-of-the-art medical and scientific information from appropriate government sources, documents from national organizations, research studies, and expert consultation. It may be helpful to use public hearings to gain input into these matters. The policy statements shall then be disseminated to all administrative levels; made available to staff, students, parents, and community leaders; and included in student and parent handbooks. They shall be reviewed at yearly intervals.

3. **Staff education and in-service training** concerning the issues of HIV infection, including transmission, prevention, civil rights, mental health, and death and bereavement, shall be carried out at least annually for all school personnel, including the school board. The program content shall be determined by a multidisciplinary team of appropriate individuals that shall include families of children with HIV infection and also persons with HIV infection. It shall aim to affect staff members' knowledge, feelings, attitudes, behavior, and acceptance of people who are HIV positive. For new employees, this education shall be built into the orientation program and offered within three months of hire. Teachers responsible for instruction of students regarding HIV infection shall receive specific in-service training.

4. **Universal precautions relating to bloodborne infections,** as adapted for schools, shall be in effect. School clinics and nursing offices shall follow OSHA guidelines for health care facilities. It is the responsibility of the school district to ensure adequate gloves, bleach, sinks, and disposal containers. There shall be systems of quality assurance or monitoring to document compliance with universal precautions in all school settings. These matters shall be featured in the staff education program.

5. The school district shall provide **education relating to the prevention of HIV infection for students in grades K–12,** within the context of a quality comprehensive school health program. Delivered by trained teachers, health educators, and nurses, it shall be developmentally, culturally, and linguistically appropriate. It shall actively promote abstinence as the best protection and shall also offer explicit information about the use and availability of condoms. Acknowledgment shall be given to the special needs of adolescents regarding emerging sexual orientation. An additional effect of this effort should be to enhance understanding of the needs of students, staff, and others who are infected with HIV.

II. The Enrollment Process

6. The parent, guardian, or student shall decide **whether or not to inform the school system** about HIV status or other health conditions. He or she may support the transfer of this information by another professional or person, including a personal physician or a case manager, but only in the context of strict informed consent procedures. It shall be recognized that disclosure of HIV status often involves revealing related facts, such as medication, parent condition, transmission, and other matters. Under no circumstances shall parents, guardians, or students be required by school personnel to obtain HIV testing or to release information about HIV test results on the student or other family members.

7. Few, if any, personnel in the school or school district shall **receive information about the HIV status** of a student. Determination of those who are to be informed is the prerogative of the parents, guardian, or student, and shall be made in the setting of consideration about special health care or social services that are needed while the student is in school. The terms *need to know* and *right to know* are usually not applicable for school staff and are best eliminated. Specific release of information by the family as they wish it is obviously acceptable, but such material should then be treated confidentially regarding further dissemination.

8. **Information about a student's HIV status** shall not be included in the educational record, usual school health records, or any other records that are accessible to school staff beyond those the parents, guardian, or student has determined should know. Documentation about specific health care given by school nurses, counselors, clinicians, or other personnel to students with HIV infection shall be put in special health records kept in locked files. If the student changes schools, a plan for the transfer of these records shall be developed with the family and student.

III. Assurance of Appropriate Services

9. The **design of an individual student's program** shall be based on educational needs and not the status regarding HIV infection. The curriculum and other activities of a student with HIV shall be modified only as required per developmental and/or personal health needs. Exclusion or segregation of students solely on the basis of HIV infection is never appropriate.

10. **In-school health services** shall be provided as needed, including special regimens required because of HIV infection, but the origin of these programs shall not be identified at the classroom level. Specific health care plans may be formulated by school health

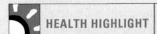

HEALTH HIGHLIGHT | **(continued)**

personnel for students with symptomatic HIV infection. Notification for families about the presence of other communicable diseases at school (e.g., chicken pox) that place students at risk shall be forwarded universally.

Particular notification will be given to families who have informed key school personnel about HIV infection. School nurses, and others with appropriate training, shall participate in counseling for students regarding HIV matters, including the availability of testing. They shall establish quality linkages with youth-serving HIV programs in the community that can provide culturally sensitive, age-appropriate medical, mental health, social, and drug treatment services.

IV. Other Elements

11. School administrators shall provide culturally sensitive information, technical assistance and consultation, and access to resources on HIV issues to the **school's parents and families** through PTAs and other parent organizations. Appropriate issues for discussion include prevention, confidentiality, classroom educational services and related supports, and community resources.

12. Relevant to existing federal and state statutes, teachers, school health professionals, and other qualified employees shall have the **right to employment and confidentiality** regardless of their own HIV status or other health conditions. If they choose to disclose their HIV status to students or other staff, this shall not have ramifications regarding employment.

Source: Crocker, Alan C., et al., "Supports for Children with HIV Infection in School: Best Practices Guidelines" from *Journal of School Health:* 64(1), 33–34. Copyright © 1994 John Wiley & Sons. Used by permission.

---

normal circumstances, these conditions do not usually lead to death, but they are uncomfortable and, in more severe cases, can cause suffering. Although medicine is used in treatment, development of a wellness lifestyle may decrease both the incidence and the effects of these diseases.

The Cardiovascular System

Chronic diseases affecting the cardiovascular system are now among the leading causes of death. The cardiovascular system is complex and is subject to a range of diseases.

▪ Anatomy and Physiology

The heart is composed of specialized muscle tissue called *cardiac muscle*. This muscle is extremely thick and strong and has amazing endurance capacity. Although the heart is only about the size of a fist and weighs a mere eight to ten ounces, it contracts an average 70 to 80 times per minute, 100,000 times per day, and nearly one billion times in an average lifespan of seventy years. It pumps thirty million to forty million gallons of blood over the lifespan. The heart is divided into two pumps by a wall called the septum. Each half is divided into an upper chamber called the atrium and a lower chamber called the ventricle. The right side of the heart receives deoxygenated blood from the body and pumps it to the lungs so that carbon dioxide can be exchanged for a new supply of oxygen. This oxygen-rich blood is then sent to the left side of the heart so that the oxygenated blood can be pumped throughout the body.

On leaving the heart, blood travels throughout the body as part of the circulatory system. Blood containing oxygen and nutrients travels away from the heart, first in arteries, then in arterioles, and then in capillaries. It is through the very thin walls of the capillaries that oxygen, carbon dioxide, nutrients, and waste products are exchanged. Even the heart receives its nourishment in this manner. The waste products and carbon dioxide that are picked up by the blood in its deoxygenated state are returned to the heart through venules (small veins) and then veins, before reentering the venae cavae to the right atrium.

The heart has its own system for controlling its rhythmic pace. This mechanism begins with a group of specialized cells called the **sinoatrial node** (SA node) or *pacemaker.* The heartbeat begins when the SA node emits electrical impulses that signal the atria to contract and simultaneously travel toward the atrioventricular node (AV node). There is a momentary pause before the electrical impulse is distributed through the **bundle of His,**

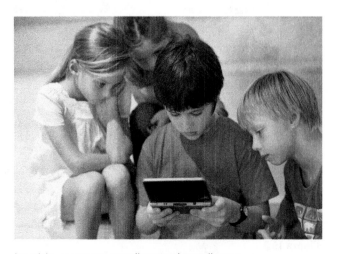

Inactivity at any age contributes to heart disease.

or AV bundle, and then throughout the Purkinje fibers, thereby causing the ventricles to contract. This conduction of electrical charge occurs slightly later in the ventricles and accounts for the characteristic "lub-dub" heart sound heard through a stethoscope (Thibodeau and Patton 2009).

Types of Cardiovascular Disease

The most common cardiovascular diseases do not originate in the heart, but in the arteries. **Arteriosclerosis** is the generic term for a collection of diseases characterized by hardening of the arteries. The most common form of arteriosclerosis is known as **atherosclerosis.** Atherosclerosis is a degenerative disease that begins early in life, perhaps as early as two years of age. Atherosclerosis is the result of a buildup of plaque, fat, and other materials that aggregate at sites of damaged cells inside arterial walls (Figure 15.3). The earliest formations are composed of fatty streaks in the inner lining of the arteries. As atherosclerosis progresses, the arteries harden and thicken. With this hardening, the arteries begin to lose their ability to dilate and constrict, an ability needed to meet all the body's requirements for oxygen in the various parts.

> **Creativity in the Classroom**
>
> Bring a stethoscope to class for lessons about cardiovascular health and let students listen to their own heartbeat.

Over time, more and more plaque accumulates, gradually narrowing the flow of blood through the arteries. This narrowing can result in **ischemia,** or diminished blood flow. Also, as channels narrow, the chances for developing a **thrombus,** or stationary blood clot, increase. If the channels become sufficiently narrow, a free-floating clot (air or gas bubble or clump of bacteria, tissue, tumor, or thrombus), known as an **embolus,** can become stuck and block blood flow, resulting in a **heart attack** (or **myocardial infarction**) or a stroke (if the blood vessel is in the brain). A heart attack may be severe enough to result in death or may be sufficiently mild so that heart function can return to normal. In either event, a certain amount of heart tissue dies, and heart tissue does not regenerate. In time, scar tissue can form, and if it is located in strategic areas (such as along the electrical conducting pathways), full recovery from a heart attack may not be possible. If atherosclerosis affects arteries going to the brain (the carotid and cerebral arteries), a **stroke** (or shortage of blood to the brain) may result. Between 70 and 80 percent of all strokes are due to either a thrombus or embolus. Figure 15.4 shows the possible effects of atherosclerosis in the arteries.

Coronary heart disease (disease of the coronary vessels, rather than of the heart itself) is the leading cause of death in the United States today. Coronary atherosclerosis is the leading form of coronary heart disease. Current research has indicated that some heart attacks may be caused by spasms (cramping) in the coronary arteries. The origin of these spasms is at present unknown, although there is the possibility of a relationship between stress, tension, and heart spasms. Other experts believe that spasms are due to overabundance of calcium in cells that are being deprived of oxygen, or that the release of chemical substances at diseased sites causes the artery to close down. When these spasms occur in cases where sufficient atherosclerosis is

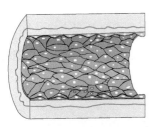

Cross section of a normal artery

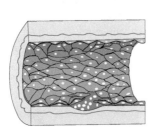

Fatty deposits form on the inner lining

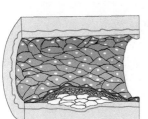

Channel narrows as fat deposits increase

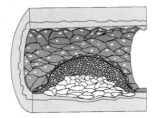

Blood clot can block narrowed channel

Figure 15.3
Progress of Atherosclerosis

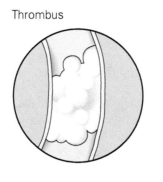

Thrombus

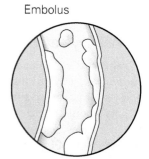

Embolus

Hemorrhage

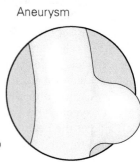

Aneurysm

Figure 15.4
Possible Effects of Atherosclerosis on Arteries

present, the chances of having a heart attack increase. An aneurysm, a ballooning in an artery or vein due to weakened or damaged arterial walls (see Figure 15.4), is another source of coronary heart disease. An aneurysm in arteries in the brain may hemorrhage and cause a stroke.

Other forms of heart disease include **congenital heart defects** that originate during the development of the fetus. These difficulties usually affect the septum or valves of the heart so that they do not function properly. In congestive heart failure, the heart has lost strength and cannot pump all the blood out of the chambers. Circulation is negatively affected. The primary reason for congestive heart failure is high blood pressure or **hypertension** that is uncontrolled, although it may also be due to a previous heart attack, atherosclerosis, or a birth defect. Hypertension usually has no symptoms and may affect people of all ages, including children. Men are more susceptible than women are to high blood pressure, and blacks are more susceptible than whites are.

The common childhood illness of strep throat is the source of an infection that can cause **rheumatic heart disease.** Undiagnosed strep can result in rheumatic fever; in a portion of these cases, rheumatic heart disease results, causing damage to one or more of the heart's valves.

Abnormal heart sounds, known as **heart murmurs,** may be indicative of turbulence in the blood flow resulting from such problems as narrowed or leaky heart valves or an incomplete closure of a congenital hole in the heart's septum (prior to birth, there is a hole, the foramen ovale, between the two atria to allow the blood to bypass the nonfunctional lungs). *Functional heart murmurs,* on the other hand, are considered normal and may be the result of changes in blood turbulence due to increased exercise; this type of murmur is especially common in young people (Spence and Mason 1992).

Angina pectoris is defined as chest pains. Angina is not a heart attack, nor is it a disease. It is a frequent symptom of coronary heart disease, however. An angina attack usually lasts less than five minutes, often after unaccustomed exercise or stress. A primary symptom is a squeezing sensation in the chest, as if a weight had been placed there. For some, it is pain elsewhere in the upper body, frequently the left arm, or a pain that feels similar to indigestion or heartburn. Angina usually subsides with rest and medication. The positive aspect of angina is that it is an early warning of progressive heart disease. For one-third of all victims, the actual heart attack is the first symptom. Recognized and properly treated, angina can lead to prevention of more serious heart disease or even a heart attack. The risk factors for cardiovascular disease are shown in Table 15.3. See Table 15.4 on page 272 for information about cholesterol levels in children. Although there

Table 15.3	**Risk Factors for Cardiovascular Disease**
Major Risk Factors that Cannot Be Changed	
Age	According to the American Heart Association, 55 percent of all heart attacks occur in people over sixty-five; this age group accounts for more than 83 percent of all fatal attacks.
Gender	Women have less heart disease than men do, particularly before menopause. After menopause the heart attack rate among women increases significantly until the mid-sixties, when women's risk is equal to that of men the same age.
Heredity	Male relatives (father, grandfather, and brothers) who die of coronary heart disease before the age of fifty-five or female relatives (mother, grandmother, and sisters) who died of coronary heart disease before the age of sixty-five indicate a strong familial tendency.
Major Risk Factors that Can Be Changed	
Cholesterol	There are several types of cholesterol. Very low-density lipoproteins (VLDL) and low-density lipoproteins (LDL) cholesterol have been referred to as the bad cholesterol or the type that enhances the depositing of plaque in the lining of the arteries. High-density lipoproteins (HDL) cholesterol, in contrast, picks up fat from the cells and linings of the arteries and delivers it to the liver, where it is degraded and eliminated or used to form other tissue.
Cigarette smoking	Tars, carbon monoxide, and nicotine adversely affect the body. The effects of these products increase heart rate, raise blood pressure, increase arterial spasms, reduce the ability of the blood to carry oxygen, and elevate cholesterol levels. Smoke destroys the alveoli in the lungs and paralyzes the cilia.
Hypertension	Systolic blood pressure is the force exerted against the arteries when the heart is contracting. Diastolic pressure is the force against the arteries when the heart is relaxed. These pressures are measured in millimeters of mercury (mm Hg). As a result of hypertension, the heart receives inadequate rest between beats that produces muscle fibers that are overstretched and lose the ability to contract. This increases pressure, damages the kidneys and arteries, and accelerates atherosclerosis.

(continued)

Table 15.3   Risk Factors for Cardiovascular Disease (*continued*)

Inactivity	Research has shown that the impact of physical inactivity on heart disease is similar in magnitude to that of cigarette smoking, high serum cholesterol levels, and hypertension; 78 percent of Americans exercise too infrequently. In addition, exercise has a modifying effect on many of the risks for cardiovascular disease.
Obesity	There is a strong positive association between obesity and abnormal cholesterol and triglycerides, hypertension, and excessive production of insulin. These factors lead to increased likelihood of coronary artery disease and type 2 diabetes.
Diabetes mellitus	Long-range complications lead to degenerative disorders of the blood vessels and nerves. Diabetics often are victims of cardiovascular lesions and accelerated atherosclerosis. The incidence of heart attacks and strokes is higher among diabetics than nondiabetics. Diabetes increases the risk of coronary artery disease by two to three times the normal rate in men and three to seven times in women.
Stress	Experts agree that chronic stress produces a complex array of physiological changes in the body. Some of these physiological responses can constrict the arteries and increase the workload of the heart.
Homocysteine	When building blocks of protein (amino acids) are found in high levels in the blood, the probability of having a heart attack increases to three times that of normal level subjects.

Table 15.4   Blood Cholesterol in Children

Total Blood Cholesterol and LDL Cholesterol Levels for Children Ages Two to Nineteen

	Acceptable	Borderline	High
Total cholesterol (mg/dL)	Less than 170	170–199	200 or greater
LDL cholesterol (mg/dL)	Less than 110	110–129	130 or greater
	HDL levels should be greater than or equal to 35 mg/dL and triglycerides should be less than or equal to 150 mg/dL.		

Source: American Heart Association, Inc., 2011.

are set blood pressure ranges for adults, normal ranges for children vary according to age, gender, and weight so that different levels of growth are considered when evaluating blood pressure for children.

Once a heart attack has occurred, the most common forms of surgical treatment are coronary bypass, angioplasty, coronary atherectomy, and coronary stents. **Coronary bypass** is designed to shunt blood around the blocked segment of a heart artery or arteries. A vein from the leg is removed and one end is sewn into the aorta and the other end is sewn into the coronary artery below the blockage—thus restoring blood flow. **Angioplasty** (also known as balloon angioplasty) uses a catheter with a balloon at the tip. The catheter is positioned at the narrow point in the artery end, and the balloon inflated, compressing the blockage against the vessel wall and thus returning blood flow to the blocked

area. **Coronary atherectomy** uses a specially tipped catheter with a high-speed rotary cutting blade to shave off plaque in the blocked area of the heart artery. Another type of catheterization is used to implant a **coronary stent** in a diseased artery. The stent is a flexible, metallic tube that maintains an open passage for blood flow through a diseased artery. This procedure is much like the angioplasty, but the supporting stent is left in place to help ensure that the artery will remain open. When the stent is placed in an artery, blood-thinning medications must be taken for two to three months. Thereafter the patient must take aspirin every day to maintain the blood thinning.

Cancer

The term **cancer** does not refer to one disease, but rather to a large group of diseases. Cancer is characterized by uncontrolled growth and spread of abnormal cells or **neoplasms.** These neoplasms often form a mass of tissue called a **tumor.** Tumors can be **malignant** (cancerous) or **benign.** Benign tumors usually cause no harm. However, if they are located in an area where they obstruct or crowd out normal tissues or organs, benign tumors can be life threatening; for example, a benign tumor in the brain could restrict the flow of blood. Benign tumors are enclosed in a fibrous capsule that prevents their spreading to other areas of the body. To determine if a tumor is malignant or benign, a **biopsy** (microscopic examination of tissue) must be done.

▪ Types of Cancer

There are four major categories of tumors: carcinoma, sarcoma, lymphoma, and leukemia. **Carcinoma** is the most common form of cancer. Cancers of the skin, breast,

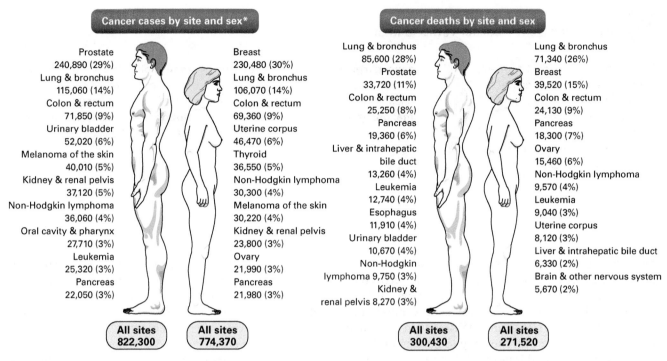

Figure 15.5

Leading Sites of New Cancer Cases and Deaths—2011 Estimates

* Excludes basal and squamous cell skin cancers and in situ carcinoma except urinary bladder.

Source: Data from American Cancer Society, 2011.

uterus, prostate, lung, stomach, colon, and rectum are examples of carcinoma. **Sarcomas** are cancers of the connective tissue and include muscle, bone, and cartilage cancers. These cancers occur less often than carcinomas but usually spread more quickly. **Lymphomas** are cancers that affect the lymph nodes. **Leukemia** is cancer of the blood-forming cells, causing an overproduction of immature white blood cells. Data on the incidence of cancer appear in Figure 15.5.

How Cancer Spreads

Malignant tumors are not contained in a fibrous capsule. Consequently, the malignant cells can spread from one part of the body to another, a process known as **metastasis.** Cancers metastasize by invading adjacent tissues or dislodging and moving through the blood and lymphatic vessels to other parts of the body. Early diagnosis is vital for any type of cancer. If the cancer metastasizes, treatment becomes much more difficult. As the malignant cells spread, they begin to disrupt the chemical functioning of the normal cells in the area they invade. The cancerous cells disrupt the ribonucleic acid (RNA) and deoxyribonucleic acid (DNA) within the normal cells. When this disruption occurs, mutant cells that differ in form, quality, and function are developed. Some cancers, leukemia for example, do not form tumors but involve the blood and blood forming mechanisms of the body.

Causes of Cancer

Cancer is a problem of cell regulation. In simplistic terms, cells fail to perform in a prescribed fashion. To control what is an orderly replacement of cells in the body there are **regulatory genes.** A failure of these genes to regulate the specialization and replication will result in the abnormal production of cells and the development of cancer. Cells also have genes that repair any mistakes in the copying of genetic material found in each cell. Normally, if genes fail to work properly and result in the development of abnormal cells, the immune system will destroy the abnormalities before cancer can develop.

The genes responsible for specialization, replication, repair, and suppression can become **oncogenes,** or cancer-causing genes. Prior to becoming oncogenes they are referred to as proto-oncogenes (Lichtenstein et al. 2000). The mechanisms that cause proto-oncogenes to become oncogenes have received much attention. Many different factors may cause cancer, but three seem to be especially important: genetic mutations, viral infections, and carcinogens. Carcinogens are environmental agents that have been associated with causing cancer. Examples include tobacco smoke, environmental pollutants (water, air, toxic wastes), food preservatives, and even high-fat foods.

In humans it appears that the same proto-oncogenes (noncancerous; normally found in the DNA) can be converted to oncogenes (cancer-inducing genes) either

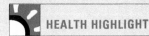

The following terms are commonly used in the language of cancer treatment. Additional terms are also included in the Glossary.

benign: a noncancerous growth

biopsy: removal and microscopic examination of tissue from a living body for diagnosis

cancer: a general term for more than 100 diseases involving abnormal and uncontrolled growth of cells

malignant: a growth of cancerous cells

remission: a lessening or stopping of symptoms of a disease when the disease is under control

tumor: a palpable mass; may be malignant or benign

---

by undergoing some form of mutation that is not associated with a virus or by passage through a **retrovirus.** A retrovirus—such as Rous sarcoma virus (RSV)—enters a cell and converts its own genetic information from RNA to DNA (RNA and DNA contain the genetic information necessary for the body to develop and function). Then the RSV adds its own DNA to that of the host cell so that it is replicated along with the normal DNA every time the host cell divides. A single change to the proto-oncogene is probably not enough to cause the cell to become cancerous—it is accumulated changes that are the likely cause, with each successive change triggering the occurrence of additional abnormalities associated with cancer (Mange and Mange 1990). (Abnormalities include cell proliferation, invasion of adjacent tissue, and metastasis.) Some genes, such as the BRCA-1 breast cancer gene, have been clearly tied to an increased tendency to develop certain kinds of cancer. Individuals in families with a high incidence of breast cancer, for example, may be tested for the presence of such proto-oncogenes and given special counseling on ways to modify their habits (i.e., environmental influences) to reduce their chances of having the oncogenes develop (Mange and Mange 1990).

Although the evidence is still under investigation, there are indications that viruses enhance the probability for the development of cancer. There is evidence that the herpes viruses may contribute to the development of Burkitt's lymphoma, Hodgkin's disease, cervical cancer, and some forms of leukemia (Crowley 2005).

Cancer Prevention and Risk Reduction

It is hoped that by putting into practice cancer prevention methods the number of deaths from cancer will be lowered. Some risk factors are not controllable, such as the part genetics can play in cancer development. Practicing healthy lifestyle and activity habits can lower some cancer risk.

Eliminating or not starting cigarette and tobacco use can decrease the risk of developing acute myelogenous leukemia, among other types of cancer. Practicing safety measures to avoid contracting Human papillomavirus (HPV) can reduce risk of developing cancer in the cervix, penis, vagina, and the anus. Certain types of radiation exposure is known to cause cancer; practicing safety measures can reduce risk. People who are physically active have a lower risk for certain cancers than those who are not (NCI 2011). Obesity is linked to a higher risk of certain types of cancer.

Identifying precancerous conditions early can also affect treatment and survival chances. In some cases medication or surgical intervention can be used to treat a cancerous condition or keep a cancer from starting (NCI 2011).

Cancer, Nutrition, and Physical Activity. Although useful as preservatives, many chemical food additives and preservatives such as cyclamate saccharin and the nitrosamines have been linked with cancer. It has been estimated that 40 to 50 percent of cancers derive from environmental chemicals such as pesticides, herbicides, preservatives, and other chemicals. The Food and Drug Administration (FDA) has developed a list of over 14,000 chemicals suspected of causing cancer.

In addition to avoiding identified cancer-causing chemicals, steps can be taken in regard to nutrition to potentially minimize cancer risk. The National Cancer Institute (NCI) (2011), based on information from multiple research studies, recommends following a healthy and varied diet to potentially reduce risk factors related to obesity and inadequate nutrient intake. The American Cancer Society (ACS) (2002) has developed some nutritional guidelines for preventing cancer, including:

- **Maintain desirable weight.** Obesity increases the risks for colon, breast, gallbladder, and uterine cancer.

- **Avoid too much fat, saturated fat, and cholesterol.** A low-fat diet may reduce the risks for cancers of the breast, prostate, colon, and rectum.

- **Eat foods with adequate starch and fiber.** Starch and fiber can be increased by eating more fruit, vegetables, potatoes, and whole-grain breads and cereals. A high-fiber diet may help reduce the risk of colon and rectal cancer.

- **Include foods rich in vitamins A and C.** Foods such as carrots, spinach, oranges, strawberries, and green peppers are high in vitamin C. Vitamin A can be found in dark green and deep yellow fresh vegetables. These foods may help reduce the risk for cancers of the larynx, esophagus, and lungs.

- **Eat salt-cured, smoked, and nitrate-cured foods in moderation.** Consuming these foods in large amounts is associated with higher incidence of cancer of the esophagus and stomach.
- **If you drink alcohol, do so in moderation.** Moderation is considered to be no more than two drinks a day for men and one drink a day for women. Heavy drinking is associated with cancer of the mouth, throat, esophagus, and liver.

Finally, all children and adults should adopt a physically active lifestyle. The recommendation for adults is to engage in moderate activity for thirty minutes or more at least five times per week. A more refined schedule requires vigorous activity on five or more days per week for forty-five minutes. This schedule may reduce the risk of breast and colon cancers. Children and adolescents are advised to engage in moderate to vigorous activity for sixty minutes at least five days a week.

▪ Warning Signs of Cancer

The National Cancer Institute states that the following warning signs should be carefully monitored.

- a change in bowel or bladder habits
- a sore that does not heal
- unusual bleeding or discharge
- thickening or lump in the breasts or elsewhere
- difficulty in swallowing
- a new mole or a change in an existing mole
- discomfort after eating
- weight gain or loss with no known reason
- feeling weak or very tired
- nagging cough or hoarseness

The chances of survival are significantly better if early detection and diagnosis take place. None of the risk factors are sure indicators of cancer, but they should be checked by a physician.

▪ Cancer Staging

Staging is the process of determining how far cancer has spread. Staging is extremely important because it is a vital step in determining what types of treatment will be used. There are several systems for staging, but a procedure called TNM is most commonly used. The system provides three key pieces of information:

1. T—Describes the size of the tumor and if cancer has spread to other tissues and organs.
2. N—Describes how far the cancer has spread to nearby lymph nodes.

3. M—Determines if cancer has metastasized to other organs of the body.

Letters or numbers after the T, N, and M provide details about each of the three factors. A tumor classified as T1, N0, and M0 is one that is very small, has not yet spread to the lymph nodes, and has not metastasized (NCI 2001; ACS 2011).

▪ Treatment of Cancer

Surgery offers the greatest chance for a cure for many types of cancer. Almost 60 percent of people with cancer will have some type of surgery. The malignant tissue and some additional noncancerous tissue are removed in an attempt to ensure that all the cancerous cells are removed. Surgery is combined with chemotherapy and/or radiation. Surgery is used most often with breast, female reproductive organ, prostate, and testicular cancers. Other treatment options for cancer include:

- *Radiation*—uses high-energy X-rays or gamma rays to destroy or damage cancer cells so that they cannot replicate. Radiation causes side-effects such as diarrhea, itching, and difficulty swallowing. Over the last few years, because of the ability to be more precise in focus and length of exposure, the damage to noncancerous cells has lessened and the potential side-effects have decreased.
- *Chemotherapy*—the use of drugs to treat cancer. Some of the most important advances in the treatment of cancer have been in this area. These advances include new drugs, as well as more effective combinations of new drugs and drugs already used in treatment. The drugs are usually given by mouth or intravenously. They enter the bloodstream and reach all areas of the body, which makes them useful in reaching cancers that have spread. Most chemotherapeutic agents work by destroying the cancer cells' ability to replicate. There are side-effects, such as suppression of the immune system, diarrhea, and hair loss.
- *Hormone therapy*—treatment with hormones that interfere with hormone production or their action. This modality is sometimes classified as chemotherapy.
- *Immunotherapy*—the use of a variety of substances to trigger an individual's own immune system to the cancer. The substances are made through genetic engineering techniques and work by attacking malignant cells or keeping them from becoming active. Among these technologies are interferon, interleukin-2, tumor necrosis factor, and bone marrow growth regulators.

Other technologies have enhanced the diagnosis and treatment of cancer. Such technologies as magnetic resonance imaging (MRI) and computerized tomography (CT) scanning help to detect and map tumors that once were hidden.

Table 15.5	Common Allergic or Sensitivity Reactions		
Reaction	**Causes**	**Symptoms**	**Relief**
Hay fever	Pollen from trees, grasses, or weeds; molds; dust mites; furry animals	Stuffy nose, sneezing, runny nose, itching eyes and nose, watering eyes	Avoidance of allergens; medications
Eczema (atopic dermatitis)	Food allergies; contact with pollen, dust mites, furry animals, makeup, soaps, detergents	Patchy, dry, red itchy rash— often in creases of arms, legs, and neck	Avoidance of allergens; medication
Food allergies and/or sensitivities	Any food, but most common are eggs, peanuts, milk, fish, soy, wheat, peas, and shellfish	Vomiting, hives, diarrhea, or breathing/circulation problem	Avoidance of products

Respiratory Disorders

The term **allergy** can be used synonymously with the term **hypersensitivity.** Both terms refer to an exaggerated response to an antibody-forming substance (**antigen**). Many people with the most common allergic disorders have an inherited tendency to develop this hypersensitivity. Although it may seem to those who suffer from allergies that the vast majority of people do experience hypersensitivity, each specific reaction is theoretically harmless to 80 percent of the population. Table 15.5 lists the more common allergic reactions.

Asthma

Asthma is characterized by spastic contractions of the air passageways, resulting in difficulty breathing. The typical cause is a hypersensitivity of the air passageways to foreign substances found in the air; for about 70 percent of people under the age of thirty, this sensitivity is the cause of their asthma, pollen being the most common culprit (Guyton and Hall 2005). Such *extrinsic asthma* is episodic or seasonal, and attacks may be provoked psychologically if the air passages have already been sensitized by antigens. Hyposensitization treatments (a form of immunotherapy in which increasingly graduated doses of an allergen are given in order to develop immunity) may be helpful for some types of antigens that trigger extrinsic asthma; medications may relieve some symptoms. For people over thirty, asthma is almost always due to hypersensitivity to such nonallergenic types of irritants as those found in smog, strong cooking odors, and paint fumes. This form of asthma, known as *intrinsic asthma*, is chronic and persistent, and it may also be triggered by

sudden inhalation of cold dry air, physical exercise, or violent coughing or laughing (Anderson, Anderson, and Glanze 1998).

Because of their small airways, children are prone to asthma. Childhood asthma tends to improve as the lung airways become larger. Older children tend to become relatively free of symptoms, yet many experience problems throughout their lives. If a child's asthma is more than mild, a proper treatment plan should be undertaken. This plan should be shared with the child's teachers so that the child can fully participate in school activities.

Other Conditions

There are several other significant conditions of which a teacher needs to be aware. Teachers need to understand not only the nature of these disorders, but also the signs and symptoms so they can help identify problems students might be experiencing. These conditions include diabetes, sickle-cell anemia, and epilepsy.

Diabetes Mellitus

Diabetes can result from the secretion of too little insulin from the pancreas, insufficient numbers of insulin receptors on target cells, or defective receptors that do not respond normally to insulin (Margolis and Saudek 2009). **Hyperglycemia** (high blood sugar) is the hallmark symptom of diabetes. Obesity is a contributing factor to the lack of receptor sites in older people. Insufficient amounts of insulin are available to metabolize sugar, the primary source of fuel. When fat is metabolized without sugar, a residue called a **ketone body** develops, increasing acid in the bloodstream. Sufficient amounts of ketone bodies produce a diabetic coma and can cause death. The earliest symptom of characteristically elevated blood glucose levels is excessive urination. Other common warning signs of diabetes include unusual thirst, irritability, blurred vision, frequent infections, extreme hunger, and sudden weight loss.

There are three types of diabetes mellitus. **Type 1 diabetes,** or insulin-dependent diabetes mellitus (IDDM), is usually caused by a lack of insulin secretion. Viral infection of the pancreatic islets or an autoimmune response that destroys the insulin-making beta cells of the pancreas may be responsible for the development of the condition. Type 1 usually appears in people under the age of thirty-five, most commonly between the ages of ten and sixteen years. Type 1 diabetics must be aware of their sugar levels at all times and take daily insulin injections. **Type 2 diabetes,** or non-insulin-dependent diabetes mellitus (NIDDM), is considered a metabolic disease in that the beta cells of the pancreas secrete too little insulin, there are insufficient numbers of insulin receptors on target cells, or defective receptors that do not respond normally to insulin (Crowley 2011). The onset is gradual and usually occurs in people over the age of forty; however, over the last few years there has been a significant increase in the number of adolescents developing type 2 diabetes. This increase has been attributed to an increase in the numbers of adolescents who are overweight or obese and who lead sedentary lifestyles. **Gestational diabetes** is the third type. This can develop in a woman during pregnancy. The condition usually disappears after childbirth, but it does put the woman at greater risk for diabetes later in her life.

Approximately 25.8 million people (8.3 percent of the population in the United States) have diabetes; an estimated 18.8 million have been diagnosed while 7.0 million people are unaware they have the disease (American Diabetes Association 2011). Breakthroughs in the ability to implant insulin monitors and insulin infusion pumps that regulate/dispense insulin as needed by the body have greatly changed the lives of diabetics. Now being tested is an insulin inhaler that would allow the diabetic to inhale rather than inject insulin when needed. These devices help to eliminate many of the potential side-effects associated with treatment and allow more normal lives for diabetics; however, they are very expensive and thus not available to all diabetics.

Insulin shock can develop when too much insulin is present. This occurs when a diabetic is either injected with too much insulin or has not eaten after an insulin injection. Disorientation, convulsions, and loss of consciousness may result.

Extra care with personal hygiene is part of treatment. Diabetics are very prone to infections, so it is important for them to maintain sterile conditions for shaving and to treat cuts and abrasions carefully. The feet and legs are particularly susceptible to infection. Long-term complications include heart disease, stroke, hypertension, blindness, kidney disease, nerve damage, dental disease, and amputations. Some newer classes of drugs work in the small intestine to inhibit the absorption of carbohydrates (which raise blood sugar levels), while others stop the liver from producing excess amounts of sugar.

Sickle-Cell Anemia

Sickle-cell anemia is an inherited blood disease that can cause pain, damage to vital organs, and, for some, early death. The effects of the disease vary greatly from person to person, but most people with the condition enjoy good health much of the time.

Normally, red blood cells are round and flexible. However, the red blood cells of a person with sickle-cell anemia may change into a rigid sickle shape within their blood vessels. The sickle cells tend to become trapped in the spleen and elsewhere and are destroyed. This results in a shortage of red blood cells, which causes the person to be pale, short of breath, easily tired, and prone to infections. Viral infection and vitamin deficiency can worsen the condition.

When the cells become stuck in the blood vessels, portions of the body lose oxygen. This loss of oxygen causes severe pain in the abdomen, chest, and joints; fever; chronic anemia; lethargy; and weakness. If the condition is long lasting, damage to the brain, lungs, or kidneys can even lead to death.

Sickle-cell anemia is not contagious, but it is inherited. Individuals may carry one gene for the disease (sickle-cell trait) but have no signs of the disease. When two persons who have the trait have a child, that child may inherit two sickle-cell genes and develop the disease. A test can identify people who either have the disease or carry the trait. Unfortunately there is no medication or therapy that will correct the effects of the disease-causing gene.

See the Health Highlight "A Student Who Has Sickle-Cell Anemia in the Classroom" on page 278 for more information and points to keep in mind if you have a child with sickle-cell anemia in your classroom.

Epilepsy

The word *epilepsy* comes from the Greek word for seizures. **Epilepsy** is a disorder of the central nervous system characterized by sudden seizures, which usually last only a few minutes. Seizures are not always convulsive,

HEALTH HIGHLIGHT | **A Student Who Has Sickle-Cell Anemia in the Classroom**

There may be a student in your class with the severe chronic disease sickle-cell anemia. Your understanding of this handicap will help him or her on the road to learning.

Such a student is often thin and small for his or her age. When not experiencing physical discomfort, the student is usually as active as any student in the class is. Intelligence is not affected. As noted in earlier chapters, the majority of those affected are African Americans, but the disease also occurs in people from Mediterranean countries, South and Central America, Caribbean countries, and southern India.

There are periods when the disease is more active (crises). These episodes often occur with colds and other infections and are more frequent in early childhood. At such times, the child becomes listless and complains of pain, usually in the back, extremities, or abdomen. The whites of his or her eyes may be slightly yellow. Most of these attacks will necessitate a week or two of absence from school. Sometimes, hospitalization and special procedures, such as blood transfusion, will be required.

The disease is due to a hereditary defect in the red blood cells, causing them to assume the crescent shape that gives the disease its name. The pains are due to aggregations of sickled cells causing a temporary blockage of the small blood vessels. These cells are subject to early destruction in the circulation, causing a chronic anemia.

Sickle-cell anemia is inherited as a recessive trait affecting both males and females. If both parents carry a recessive sickle-cell gene, the affected child receives one such gene from each parent. When both parents have sickle-cell trait, their offspring has a 25 percent chance of being normal, a 25 percent chance of having sickle-cell anemia, or a 50 percent chance of having sickle-cell trait. An examination of the blood by laboratory tests will show whether a person has sickle-cell anemia or sickle cell trait. Individuals who have the trait have a very small percentage of sickled cells in their blood. They never develop sickle-cell anemia per se, and as a rule, they are free of symptoms that could be attributed to the presence of abnormal hemoglobin in their red blood cells.

Points for the Teacher to Keep in Mind

1. Sickle-cell anemia is a chronic hereditary handicapping illness.
2. Crises cause frequent absence from school, especially in younger students.
3. Colds and other infections may precipitate crises.
4. Between crises, a student who has sickle-cell anemia may carry on the usual activities of his or her peer group, with the exception of strenuous sports.
5. The disease does not affect intelligence.
6. Education should be encouraged because this handicap will necessitate a sedentary occupation as an adult.
7. When long hospitalizations are required, students should be able to continue schoolwork in the hospital with the help of a visiting teacher.
8. Psychological problems may arise from adjustment to the handicap and the environment.
9. It is important that there be some activity in which the student can excel to gain acceptance with the peer group. This could be music, art, handicrafts, games, and so forth.
10. The disease tends to become milder as an individual grows into adulthood. Crises become less frequent and less severe after adolescence.

Source: Based on Scott and Kessler 1988, 1–4

---

and, even when they are, they are not as dangerous as they look. Epilepsy is not contagious, and, between seizures, epileptic children function normally. Seizures occur when there are excessive electrical discharges in some nerve cells of the brain. When this happens, the brain loses conscious control over certain body functions and consciousness may be lost or altered.

There are more than twenty different kinds of seizures. Only three will be described here.

General Tonic Clonic Seizures (Grand Mal). These are the most disruptive type of seizures that might occur in the classroom. The child becomes stiff and slumps to the floor unconscious. Rigid muscles give way to jerking, breathing is suspended, and saliva may escape from the lips. The seizure may last for several minutes, and the child will regain consciousness in a confused or drowsy state but is otherwise unaffected.

For tonic clonic seizures:

- Keep calm. Ease the child to the floor, and loosen his or her collar. You cannot stop the seizure. Let it run its course, and do not try to revive the child.

- Remove hard, sharp, or hot objects that may injure the child, but do not interfere with his or her movements.

- Do not force anything between his or her teeth.

- Turn the child on one side to release saliva. Place something soft and flat under his or her head.

- When the child regains consciousness, let him or her rest.

- If the seizure lasts beyond a few minutes or the child seems to pass from one seizure to another without gaining consciousness, call for medical assistance and notify his or her parents. This rarely happens but should be treated immediately.

Generalized Absence (Petit Mal) Seizures.
The most common seizures in children, generalized absence seizures usually last for only five to twenty seconds. They may be accompanied by staring or twitching of the eyelids and are frequently mistaken for daydreaming. The child is seldom aware he or she has had a seizure, although he or she may be aware that his or her mind "has gone blank" for a few seconds.

Complex Partial (Psychomotor or Temporal Lobe) Seizures.
The most complex behavior patterns occur with these seizures and may include constant chewing or lip smacking, purposeless walking or repetitive hand and arm movements, confusion, and dizziness. The seizure may last from a minute to several hours. The person should not be restrained, but also should not be allowed to harm himself or herself. Medical assistance is required if the seizure lasts more than a few minutes or if it is the first time such a seizure has occurred.

Chapter In Review

Summary

- Microorganisms (microbes) are living agents. Microbes that cause disease in humans are called *pathogens*.
- There are six general types of pathogenic microbes: viruses, bacteria, rickettsias, fungi, protozoa, and helminths.
- Every illness follows a pattern from the time the pathogen enters the body to the incubation period, prodromal period, typical illness, convalescence, and recovery.
- The immune system protects against disease.
- Body defenses include the skin, body secretions, mucous membranes, enzymes, blood compounds, and interferon.
- Common diseases that can impact children include the common cold, streptococcal throat infection, influenza, infectious mononucleosis, and the various types of hepatitis.
- HIV is the virus responsible for AIDS. It cannot be contracted through casual contact.
- There are no cures for HIV/AIDS, but a combination of drug therapy can be used to treat existing cases.
- Teachers must be aware of the emotional, social, and legal support an HIV-positive child needs.
- The risk factors for cardiovascular disease include heredity, sex, age, tobacco use, high cholesterol, hypertension, inactivity, obesity, diabetes, and stress.
- Conditions of the heart and cardiovascular system include congenital heart defects, congestive heart failure, myocardial infarction, angina pectoris, hypertension, and rheumatic heart disease.

- The term *cancer* is used to describe conditions characterized by uncontrolled cell growth.
- Neoplasms (tumors) can be benign (noncancerous) or malignant (cancerous).
- Types of cancer include carcinomas, sarcomas, lymphomas, and leukemia.
- Cancer spreads through a process called *metastasis*.
- Sickle-cell anemia is an inherited blood disease that can cause extreme pain, damage to vital organs, and possible early death.
- Epilepsy is one of more than twenty types of disorders of the central nervous system.
- The three most common types of epilepsy are general tonic clonic (grand mal); generalized absence (petit mal); and complex partial (psychomotor).

Discussion Questions

1. List and describe six types of pathogens.
2. Discuss immunity and the various protective mechanisms the body has to protect itself against disease.
3. Trace the stages through which a communicable disease typically progresses.
4. Describe the antigen-antibody response.
5. List the possible physiological effects experienced by an HIV-positive person.
6. Trace the blood through the heart and circulatory system.
7. Distinguish between angina pectoris, heart attack, and stroke.

8. Describe the major risk factors for cardiovascular diseases.
9. What are four types of cancer?
10. Describe how IDDM differs from NIDDM.
11. What considerations are necessary for a child with sickle-cell anemia?

Critical Thinking Questions

1. Reflect on the HIV/AIDS epidemic in the United States. Select a grade level, and outline the types of content that should be covered.

2. What types of guidelines and protocols do your state and local school district have regarding protecting teacher and school personnel against bloodborne pathogens?

3. What guidelines would you establish in your classroom for the prevention of diseases?

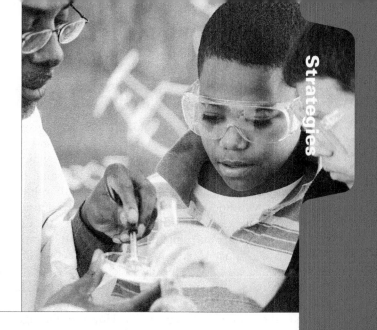

16 Strategies for Teaching Infectious and Noninfectious Conditions

Valued Outcomes

After completion of this chapter, you should be able to convey the following to your students:

- Discuss the diseases that are the leading causes of deaths.

- Identify how pathogens cause disease.

- Describe how the immune system protects against disease.

- Identify how the heart works.

- Discuss how noninfectious diseases often develop over time and are affected by lifestyle.

Reflections

Using the content information for infectious and noninfectious diseases, select one disease or condition and develop the concepts that should be taught at a selected grade level. If you feel more emphasis should be placed on a particular content area, justify your feelings and outline the conceptual framework for that grade level.

There is no shortage of good days, it is good lives that are hard to come by.

—Annie Dillard

NATIONAL HEALTH EDUCATION STANDARDS

1. Students will comprehend concepts related to health promotion and disease prevention to enhance health.

2. Students will analyze the influence of family, peers, culture, media, technology, and other factors on health behaviors.

3. Students will demonstrate the ability to access valid information and products and services to enhance health.

5. Students will demonstrate the ability to use decision-making skills to enhance health.

7. Students will demonstrate the ability to practice health-enhancing behaviors and avoid or reduce risks.

8. Students will demonstrate the ability to advocate for personal, family, and community health.

Teaching Children about Disease

Many of the values that protect and direct us as we grow are fostered during the elementary years. Learning at an early age about pathogens, the stages through which diseases progress, and lifestyles that are detrimental to high-level wellness can establish positive health values and habits. In addition, many chronic conditions detract from the quality of life for children. Awareness on the part of every teacher and child that children with chronic conditions can function effectively in the school setting improves the quality of life for the affected child.

As with other strategy chapters, the suggested grade level(s) for which the activity might be appropriate is shown to the right of each activity title. However, through modification, many of the suggested activities could be used at various grade levels. This modification could include changing the questions to be more age appropriate for the activity than those provided.

Information Assessment Activities

Facts and Myths   Grades 2–5

Valued Outcome: Students will determine what is true and false concerning various diseases and conditions.

National Health Education Standard: 1

Description of Strategy: The following are questions that students can be asked to vote on concerning heart disease, cancer, or infectious diseases. Other questions can be formulated for other topics. Have the students put their thumbs up if they agree and thumbs down if they disagree. Students can fold their hands if they have no opinion.

- Do you think exercise is good for your heart?
- Do you think your diet affects your heart?
- Do you think exercise is good for your health?
- How many think that there is no cure for cancer?
- Can you get cancer from another person?
- Can you get cancer from overexposure to the sun?
- Can infectious diseases be spread by sneezing?
- Do you think you should be around someone who is ill?
- Does washing your hands help prevent disease?

Processing Questions:

1. Why is exercise good for you?
2. How can you avoid the germs of someone who is sick?
3. When should you wash your hands?

○ **Integration:** Science

✓ **Assessment:** Students can state three healthy habits that will help them avoid illness.

How Did I Get It?   Grades 4–6

Valued Outcome: Students will be able to identify the risk factors associated with contracting disease.

National Health Education Standards: 1, 7

Description of Strategy: Ask the students to think of someone who is seriously ill. Then ask them to identify some factors that may have been associated with the sick person's illness. Write the responses on the board. Make two lists, one for uncontrollable factors and one for factors that could have been better controlled if the person had followed a wellness lifestyle. Have students identify in which column each of their responses belongs. Do this for several different illnesses. You may also assign students to further research some of the conditions identified and how the illness can be prevented.

Materials Needed: board and markers

Processing Questions:

1. How many of the illnesses/conditions are related to lifestyle?
2. What lifestyle factors may have put the individual at greater risk for developing the condition?
3. Are there factors that cannot be controlled? (Point out that a wellness lifestyle can delay or prevent some of the genetic predispositions we have for certain diseases.)
4. Name some things you can do to prevent diseases.
5. What type of diseases/conditions would fall under the category of uncontrollable (hemophilia, for example)?

✓ **Assessment:** Students can differentiate between controllable and uncontrollable risk factors for disease.

Values Statements   Grades 4–8

Valued Outcome: Students will examine issues and lifestyle factors associated with various conditions.

National Health Education Standards: 1, 7

Description of Strategy: utilize unfinished sentences that can help initiate discussion. Use the list in Worksheet 16.2 (on page 491) or design your own questions to meet the individual needs of the students.

Materials Needed: pencils, a copy of Worksheet 16.2 for each student

Processing Questions:

1. What are three lifestyle habits you can adopt to help you stay healthy?
2. How can we help our friends or family members if they have a disease?
3. When should you go to the doctor?

TEACHING IN ACTION | **Daily Lesson Plan**

Lesson Title: Wash Those Hands

Date: March 5, 2012   **Time:** 9:00 A.M.   **Grade:** Two   **Teacher:** Ling

I. National Health Education Standards

Health Education Standard 1: Students will comprehend concepts related to health promotion and disease prevention to enhance health.

II. National Health Education Standards Performance Indicator

1.2.3 describe ways to prevent communicable diseases.

III. Valued Outcomes

- Students will be able to discuss how germs are spread from person to person.
- Students will be able to list times when hands should be washed.
- Students will be able to demonstrate proper hand-washing technique.

IV. Description of Strategy

1. Begin by stressing to students when hands should be washed—before eating or touching food, before setting the table, and after using the restroom, just to name a few.
2. Have students spray water on a dark colored piece of paper and explain that sneezes and coughs spray germs in the same manner. Tell students that this is why the mouth should be covered when a person sneezes or coughs. Give students other examples of how germs are spread.
3. Tell students that even when hands might look clean germs can still be present. Then demonstrate the proper way to wash hands. Describe washing the front and back of hands as well as between fingers and under nails with soap and water.
4. Explain that singing "Happy Birthday" twice is the amount of time it should take to thoroughly wash hands. Include this in your demonstration, and have students take turns washing their hands.

V. Materials Needed

- spray bottle of water
- dark-colored paper
- soap and paper towels

VI. Formative Evaluation

Benchmarks

- Level 1: Student was able to identify some occasions when hands should be washed.
- Level 2: Student was able to identify many occasions when hands should be washed.
- Level 3: Student was able to identify many occasions when hands should be washed and demonstrate proper hand-washing technique.
- Level 4: Student was able to identify many occasions when hands should be washed and demonstrate proper hand-washing technique. Student was able to explain how germs spread.

VII. Points of Emphasis

1. Explain where germs come from and the many ways that they can be spread.
2. Explain how washing hands properly and regularly can keep people from getting sick.
3. Explain the importance of proper hand-washing, not just running hands under the water.

Teacher Evaluation

1. Keep the lesson as taught?   yes _____   no _____

2. What I need to improve _____

3. Next time make sure _____

4. Strengths of lesson _____

| **Daily Lesson Plan**

Lesson Title: The "Bert Bird Knows" Mobile

Date: March 12, 2012   **Time:** 10:00 A.M.   **Grade:** Three   **Teacher:** Caen

I. National Health Education Standards

Health Education Standard 1: Students will comprehend concepts related to health promotion and disease prevention to enhance health.

II. National Health Education Standards Performance Indicator

1.5.1 describe the relationship between healthy behaviors and personal health.

III. Valued Outcomes

- Students will identify risk factors for cardiovascular disease.
- Students will differentiate between risk factors that can and cannot be changed.
- Students will identify other diseases that these risk factors may be associated with.

IV. Description of Strategy

1. Have the students construct the "Bert Bird Knows" mobile from **Worksheet 16.1** (on page 490). Provide students with yarn and cardboard.
2. Have students use yarn to suspend risk factors from the "Risk Factors for Cardiovascular Disease" card. Each suspended card should be a risk factor for heart disease (i.e., no exercise, family history, smoking, high blood pressure, diabetes, poor diet, gender, age, high cholesterol, obesity, and stress).
3. Have students use square cards for risk factors that cannot be changed (age, family history, and gender) and oval cards for risk factors that can be changed (no exercise, smoking, high blood pressure, etc.).
4. Describe some ways to change the risk factors for disease.
5. Have the students give examples of other diseases for which these might be risk factors.

V. Materials Needed

- cardboard and yarn
- list of risk factors

VI. Formative Evaluation

Benchmarks

- Level 1: Student was able to identify some risk factors for heart disease.
- Level 2: Student was able to identify all risk factors for heart disease and classify them as changeable or not changeable.
- Level 3: Student was able to identify all risk factors for heart disease and classify them as changeable or not changeable. Student was able to describe ways to change some risk factors.
- Level 4: Student was able to identify all risk factors for heart disease and classify them as changeable or not changeable. Student was able to describe ways to change some risk factors and listed other diseases for which these might be risk factors.

VII. Points of Emphasis

1. Explain how things we do in our everyday lives affect these risk factors.
2. Explain the importance of making wise health decisions to prevent heart disease later in life.
3. Give examples of things that can be done to change each risk factor.

Teacher Evaluation

1. Keep the lesson as taught?   yes _____   no _____

2. What I need to improve _____

3. Next time make sure _____

4. Strengths of lesson _____

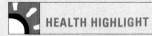 **HEALTH HIGHLIGHT** | **A Most Preventable Situation**

Chronic disease has replaced infectious or communicable disease as the leading cause of death in the United States. At the same time, however, some communicable diseases have been appearing more often. One such disease is measles, which has made a dramatic comeback. The major reason for the increase in the incidence of measles is the failure to immunize children at the recommended age intervals. This particular disease should be totally preventable in the United States if parents have access to the health care system.

○ **Integration:** Social Studies

✓ **Assessment:** Students can list three lifestyle factors that can help prevent chronic diseases, such as heart disease and diabetes.

The Help I Get   Grades 5–8

Valued Outcome: Students will appreciate the many defenses the body uses to protect them from disease.

National Health Education Standard: 1

Description of Strategy: Provide the students with a copy of Worksheet 16.3 on page 492. Have students write a brief description of how each defense listed on the handout helps protect their bodies. (*Example:* C. Sweat helps our body maintain a constant temperature.) The various body defenses can be discussed in class or assigned as a group or individual activity for reporting findings back to the class.

Materials Needed: one copy of worksheet for each student, pens or pencils

Processing Questions:

1. What happens to our body defenses if we do not take care of our bodies?
2. Can you name all the body defense mechanisms?
3. How can we make sure our body defenses are operating at the highest level possible?
4. What are some lifestyle habits that inhibit our body defenses from operating at peak performance?

○ **Integration:** Writing

✓ **Assessment:** Students can list the body's defense systems and describe how they help protect the body from injury or disease.

Decision Stories

(Follow the procedures outlined in Chapter 4 on pages 60–62 for Decision Stories.)

For each of the decision stories, write a list on the board of ideas generated by the class for how each situation should be dealt with. Ask the students to discuss the merits of the methods suggested.

Assessment for Decision Stories: Students can identify health-enhancing behaviors and exhibit positive decision-making skills.

Play Ball   Grades 2–5

Sam has allergies in the spring. This year he is ten years old and wants to try out for the school baseball team, but tryouts occur when his allergies bother him the most. His parents told him he should just stay inside during the spring and wait until his allergies clear up. Sam says that playing baseball is really important to him. All his friends play on teams, and they have a really great time. Besides, Sam doesn't have anyone to play with because all his friends are involved in sports.

Focus Question: Should Sam try out for the baseball team or stay inside as his parents suggest?

National Health Education Standards: 1, 5

Moles Can Change   Grades 3–6

Juan's dad has a mole on his foot that has been changing in appearance. It is growing and is an unusual black color. The mole has been on his dad's foot for as long as he can remember, but it has only recently changed in looks. Juan's dad insists that it is only because of the way his shoe has been rubbing his foot. Juan's mom has expressed some concern due to the changes. Juan knows that an obvious change in a wart or mole is one of the warning signals of cancer.

Focus Question: What should Juan's dad do?

National Health Education Standards: 5, 8

Your Heart's Eating Habits   Grades 4–6

Jenny's grandmother recently had a myocardial infarction, or heart attack. The grandmother was only fifty-four years old. The heart attack was precipitated by the presence of atherosclerosis. Jenny's great-aunt, her grandmother's sister, died of heart disease when she was only sixty-one.

Jenny's family eats a lot of food high in fat, and they all tend to be overweight. Jenny's mom and dad are concerned about the grandmother, and they are worried about Jenny's mom, who is thirty-four, and even Jenny, who is only eleven. The doctor has indicated that Jenny's family needs to change their eating habits, but they all really enjoy eating. Diets have never been successful in this family.

Focus Question: What are some options that Jenny and her family have in dealing with this problem?

National Health Education Standards: 3, 8

Dramatizations

Two examples of dramatization are provided. These can be modified according to need and grade level.

Betty Bacteria   Grades 3–5

Valued Outcome: Students will be able to describe how communicable diseases are spread through lack of sanitary habits.

National Health Education Standard: 1

Description of Strategy: Younger students can act out a skit stressing the importance of cleansing wounds. Discussion can include topics such as the importance of washing all wounds, cuts, and scrapes, as well as preventive care and washing hands at appropriate times. Ask the students to identify how germs are spread. Question the students on how they felt when they were becoming ill—list the symptoms on the board. Ask the students if they know how they "caught" their disease. Introduce the skit by telling the students they are going to see one way diseases can be contracted. The characters for the skit include Betty Bacteria; Zach, the little boy; Mother; and the Narrator.

Narrator:	*It is Saturday afternoon. Mother is outside washing the car when Zach comes running up.*
Zach:	Mom! Mom! *(Zach is crying.)* I hurt my leg, and it's bleeding very badly! Mom, make it stop hurting! *(Zach sits down and shows his mother his knee. Betty Bacteria is standing beside Zach's knee. She starts laughing.)*
Betty:	Now is my chance! I am going to get inside Zach's cut and infect it! I love to make people hurt! *(Betty moves closer and closer to Zach's cut.)*
Mom:	I know just what to do, Zach. First, we are going to wash it so that no germs will get inside of it and make you sick. Wait here while I get the soap and some medicine and a bandage.
Betty:	No! No! Don't use soap and water on me! I don't like soap and water! I can't live if soap and water

are around and a cut is all clean. I better start making Zach's cut sick as quickly as I can. *(Betty touches Zach's knee with her hand as Zach's mom returns. Mom picks up the hose and washes off Zach's knee. Betty jerks her hand back.)*

Betty:	Stop! Stop! I don't like water. Water will make me go away, and I want to hurt Zach! *(Mom rubs the soap over Zach's knee and then rinses it off. Using a towel, she dries it and proceeds to put an antibiotic on the cut. Betty is crying and starts to shrivel up and go away.)*
Betty:	This is no fun. I can't live with soap and water. Soap and water are the end of me. *(Betty disappears offstage.)*
Mom:	Now your cut is nice and clean, and the medicine will keep any new germs from trying to hurt you. Do you feel better?
Zach:	I feel much better now, Mom. Thanks for taking care of my cut.

Materials Needed: a copy of the script for each actor, props for the skit (medicine container, bandage, piece of hose, and soap)

Processing Questions:

1. What did you learn from today's lesson?
2. Can someone explain how disease germs are spread?
3. How can we prevent the spread of disease germs?

✓ **Assessment:** Students will be able to explain why cleaning cuts and scrapes is important.

"Catching" Cold   Grades 4–6

Valued Outcome: Students will describe how sneezing can spread disease.

National Health Education Standard: 1

Description of Strategy: Students role-play the following situation. Bill and Jay are eating lunch together. Bill has a cold. Bill sneezes (sprays a short squirt of water from a spray bottle) and doesn't cover his nose and mouth while sitting beside Jay. Jay is wiping himself off when Aimee comes up and sits down beside them. She asks Jay why he is so upset.

Materials Needed: one spray bottle of water that can be used as the "sneeze"

Processing Questions:

1. Why do you think Jay is upset?
2. What should Bill have done when he had to sneeze?
3. Do you think Jay can catch a cold from Bill? Why?
4. Can Aimee catch the cold from Bill, since he just sneezed?

✓ **Assessment:** Students can explain how coughing and sneezing can spread infectious diseases.

Discussion and Report Techniques

Name that Disease   Grades 4–8

Valued Outcome: Each student will be able to discuss the important signs and symptoms of various diseases.

National Health Education Standard: 1

Description of Strategy: Students working in groups can select a disease (infectious or chronic) and research the causes, signs or symptoms, and methods of treatment for the disease. The information should be placed on large sheets of paper and posted on the walls for each student to read. Oral reports may be given, using the large sheets as teaching aids.

Materials Needed: markers, butcher paper, and references for students to research the various diseases

Processing Questions:

1. What were some important points we learned about diseases in general?
2. For the diseases each of you read about, what were some facts that surprised you?
3. How are diseases treated?

✓ **Assessment:** Students will be able to explain the causes, symptoms, and treatment options for the disease that they research.

Disease Search   Grades 6–8

Valued Outcome: Students will be able to identify the most common diseases and discuss how they might have been prevented.

National Health Education Standards: 1, 7

Description of Strategy: Have the students ask their parents which chronic and communicable diseases have been experienced within the immediate family (parents, grandparents, aunts, and uncles). These diseases probably would include heart disease, cancer, arthritis, allergies, measles, chicken pox, mumps, and so on. Students can then bring in lists of these diseases and turn them in to be placed on the board. Going down the list, have students raise their hands if someone in their family has had the disease and record the totals for each disease on the board. When finished, note the diseases that have been experienced the most, ranking from least to most common.

Materials Needed: board, overhead projector, or butcher paper; markers

Processing Questions:

1. What are the diseases experienced most often by our group?
2. How many of the diseases listed have you personally had?
3. How could some of these diseases have been avoided?

✓ **Assessment:** Students can list the most common diseases in their families and discuss whether these also apply to the general population.

What Should Be Done?   Grades 6–8

Valued Outcome: Students will be able to discuss the school policy concerning illness.

National Health Education Standards: 2, 7

Description of Strategy: Allow the students to investigate the school policy on illness. Hold a discussion on appropriate actions to take when someone becomes ill. What should the teacher do? What should the students do? What is the responsibility of the school? How can the school nurse help (if one is available)?

Materials Needed: copy of the school policy on illness for each student

Processing Questions:

1. Do you think the policies cover everything needed?
2. What would you do if a friend became ill?
3. What should be done if the school nurse is not at school when someone becomes ill?

✓ **Assessment:** Students can describe the school health policy and appropriate actions to take when someone becomes ill at school.

Experiments and Demonstrations

Draw a Bug   Grades 3–6

Valued Outcome: Students will be able to identify what pathogens cause various diseases.

National Health Education Standard: 1

Description of Strategy: Show pictures of the various pathogens (viruses, bacteria, fungi, and so on; see Table 15.2 on page 260). Have the students draw one of the pathogens. On the board or overhead projector, list the names of various diseases. On their paper, have the students list the diseases caused by the pathogen they drew.

Materials Needed: pictures or drawings of the various pathogens, list of diseases, board or overhead projector and markers

Processing Questions:

1. How many of the listed diseases did the pathogen you drew cause?
2. Are some of them more serious than others?
3. How can a certain pathogen cause so many illnesses?

○ **Integration:** Art

✓ **Assessment:** Students will be able to list the types of pathogens and name the diseases caused by each type.

Things I Know, Things I'd Like To Know
Grades 4–6

Valued Outcome: Students will identify and answer areas of concern for various diseases.

National Health Education Standards: 1, 3

Description of Strategy: Select several diseases or conditions for students to investigate. Students must write down what they think is true concerning each disease. Students can then list some questions (establish a minimum number) they have concerning each disease. During investigation, they can determine the accuracy of their ideas on their specific disease and learn the answers to the questions they have written. Use the form in Worksheet 16.4 (page 493).

Materials Needed: one copy of the Worksheet 16.4 for each student, pencils

Processing Questions:

1. Was any of the information you thought you knew incorrect?
2. What was one new thing you learned from the activity?

✓ **Assessment:** Students will be able to describe what they knew and what they learned about the disease they researched.

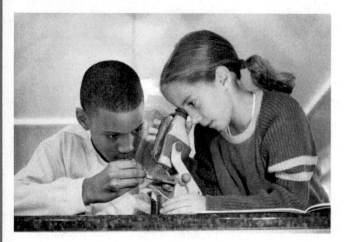

A microscope is an invaluable learning tool for students studying pathogens.

The Anatomy of the Heart
Grades 4–8

Valued Outcome: Students will be able to identify the various structures of the heart and explain the function of each.

National Health Education Standard: 1

Description of Strategy: Ask the meat department at the local grocery to donate a beef heart for dissecting purposes. (You should wear protective gloves while performing the dissection and handling the heart.) The class can observe as various structures and functions of the structures of the heart are noted. The atria, ventricles, aortas, and various valves can be pointed out.

Materials Needed: beef heart, rubber gloves, scalpel, paper towels, chart of the structures of the human heart

Processing Questions:

1. How many chambers does the heart have?
2. What function does each part of the heart fulfill?
3. How does the blood get to the heart muscle?

○ **Integration:** Science

✓ **Assessment:** Students will be able to name the four chambers of the heart and at least two other main structures and their functions.

Using Technology to Understand Infectious Diseases
Grades 5–8

Valued Outcome: The student will identify the factors that influence the development of infectious diseases and how they spread.

National Health Education Standards: 1, 2, 3, and 8

Description of Strategy: This activity is adapted from the website *BAM! Body and Mind.* (The site created by the CDC for kids nine through thirteen years old is intended to give kids the information they need to make healthy lifestyle choices.) Students will become interested in infectious diseases by discussing and charting their own experiences and will, without knowing it, act like young epidemiologists. The activity also will help you teach about the scientific concept of the epidemiologic triangle using an infectious disease example. Once students understand the triangle, they can apply it to other diseases they encounter.

The epidemiologic triangle (Worksheet 16.5 on page 494) should be explained to students to show them how it helps organize information about a specific disease. Describe and define each component. The students should then be asked to identify the infectious diseases they have had (common cold, flu, chicken pox, etc.). List these diseases on the board/overhead/PowerPoint. Each student should then go online to research one of the diseases they identified. Once the information is gathered, each student examines the epidemiological triangle and identifies the factors that could have influenced their developing the disease. This exercise should help students refine research, reasoning, and problem solving skills.

Materials Needed: computer, Internet, copy of epidemiological triangle (Worksheet 16.5)

Processing Questions:

1. What are the ways a disease can be spread?
2. What factors did you identify under the epidemiological triangle?
3. What conclusions can you make from the results of your investigation?

○ **Integration:** Science

✓ **Assessment:** Students can identify pathogenic agents and factors that can influence whether a disease develops.

Analyzing Cigarette Smoke   Grades 6–8

Valued Outcome: Students will be able to list the many harmful materials found in cigarettes.

National Health Education Standard: 1

Description of Strategy: This activity was developed by Dr. David White and Linda Rudisill. Due to the danger inherent in the chemicals involved, actual ingredients are not used. All ingredients represent by-products of cigarette use. Students are not informed about what the ingredients represent. They are to guess, based on their knowledge. The entire script is provided for the activity.

Lesson Focus: How many of you have ever received products in the mail to sample, such as soap, shampoo, or toothpaste? The makers provide a small amount for us to try, and then we decide if we want to purchase the product. Suppose we could sample one of these products by breaking it down and trying the main ingredients, or analyzing it. (Teacher may want to discuss the meaning of analyze.) We might know much more about a product if we could analyze it, rather than simply trying a sample. The purpose of this lesson is to help you analyze a product that is used by millions of people in the United States. Its popularity, however, has been declining for several years. (Emphasize here that it is important not to comment on what the product is until instruction is complete. Have students write the name of the product on a sheet of paper when they think they have guessed correctly.)

Teacher Input: I will NOT ask you to sample these items as I describe them. When I have completed the discussion, you can then decide if you want to try them. Remember, if you do not want to try it, your grade will NOT be affected.

Point to [two] balloons: The product that we are analyzing is associated with over 500 gases and

several thousand chemicals. Since I would have to go to a lot of trouble to bring you over 500 gases, I just brought two of them in balloons. This balloon contains some *carbon monoxide*. Joe, after I describe the other chemicals, would you please inhale the gas in this balloon? This gas is odorless, colorless, and although this amount should not hurt you, this gas is deadly. When you use this product, your blood transports five to ten times more carbon monoxide than normal [and carries the carbon monoxide instead of oxygen]. This is because carbon monoxide binds to hemoglobin about 240 times more strongly than oxygen.

Now, Joe, I know what you are thinking. Why should only a guy try this? Sue, I would like you to choose a balloon and try it, too. Remember, if you use the average amount of this product daily, you will lose 6 to 8 percent of your body's oxygen-carrying capacity.

Point to [next two] other balloons: I have put another of the gases from this product in these balloons. This gas is *hydrogen cyanide*. Hydrogen cyanide is a gas that has been used in the gas chamber. When you use the product we are analyzing, the hydrogen cyanide paralyzes your cilia for 20 to 30 seconds. (Teacher may need to explain the functions of the cilia here.) Now, Carl, would you and Judy sample this ingredient by breathing the gas in these balloons? I'm fairly sure that the amount I have in here will not hurt you; however, remember that this gas paralyzes your cilia for 20 to 30 seconds each time you use it.

Hold up the jar of flour (arsenic): In this jar I have a little arsenic. Kathy, would you sample this for us later? I have clean spoons for both you and Tom. Arsenic is a silvery-white, tasteless, poisonous chemical used in making insecticides. It looks like flour, and that is what it is mixed with in this jar. Arsenic is associated with the product we are analyzing.

Hold up a glass jar (about one cup) of chocolate syrup (tar): In this jar I have a brown sticky substance. If you use the average amount of the product we are analyzing, your body will collect about a cup of this brown, sticky substance a year. Tom, would you put your finger in this jar and then lick your finger?

Refer students to jar of clear syrup (nicotine): This substance is a poison. It can kill instantly in its pure form, but I have mixed it so that it will not kill you. It looks like clear syrup, so that is what it is mixed with. This poison is habit forming. It speeds the heart rate an extra 15 to 25 beats per minute, or as many as 10,000 extra beats a day. Also, it constricts the blood vessels and quickens breathing. George, would you sample this for us? Remember, a one-drop injection of this substance would cause death! Jean, you are so cooperative in class, would you mind doing this with George so he won't feel so uneasy? Also, when you use this product, this poison reaches your brain in only seven seconds. If it were not for this ingredient, people would probably not be interested in long-term use of the product we are analyzing.

Now, are you all ready to sample a few of the ingredients in this product? Before you answer, I want to give you some facts about this product. (Teacher can discuss or delete from this list, as is desirable.)

- If you start using this product now and continue, you can expect to lose six and one-half years of your life.
- If you use it a lot, your chances of dying between the ages of 26 and 65 are about twice as great as for those who do not use this product.
- Over 100,000 physicians have quit using this product.
- Before this day is over, approximately 4,500 young people will have tried or started using this product. By the time they graduate from high school, half the nation's teenagers will have used this product, 18 percent on a daily basis.
- About 1.5 billion of these products are used by 54 million Americans for an average of about 27 each day. The substances in this product are the primary cause of 360,000 known deaths a year, an average of 1,000 deaths a day.
- Using this product is one of the largest self-inflicted risks a person can take. It is responsible for more premature deaths and disability than any other known agent.
- More people die from using this product than seven times our annual death toll from highway accidents.
- A pregnant woman who uses this product may be affecting the health of her unborn child. Comparing users with nonusers, users have a higher percentage of stillbirths, a greater number of spontaneous abortions and premature births, and more of the infants die a few weeks after birth. The child's long-term physical and intellectual development may be adversely affected.
- This product will stain your teeth, and users often have bad breath.

You might say, "Surely a person can stop using this product whenever he or she wants to." My reply is "not necessarily." Remember the habit-forming substance we mentioned. Withdrawal symptoms for using this drug often include tension, irritability, restlessness, depression, anxiety, difficulty in concentrating, overeating, constipation, diarrhea, insomnia, and an intense craving for the product.

A few of the things I have not mentioned are:

- If you use this product, you are 1,000 percent more likely to die from lung cancer than those who do not use it.

- You are 500 percent more likely to die of chronic bronchitis and emphysema if you use it.
- Average users of this product are 70 percent more likely to die of coronary artery disease. They also tend to suffer from more respiratory infections, such as colds, than nonusers.
- Finally, this product is so dangerous that warning labels are required by law to be on the package.

If you were sent this product in the mail to sample, would you be likely to try it? If you received a box in the mail and, on the outside, these facts were printed, would you try it?

Ask students to tell you what they think the product is. End the lesson with a statement about the importance of making wise decisions that influence your life in positive ways. For example, you might say, "You have the power to influence your future in vital ways. The choice is up to you. No one can keep you from smoking, and it definitely will affect your entire life, however short or long it may be. Why start and get hooked? If you want to smoke, it is your life. But it is the only one you will ever get."

Materials Needed: four blown-up balloons (two representing carbon monoxide and two representing hydrogen cyanide), one small glass jar of flour (representing arsenic), two spoons, one cup of chocolate syrup (tar), and one cup of clear syrup (nicotine)

Processing Questions:

1. Who is responsible for your using or not using cigarettes?
2. What are some of the bad things found in cigarettes?
3. What are some of the scariest things about cigarettes?

○ **Integration:** Science

✓ **Assessment:** Students will be able to name at least three harmful chemicals found in cigarettes and explain how the chemicals affect the body.

Source: White and Rudisill 1987. Used with permission.

Mini-Documentary for Noninfectious and Infectious Diseases Grades 6–8

Valued Outcome: Students will be able to discuss cancer and the many forms it can take.

National Health Education Standards: 1, 3

Description of Strategy: The concept is for each child to be a "star" of his or her own television show. Set the activity up like the *60 Minutes* or *20/20* television programs, with students playing the roles of different "experts" who will be interviewed about a specific cancer topic. Videotaping the show allows everyone to see the production again. The videotape would be good for showing at Parent–Teacher Association functions.

Each student chooses a notecard that lists one particular topic on cancer. On this card are several questions that the student will research and discuss. They are also given a title for themselves and may choose their own names. As an example, a student chooses "cancerous tumors." Her card will read:

Dr. _____, a leading oncologist from Harvard.

1. What are tumors?
2. What are two different types of tumors?
3. Are there any special tests to detect tumors?
4. Do tumors exhibit any special symptoms?

The student must find the correct answers and be able to report her findings on "television." The following is a list of other potential cancer topics.

physiology of cancer cells	cancer of the prostate gland
most common causes of cancer	cancer of the testes
carcinogens	cancer of the larynx
warning signals of cancer	oral cancer
tests for cancer	skin cancer
treatments for cancer	cancer of the esophagus
most common cancers in women	cancer of the stomach
breast cancer	colorectal cancer
cancer of the uterus	thyroid cancer
most common cancers in males	Hodgkin's disease
lung cancer	leukemia
	cancer in children
	the American Cancer Society

Two students must be chosen to fill the spots of commentator and interviewer. (Students who have the most enthusiasm and originality seem to be best suited for these roles.) The commentator's job is to introduce the show and make some concluding statements at the end, whereas the interviewer is responsible for accepting the notecards from the specialists, introducing them, and asking the questions. A small "set" consisting of chairs, a table, and a lamp could be constructed so that the camera operator can focus on both of the "stars" at once. To avoid confusion and allow continuity of the show while videotaping, a list should be posted so that everyone knows when her interview is coming up. The specialist takes her seat on the "set," gives her notecard to the interviewer, and when all is quiet, the camera operator says "ready...action!"

As soon as the interview is finished, the next specialist comes up and gets ready to go. The interviewee may also wear a lab coat and a stethoscope to add to the total effect. If each interview lasts one to two minutes, the whole show can be completed in a single class period. Students may be evaluated on their degree of research and their ability to answer the questions correctly.

Even though cancer is a prime example of the topics that could be used, the mini-documentary does not need to be limited to cancer only. The same activity can be done using a variety of topics. The following is a list of possible topics for infectious diseases.

viruses	poliomyelitis
bacteria	measles
fungi	German measles
protozoa	mumps
pathogens	chicken pox
incubation period	common cold
active immunity	influenza
passive immunity	tuberculosis
diphtheria	infectious
whooping cough	mononucleosis
tetanus	infectious hepatitis

Materials Needed: videotaping equipment, books and pamphlets for students to research the various topics, small set for videotaping (students can make this)

Processing Questions:

1. What new information did you discover from the television program?
2. What do the various conditions discussed seem to have in common?
3. What are some things we might do to protect ourselves against such diseases?

✓ **Assessment:** Students will demonstrate knowledge about the cancer topic they researched.

Puzzles and Games

Listed here are several suggestions for supplementing or building a lesson. Obviously you must design and develop these activities to fit your students' abilities. They are great fun and provide excellent learning tools.

Heart Word Search   Grades 4–6

Valued Outcome: Students will be familiar with terms that relate to the anatomy of the heart and various conditions that affect it.

National Health Education Standard: 1

Description of Strategy: Instruct students to find and circle the terms listed in a word search.

Materials Needed: copy of word search worksheet and pencil for each student (sample word search available at www.pearsonhighered.com\anspaugh)

Processing Questions:

1. What are the names of the structures of the heart?
2. What are some common conditions that can affect the heart or circulatory system?

✓ **Assessment:** Students will be able to list anatomical terms for the heart and common conditions that can afflict the heart and circulatory system.

Cancer Crossword Puzzle   Grades 4–6

Valued Outcome: Students will be familiar with various cancer terms and definitions.

National Health Education Standard: 1

Description of Strategy: Distribute copies of a crossword puzzle and have each student complete one.

Materials Needed: copy of crossword puzzle worksheet and pencil for each student (Sample puzzle available at www.pearsonhighered.com\anspaugh)

Processing Questions:

1. What is one new term you learned from doing this puzzle?
2. What is one new definition you learned from doing this puzzle?

✓ **Assessment:** Students will demonstrate familiarity with cancer-related terms, such as tumor, malignant, benign, biopsy, carcinogen, and leukemia.

Hidden Message to Help Prevent Heart Disease   Grades 5–7

Valued Outcome: Students will understand various cardiac terms and health problems.

National Health Education Standards: 1, 7

Description of Strategy: Prepare a worksheet from the material here. Have each student complete the worksheet based on the following directions: Use the word list to fill in the blanks in the sentences. Then place each answer in the corresponding spaces in the right column of this page. The letters in the box reveal a hidden message.

pacemaker	hypertension	embolus
tobacco	cardiac	arteriosclerosis
aneurysm	veins	stroke

1. The heart is called the _____ muscle.
2. Cigarettes are made from _____.
3. Blood returns to the heart through the _____.
4. When a clot or vessel breakage occurs in the brain, that event is called a(n) _____.
5. High blood pressure is known as _____.
6. A free-floating blood clot is called a(n) _____.
7. _____ is the term for the collection of diseases characterized by hardening of the arteries.
8. The specialized group of cells called the sinoatrial node is also called the _____ of the heart.
9. Ballooning that occurs in weakened or damaged arterial walls is a(n) _____.

Place your answers here for the secret message.

1. — — — — — —
2. — — — — — —
3. — — — — —
4. — — — — —
5. — — — — — — — — — — — —
6. — — — — —
7. — — — — — — — — — — — —
8. — — — — — — — —
9. — — — — — — —

Materials Needed: copy of questionnaire and pencil for each student

Processing Questions:

1. What are two potentially life-threatening events that can occur in the cardiovascular system
2. What is the hidden message in the puzzle?

✓ **Assessment:** Students will be able to define five terms related to cardiac health.

17 Nutrition

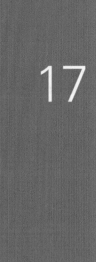

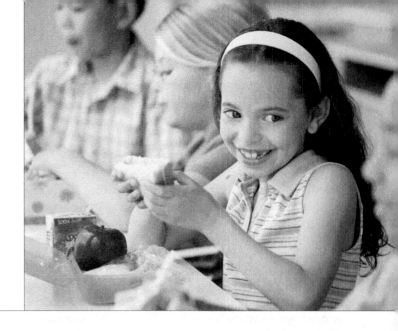

Valued Outcomes

After completion of this chapter, you should be able to:

- Discuss the *Healthy People 2020* objectives for nutrition.
- Describe children's eating patterns.
- Explain the economic, personal, and lifestyle factors that determine our food choices.
- Discuss the *Dietary Guidelines for Americans, 2010*.
- Discuss categories of nutrients.
- Understand and use the Nutrition Facts panel.
- Discuss vitamins and minerals.
- Compare food selections from fast-food restaurants.
- Discuss USDA's MyPlate and ChooseMyPlate.gov.
- Describe nutritional problems, such as undernutrition, anorexia nervosa, and bulimia.
- Explain the factors that have led to an increase in childhood obesity.
- Read and understand a food label.
- Discuss food quackery.

Reflections

As you read this chapter, keep in mind the myriad factors (physical, social, emotional, and cultural) that affect nutritional health and fitness. Use this information to compose a complete plan for your fitness and wellness, including diet, exercise plan, change of any negative habits, stress reduction, and so on.

The Food and Nutrition Service (FNS) identifies schools that have made changes to
1. improve the quality of the foods served,
2. provide students with nutrition education, and
3. provide students with physical education and opportunities for physical activity.

—USDA, 2011

NATIONAL HEALTH EDUCATION STANDARDS

1. Students will comprehend concepts related to health promotion and disease prevention to enhance health.
2. Students will analyze the influence of family, peers, culture, media, technology, and other factors on health behaviors.
3. Students will demonstrate the ability to access valid information and products and services to enhance health.
4. Students will demonstrate the ability to use interpersonal communication skills to enhance health and avoid or reduce health risks.
5. Students will demonstrate the ability to use decision-making skills to enhance health.
7. Students will demonstrate the ability to practice health-enhancing behaviors and avoid or reduce risks.
8. Students will demonstrate the ability to advocate for personal, family, and community health.

Knowledge and Nutrition

Today, more is known about nutrition than at any other time in history, yet this knowledge has not translated into proper nutritional and/or lifestyle behavior for many people. The United States is a food-affluent society, yet many living here—and not just the poor—are malnourished (i.e., they have imbalanced nutrition from poor diet, overeating, or improper absorption). An unwillingness to alter one's lifestyle to meet sound nutritional standards and concessions to convenience are often at the heart of the problem. In our fast-paced society, people frequently skip meals, especially breakfast, or opt to eat a poorly balanced meal at a fast-food restaurant. Despite the fact that a well-nourished student is more apt to reach his or her full potential—physically, mentally, and intellectually—many parents and teachers fail to provide good examples for their students concerning nutritional habits.

Nutrition education has been included as a priority by the U.S. Department of Health and Human Services in the Year 2020 Health Objectives for the Nation, as listed by the U.S. Surgeon General (2011). (See the Health Highlight box on page 295.) School nutrition programs can positively affect student's eating habits, leading to healthy eating patterns that allow students to achieve their full potential, optimal development, and lifelong health and well-being (USDA 2011). Refer to the Health Highlight box on page 297 for detailed information on the *Dietary Guidelines for Americans*, 2010. Helping students develop sound nutritional habits should be a major goal in elementary health instruction. To accomplish this, teachers must do more than simply provide information; they must counter the impact of television commercials and other sources. Also, they must help students recognize that although the food they eat is strongly influenced by their culture and their lifestyle, they can learn to control these influences. Teachers must also dispel misconceptions associated with food and nutrition, help students become informed consumers, and help them develop a sense of the importance of nutrition.

Food Habits and Customs

Every culture has its own food habits and customs. Approaches to nutrition are based in part on the food resources available. Food habits and customs in the United States reflect the multicultural nature of our society. At one time, there were significant regional differences in cooking and food preferences. Seafood was a major part of the diet on the East Coast. Wild game provided much of the meat eaten in the rural South. Mexican and Indian cultures influenced the cuisine of the Southwest. Today, these regional differences have faded, largely as a result of refrigeration and modern transportation. It is now almost as easy to get fresh seafood in Kansas as it is in Massachusetts. Cultural intermixing has also diminished regional differences, while at the same time expanding the range of dishes commonly eaten. Pasta, for instance, is no longer eaten only by Americans of Italian heritage. Chinese, French, German, Mexican, and Middle Eastern dishes have also become popular.

■ Economic, Personal, and Lifestyle Factors

As an affluent, multiethnic nation, we have a greater variety of foods and dishes to choose from than almost any other people on earth. This does not mean, however, that Americans can afford to eat anything they like. Inflation has influenced the eating habits of all Americans, rich and poor alike—but especially the poor. Those living near or below the poverty level often must subsist on cheap starchy foods, which are filling but not particularly nutritious.

Although economics influences the U.S. diet, as it does the diet of every nation, most Americans cannot blame lack of money for poor nutritional habits. Instead, we must look for the reasons in personal preferences and lifestyles. Personal preference for a food often is formed by reasons that have little or nothing to do with the nourishment that will be provided by that food. For example, parents typically pass their food preferences on to their children. People develop dislikes for foods because of bad experiences, such as an allergic response or gastrointestinal upset. The most popular foods eaten by one's subculture and peer group also influence food choices. Finally, a food might be chosen because of the way it looks, smells, and tastes.

The national lifestyle also influences our nutritional habits. When the United States was mostly a rural, agrarian society, breakfast was a major meal, and the main meal of the day was served at noon. These two meals provided the necessary energy for performing farm labor and chores. Evening dinner was typically a lighter meal. Today, the reverse is true. Most Americans eat a light breakfast, and some skip breakfast entirely. Lunch is also a light meal, often eaten in haste. The largest meal of the day is consumed in the evening, because there is more time to prepare and eat it. Unfortunately, this meal is usually followed by general physical inactivity and sleep. This is one reason why so many Americans are overweight. In addition, many overspice their foods, especially with salt and sugar.

Breakfast seems to be the most frequently missed meal of the day, even though research has suggested that missing breakfast can affect concentration, ability to learn, and overall health. Recent studies have confirmed that eating breakfast helps children learn better. Students who eat breakfast demonstrate improved math, reading, and standardized test scores. They are also more likely to behave better in school and get along with their peers, find it easier to pay attention and to perform problem-solving tasks, and are less likely to have absences and incidents of tardiness than those who do not eat breakfast (USDA 2011).

Various lifestyle habits, including many behavioral and environmental factors, have led to an enormous increase in childhood obesity. In fact, childhood obesity has more than tripled in the past thirty years. According to

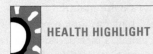

Healthy People 2020 Objectives for Nutrition: Select Nutrition and Weight Status Objectives

Healthier Food Access

- Increase the number of states with nutrition standards for foods and beverages provided to preschool-aged children in child care.
- Increase the proportion of schools that offer nutritious foods and beverages outside of school meals.
- Increase the proportion of schools that do not sell or offer calorically sweetened beverages to students.
- Increase the proportion of school districts that require schools to make fruits or vegetables available whenever other food is offered or sold.

Health Care and Worksite Settings

- Increase the proportion of primary care physicians who regularly measure the body mass index of their patients.
- Increase the proportion of physician office visits that include counseling or education related to nutrition or weight.
- Increase the proportion of physician visits made by all child or adult patients that include counseling about nutrition or diet.
- Increase the proportion of worksites that offer nutrition or weight management classes or counseling.

Weight Status

- Increase the proportion of adults who are at a healthy weight.
- Reduce the proportion of adults who are obese.
- Reduce the proportion of children and adolescents who are considered obese.

Food Insecurity

- Eliminate very low food security among children.
- Reduce household food insecurity and in so doing reduce hunger.

Food and Nutrient Consumption

- Increase the contribution of fruits to the diets of the population aged two years and older.
- Increase the variety and contribution of vegetables to the diets of the population aged two years and older.
- Increase the contribution of whole grains to the diets of the population aged two years and older.
- Reduce consumption of calories from solid fats and added sugars in the population aged two years and older.
- Reduce consumption of saturated fat in the population aged two years and older.
- Reduce consumption of sodium in the population aged two years and older.
- Increase consumption of calcium in the population aged two years and older.

(*Source:* U.S. Department of Health and Human Services 2011. *Healthy People 2020*: Nutrition and Weight Status. Full text available at www .healthypeople.gov/2020/topicsobjectives2020/ pdfs/NutritionandWeight.pdf)

---

the Department of Health and Human Services (2010), the prevalence of obesity among children aged six to eleven years increased from 6.5 percent in 1980 to 19.6 percent in 2008 and the prevalence of obesity among those aged twelve to nineteen years increased from 5.0 percent to 18.1 percent during the same period. Health impacts of childhood obesity include increased risk factors for cardiovascular disease, greater risk for bone and joint problems, sleep apnea, and social and psychological problems. It is also more likely for an obese youth to become an overweight or obese adult who is at higher risk for health problems such as heart disease, type 2 diabetes, stroke, and several types of cancer. Healthy lifestyle habits can lower the risk of obesity and related diseases (U.S. Department of Health and Human Services 2010).

Teachers should emphasize the value of a balanced, nutritious lunch and a reasonable evening meal. This is not to suggest that teachers should criticize the eating patterns of any student's family or any religious dietary restrictions a family might have, but they can be a source of information about sound nutritional practices and encourage students to consider changes in their diet that could lead to improved nutrition. Teachers can also stimulate students' curiosity about trying new dishes that could add needed variety to their diets.

Further, teachers should emphasize that snacking on junk food, such as candy, may spoil a student's appetite for a regular meal as well as contribute to tooth decay. Although children can benefit from snacking, they often fall into the habit of constantly eating the same foods. Snacks sometimes even substitute for, rather than supplement, children's regular meals, and these snacks may not provide the variety of nutrients these youngsters need. Thus, while snacking is regarded as a potential asset to the child's diet, it can become a liability if it results in more calories than are needed. Most commercial snacks are high in fat, sugar, or salt and have few healthful nutrients.

According to the U.S. Department of Agriculture (USDA 2011), in 2009 over 11.1 million children participated in the school breakfast program every day. Of those, 9.1 million children received their meals free or at a reduced price.

Food is one of the delights of every civilization. In many cultures, preparation of some dishes is an art. Eating a fine meal is an aesthetic experience, not just fulfillment of nutritional requirements, and even the simplest dish can provide great pleasure. Teachers can use this positive approach in presenting nutritional concepts. Too often nutrition is taught as a grim and dry subject, divorced from the human perspective. No wonder students often emerge from health education with scorn for nutritional principles; they associate nutrition with the imagined somber atmosphere of a health food store!

Nutrients

The most basic function of food is to provide nutrients to the body. **Nutrients** are the substances in food needed to support life functions.

There are six classes of essential nutrients: carbohydrates, protein, lipids, vitamins, minerals, and water. One vital role of nutrients is to provide energy that the body needs. This energy, produced as a by-product of food consumption, is measured in calories. A **kilocalorie** (or **Calorie**) is the amount of heat energy required to raise the temperature of one kilogram of water one degree Celsius. All foods have specific caloric values, and a given amount of food will produce a certain number of calories when broken down by the body.

The number of calories needed daily by the body depends on two factors: (1) the individual's basal metabolism and (2) the amount of energy expended in daily activities. **Basal metabolism** is the minimum amount of energy required by the body to maintain essential body functions (e.g., to maintain a normal body temperature, muscle tone, respiration) when at rest. The amount of energy expended by an individual varies, depending on his or her activities. Thus, someone who engages in heavy physical labor each day needs more calories than someone who works in an office. Young students need fewer calories per day than active adults because of the difference in body sizes.

During periods of rapid growth, children also need more calories. For example, a ten-year-old boy requires an average daily intake of about 2,200 calories, with this amount rising to 2,900 calories by age thirteen. A girl requires an average daily intake of 2,200 calories at age ten and 2,400 calories at age thirteen.

Three categories of nutrients provide caloric energy: carbohydrates, lipids, and proteins. Together, they comprise most of the foods we eat.

▪ Carbohydrates

Foods rich in carbohydrates form about half of the typical American diet. Carbohydrates are either simple sugars, derived from such foods as sugar and honey, or more complex compounds, derived from such foods as cereals and potatoes. For example, the sweet taste of corn and peas is due to the presence of carbohydrate compounds.

Carbohydrates are found in foods as monosaccharides, disaccharides, and polysaccharides. The *monosaccharides* are glucose, galactose (found in human breast milk), and fructose, all of which are found in fruits and honey.

The *disaccharides* are sucrose (a combination of glucose and fructose found in table sugar, bananas, green peas, and sweet potatoes), lactose (a combination of glucose and galactose found in milk and milk products), and maltose (a combination of two glucoses used in candy flavor and brewing beer). Many adults, especially Asian Americans and African Americans, suffer from *lactose intolerance*. In other words, undigested lactose is not absorbed and remains in the gastrointestinal tract, resulting in bloating, a large amount of gas, and abdominal cramping. Individuals with lactose intolerance may find that consuming dairy products in small amounts, or using digestive aids that help break down lactose, can help them avoid these uncomfortable symptoms.

The *polysaccharides* are composed of many monosaccharide molecules and are categorized as: (1) glycogen (which is synthesized in the liver and muscles and serves as a reserve source of blood glucose), (2) cellulose (found in many vegetables but indigestible by humans), and (3) starch (found in plant seeds, cereal grains, and some vegetables).

Carbohydrates are broken down into their components, and the metabolism of glucose is the most significant source of energy. (Glucose is the *only* energy source used by brain cells and acts as the most common energy "currency.") Four calories are produced per gram of carbohydrates. If carbohydrates are not abundant in the diet, protein and fat have to be metabolized to produce needed energy. Carbohydrates must be constantly replenished in the blood, either by eating or by breaking down glycogen that is stored in the liver and muscles.

Carbohydrates are important in a child's diet and should comprise approximately 60 percent of total caloric intake. Foods rich in carbohydrates include rice, pasta, noodles, bread, breakfast cereals, and potatoes. Many vegetables, fruits, and fruit juices are primarily carbohydrates. Although candy and cookies are sources of carbohydrates, the refined sugar they contain contributes to tooth decay and gum disease and does not provide additional nutrients; they also contain a high proportion of fat. Fruits, vegetables, juices, and milk make healthier snacks, but even these foods contain sugar. Thus, the individual should brush and floss immediately after the meal or at least rinse out the mouth with water. Brushing and flossing before bedtime are especially important in reducing tooth decay.

Dietary Fiber. **Dietary fiber** is a generic term for nondigestible carbohydrates (including cellulose, lignin, and pectin) found in plants; it has important health benefits in childhood, especially in promoting normal laxation (bowel movements). The American Dietetic Association (2009) recommends that children consume dietary fiber from a variety of plant foods; following this recommendation will lead to less likelihood of developing several chronic diseases. The appropriate kinds and amounts of dietary fiber for children are unknown, but the "age plus 5" rule (the child's age plus 5 grams per day of fiber) is commonly used to determine the recommended amount (ADA 2009).

The *Dietary Guidelines for Americans* is published jointly by the Department of Health and Human Services (HHS) and the Department of Agriculture (USDA). The following outlines some of the general guidelines.

Balancing Calories to Manage Weight

- Prevent and/or reduce overweight and obesity through improved eating and physical activity behaviors.
- Control total calorie intake to manage body weight. For people who are overweight or obese, this will mean consuming fewer calories from foods and beverages.
- Increase physical activity and reduce time spent in sedentary behaviors.
- Maintain appropriate calorie balance during each stage of life—childhood, adolescence, adulthood, pregnancy and breastfeeding, and older age.

Foods and Food Components to Reduce

- Reduce daily sodium intake to less than 2,300 milligrams (mg) and further reduce intake to 1,500 mg among persons who are fifty-one and older and those of any age who are African American or have hypertension, diabetes, or chronic kidney disease.
- Consume less than 10 percent of calories from saturated fatty acids by replacing them with monounsaturated and polyunsaturated fatty acids.
- Consume less than 300 mg per day of dietary cholesterol.
- Keep *trans* fatty acid consumption as low as possible by limiting foods that contain synthetic sources of *trans* fats, such as partially hydrogenated oils, and by limiting other solid fats.
- Reduce the intake of calories from solid fats and added sugars.
- Limit the consumption of foods that contain refined grains, especially refined grain foods that contain solid fats, added sugars, and sodium.
- If alcohol is consumed, it should be consumed in moderation—up to one drink per day for women and two drinks per day for men—and only by adults of legal drinking age.

Foods and Nutrients to Increase

Individuals should meet the following recommendations as part of a healthy eating pattern while staying within their calorie needs.

- Increase vegetable and fruit intake.
- Eat a variety of vegetables, especially dark-green and red and orange vegetables and beans and peas.
- Consume at least half of all grains as whole grains. Increase whole-grain intake by replacing refined grains with whole grains.
- Increase intake of fat-free or low-fat milk and milk products, such as milk, yogurt, cheese, or fortified soy beverages.
- Choose a variety of protein foods, which include seafood, lean meat and poultry, eggs, beans and peas, soy products, and unsalted nuts and seeds.
- Increase the amount and variety of seafood consumed by choosing seafood in place of some meat and poultry.
- Replace protein foods that are higher in solid fats with choices that are lower in solid fats and calories and/or are sources of oils.
- Use oils to replace solid fats where possible.
- Choose foods that provide more potassium, dietary fiber, calcium, and vitamin D, which are nutrients of concern in American diets. These foods include vegetables, fruits, whole grains, and milk and milk products.

Recommendations for Specific Population Groups

Women capable of becoming pregnant:

- Choose foods that supply heme iron, which is more readily absorbed by the body, additional iron sources, and enhancers of iron absorption such as vitamin C-rich foods.
- Consume 400 micrograms (mcg) per day of synthetic folic acid (from fortified foods and/or supplements) in addition to food forms of folate from a varied diet.

Women who are pregnant or breast-feeding:

- Consume 8 to 12 ounces of seafood per week from a variety of seafood types.
- Due to their high methyl mercury content, limit white (albacore) tuna to 6 ounces per week and do not eat the following four types of fish: tilefish, shark, swordfish, and king mackerel.
- If pregnant, take an iron supplement, as recommended by an obstetrician or other health care provider.

Individuals aged fifty years and older:

- Consume foods fortified with vitamin B12, such as fortified cereals, or dietary supplements.

Building Healthy Eating Patterns

- Select an eating pattern that meets nutrient needs over time at an appropriate calorie level.
- Account for all foods and beverages consumed and assess how they fit within a total healthy eating pattern.
- Follow food safety recommendations when preparing and eating foods to reduce the risk of foodborne illnesses.

(*Source:* United States Department of Agriculture, May 2011. Dietary Guidelines 2010, http://www.cnpp.usda.gov/Publications /DietaryGuidelines/2010/PolicyDoc/ExecSumm .pdf.)

Despite intensive efforts by nutritionists, manufacturers, and others in the health care industry to promote the virtues of fiber, intakes remain below the recommended level. Research has established that diets low in fat and high in fiber-containing grain products, fruits, and vegetables can reduce some types of cancer. Unfortunately, U.S. diets tend to be high in fat and low in grain products, fruits, and vegetables. The dietary goals promoted by the U.S. Food and Drug Administration (FDA) and other federal government agencies and professional health organizations recommend decreased consumption of fats; maintenance of desirable body weight; and an increased consumption of fruits, vegetables, and grain products (USDA 2011).

▪ Proteins

Protein means primary, and no organism can live, and almost no biological process can take place, without it. A protein molecule is composed of smaller structures called *amino acids*. Eight amino acids (nine in infants) are termed *essential*, which means they must be provided by the diet; the remainder are termed *nonessential*, which means they are synthesized by the body. (All twenty amino acids are required by the body for proper nutrition.) These amino acids are building blocks necessary for performing many body functions. Proteins are present in every cell, in enzymes, and in body secretions. Proteins provide calories but also serve other important and complex functions. They help build new cells and tissues in growing children; repair damaged tissues; maintain tissues that are already built; and play a role in the manufacture of blood, enzymes, hormones, and human milk. Even antibodies, which combat infection, are synthesized from proteins in response to infectious agents.

Proteins provide four calories per gram. Proteins should constitute about 10 to 12 percent of a child's total caloric intake. Most children require approximately 60g of protein daily. Milk and meat products (including poultry) are excellent sources of protein.

If a person eats a vegetarian diet, enough protein must be ingested to support normal growth and development. This requires **complementary protein ingestion**, a dietary strategy that ensures that each food supplies some amino acids that the others lack. For example, corn is deficient in the amino acids isoleucine and lysine, so it is often eaten with beans (which lack the tryptophan and methionine found in corn); similarly, wheat is deficient in lysine, so it may be combined with beans for nutritional completeness. Cereal grains, vegetables, and fruits contain vegetable protein, which must be augmented by other protein sources, as in tortillas and beans combined. Peanut protein is combined with wheat, oats, corn, rice, or coconut, and soy protein is combined with corn, wheat, rye, or sesame. Non-meat sources of protein include soybeans, dried beans, nuts, and dairy products.

▪ Lipids

Lipids are an important part of our diet and are required for good health. **Lipids** are organic compounds that do not readily dissolve in water; based on their solubility, they are classified into triglycerides (more commonly known as fats), phospholipids, and sterols. The energy of *triglycerides* provides much of the stored energy of the body, and the fat deposits insulate body organs against changes in environmental temperature and protect the organs and underlying tissues by acting as a shock absorber. Fats in foods provide flavor and even contribute to satiety because the rate at which a meal is emptied from the stomach is related to the fat content, and the higher the fat content of a meal, the slower the food empties from the stomach.

Phospholipids are an essential component of all cell membranes and thus are ubiquitous throughout the human body. The most well known **sterol** is cholesterol, which, despite its reputation, plays several important roles in the body.

Triglycerides (Fats). The triglycerides are commonly called **fats** (which are solid at room temperature) and **oils** (which are liquid at room temperature). They are a group of chemical compounds that contain fatty acids, often in very long strands, and at 9 calories per gram, are the most concentrated source of energy in the diet. Some fat is needed in the diet to supply essential fatty acids to build new fat molecules, and these fat molecules are stored in deposits throughout the body, including a layer just below the skin, where they can be accessed when energy is needed for growth or body maintenance.

There are two main types of fatty acids: saturated and unsaturated (the latter is further categorized into monounsaturated and polyunsaturated fatty acids). All fatty acids are molecules composed mostly of carbon and hydrogen atoms. A **saturated fatty acid** has the maximum possible number of hydrogen atoms attached to every carbon atom, so it is said to be saturated with hydrogen atoms; there are only single bonds between the carbon atoms. Some fatty acids have a double bond between two of the carbons and thus lack a pair of the hydrogen atoms found in saturated fatty acids; these double-bonded carbons are called units of unsaturation (since some hydrogen atoms are missing). If only one pair of hydrogen atoms is missing, the molecule is a **monounsaturated fatty acid**; if more than one pair of hydrogen atoms is missing, the molecule is a **polyunsaturated fatty acid**. Two types of polyunsaturated fatty acid, omega-3 and omega-6, are identified on the basis of where these double bonds and missing hydrogen atoms occur. The more saturated a fat is (i.e., the more hydrogen atoms and the fewer the double bonds between carbon atoms that it has), the more solid it is at room temperature.

***Trans* fatty acids** are by-products of partial hydrogenation, a process by which some of the missing hydrogen atoms are put back into polyunsaturated fats during food processing. Some of the hydrogenated fatty acids take on a straighter structure as hydrogen atoms are added on diagonally opposite ends of the double carbon bond: these are the *trans* fatty acids. The straightened fatty acids pack more tightly together, so the resulting hydrogenated vegetable oils (such as vegetable shortening and margarine) are solid at room temperature.

Saturated fatty acids are mostly found in foods of animal origin such as animal fat, beef, butter, chicken eggs, and whole milk. Unsaturated fatty acids are mostly found in foods of plant origin, including vegetable oils (corn, olive, soybean, peanut, and safflower oils) and some seafoods. Olive and canola oils are particularly high in monounsaturated fats; most other vegetable oils, nuts, and high-fat fish are sources of polyunsaturated fats.

Cholesterol. All the cholesterol the body needs is made by the liver. Cholesterol is used to build cell membranes and brain and other nervous tissue. Among other functions, cholesterol helps the body produce steroid hormones needed for the regulation of blood sugar, salt and water balance, production of bile acids needed for digestion, and reproduction.

A person's cholesterol number refers to the total amount of cholesterol in the blood. Cholesterol is measured in milligrams per deciliter (mg/dL) of blood. (A deciliter is a tenth of a liter.) According to the American Heart Association, if an adult has no other risk factors for heart disease, a desirable total blood cholesterol level is below 200 mg/dL. A total of 200–239 mg/dL of total cholesterol is considered borderline-high risk, and the levels of low-density cholesterol, high-density cholesterol, and triglycerides would need to be examined. A total score of 240 mg/dL or higher is considered to be a high risk, meaning that you have twice the risk of coronary heart disease as people whose cholesterol level is desirable (200 mg/dL) (American Heart Association 2011).

Cholesterol is transported in the bloodstream in large molecules of fat and protein called **lipoproteins**. Cholesterol carried in low-density lipoproteins is called **LDL cholesterol**; most cholesterol in the blood is of this type. Cholesterol carried in high-density lipoproteins is called **HDL cholesterol**. LDL cholesterol and HDL cholesterol act differently in the body. A high level of LDL cholesterol in the blood increases the risk of fatty deposits forming in the arteries, which in turn increases the risk of a heart attack; thus, LDL cholesterol is often referred to as the bad cholesterol. On the other hand, an elevated level of HDL cholesterol seems to have a protective effect against heart disease, so HDL cholesterol is often called "good" cholesterol. A common misconception is that people can improve their cholesterol numbers by eating good cholesterol; however, in food, all cholesterol is the same. In blood, whether cholesterol is good or bad depends only on the type of lipoprotein (HDL or LDL) that is carrying it.

Recommended Blood Levels of Lipoproteins and Triglycerides. In 1992, a panel of medical experts convened by the National Institutes of Health (NIH) recommended that individuals should have their HDL levels checked along with their total cholesterol. According to the National Heart, Lung, and Blood Institute (NHLBI), part of NIH, a healthy person who is not at high risk for heart disease and whose total cholesterol level is in the normal range (around 200 mg/dL) should have an HDL level of more than 40 mg/dL and an LDL level of less than 130 mg/dL in order to minimize the risk of heart disease.

The NIH panel also advised that individuals with high total cholesterol or other risk factors for coronary heart disease should have their triglyceride levels checked along with their HDL levels. NHLBI considers a triglyceride level below 200 mg/dL to be normal. It is not clear whether high levels of triglycerides alone increase an individual's risk of heart disease. However, they may be an important clue that someone is at risk of heart disease for other reasons. Many people who have elevated triglycerides also have high LDL or low HDL levels. People with diabetes or kidney disease—two conditions that increase the risk of heart disease—are also prone to having high triglycerides.

Health Implications and Diet. The vital roles of lipids are sometimes overlooked because of the association of fats with cardiovascular problems. Most people are aware that high levels of saturated fat and cholesterol in the diet are linked to increased blood cholesterol levels and a greater risk for heart disease and certain cancers. In countries where the average person's blood cholesterol level is less than 180 mg/dL, very few people develop atherosclerosis or have heart attacks. In many industrialized countries where diets are heavy with meat and dairy products (and thus contain a lot of saturated fats) and a lot of people have blood cholesterol levels above 220 mg/dL, coronary heart disease is the leading cause of illness and death and there is a high rate of certain cancers that have been linked to high fat intake. Blood lipids are major risk factors for heart disease, and their concentrations are modulated by both genetic and environmental factors. Among the latter, dietary habits (most specifically the consumption of large quantities of dietary fat and cholesterol) play an important role.

However, high-fat diets and high rates of heart disease don't inevitably go hand-in-hand. More Americans are now eating less fat, less saturated fat, and fewer cholesterol-rich foods than in the recent past, and fewer people are dying from the most common form of heart disease. Still, many people continue to eat high-fat diets, the number of overweight people has increased, and the risk of heart disease and fat-related cancers remains high.

Fat, whether from plant or animal sources, contains twice the number of calories of an equal amount of carbohydrate or protein (9 calories per g of fat as compared with 4 calories per g of protein or carbohydrate). By the time a person reaches the age of two, fat should comprise only 30 percent of the total calories consumed. (Infants and young children should not restrict dietary fat intake.) The upper limit on the grams of fat in a diet will depend on the actual amount of calories needed, and cutting back on fat can help reduce the number of calories consumed.

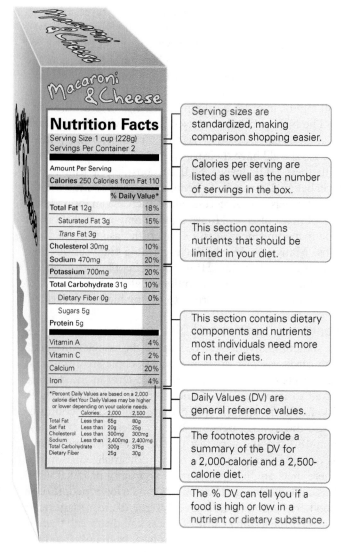

Nutrition Facts
Serving Size 1 cup (228g)
Servings Per Container 2

Amount Per Serving
Calories 250 Calories from Fat 110

	% Daily Value*
Total Fat 12g	18%
Saturated Fat 3g	15%
Trans Fat 3g	
Cholesterol 30mg	10%
Sodium 470mg	20%
Potassium 700mg	20%
Total Carbohydrate 31g	10%
Dietary Fiber 0g	0%
Sugars 5g	
Protein 5g	
Vitamin A	4%
Vitamin C	2%
Calcium	20%
Iron	4%

*Percent Daily Values are based on a 2,000 calorie diet. Your Daily Values may be higher or lower depending on your calorie needs.

		Calories:	2,000	2,500
Total Fat	Less than		65g	80g
Sat Fat	Less than		20g	25g
Cholesterol	Less than		300mg	300mg
Sodium	Less than		2,400mg	2,400mg
Total Carbohydrate			300g	375g
Dietary Fiber			25g	30g

Serving sizes are standardized, making comparison shopping easier.

Calories per serving are listed as well as the number of servings in the box.

This section contains nutrients that should be limited in your diet.

This section contains dietary components and nutrients most individuals need more of in their diets.

Daily Values (DV) are general reference values.

The footnotes provide a summary of the DV for a 2,000-calorie and a 2,500-calorie diet.

The % DV can tell you if a food is high or low in a nutrient or dietary substance.

Figure 17.1
Interpreting Nutrition Labels

For example, at 2,000 calories per day, the suggested upper limit of calories from fat is about 600. Sixty-five grams of fat contribute about 600 calories (65 g of fat × 9 calories per g = 585 calories). On the Nutrition Facts panel (see Figure 17.1), 65 g of fat is the maximum Daily Value for a 2,000 calorie intake.

Fats contain both saturated and unsaturated (monounsaturated and polyunsaturated) fatty acids. Saturated fat raises blood cholesterol more than other forms of fat. Reducing saturated fat to less than 10 percent of the total calories will help lower blood cholesterol level; on the Nutrition Facts panel, 20g of saturated fat (9 percent of caloric intake) is the recommended Daily Value for a 2,000 calorie diet. The fats from meat, milk, and milk products are the main sources of saturated fats in most diets. Many bakery products are also sources of saturated fats, and vegetable oils supply smaller amounts as well. Polyunsaturated and monounsaturated fats do not promote the formation of artery-clogging fatty deposits

the way saturated fats do. Both kinds of unsaturated fats reduce the levels of LDL cholesterol when they replace saturated fats in the diet; however, today many researchers believe that polyunsaturated fats may simultaneously decrease the beneficial HDL cholesterol levels. For example, omega-6 polyunsaturated fatty acids have been found in some studies to reduce both LDL and HDL levels in the blood. Linoleic acid, an essential nutrient (one that the body cannot make for itself) and a component of corn, soybean, and safflower oil, is an omega-6 fatty acid. Partially hydrogenated vegetable oils containing polyunsaturated *trans* fatty acids may raise blood cholesterol levels, though not as much as saturated fat.

Oils rich in monounsaturated fats, such as olive and canola oil, tend to lower LDL cholesterol without affecting HDL cholesterol levels. The fats in most fish are low in saturated fatty acids, and fish such as mackerel and salmon (as well as soybean and canola oil) contain omega-3 fatty acids, which are polyunsaturated fatty acids that lower LDL and triglyceride levels and decrease the risk of heart disease.

The Nutrition Facts panel lists the Daily Value for dietary cholesterol at less than 300 mg. Because dietary cholesterol comes largely from animal sources, many of which are also high in saturated fats, an individual generally can keep cholesterol intake at or below this level by eating more grain products (the less processing, the better), vegetables, and fruits, and by limiting intake of animal-based products.

Research focusing on the effects of different combinations of dietary fats and cholesterol on blood lipid levels and removal of cholesterol from cells indicates that, when consuming diets low in cholesterol, the lipid levels in blood are better in subjects consuming high levels of oleic acid (a monounsaturated fatty acid found in almost all natural fats and promoted in the Mediterranean diet) than in those consuming low-fat diets. (The Mediterranean diet promotes the use of monounsaturated fatty acids, olive oil, and seafoods.) This suggests that reducing the intake of dietary cholesterol can lower blood lipids.

What, then, *is* a healthy diet? Scientific evidence shows that reducing the consumption of saturated fat, *trans* fat, and dietary cholesterol produces a healthier diet and reduces the risk of coronary heart disease (FDA 2005). Select foods that are lower in total fat, solid fat, saturated fat, and cholesterol, which means eating fewer foods of animal origin (such as meat and whole-milk dairy products) and replacing those dietary calories by eating more grain products, fruits, vegetables, low-fat milk products or other calcium-rich foods, and more beans, lean meat, poultry, fish, and other protein-rich foods.

▪ Water

In considering nutrition, water is often overlooked, but it is second only to oxygen in importance to body functioning. A person can survive longer without food than without water; there can be no life without water.

Water is an essential component of body structure. It also acts as a solvent for minerals and other physiologically important compounds. In the body, it transports nutrients to and waste products from the cells and helps regulate body temperature. Water comes from fluids and solids in the diet and also is produced by the metabolic processing of energy nutrients within the tissues. Foods high in water content include fruits and vegetables; foods with low water content include meat. The amount of activity and the climate are important factors influencing the amount of water a person needs. Because children usually participate in more physical activities, they perspire more and therefore need more water than do many adults. Water is also lost through exhaled air. The recommended daily intake is the equivalent of six to eight glasses of water. Much of this is gained from solid foods.

▪ Minerals

The body needs organic compounds, such as carbohydrates, fats, and proteins, for proper nutrition, but it also needs inorganic materials such as minerals. These inorganic elements are present in the body in small amounts, but they play a vital role in nutrition. The **major minerals** needed by the body are calcium, phosphorus, potassium, sulfur, sodium, chloride, and magnesium. Food sources for these major minerals are:

- **calcium**—milk, cheese, sardines, salmon, green vegetables
- **phosphorus**—milk, cheese, lean meat
- **potassium**—oranges, bananas, dried fruits
- **sulfur**—eggs, poultry, fish
- **sodium**—table salt, beef, eggs, cheese
- **chloride**—table salt, meat
- **magnesium**—green vegetables, whole grains

Trace minerals are required in lesser amounts, and include iron, zinc, selenium, magnesium, copper, iodine, fluorine, chromium, molybdenum, and manganese.

Minerals function in the body in several ways. After the organic compounds have been oxidized, minerals remain to form actual body parts. For example, calcium, magnesium, and phosphorus are components of the bones and teeth. Minerals also act as regulators by contributing to the water and electrolyte balance of the body and are necessary to certain body functions, such as the transmission of nerve impulses. Minerals contribute to the osmotic pressure of body fluids and to the maintenance of neutrality—the acid–base balance of the blood and body tissues. Finally, they make possible the normal rhythm in the heartbeat.

Elevated amounts of some minerals may cause health problems. For example, elevated levels of sodium are associated with high blood pressure and cardiovascular disease.

Sodium. Salt and other sodium compounds are used to preserve, flavor, and stabilize other ingredients when food is being processed; they also occur in smaller amounts in unprocessed food. As a result, many processed foods already contain the amount of sodium the Nutrition Facts panel recommends for daily intake.

In the body, sodium plays an essential role in the regulation of fluids and blood pressure. Studies of diverse populations have shown that a high sodium intake is associated with higher blood pressure. Although there is no way at present to tell who might develop high blood pressure from eating too much sodium, individuals can reduce their risk of high blood pressure by reducing their consumption of sodium. According to the FDA, most Americans consume more salt than they need. The current recommendation is to consume less than 2,300 milligrams of sodium a day; that equals about 1 teaspoon of table salt a day. Sodium, rather than salt, is the term that will generally appear in dietary recommendations and food labels because it is the sodium component of salt that is most relevant for human health (USDA 2011). Fresh fruits and vegetables have very little sodium. Use herbs and spices to flavor food, and read the Nutrition Facts panels to compare and help identify foods lower in sodium. Table 17.1 below provides some tips on cutting down salt intake.

Other factors may interact with sodium to affect blood pressure, so reducing sodium intake alone may not be sufficient to control high blood pressure. Consuming less salt or sodium is not harmful and therefore can be recommended for the healthy normal adult.

Iron. Iron is an essential mineral needed for the proper functioning of the human body. This mineral is used in many cell functions and helps carry oxygen from the lungs throughout the body. Without proper iron intake,

Table 17.1 **Low-Sodium Alternatives**	
Instead of:	**Eat:**
smoked, cured, salted, and canned meat, fish, and poultry	unsalted fresh or frozen beef, lamb, pork, fish, and poultry
regular hard and processed cheese	low-sodium cheese
regular peanut butter	low-sodium peanut butter
salted crackers	unsalted crackers
regular canned and dehydrated soups, broths, and bouillons	low-sodium canned soups, broths, and bouillons
regular canned vegetables	fresh and frozen vegetables and low-sodium canned vegetables
salted snack foods	unsalted tortilla chips, pretzels, potato chips, and popcorn

a deficiency can result that may lead to anemia and affect the functioning of organ systems. An iron deficiency can cause fatigue, affect memory or other mental function, and lead to other serious health problems including slowed development during childhood. Pregnant mothers have higher iron needs than other adults, infants and toddlers need more iron than older children due to their rapid growth, and adolescent girls and women are at risk of deficiency due to menstruation (CDC 2011). As many as 80 percent of the world's population may be iron deficient, while 30 percent may have iron deficiency anemia (NIH 2007).

▪ Vitamins

No group of nutrients has captured the imagination of the public more than vitamins. Vitamins were discovered fairly recently, when physicians sought the cause of certain diseases, such as scurvy. They concluded that the chemical compounds called *vitamins* can make a great deal of difference to health. These vitamin-related discoveries led people to equate good nutrition with vitamins, and some even thought vitamins contained the essential element for life.

Vitamins are organic compounds required by every part of the body to maintain health and prevent disease. They are classified as either fat-soluble or water-soluble. Unlike minerals (such as calcium, which is integrated into bones), vitamins do not become part of the body. Only small amounts of vitamins are needed, but these must be provided by the diet because the body is not able to synthesize them in the required quantities for proper nourishment and body function. Vitamins foster growth, promote the ability to produce healthy offspring, maintain health, aid in the normal function of the digestive tract and appetite, and help maintain immune system functions.

Some vitamins can be a potential health hazard; some are particularly problematic if taken incorrectly or in excess. While vitamins are essential nutrients, overdosing (taking them far in excess of Recommended Dietary Allowances or individual needs) can result in toxicity and can be a danger to good health (National Institute of Health 2011). Overdosing on vitamins can cause serious side effects: loss of coordination, nausea, rashes, diarrhea, and fatigue. Excess amounts of fat-soluble vitamins, which are stored in the body, can reach toxic levels. Even water-soluble vitamins, taken to extreme, can be dangerous. The key is moderation and a well-balanced diet featuring a range of healthful, vitamin-rich foods.

Food sources for some of the vitamins are:

- **A**—liver; dark green, leafy vegetables, and orange vegetables such as carrots and sweet potatoes, which contain the vitamin A precursor *beta carotene*.
- **C**—citrus fruits, broccoli, tomatoes, potatoes
- **D**—eggs, liver, fortified milk
- **E**—margarine, salad dressing, sunflower seeds, almonds
- **K**—egg yolk, liver, milk, cabbage, spinach, kale

- **thiamin** (B_1)—pork, beef, liver, eggs, fish, whole grains, legumes
- **riboflavin** (B_2)—milk, green vegetables, cereals, liver
- **pyridoxine** (B_6)—pork, milk, eggs, legumes
- **cobalamin** (B_3)—seafood, meats, eggs, milk
- **niacin**—fish, poultry, enriched grain products
- **folic acid**—spinach, asparagus, broccoli, kidney beans, orange juice
- **biotin**—milk, liver, mushrooms, legumes

Fat-Soluble Vitamins. Fat-soluble vitamins are found in the fatty parts of food and body tissues. They are stored in the body until needed, so it is not necessary to consume them every day. The fat-soluble vitamins transported by lipids through the body are A, D, E, and K. Vitamin A is important in promoting growth and health of body tissues as well as enhancing the function of the immune system. This vitamin also enhances vision by helping the retina function properly, permitting us to distinguish between light and shade and to see various colors distinctly. A form of vitamin A is used by dermatologists to treat acne and other skin disorders. Overdoses of vitamin A may result in yellowish, dry, scaly skin and dry, irritated eyes.

Vitamin D is essential for calcium absorption and thus is needed to prevent and cure rickets, a deficiency disease in which bones fail to harden. Vitamin E is an activator in certain enzyme reactions, and it protects vitamins A and C from being used up too quickly. Vitamin K is essential for the synthesis of prothrombin, a substance needed for normal blood coagulation.

Water-Soluble Vitamins. Water-soluble vitamins are associated with the watery parts of food and body tissues. These vitamins are not stored by the body. Excess amounts are usually excreted in the urine and, therefore, should be provided in the diet on a regular basis. The water-soluble vitamins include the B vitamins and vitamin C (ascorbic acid). The B vitamins are essential to daily human nutrition. Known as the B-complex group, they help body systems combat stress and maintain energy reserves. The B-complex group consists of vitamin B_1 (thiamin), vitamin B_2 (riboflavin), vitamin B_3 (niacin), vitamin B_6 (pyridoxine), vitamin B_{12} (cobalamin), folic acid, and biotin.

Thiamin is necessary for carbohydrate metabolism. It aids in the release of energy from food. Riboflavin helps body cells use oxygen, promotes tissue repair, and helps the nervous system function properly. Niacin is essential to growth; without niacin, thiamin and riboflavin could not function properly in the body. Pyridoxine is necessary for healthy teeth and gums and helps maintain normal body cholesterol. Further, it aids in the production of antibodies. Cobalamin works in conjunction with folic acid and iron to build normal blood cells and prevent pernicious anemia. Folic acid aids in the proper growth and reproduction of blood cells and contributes to healthy skin. It also helps prevent neural tube defects in the fetus during pregnancy. Biotin is necessary for the proper use of fats, carbohydrates, and protein and helps produce antibodies. Vitamin C is vital in preventing scurvy, in the formation and maintenance of collagen (the cementing material that holds cells together), in the normal metabolism of some amino acids, and in the function of the adrenal glands.

Antioxidants

Chemical reactions occur continuously in the world around us and in our bodies. One of the most common types of reaction is oxidation. Some more familiar and visible examples of the damage caused by oxidation include rust, brittle rubber, and food spoilage. In our bodies, the energy-yielding reactions within cells are also **oxidation reactions**; that is, they are reactions in which either an oxygen atom adds an electron to or a hydrogen atom removes an electron from a substrate (a group of atoms or molecule)—the net result is a substrate that has had a partial or complete loss of a negatively charge particle, an electron. Two partially charged atoms or groups of atoms, one positively charged and the other negatively charged, now exist. Any atom or group of atoms that has an unpaired electron is called a **free radical**, or oxidant. Because electrons typically function in pairs, the free radicals are very prone to binding to other substrates in an effort to regain this paired status. When this happens in the human body, there is potential for a great deal of damage.

In the human body, this problem is mostly avoided because oxidation reactions are paired with reduction reactions so that the reduction reactions pick up the electrons that are lost during the oxidation reactions. Our bodies actually rely on these reactions occurring properly all the time. Whenever our bodies use glucose (recall this is the most common energy-containing molecule in the body), it is oxidation that releases the energy for our bodies to use. When more energy is needed than can be supplied by glucose in the blood, then our bodies start to tap into the stored energy supplies—especially those stored as fat. Oxidation of triglycerides, notably the fatty acid components, provides this energy. (Our bodies also oxidize glycogen, a storage form of glucose found in the liver and in muscle.)

When the free radicals are not incorporated immediately into other reactions, they may bind to inappropriate molecules or atoms and disrupt their normal function. For example, partially charged atoms or molecules often exist temporarily as intermediate steps in chemical reactions, so chemical reactions that are essential for normal body function may be interrupted if a free radical binds to one of the charged intermediates.

Oxidation and the resulting free radicals accelerate the aging process and contribute to organ and tissue damage. LDL oxidation has been linked to atherosclerosis (and thus contributes to heart disease). Oxidation processes contribute to the development of cancer. As research continues, free radical damage from oxidation appears more likely to be associated with chronic conditions. **Antioxidants** act as scavengers by binding to free radicals, thus preventing them from causing damage. Free radical damage may lead to cancer, but antioxidants such as beta-carotene, lycopene, selenium, and vitamins C, E, and A can interact with and stabilize free radicals and may prevent some of the damage free radicals might otherwise cause (National Cancer Institute 2004).

Another possible way to minimize free radical damage is by eating foods that boost antioxidant defenses. Vitamin C is found in fruits and vegetables. Beta-carotene is found in carrots, cantaloupe, dark green leafy vegetables, and vegetable-based soups. Vitamin E is found in vegetable oils, wheat germ, nuts, and green leafy vegetables. Natural foods likely do not provide too much of these vitamins, but large doses of vitamin C or vitamin E used as a dietary supplement may actually promote free radical damage.

Trace minerals—copper, zinc, and selenium—act as antioxidants because they are necessary components of specific antioxidant enzymes and thus are essential to life. Organ meats such as liver, seafoods, nuts, and seeds are good dietary sources of copper and selenium. Zinc is found in meat, liver, eggs, and seafood. Trace minerals, like vitamins, should be consumed in proper amounts. Large amounts not associated with enzymes may promote free radical formation.

Nutritional Needs

About fifty different nutrients are needed to maintain health. No food contains all the nutrients needed, not even fortified milk, which is highly regarded in our society. Therefore, a variety of foods are required to satisfy nutritional needs. One way to assure this variety and to establish a balanced diet is to select foods each day from the types identified in MyPlate (see Figure 17.2) by the USDA.

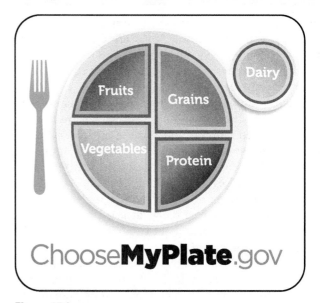

Figure 17.2
MyPlate

In 2010, the MyPyramid Food Guidance System, which used the "pyramid" concept for food guidance based on the ideas of variety, moderation, and proportion, was replaced by the new MyPlate food guidance system. The MyPlate system incorporates information from the updated *Dietary Guidelines for Americans, 2010.* The new icon is intended to serve as a reminder to eat more healthfully and proportionally. The icon also references the new website www.ChooseMyPlate.gov, a resource that continues to offer online resources and tools to make it easier for people to personalize their health and nutrition and make healthier food choices for themselves and their families (U.S. Department of Agriculture 2011).

Nutritional Needs for School-Age Children

Caloric needs vary widely for elementary school children. They should eat at least the lower number of servings from each of the five major food groups daily. Most children will need more calories for growth and activity; they should eat larger portions of foods from the major food groups and some nutritious snacks while following the percentages of each nutrient as recommended by the USDA. Go easy on fatty and sugary foods such as butter, margarine, salad dressings, candies, and soft drinks, but don't forbid them. Have these as occasional treats, not everyday fare. Many children gain unwanted weight due to a sedentary lifestyle. Encourage physical activity, including outdoor play, to promote strength and fitness.

Nutrient Characteristics of Types of Food

Fruits are usually good sources of vitamins A and C, carbohydrates, and fiber. Citrus fruits are especially good sources of vitamin C. Two to four servings daily (at least one of which provides vitamin C), each about equal in size to an orange, are recommended.

Vegetables are usually good sources of vitamins A and C, carbohydrates, and fiber. Vegetables are low in calories if served without added fat. Dark green, leafy vegetables such as spinach, kale, collard greens, mustard greens, and broccoli are high in calcium and vitamins A and C. Orange vegetables such as carrots, sweet potatoes, and squash are also high in vitamin A. Three to five servings of vegetables daily (at least one of which provides vitamin A), each about equal in size to a small potato, are recommended.

Dried beans and peas are high in protein and iron. This food type also includes nuts, lentils, peanut butter, and tofu. They are usually low in cost and can be prepared a variety of ways. Nuts and peanut butter are high in fat and therefore high in calories. A combined total of two to three servings per day from this group and/or the meat, poultry, fish, and eggs group is recommended.

Meat, poultry, fish, and eggs are high in protein and iron. Lean meats, poultry without skin, and most fish are lower-calorie choices. A serving of this group is 3 ounces. A combined total of two to three servings per day from this group and/or the dried beans and peas group is recommended.

Bread, cereal, and pasta are high in iron, carbohydrates, and some B vitamins. Although the actual amount of protein is small in each serving, if many grain foods are eaten each day, part of the daily need for protein can be met. However, if these are the only sources of protein, they need to be combined with nuts and legumes to fulfill the needs for the required essential amino acids. Whole-grain products contain more fiber, vitamins, and minerals than refined products. Six to eleven servings daily, each about equal to the size of a slice of bread, are recommended.

Milk and cheese are good sources of calcium and protein. Low-fat milk and cheese made from low-fat milk are lower-calorie choices. These low-fat products have the same amount of vitamins and minerals but a lower percentage of fat. Two to three servings are recommended daily for this food group.

Sweets and fats are added to other foods, thus increasing the number of calories. These foods supply few nutrients for the calories they contain. Beverages such as alcohol and soft drinks should be limited in the diet.

Food Problems

Problems concerning food have been a part of human life from the earliest times. In past ages, crop failures have led to famine and war. Even today, starvation kills hundreds of thousands of children and adults in very poor nations each year. Although there is also poverty in the United States, few children actually face the threat of starvation. Unfortunately, this does not mean that our nation does not have food problems. Many Americans are undernourished or malnourished. Overweight and obese individuals are also common.

▪ Undernutrition

Typically, an undernourished person is also underweight, but this is by no means always the case. **Undernutrition** implies that the individual is not getting enough nutrients. This can occur even if the person is consuming more than enough calories. Thus, personal weight is not necessarily an indication of nutritional status. In the United States, **malnutrition** (an imbalance of proper nutrients) due to undernutrition is most likely to occur in infants, children, and adolescents, when nutritional requirements for tissue growth and development are high. When one is undernourished, the available proteins and carbohydrates are depleted, and the body begins to burn

HEALTH HIGHLIGHT | **Diagnosis, Warning Signs, Treatment, and Prevention of Anorexia Nervosa**

To be diagnosed with anorexia, a person must:

- Have an intense fear of gaining weight or becoming fat, even when she or he is underweight
- Refuse to keep weight at what is considered normal or acceptable for her or his age and height (15 percent or more below the expected weight)
- Have a body image that is very distorted, be very focused on body weight or shape, and refuse to admit or acknowledge the seriousness of weight loss
- Have not had her period for three or more cycles

Warning signs and symptoms

People with anorexia may severely limit the amount of food they eat, or eat and then make themselves throw up. Other behaviors include:

- Cutting food into small pieces or moving them around the plate rather than eating
- Exercising all the time
- Going to the bathroom right after meals
- Refusing to eat around others
- Using pills to make themselves urinate (water pills or diuretics), have

a bowel movement (enemas and laxatives), or to decrease their appetite (diet pills)
- Blotchy or yellow skin that is dry and covered with fine hair
- Confused or slow thinking, along with poor memory or judgment
- Depression
- Extreme sensitivity to cold (wearing several layers of clothing to stay warm)
- Loss of bone strength
- Wasting away of muscle and loss of body fat

Treatment

- Most persons with anorexia nervosa deny that they have an eating disorder.
- The goals of treatment are to first restore normal body weight and eating habits.
- Sometimes weight gain is achieved using schedules for eating, decreased physical activity, and increased social activity.
- Individual cognitive behavioral therapy, group therapy, and family therapy have all been successful.
- Although some medications may help, no drug has been proven to decrease the desire to lose weight.

- Treatment is often very challenging, and it requires hard work by patients and their families.
- Patients may drop out of programs if they have unrealistic expectations of being "cured" with therapy alone.

Although a short hospital stay is a common way to start treatment, a longer hospital stay may be needed if:

- Severe and life-threatening malnutrition requires feedings through a vein or stomach tube
- Weight loss continues despite treatment
- Medical complications, such as heart problems, confusion, or low potassium levels develop
- The person has severe depression or thinks about committing suicide

Prevention

- In some cases, prevention may not be possible.
- Encouraging healthy, realistic attitudes toward weight and diet may be helpful.
- Sometimes, talk therapy can help.

(*Source:* National Institutes of Health. National Library of Medicine 2011. Anorexia Nervosa. Full text available at www.nlm.nih.gov/medlineplus/ency/article/000362.htm.)

---

fat reserves. This can lead to a process known as *ketosis*. Undernutrition may retard growth and affect a student's ability to learn.

The causes of undernutrition are many; poverty and lack of nutrition education are two major factors. Many Americans are undernourished because they resist changing nutritionally deficient eating habits and patterns. Other practices dictated by cultural taboos, religious beliefs, and cultural patterns also sometimes lead to nutritional health problems. Occasionally the cause is physiological. A poorly functioning body might fail to use nutrients supplied to it. For example, a disease such as hyperthyroidism can affect growth regardless of the quality of diet.

Psychological factors can also lead to undernutrition. Hurried meals in haphazard settings may be harmful because of the type and amount of food as well as how the food is eaten.

▪ Eating Disorders

Anorexia Nervosa. An inaccurate perception of one's own nutritional state can bring on health problems such as anorexia nervosa. **Anorexia nervosa** literally means loss of appetite, but this is a misnomer: A person with anorexia nervosa is hungry, but he or she denies the hunger because of an irrational fear of becoming fat. Self-starvation, food preoccupation and rituals, compulsive exercising, and often an absence of menstrual cycles in women typically characterize anorexia nervosa. She or he may occasionally binge on large quantities of a particular food, then make her- or himself vomit, and may regularly use large quantities of laxatives. (If these bingeing and purging behaviors are dominant, then she or he is diagnosed with *bulimia*.) This condition is more than a simple eating disorder: It refers to a distinct psychological disorder in which a drive for thinness and a fear of fatness result in life-threatening emaciation and a host of other problems. Untreated, anorexia nervosa can be fatal. It is not a fad that the victim will outgrow if left alone. The most common cause of death in a long-time anorexic is a low level of potassium in the blood, which can cause an irregular heartbeat; other causes of death are starvation, infections due to poor nutrition, dehydration from overuse of laxatives, and suicide due to depression. It occurs primarily in adolescents and may affect both sexes, but most often it is girls who become anorexic.

The symptoms of anorexia nervosa are difficult to specify because the disorder emerges over time as a complex mixture of the relentless drive for thinness, the effects of starvation, and commonly associated psychological disturbances (such as low self-worth and mistrust of others). A significant weight loss is one of the classic symptoms of anorexia nervosa. The anorexic individuals approach weight loss with a fervor, convinced that their bodies are too large. Lost weight is viewed as an accomplishment. The fact that slenderness is highly valued in our culture contributes to these attitudes. This drive for thinness is coupled with an extreme fear of becoming fat. This phobic fear of weight gain may express itself as excessive anxiety over any weight increase. An anorexic individual may have a distorted body image. This can be shown by the person thinking she or he is fat, wearing baggy clothing, or weighing him or herself many times a day (USDHHS 2011).

Anorexics are typically compulsive, perfectionistic, and very competitive. The anorexic sometimes suffers from a low self-image due to a feeling of incompetence, so she or he becomes consumed with losing weight to demonstrate to her- or himself and others that she or he is in total control. Therefore, if a friend, parent, or teacher admonishes the anorexic for looking too thin, the anorexic may take this as a compliment, for it means others are aware of her or his disciplined approach to weight loss. Therapy consists of psychological counseling and family therapy, as well as steps to improve nutrition.

The long-term effects of anorexia nervosa include psychological problems such as obsessions, compulsions, paranoia, social withdrawal, and depression. Anorexic individuals may become irritable, hostile, indecisive, depressed, defiant, and resistant to change. The arguments with parents and other authorities over eating habits become power struggles for control. Starvation can interrupt normal brain–body functions such as sleep, maintenance of proper blood pressure, muscle weakness, immunity to disease, and sexual drive. Vomiting disrupts the potassium–sodium balance necessary for proper functioning of nerves and muscles (including the heart) and produces enamel erosion, tooth degeneration, and lesions in the esophagus. The Health Highlight box shows the warning signs and problems associated with anorexia nervosa.

Bulimia Nervosa. **Bulimia nervosa** is characterized by recurring periods of binge eating, during which large amounts of food are consumed in a short period of time—

sometimes as many as 20,000 calories during the course of a single binge. The bulimic is aware that his or her eating is out of control. He or she is fearful of not being able to stop eating and is afraid of being fat. The bulimic usually feels depressed and guilty after a binge. Frequently, purging (through self-induced vomiting, abuse of laxatives and/or diuretics, or periods of fasting) follows the binges. The bulimic's weight is usually in a normal or somewhat above normal range; it may fluctuate more than ten pounds due to alternating binges and fasts. The Health Highlight box shows warning signs and problems associated with bulimia.

Treatment. Treatment can save the life of someone with an eating disorder. Friends, relatives, teachers, therapists, dietitians, peer support groups, and physicians all play an important role in helping the ill person start and stay with a treatment program. Encouragement, caring, and persistence, as well as information about eating disorders and their dangers, may be needed to convince the ill person to get help, stick with treatment, or try again.

Hunger and Learning

Hunger is a physiological and psychological state that occurs when food needs are not met satisfactorily. Research has shown that hunger definitely has an effect on learning behavior. Hunger increases nervousness, irritability, and disinterest in a learning situation. Students who are hungry will demonstrate a lack of interest in what is being taught and an inability to concentrate.

Hunger and malnutrition lead to weakness and illness. A variety of avitaminoses (vitamin deficiency disorders) can result from malnutrition. A person's development and brain function can be severely affected by hunger. Malnourished individuals are also more susceptible to infections, which can further lead to impaired growth.

Obesity

Obesity is prevalent among children and adolescents in the United States. Evidence gathered over the past three decades indicates that it is increasing. Data show that 13 percent of children age six to eleven and 14 percent of adolescents age twelve to nineteen in the United States are overweight. This is nearly double for children and triple for adolescents from twenty years ago. Overweight children, especially adolescents, are likely to become overweight or obese adults at risk for serious health problems such as type 2 diabetes, hypertension, heart disease, stroke, and some types of cancer.

Lifestyle Habits Contribute to Obesity. Poor eating habits and inactive lifestyles, rather than heredity, are contributing to the prevalence of obesity among children and adolescents, particularly African Americans and Hispanics. Poor dietary patterns include increased intake of sugars in sweetened soft drinks, foods and meals of high energy but low nutrient density, and large portion sizes.

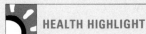

HEALTH HIGHLIGHT | **Causes, Symptoms, Treatment, and Prevention of Bulimia**

Bulimia is an illness in which a person binges on food or has regular episodes of significant overeating and feels a loss of control. The affected person then uses various methods (such as purging) to prevent weight gain. Many people with bulimia also have anorexia nervosa.

Causes

- The exact cause of bulimia is unknown.
- Genetic, psychological, trauma, family, society, or cultural factors may play a role.
- Bulimia is likely due to more than one factor.

Symptoms

- Eating binges may occur as often as several times a day for many months.
- People with bulimia typically eat large amounts of high-calorie foods, usually in secret. The person generally feels a lack of control over their eating during these episodes.
- These binges cause a sense of self-disgust, which leads to what is called purging, in order to prevent gaining weight. Purging may include: making oneself vomit, excessive exercise, and use of laxatives, enemas, or diuretics (water pills). Purging often brings a sense of relief.
- Body weight is often in the normal range, although people with bulimia often see themselves as being overweight. Because weight is often normal, this eating disorder may not be noticed by others.

Symptoms or behaviors that may be noticed include:

- Compulsive exercising
- Evidence of discarded packaging for laxatives, diet pills, emetics, or diuretics
- Regularly going to the bathroom right after meals
- Suddenly eating large amounts of food or buying large quantities of food that disappear right away
- Eroded or pitted enamel of the teeth due to excessive exposure to the acid in vomit
- Broken blood vessels in the eyes from the strain of vomiting
- Pouch-like appearance to the corners of the mouth due to swollen salivary glands
- Rashes and pimples
- Small cuts and calluses across the tops of the finger joints due to self-induced vomiting

Treatment

People with bulimia rarely need to be hospitalized, unless:

- Binge-purge cycles have led to anorexia

- Drugs are needed for withdrawal from purging
- Major depression is present

Most often, a stepped approach is taken for patients with bulimia:

- Support groups, cognitive-behavioral therapy (CBT), or nutritional therapy may be effective.
- Drugs used for bulimia are typically antidepressants known as selective serotonin-reuptake inhibitors (SSRIs).
- Patients may drop out of programs if they have unrealistic expectations of being "cured" by therapy alone.
- Self-help groups like Overeaters Anonymous may help some people with bulimia.
- People with fewer medical complications of bulimia, and who are willing and able to engage in therapy, tend to have a better chance of recovery.

Prevention

- Less social and cultural emphasis on physical perfection may eventually help reduce the frequency of this disorder.

(Source: National Institutes of Health. National Library of Medicine 2011. *Bulimia.* Full text available at www.nlm.nih.gov/medlineplus/ency /article/000341.htm.)

Researchers suggest that intake of soft drinks may promote obesity because of their high glycemic index (ability to raise blood sugar). Milk, on the other hand, which was once commonly consumed, may protect against obesity because of its low glycemic index.

The data available for the years 1994–1996 shows that only 2 percent of children met food serving recommendations for all five major food groups. When further examined, it was found that the percentages of children meeting the recommended number of food group servings were 14 percent for fruit, 17 percent for meat, 20 percent for vegetables, 23 percent for grain, and 30 percent for milk. Those children who participated in the National School Lunch Program were more likely to meet the recommended servings and to consume less added sugar (Food and Nutrition Service 2010).

Increased Sedentary Living and Obesity Rates. Many children are less physically active than recommended. The U.S. Department of Health and Human Services (USDHHS) reports that "overweight in children and adolescents is generally caused by lack of physical activity, unhealthy eating patterns, or a combination of the two, with genetics and lifestyle both playing important roles in determining a child's weight." The prevalence of television and computer and video games contribute to inactive lifestyles (USDHHS 2007). School physical education programs can help combat sedentary habits and promote healthy lifetime habits. According to the USDHHS, the percentage of districts that required elementary schools to teach physical education increased from 82.6 percent in 2000 to 93.3 percent in 2006 and the percentage of states that required elementary schools to provide students with regularly scheduled recess increased from 4.1 percent to 11.8 percent and the percentage of districts with this requirement increased from 46.3 percent to 57.1 percent (USDHHS 2010). School administrations and teachers are also now strongly discouraged from using physical activity to punish students; this prohibition removes a negative influence that may affect lifetime physical activity habits

Health Risks of Obesity.

The health risks of obesity, such as degenerative diseases and shorter life span, may not be of immediate concern to elementary school students, but there are many other reasons for maintaining a healthy weight. Obesity can be considered a physical handicap at any age because it affects physical activity. Also, overweight students face many emotional problems. In a society where thinness is emphasized, overweight students may be shunned, ridiculed, stared at, and rejected socially. As a result, overweight students may lose their sense of self-worth and withdraw from others. A complicating problem occurs when overweight students find satisfaction in nothing else except eating, which causes them to gain even more weight, further alienating them from peers.

Being overweight becomes a health problem when the person is 15 to 20 percent above normal weight. Of course, body build and an individual's lean-to-fat ratio also have to be taken into consideration. Different people gain weight in different places in the body. Those who typically gain weight in the lower portions of the body (hips and thighs, usually females) do not have as many health risks posed as those who gain weight in the upper body (abdomen, usually males). A person might have a stocky build and be over the desired weight for his height and age, but the percentage of body fat might be within the normal range. More often than not, however, obesity is self-evident.

Weight Control.

Weight reduction demands self-discipline and commitment. An overweight or obese individual must accept personal responsibility for the condition. If an emotional problem is the cause, that problem must be treated first to ensure long-lasting success at weight control because the overweight condition is only a symptom of a deeper problem. Before any weight loss plan is implemented, a physician should be consulted.

Obese persons must consume fewer calories than they expend daily, but this is easier said than done. Dieters should use a diet that is similar to the one to which they are accustomed so they do not feel as restricted and tempted to quit dieting. Other techniques that have helped people lose weight are to:

- arrange to eat in one place only
- remove all unnecessary fat when cooking and eating meat
- avoid gravies and use herbs and spices for seasoning instead
- start meals with filling, low-calorie dishes such as a salad or broth-based soup

- eat fresh fruit instead of canned fruit
- eat regular meals—missed meals may make you even hungrier during the day
- eat raw vegetables for snacks
- eat baked, broiled, or boiled foods without adding fat
- use a salad-sized plate rather than a dinner plate so the portions look larger
- cut food into small bites and eat slowly
- brush the teeth after each meal; sometimes the aftertaste of food can stimulate the appetite
- exercise moderately and regularly
- develop hobbies; sometimes people substitute food for friends and outside activities

Care should be taken not to lose weight too rapidly. Rapid weight loss may result in exhaustion, kidney problems, dehydration, reduced cardiovascular output, decreased strength, decreased growth, and decreased endurance.

One point that should be kept in mind regarding an individual's weight is ideal weight versus average weight. Some weight tables will provide data on average weight; but, as noted earlier, trends for the average American child are moving toward overweight. Ideal weight tables should be used as the standard for evaluating weight.

Further, weight alone should not be the total issue. The child's body fat (or lean-to-fat ratio) is even more critical. If a child is "big boned," he or she may appear overweight, yet his or her body fat may be very acceptable. Conversely, a child with small bones may weigh within an acceptable range but actually have a body fat percentage that is unacceptable. Also, if a person couples a dieting program with an exercise program, that person may be losing fat and gaining muscle. The result may not be lost pounds but rather lost fat—a healthy condition. However, since most dieters are concerned only with how much they weigh, they may be disappointed that they are not losing weight. Again, the focus for a dieter should be on the lean-to-fat ratio, not on weight alone.

> **TEACHING TIP**
>
> Have your students go to www.ChooseMy Plate.gov and complete the MyPlate Plan to generate food plans that fit their age, sex, weight, height, and amount of physical activity. Students can print their results and bring them home, and they can also explore the other tools on the site, such as the Meal Tracking Worksheet.

The Role of the Teacher.

Teachers should provide accurate information concerning nutrition and teach students how to make wise food decisions. They need to emphasize the importance of eating a good breakfast and lunch, as well as encourage sociability among students when they are eating. Teachers can help the students enjoy the taste, smell, color, and texture of food and thereby increase interest in it. In addition, teachers have an excellent chance to be exemplary role models by eating the right foods in the right way while at school.

Weight reduction is usually more successful when using a "buddy system" or peer support groups. Teachers can help by getting together several students who have a similar goal of weight reduction and having them eat together and share their concerns and problems. Teachers can also educate obese and overweight students about proper nutrition and encourage physical activity. To nurture the emotional health of the obese student, teachers need to offer security and acceptance without pitying or overprotecting the student. Being supportive will produce much better results than constant harassment or criticism. Trying to reduce the student's anxiety while helping build self-esteem and independence are also important.

Other Food-Related Issues

▪ Fad Diets

Obese individuals may understand the need to diet but may want to do so as painlessly as possible. Such individuals are vulnerable to fad diets advertised to help a person lose weight quickly. Some of these fad diets are restricted in variety, expensive, useless, and sometimes even detrimental to health. Most fad diets are directed at adults, rather than children, of course, but children are impressionable. It is important to put these diets into proper perspective. The fact is that most people who are overweight do not need to read a book on what to eat to lose weight. Simply eating somewhat less of everything will usually produce results, if the diet is followed conscientiously.

Although it took several months and years to put on the extra weight, many overweight and obese individuals are looking for a quick way to lose that weight. This attitude results in choosing quick-weight-loss diets that are not effective and may be harmful.

Some try metabolic products, such as herbs or caffeine, to lose weight. Herbs have not been shown to speed the loss of fat, and caffeine shows little promise as a weight-loss aid.

Others go on very-low-calorie diets, which severely restrict nutrients and can result in serious metabolic imbalances. Weight can be lost on this type of diet, but much of the weight lost will be lean protein tissue and/or water, not fat. This results in harm to the muscles (including the heart), loss of essential vitamins and minerals through the water loss, and dizziness and fatigue. Further, if one cuts calories, this slows the metabolism; and once this person goes off the diet, the metabolism remains slow and the body continues to use few calories—and the pounds come back.

Highprotein diets (low-carbohydrate diets) operate on the theory that insulin is controlled and therefore more fat is burned. With this type of diet, ketosis (ketones formed and released into the bloodstream) will result. Ketosis will increase blood levels of uric acid, a risk factor for gout and kidney stones. There is no research evidence that carbohydrates lead to fat storage and weight; and further, the excessive protein in this diet can damage the kidneys and cause osteoporosis.

Over-the-counter diet aids act as mild stimulants and suppress the appetite, usually by providing fiber and thereby providing a feeling of fullness. The FDA has found no evidence to support fiber as an aid in weight control or as an appetite suppressant.

Prescription drugs, such as Redux and Pondimin (fen-phen), curb hunger by increasing the level of serotonin in the brain. These were intended for the obese, but were banned in 1997 after the FDA found strong evidence that they could seriously damage the heart.

Some people try crash diets to lose a moderate amount of weight in a very short period. These types of diets can damage several body systems, and have been proved not to work because most of these individuals regain their weight. One popular diet (the "grapefruit diet" or "Hollywood diet") assumes that grapefruit contains fat-burning properties; although there is no research to support this theory, people still follow this diet to lose weight quickly. Those who follow this limited diet eat grapefruit with multiple meals during the day and limit intake of certain other foods. Most plans based around the premise of the grapefruit diet tend to be lacking essential vitamins and minerals, making the diet unhealthy and unrealistic (University of Pittsburgh 2011).

Animal studies have found that yo-yo dieting (or weight cycling) can cause one to gain more body fat than those with a steady caloric intake. The research suggests that animals and people adapt to a reduction in calories by storing more fat in times of higher caloric intake to prepare for the next crash diet (USDA 2008). The best way to lose weight is to eat a variety of healthy foods in moderation and to exercise.

▪ Fast Foods

Preparing meals at home allows preplanning of balanced meals, control of portion sizes, limiting of less healthy ingredients, and likely financial savings. An entire family, from parents to children, can be involved in planning and preparing meals. Research shows that children are more likely to try a new dish when they helped prepare it (NIH 2011). Although there are many benefits to preparing and eating food at home, Americans are consuming a large portion of their meals away from the home; daily caloric intake from foods eaten away from home increased from 18 percent in the 1970s to 32 percent in the 1990s (USDA 2006). Foods eaten in restaurants or as take-away tend to be more calorie dense and nutritionally poorer than foods people prepare at home. Table 17.2 shows a comparison of the nutrition facts of some standard foods from various popular fast-food restaurant chains.

Eating away from home doesn't have to be unhealthy. The American Heart Association (2010) recommends planning ahead and making smart choices to reduce calorie and unhealthy nutrient intake: visit the chain's website to identify in advance the healthiest choices; pass on "super-size" servings; skip standard side dishes or replace them with salad or fruit; select a plain baked potato over French fried; choose grilled chicken sandwiches often; add zero-calorie condiments to sandwiches (skip the bacon!); and drink water, diet soda, or low-fat milk.

Table 17.2 Recommended Daily Intake* vs. Fast Food Nutrition Facts
Recommended daily intake:
2,000–2,700 calories
No more than 50–80 g
No more than 300 mg
No more than 1,100–3,300 mg
Quarterpound Cheeseburger, Large Fries, 16 oz. soda (McDonald's)
1,166 calories
51 g fat
95 mg cholesterol
4 slices Sausage and Mushroom Pizza, 16 oz. soda (Domino's)
1,000 calories
28 g fat
62 mg cholesterol
2,302 mg sodium
Fried Chicken (Breast and Wing), Buttermilk Biscuit, Mashed Potatoes and Gravy, Corn-on-the-Cob, 16 oz. soda (KFC)
1,232 calories
57 g fat
157 mg cholesterol
2,276 mg sodium
Taco Salad, 16 oz. soda (Taco Bell)
1,057 calories
55 g fat
80 mg cholesterol
1,620 mg sodium

*For most adults

Source: From Missouri Department of Health and Senior Services, Healthy Living: Education Components. Used by permission.

Food Quackery

Food quackery is by no means confined to diet books or diet clinics that employ dubious methods. The whole natural and health foods industry is considered quackery by many nutritional experts. Both of these areas prey on natural fears and uncertainties about foods and nutritional requirements. There is no accepted legal definition of what natural foods actually are and no way to keep entrepreneurs from selling granola, dried fruits, and so on at inflated prices, all the while hinting that these products are somewhat healthier for a person to eat. So-called health foods, such as bee pollen and algae extracts, fall into the same category. Such foods are not harmful to health, but they are no better than foods obtained from ordinary sources. Advocates of natural, organic, and health foods claim that additives or pesticide residues in regular foods can cause disease or even lower the nutritional value of the food, but these claims may be highly exaggerated. By and large, the FDA and other supervisory agencies do a good job in preventing possibly harmful or unsafe foods from reaching the market. Teachers can help students become informed consumers of food products and develop a good knowledge of nutritional principles. But nutrition should not become an obsession, as it is with many food faddists. Students should also be taught to recognize the difference between nutrition and food panacea.

Food Labeling

A tremendous amount of nutritional information is available today, but many Americans are still misinformed and confused about the foods they buy and eat. Some FDA regulations have resulted in improved labeling designed to give a listing of nutrients in the product and to make the information on food labels more meaningful to consumers (see Figure 17.1 on page 300). For example, ingredients are listed on the label in order, beginning with the largest quantity. Typically, the label provides nutritional information based on one serving of the food product rather than on the entire can or package.

Manufacturers must use nutritional labeling when they add any nutrient to packaged food or when they make some nutritional claim for their products. Labeling is also meant to stop unsupported generalizations and fraudulent statements. Nutritional labeling of food products is being sought for nearly all foods. This would be difficult for some foods, such as fresh fruits, but labeling of all food products would be beneficial to the consumer.

As outlined by the U.S. Food and Drug Administration, there are two sets of reference values for reporting nutrients in nutrition labeling: 1) Daily Reference Values (DRVs) and 2) Reference Daily Intakes (RDIs). These values are available to consumers so that they may more easily interpret information about nutrient amounts present in foods and compare nutritional values of food products. DRVs are established for adults and children aged four and older, as are RDIs, with the exception of protein. DRVs are provided for total fat, saturated fat, cholesterol, total carbohydrate, dietary fiber, sodium, potassium, and protein. RDIs are provided for vitamins and minerals and for protein for children less than four years of age and for pregnant and lactating women (FDA 2011). Only the DV term appears on the food label, though, to make label reading less confusing.

Under regulations from the FDA of the U.S. Department of Health and Human Services and the Food Safety and Inspection Service of the USDA, food labels include:

- formats that enable consumers to quickly find the information they need to make healthful food choices
- information on the amount per serving of saturated fat, cholesterol, dietary fiber, *trans* fat, and other nutrients of major health concern
- nutrient reference values, expressed as % Daily Values, that help consumers see how a food fits into an overall daily diet
- uniform definitions for terms that describe a food's nutrient content—such as "light," "low-fat," and "high-fiber"—to ensure that such terms mean the same for any product on which they appear
- claims about the relationship between a nutrient or food and a disease or health-related condition, such as calcium with osteoporosis and fat with cancer (helpful for people who are concerned about eating foods that may help keep them healthier longer)
- standardized serving sizes to make nutritional comparisons of similar products easier
- declaration of total percentage of fruit or vegetable juice in juice drinks

▪ The School Lunch Program

School lunch programs began with the enactment of the National School Lunch Act in 1946. This federal legislation provided surplus agricultural commodities and federal funds to local school districts for the purpose of providing nutritious meals to children through a school lunch program. Federal government management of this program is the responsibility of the USDA.

The National School Lunch Program (NSLP) provides nutritionally balanced low-cost or free lunches and after school snacks to more than thirty-one million children each school day. NSLP operates in over 101,000 schools and residential child care institutions. The meals served within the program must meet federal nutrition requirements (USDA 2011). The Hunger-Free Kids Act of 2010, the school lunch program championed by First Lady Michelle Obama, presents new legislation to continue programs offering food options to children of low-income families, to offer more nutritious food options to children, educate them about healthy food choices, and teach children healthy lifetime habits. The act grants the USDA the authority to set nutritional standards for *all* food sold in schools during the school day, provides additional funding to schools so they can meet updated nutritional standards for federally-subsidized lunches, encourages use of local foods in schools, expands access to drinking water in schools, sets basics standards for school wellness policies, promotes nutrition and wellness in child care settings, and expands support for breast-feeding through the WIC program. School districts are also given increased standards for accountability under the program.

Though the school lunches provided through federal programs may be nutritious, several factors prevent children from eating wisely at school. Many schools offer foods that are not as nutritious but are sold in competition to the regular school lunch. Also, many schools sell soft drinks and snacks through vending machines, and some children consume these instead of the regular cafeteria meal. As reported by the CDC in 2009, 77 percent of high schools still sell soda or fruit drinks that are not 100 percent juice, and 61 percent sell salty snacks not low in fat in their vending machines or school stores (CDC 2009). An increasing number of states are prohibiting schools from offering junk foods in vending machines (increased from 8 percent in 2000 to 32 percent in 2006), and a number of individual school districts also prohibit the sale of junk food in vending machines. Schools that sold cookies, cake, or other high-fat baked goods in vending machines or school stores decreased from 38 percent in 2000 to 25 percent in 2006 (CDC 2009).

Nutrition Education

The educational impact of a lunch program can be important if it is used correctly. For students who bring their lunches from home, teachers need to provide several examples of nutritious sack lunches (for example, a sandwich including some type of lean meat and lettuce on whole-wheat bread, banana, raisins, and milk). The new MyPlate icon can be used to emphasize food groups and proportionality (see the Health Highlight on page 312).

The cafeteria can be used as a place in which to help students learn table manners, sitting posture, and appropriate social behavior. The planning, preparation, and serving of meals by the cafeteria staff can also provide excellent learning opportunities for students.

In emphasizing sound nutrition to students, teachers need to make sure that the learning opportunities provided are interesting and personalized. Students should be taught to make responsible food choices. The home and school have to work together to make the nutrition education of the student a success.

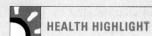 **HEALTH HIGHLIGHT** | **MyPlate and ChooseMyPlate.org**

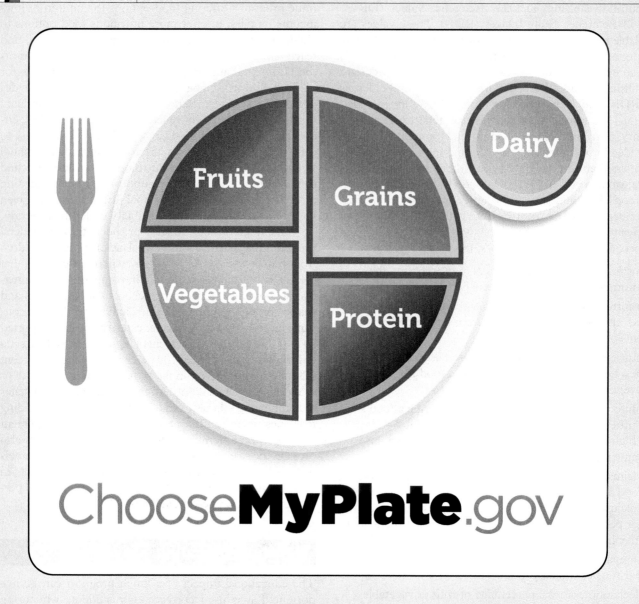

MyPlate is a food guidance system based on the *Dietary Guidelines for Americans, 2010,* replacing the previously used MyPyramid. Through the illustration of a familiar place setting, this new **MyPlate** icon is intended to remind you to eat healthfully. Visit **www.ChooseMyPlate.gov** to assess your current diet and physical activity levels and also access an interactive and personalized food plan. Tips are available on the website to help you make healthy changes in your current food choices and physical activity patterns.

Reflective of the *Dietary Guidelines for Americans, 2010,* **MyPlate** encourages you to eat for health through three general areas of recommendation:

1. **Balance calories:**
   - Enjoy your food, but eat less
   - Avoid oversized portions
2. **Foods to increase:**
   - Make half your plate fruits and vegetables
   - Make at least half your grains whole
   - Switch to fat-free or 1% milk

3. **Foods to reduce:**
   - Compare sodium in foods like soup, bread, and frozen meals— and choose the foods with lower numbers
   - Drink water instead of sugary drinks

The new **MyPlate** takes into consideration the dietary and caloric needs for a wide variety of individuals, such as pregnant or breastfeeding women, those trying to lose weight, and adults with different activity levels.

Source: U.S. Department of Agriculture, Center for Nutrition Policy and Promotion, 2011.

Chapter In Review

Summary

- Although food is basic to human existence, food choices often have little to do with good nutrition.

- Socioeconomic factors, personal preferences and habits, cultural customs, and religious beliefs are all determining factors in the food we select.

- The eating habits of American students are often poor. This is due primarily to the habits of their parents, hurried life-styles, and lack of nutrition education.

- The development of positive lifetime eating habits in students is a critical issue.

- Food's basic function is to provide nutrients to the body.

- All foods contain calories.

- The USDA's MyPlate and the Daily Values can be used to plan a healthy diet.

- Food problems abound among students.

- Hunger and malnutrition affect a student's growth and learning.

- The number of overweight students is increasing.

- Pressure from peers to be thin or to look good in order to be accepted can encourage disordered eating patterns. These conditions are physical and emotional disorders. Sometimes therapy and counseling are needed to correct these problems.

- Food quackery preys on the fears and uncertainties people have regarding foods.

- Students should be taught to distinguish between truth and misleading statements.

- Food labels are provided on most foods to help determine the nutritional value of a food.

- Students should be taught to make responsible choices about food.

- Teachers and parents have to work together for nutrition education to be successful.

Discussion Questions

1. Describe why U.S. diets are often insufficient even though we live in an affluent country.
2. What factors determine one's selection of foods?
3. Discuss the importance of complex carbohydrates in the diet.
4. Discuss some healthy ways to snack to enhance your diet.
5. List the food sources for proteins.
6. Differentiate between saturated and unsaturated fats.
7. Describe the importance of water to the body.
8. What beneficial roles do minerals play in body function?
9. Discuss the role of antioxidants in enhancing health.
10. Describe the use of the USDA's MyPlate in selecting proper foods.
11. Discuss the typical characteristics of a person with anorexia nervosa.
12. Describe obesity as an emotional and physical disorder.
13. How can food labels be helpful to consumers?
14. Discuss the importance of the school lunch program.

Critical Thinking Questions

1. What strategies should school administrators use to encourage children to eat more nutritious and balanced meals and snacks while at school?
2. Devise a strategy that will help young children interpret food labels properly.
3. Compare the relative benefits and disadvantages of selling nonnutritious foods from vending machines in schools.
4. Consider the typical diet of Americans as described in the text. What economic factors contribute to this type of diet?
5. What would you consider the ideal diet plan? Consider MyPlate in your answer.

Access more material online at www.pearsonhighered.com/anspaugh. At this companion website for *Teaching Today's Health,* **you'll find chapter quizzes, web links, flashcards, a glossary, additional Worksheets, and more to help you succeed.**

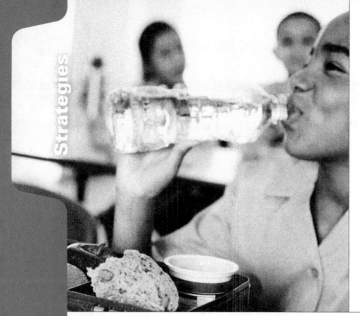

Strategies for Teaching Nutrition

Students need to internalize nutrition information and recognize its relevance to their health. To help the students do this, teachers should present learning opportunities that relate nutritional information to the students' daily lives.

NATIONAL HEALTH EDUCATION STANDARDS

1. Students will comprehend concepts related to health promotion and disease prevention to enhance health.

2. Students will analyze the influence of family, peers, culture, media, technology, and other factors on health behaviors.

3. Students will demonstrate the ability to access valid information and products and services to enhance health.

4. Students will demonstrate the ability to use interpersonal communication skills to enhance health and avoid or reduce health risks.

5. Students will demonstrate the ability to use decision-making skills to enhance health.

7. Students will demonstrate the ability to practice health-enhancing behaviors and avoid or reduce risks.

8. Students will demonstrate the ability to advocate for personal, family, and community health.

Valued Outcomes

After the completion of this chapter, you should be able to convey the following to your students:

- There is a close relationship between dietary practices and overall health.
- Food serves several functions in meeting body needs.
- Food fads and fallacies can affect an individual's food behavior.
- Caloric intake should be balanced with energy needs.
- Physical, psychological, and social factors affect personal food behavior.
- There are healthy and unhealthy ways of losing weight.
- The essential nutrients in food are carbohydrates, lipids, proteins, water, minerals, and vitamins.
- Eating a variety of carefully selected foods is the best way to ensure that the body receives the proper amounts of the nutrients it needs.
- MyPlate with ChooseMyPlate.gov can serve as an aid in planning balanced meals.
- The lack of certain nutrients can lead to certain diseases.
- Being underweight or overweight can lead to physical and emotional problems.
- Maintaining a proper weight is an individual responsibility, but others can help if there is a weight problem.
- A person who does not have a weight problem can be malnourished.
- Many people in the world do not have enough to eat.
- Food labels can provide useful nutritional information.

Reflection

The Surgeon General of the United States has called attention to the problem of childhood obesity in our country. As you read through this chapter, and as you select strategies for your classroom, reflect on how you can help students reduce their risk of obesity.

A Flexible Approach to Nutrition

Teachers have the responsibility of helping students learn the basic principles of nutrition so that they will understand the important relationship between nutrition and health and increase their skills in solving food- and nutrition-related problems. The concept of nutrition is quite abstract to younger elementary school children and is often seen as connected with, yet divorced from, eating. Your job in teaching nutrition is to make that concept more concrete to your students by presenting learning opportunities that relate nutritional information to daily life. In other words, you must personalize the information so that students will internalize it and recognize its relevance to their health.

Avoid a rigid, by-the-rules approach, and do not reduce nutrition education to a set of rules. Not only will a rule-based approach make nutrition seem grim, but it will also cause students to reject sound principles as unrealistic. Help students to understand the motivations for choosing and eating certain foods and that some of these motivations have little to do with the amount of nutrients to be attained from that food. For example, a person might be choosing a certain midafternoon snack because it was the one always offered by his or her parents. But that snack might not be as nutritious as another readily available snack.

Children and adults will change their habits only when they personally recognize the importance of doing so. Do not expect changes overnight. Encourage introspection, and foster positive decision-making skills. Act as a role model for changes you wish to bring about. Respect differences in tastes, likes, and dislikes.

Shown to the right of each activity title in this chapter is the suggested grade level(s) for which the activity might be appropriate. However, many of the suggested activities could be modified for use at various grade levels. Many of the strategies in this chapter reference MyPlate which can be found on page 303 or online at www.ChooseMyPlate .gov. When doing activities in which students are asked to taste or consume foods (milk, cheese, peanut butter, etc.), be sure to confirm that students are not allergic to those foods.

Information Assessment Activities

Nutrition Self-Portraits   Grades K–2

Valued Outcome: Students will be able to draw a picture and describe how the foods they eat help them become healthy.

National Health Education Standard: 1

Description of Strategy: Have each student draw a picture of himself or herself in the center of a piece of paper. Then have the students draw around their pictures all kinds of nutritious foods that they like to eat. Display the self-portraits around the room.

Materials Needed: paper and crayons or markers for each student

Processing Questions:

1. Why is it important to eat nutritious foods?
2. How do nutritious foods enhance our health?
3. What activities could we do besides eating nutritious food to keep us healthy?

○ **Integration:** Art

✓ **Assessment:** Students will be able to draw and name at least three nutritious foods that they like to eat.

Healthy Food Voting   Grades K–5

Valued Outcome: Students will be able to determine if their favorite foods are healthy or unhealthy.

National Health Education Standards: 1, 3, 7

Description of Strategy: Start by asking the students what their favorite foods are. List them on the board. After making these lists, make two separate columns and label one Healthy and the other Unhealthy. Then call out the list of favorite foods, and have the students vote whether each of the foods should go in the Healthy or the Unhealthy column.

Materials Needed: board and markers

Processing Question: How can I change my diet if most of my favorite foods are unhealthy?

✓ **Assessment:** Students will be able to name three healthy and three unhealthy foods that they like to eat.

Rank-Ordering Favorite Foods   Grades 3–5

Valued Outcome: Students will be able to clarify their values regarding their favorite foods.

National Health Education Standards: 3, 4

Description of Strategy: Have each student prepare a list of three or four favorite foods or dishes from each food group of MyPlate. Then tell the students to rank-order each food or dish, with the most favorite being labeled "1." Now have the students compare their lists. What class preferences seem to emerge? What are some individual preferences? Follow with a discussion of personal likes and dislikes.

Materials Needed: paper and pencils for each student

Processing Question: Do several of the students have the same favorite foods as you do? If they do not, why do you think that is true?

✔**Assessment:** Students will be able to name the food groups depicted in MyPlate and rank their favorite two foods from each group.

What's for Lunch?   Grades 3–5

Valued Outcome: Students will be able to analyze the nutritional quality of their school lunches.

National Health Education Standards: 1, 7

Description of Strategy: Have the students write down and analyze their school lunches for three days. After three days, have the students share what they thought about the school lunches. Discuss which food groups were poorly represented and which food groups were well represented. Have the students give their own opinions about the school lunches. As an instructor, make sure good things are said as well as bad.

Materials Needed: paper and pencils for each student

Processing Questions:

1. Did you enjoy these lunches?
2. Were you able to eat the types of foods you enjoy?
3. Did your analysis determine that your lunches were healthy? Unhealthy?

✔**Assessment:** Students will be able to describe the healthy and unhealthy foods they ate for lunch during the three-day period.

A Healthy Breakfast   Grades 4–5

Valued Outcome: Students will be able to decide which breakfast foods are healthful and which are not.

National Health Education Standards: 5, 7

Description of Strategy: Divide the class into groups of four to six students. Have the students get out two sheets of paper for the group. On one sheet of paper, write Nutritious; on the other sheet of paper, write Not Nutritious. Have the group decide what a nutritious breakfast is and write it down. Label the foods by their food groups as given on MyPlate. Then have them make up a breakfast that is not nutritious and label the foods by their food groups. Have a group discussion about their answers. After the discussion, do the same concept for lunch and dinner.

Materials Needed: paper and pencils for each student

Processing Questions:

1. What do you think are the most popular, nutritious breakfast foods?
2. What do you think are the most popular, nonnutritious breakfast foods?
3. Why is it important to eat a nutritious breakfast?

✔**Assessment:** Students will be able to list three nutritious and three nonnutritious breakfast foods.

Nutrition Sentence Completion   Grades 4–5

Valued Outcome: Students will be able to complete nutrition-related statements with their own feelings and beliefs.

National Health Education Standards: 4, 7

Description of Strategy: Create a handout of the following statements. Have the students complete the handout with phrases that come to mind immediately on hearing the key phrase beginning the statement:

- The most important meal of the day for me is…
- Eating a good breakfast is…
- My favorite foods are…
- Eating right means…
- I think that my present diet is…
- Between-meal snacks should be…
- One problem about nutrition for me is…

Materials Needed: handouts and pencils for each student

Processing Question: Who can help you determine what is included in a good breakfast and/or snack?

✔**Assessment:** Students will demonstrate the ability to evaluate the quality of their diet.

Nutrition Podcasts   Grades K–5

Valued Outcome: Students will be able to describe the main concepts covered in the nutrition-related podcasts.

National Health Education Standards: 1, 2, 3

Description of Strategy: Students access and listen to the various nutrition-related podcasts. The listening can be done as homework, or as a classroom activity. After listening to the podcasts, each student should write a reflective essay related to the nutrition podcast. Recommended podcasts include:

- PodcastDirectory.com: *Kids, Sports and Nutrition* episode. This podcast discusses: 1) how much exercise is healthy? and 2) what should a young athlete eat?

  Accessed at: www.podcastdirectory.com/podshows/1419765

- Medical University of South Carolina (MUSC) Health Audio Podcasts: *Overweight: Nutritional Guidance for Overweight Children.* This podcast discusses helping overweight children either by behavior change or diet modification, and emphasizes the critical role of exercise in a healthy lifestyle.

  Accessed at: www.muschealth.com/multimedia/Podcasts/displayPod.aspx?podid=582&autostart=false

☼ TEACHING IN ACTION	**Daily Lesson Plan**

Lesson Title: MyPlate Collage

Date: March 19, 2012   **Time:** 11:00 A.M.   **Grade:** Four   **Teacher:** Lerato

I. National Health Education Standards

Health Education Standard 7: Students will demonstrate the ability to practice health-enhancing behaviors and avoid or reduce health risks.

II. National Health Education Standards Performance Indicator

7.5.1 identify responsible personal health behaviors.

III. Valued Outcomes

- Students will be able to describe the areas of MyPlate.
- Students will be able to explain why MyPlate is a valid source of information about nutrition.
- Students will be able to demonstrate the ability to make good food choices.

IV. Description of Strategy

1. Have students collect food pictures from magazines, newspapers, or grocery store advertisements.
2. Divide the class into groups of four or five students, and give each group a poster board. Display a copy of MyPlate. Tell students to cut the poster board into the shape of a place setting, draw the sections of MyPlate onto the shape, and paste the food pictures onto the appropriate section to make a collage. The number of pictures in each section should represent the suggested number of servings.
3. Have each group present their collage to the class and explain which foods they put in each of the different food groups. Each group should relate why MyPlate is a good source of information.
4. Ask students to use their posters as a reference and draw a healthy meal on a paper plate.

V. Materials Needed

- large copy of MyPlate (poster can be obtained from www.ChooseMyPlate.gov)
- magazines, newspapers, and grocery store flyers
- poster board, glue, tape, crayons, and scissors
- paper plates

VI. Formative Evaluation

Benchmarks

- Level 1: Student was able to identify some of the parts of MyPlate.
- Level 2: Student was able to identify all of the parts of MyPlate.
- Level 3: Student was able to identify all of the parts of MyPlate and describe why it is a good source of nutrition information.
- Level 4: Student was able to identify all of the parts of MyPlate and describe why it is a good source of nutrition information. Student was able to choose items in a healthy meal.

VII. Points of Emphasis

1. Explain the importance of having foods from every part of the plate in each meal.
2. Explain how making healthy food choices leads to better health and less sickness.
3. Explain why MyPlate is a reliable source of nutrition information.

Teacher Evaluation

1. Keep the lesson as taught?   yes _____   no _____

2. What I need to improve _____

3. Next time make sure _____

4. Strengths of lesson Strategies _____

TEACHING IN ACTION | **Daily Lesson Plan**

Lesson Title: Do You Want to Eat This Food?

Date: March 26, 2012   **Time:** 1:00 P.M.   **Grade:** Six   **Teacher:** Anneta

I. National Health Education Standards

Health Education Standard 3: Students will demonstrate the ability to access valid information and products and services to enhance health.

II. National Health Education Standards Performance Indicator

3.8.2 access valid health information from home, school, and community.

III. Valued Outcomes

- Students will be able to read food labels for various products.
- Students will be able to interpret food labels.
- Students will be able to compare food labels to make wise food choices.

IV. Description of Strategy

1. Describe to students the parts of a Nutrition Facts panel. Tell students what information is required on the Nutrition Facts panels by the Food and Drug Administration for all foods. Make sure to tell students how reading Nutrition Facts panels can make them a more informed consumer. Also, point out to students the ingredients list on food labels.
2. Show students labels from various foods, such as bread, potato chips, soup, yogurt, and ice cream. Help students compare the nutrients in each of the foods.
3. Have students decide which food would be a better choice to eat according to the Nutrition Facts panel. Remind the students of the items to consider, such as fat content, caloric content, or any key vitamins that should be plentiful in one's diet.
4. Have the students write an essay to reinforce what they learned about the Nutrition Facts panel.

V. Materials Needed

- food labels from various products
- Worksheet 18.1

VI. Formative Evaluation

Benchmarks

- Level 1: Student was able to read some of the items on a food label.
- Level 2: Student was able to read all of the items on a food label.
- Level 3: Student was able to read all of the items on a food label. Student could interpret information and describe the food's nutritional value.
- Level 4: Student was able to read all of the items on a food label. Student could interpret information and describe the food's nutritional value. Student was able to compare food labels from various foods and choose the most nutritious item.

VII. Points of Emphasis

1. Explain the importance of serving size and servings per container in judging the nutritional value.
2. Explain how reading food labels can help students make informed decisions regarding food choices.
3. Explain how to interpret the percentage of daily value and why that is an important part of the label.

Teacher Evaluation

1. Keep the lesson as taught?   yes _____   no _____

2. What I need to improve _____

3. Next time make sure _____

4. Strengths of lesson _____

Materials Needed: computer with speakers or personal music player with capability to play podcasts (each student)

Processing Question:

1. Were you able to identify the main nutrition-related concepts covered in the podcast?
2. What nutrition or exercise discussion do you remember most from the podcast?
3. Was there information you think should have been talked about in the podcast that wasn't covered?

✓ **Assessment:** Students will demonstrate the nutrition-related knowledge they gained from the podcast(s) by completing a one-page reflective essay covering at least two major nutrition-related concepts they learned from the podcast(s).

Values Continuum   Grades 4–5

Valued Outcome: Students will be able to explain how different eating lifestyles can affect one's nutrition.

National Health Education Standards: 1, 7

Description of Strategy: Pass out continuum sheets. One end of the continuum represents a lifestyle in which every meal is eaten at home under relaxed conditions. The other end of the continuum represents a lifestyle in which every meal is eaten outside the home under hurried or hectic conditions. Have each student place an *X* on the continuum that represents his or her assessment of eating lifestyle. Follow with a general discussion of how eating lifestyle may affect growth and development as well as emotional state. Sample continuum:

All meals eaten at home   All meals eaten outside the
(relaxed conditions)   home (hectic conditions)

⟵─────────────────────────────────────⟶

Materials Needed: continuum sheets and pencils for each student

Processing Question: How does a hurried or relaxed eating lifestyle affect the digestion of the food we eat?

✓ **Assessment:** Students will be able to describe the benefits of eating in a relaxed environment and the drawbacks of eating in a rushed or stressed environment.

Decision Stories

(Follow the procedures outlined in Chapter 4, pages 60–62, for presenting decision stories.)

For each of the decision stories, write a list on the board of ideas generated by the class for how each situation should be dealt with. Ask the students to discuss the merits of the methods suggested.

✓ **Assessment for Decision Stories:** Students can identify health-enhancing behaviors and exhibit positive decision-making skills.

What to Drink?   Grades K–2

Al has just come inside from playing a game of football with his friends and is very thirsty. He opens the refrigerator and finds water, soda pop, and fruit juice.

Focus Question: Which would be best for Al to drink? Why?

National Health Education Standards: 5, 7

Fast Food   Grades K–5

Tim doesn't like the food they serve in the school cafeteria. Some of his friends go to a fast-food restaurant near the school instead. He would like to go with them, but he knows that his parents want him to eat in the cafeteria.

Focus Question: What should Tim do?

National Health Education Standards: 2, 5

Dramatizations

Foods that Keep the Body Healthy   Grades K–3

Valued Outcome: Students will be able to identify certain foods that help keep the body healthy.

National Health Education Standards: 1, 7

Description of Strategy: On butcher paper, draw an outline of three types of bodies: heavy, average, and thin. Have the students attach pictures of foods to each body type that might result from a diet of these foods. Discuss with the students why an excess of certain foods can have a negative effect on the body. (It is important to point out that some diseases may also affect body shape, so diet *is not* the only factor that may be involved.)

To show the positive effect foods have on the body, have students role-play a race. Let two students who are going to run in a race role-play different ways of eating in preparation for the event. For example, one eats very nutritious light meals, whereas the other eats high-calorie junk food. Let the two students enact what they would feel like while running in the race.

Materials Needed: drawing of the three body types on butcher paper, pictures of body types from magazines, food photos from magazines

Processing Questions:

1. What effect does food have on our body build?
2. What effect does food have on our energy level?
3. What foods should you eat to prepare for a race or other endurance activity?
4. What effect would poor food choices have on one's endurance?

✓ **Assessment:** Students will be able to name at least five foods that keep the body healthy and five foods that may have a negative health effect on the body.

Role-Playing Nutrients   Grades 3–6

Valued Outcomes: Students will be able to describe the significance of nutrients, vitamins, and minerals through role-playing.

National Health Education Standards: 1, 3, 7

Description of Strategy: Assemble the students in cooperative groups. Assign each group a category—carbohydrate, protein, fat, vitamin, mineral, or water. Then have each group research and dramatize characteristics of their category. Students may use food representations to dramatize characteristics of different nutrients; for example, for the carbohydrates in a fruit, the student could simulate planting, growing, harvesting, shipping, buying, eating, and digesting the food. Each group will present its dramatization to the class and explain why they chose to dramatize the way they did. They will explain the significance of their nutrient and its relationship to a healthy diet.

Processing Questions:

1. What are the important characteristics of each category of nutrient?
2. Why is it important to know these characteristics?

✓ **Assessment:** Students will be able to name the six classes of nutrients and provide three facts about each.

Garden Puppet Show   Grades K–3

Valued Outcome: Students will be able to demonstrate different foods that are grown in the garden and be able to tell the benefit of each food to the body.

National Health Education Standards: 1, 7

Description of Strategy: Have students make puppets of different fruits and vegetables. Let them enact a scene in a garden in which the various foods tell what they will do for the body when they are eaten.

Materials Needed: paper lunch bag or cloth; craft items (construction paper, glue, wire, etc.) for each student

Processing Question: How do various garden-grown foods help our bodies function better?

✓ **Assessment:** Students will be able to name five foods commonly grown in a garden and will understand that fresh foods from a garden are good for the body.

Dieting Puppets and Eating Disorders   Grades K–3

Valued Outcome: Students will be able to demonstrate the problems some individuals have in gaining weight and losing weight.

National Health Education Standards: 1, 7

Description of Strategy: Prepare several puppets, some to represent thin people trying to gain weight, others to represent overweight persons trying to lose weight, and some to represent persons with an eating disorder (anorexia nervosa or bulimia). Have the puppets sitting at a table during a meal and discussing why they are eating (or not eating) various foods.

Materials Needed: paper lunch bags or cloth and markers or crayons for each student

Processing Question: Why do some thin people try to lose weight? How can such behavior affect that person's health?

✓ **Assessment:** Students will be able to explain the challenges of attempting to gain or lose weight.

Star Search   Grades K–5

Valued Outcome: Students will be able to describe various nutritional problems.

National Health Education Standard: 1

Description of Strategy: Divide the class into groups of four to six students. Have them make up a song, poem, dance, or skit about a nutritional problem, such as eating too much junk food or not eating foods from MyPlate. Students then present their work to the class, and the audience should try to guess what the problem is and then discuss it. At the end of the class, reward everyone with stickers or a snack.

Materials Needed: pencils and paper for each student, rewards

Processing Question: Why do so many people in our country have nutritional problems when we have such a plentiful supply of food? How can such nutritional problems affect our overall health?

✓ **Assessment:** Students will be able to describe and then list potential causes for one nutritional problem.

Caffeine and Sleeping   Grades K–5

Valued Outcome: Students will identify effects that caffeine has on the body.

National Health Education Standards: 1, 7

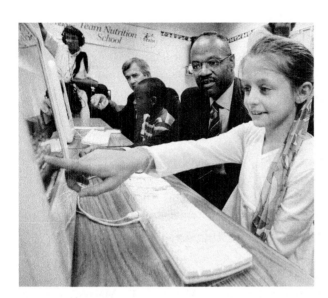

Hands-on activities enhance the learning of health concepts.

Description of Strategy: Ask the students what they know about sleep. Introduce caffeine by showing the students pictures of chocolate, cola, tea, and coffee. Ask them if they know what the objects in the pictures have in common. Explain that each of the objects contains caffeine. Ask the students if they know what caffeine is. Explain that caffeine is a drug called a stimulant, so it speeds up the nervous system and makes a person jittery or hyperactive. Let the students know that when they eat or drink something that contains caffeine and it makes them hyperactive, it is hard to sleep.

Tell the students that they will play a role-playing game. Divide the class in half: One half will be the actors; the other half will be the guessers. Tell the actors the situation: They are at a friend's birthday party, and they will be spending the night. The friend's mom said that the students could eat as much chocolate and drink as much cola as they like, as a special treat. Give each actor a card that says one of the following: "You said 'No, thank you,' and only ate milk and cookies"; "You ate one piece of chocolate and drank half of a cola"; and "You ate as much chocolate and cola as you could." The actors will demonstrate trying to go to sleep, without saying what they did or didn't eat. After the actors have finished, it is the job of the guessers to decide how much caffeine each actor consumed.

Materials Needed: pictures of chocolate, cola, tea, and coffee; note cards of responses for the game

Processing Questions:

1. What foods typically contain caffeine?
2. What happens when you try to go to sleep after you've had too much caffeine?

✓ **Assessment:** Students will be able to explain how caffeine might impact sleep.

Cafeteria Selection   Grades K–5

Valued Outcome: Students will be able to select a meal by choosing foods from each group on MyPlate.

National Health Education Standards: 1, 3, 5, 7

Description of Strategy: Using food pictures, set up a "cafeteria line" from which students will choose a meal to place on a tray. Have students take turns being the cashiers—checking to see that choices include food from each of the five main food groups on MyPlate.

Materials Needed: food pictures from magazines, scissors, glue, paper

Processing Questions:

1. What are the food groups shown in MyPlate?
2. What are two foods in each food group?

✓ **Assessment:** Students will be able to name the food groups of MyPlate, and list two foods from each group.

Choosing from a Menu   Grades 3–6

Valued Outcome: Students will be able to select foods from a restaurant menu.

National Health Education Standards: 1, 5, 7

Description of Strategy: Bring several menus from area restaurants or let students make menus. Have several students enact a situation in which they are seated in a restaurant and must make choices from the menu. Have others play the role of waiter or waitress to help guide the diner's choices.

Materials Needed: menus from restaurants, paper and pencils for each student

Processing Questions:

1. How did you decide which foods to order?
2. How did you decide which foods to avoid?

✓ **Assessment:** Students will be able describe how to select healthy foods from a restaurant menu.

Eating for Special Needs   Grades 4–5

Valued Outcome: Students will be able to plan meals for people with special needs.

National Health Education Standard: 8

Description of Strategy: Have a couple of students in the class role-play patients in the hospital. Example: The first patient is a sixty-seven-year-old man who has no teeth and an ulcer. The second patient is a seven-year-old girl who has had her tonsils removed and has a sore throat. The third patient is a forty-five-year-old man who is overweight and has a serious heart ailment. Make or plan a breakfast, lunch, and dinner for all the patients and then discuss the results.

Processing Questions:

1. Why do some people need to avoid or include certain foods in their diets?
2. What would happen to these patients if they ate or avoided certain foods such as foods that were hard to chew?

✔ **Assessment:** Students will correctly design a meal for a special needs patient and be able to explain why their meal is appropriate for the patient.

Selling a Product Grades 4–5

Valued Outcome: Students will create nutritional advertisements.

National Health Education Standards: 3, 8

Description of Strategy: Divide the students into groups of three to five. Give each group a product (some products should be nutritious and others nonnutritious). Have each group work together to think of a way to sell the product, and then come up in front of the class and try to sell their products. Discuss the product and the food group to which it belongs.

Materials Needed: different food products for each group of students

Processing Questions:

1. Why do companies use advertisements to sell their products?
2. How should we evaluate such advertisements to make sure we make wise nutritional decisions?

✔ **Assessment:** Students will demonstrate understanding of how food advertising works and how to evaluate it.

Nutrients on Trial Grades 4–5

Valued Outcome: Students will be able to determine essential functions of the nutrients in the body.

National Health Education Standard: 1

Description of Strategy: Have the students conduct a mock court with nutrients on trial. Give the students situations in which the nutrients are accused of not being useful to the body. The nutrients' defendants must defend their essential function in the body.

Materials Needed: judge's gavel and robe (optional)

Processing Questions:

1. Why are the nutrients essential?
2. What is one function of each nutrient?

✔ **Assessment:** Students will be able to name the six classes of essential nutrients and explain one function of each.

Stranger in a Strange Land Grades 4–5

Valued Outcome: Students will be able to discuss typical foods eaten in different countries.

National Health Education Standard: 2

Description of Strategy: Divide the class into small groups. Have each research the foods and dishes eaten in a different nation, such as Mexico, India, Malaysia, Germany, Japan, and Greece. Then have the students in each group prepare models or drawings of different typical dishes served in their assigned nation. You act the part of a traveler who has just arrived in the country and is very hungry. Ask about each dish the students have to offer. What is it made of? How is it prepared? How does it taste? How does one eat it? Follow with a general discussion of different ethnic foods.

Materials Needed: paper, markers, modeling clay, and paint for each student

Processing Questions:

1. What foods do people in other countries eat that we may not eat here?
2. What foods do we often eat that are not commonly found in other countries?
3. What is one dish you learned about that you would like to try?

◯ **Integration:** Social Stucdies

✔ **Assessment:** Students will describe two common foods found in at least two other countries and state whether those foods are common in the United States.

Discussion and Report Techniques

Classifying Nutritious and Nonnutritious Snacks Grades K–2

Valued Outcome: After completing the week's activity centers, the students will be able to categorize healthy and unhealthy snacks.

National Health Education Standards: 1, 7

Description of Strategy: Introduce each center as follows:

First we have the Book Center. There are many books to read and look at. There will also be a couple of books you can listen to.

Next we have the Block Center. Here I encourage you to use your imagination and relate something you build to healthy and unhealthy snacks.

Next we have the Writing Center. Here you can make your own nutrition journal by tying some decorative paper together. Today's topic is to draw or tell about the snacks that you like to eat.

Next we have the Cooking Center, where you can mix your own healthy snack. After you mix together the appropriate ingredients, you can take your mix to the eating area and enjoy it. You will be mixing things like Chex cereal, pretzels, peanuts, raisins, and popcorn in a little bag and shake it all together. Then it is ready to eat.

Next we have the Art Center. In art today we are going to make a collage of nutritious (good for you) and nonnutritious (not so good for you) snacks. Look through the magazines and find pictures of either nutritious snacks or nonnutritious snacks. Then glue them on your piece of paper. Try choosing only pictures of nutritious and nonnutritious snacks for your collage.

In the Math Center, you will sort the pictures of snacks into two piles of nutritious and nonnutritious snacks.

In the Language Arts Center, there is a worksheet, and on the worksheet there are both nutritious and nonnutritious snacks. Color the nutritious snacks.

In the Science Center, you will taste nutritious and nonnutritious snacks and chart how well you liked each snack. Then as a class we will look at the results to see who liked what the best.

In the Game Center there will be several games to play, such as Xs and Os, Hangman using the Alphabits cereal, and the usual games that are there.

Materials Needed: nutrition books, building blocks, decorative paper, crayons or markers, nutritious and nonnutritious snacks; sandwich bags, magazines, construction paper, glue, title cards, worksheet for Language Center that has pictures of both nutritious and nonnutritious foods; Alphabits cereal

Processing Question: What types of food provide the healthiest snacks?

○ **Integration:** Art

✓ **Assessment:** Students will demonstrate the ability to categorize a specific snack food as nutritious or nonnutritious.

Grocery Shopping　　　　　　　　　Grades K–3

Valued Outcome: Students will be able to purchase foods efficiently from a "grocery store."

National Health Education Standards: 1, 7

Description of Strategy: Tell the students that they are each to pretend they have $50. Have a variety of food labels set up on a table with their prices. Make note cards for fruits and other products for which you don't have labels. Tell the students that they need to purchase food for two people for three days. Have them shop for the food they'll eat by writing down the food item and its cost. Discuss the results by asking a variety of questions, such as: Who here has bought enough food for three meals a day? Who has bought something from each category of MyPlate?

Materials Needed: food labels with prices, note cards representing fruit and other products without labels pencils, paper

Processing Questions:

1. Why is it important to plan a budget for buying food?
2. What can you learn about a food from reading the label?

○ **Integration:** Math

✓ **Assessment:** Students will demonstrate the ability to "shop" for healthy foods while sticking to a budget.

Healthy Breakfasts　　　　　　　　　Grades K–3

Valued Outcome: Students will be able to explain why we need a good breakfast and will be able to choose healthy breakfast foods.

National Health Education Standards: 5, 7

Description of Strategy: Give each student a magazine containing food pictures that he or she can cut out. Students will cut out enough pictures to create a balanced breakfast. They will glue these pictures onto a sheet of construction paper labeled "A Healthful Breakfast."

Materials Needed: magazines, glue, scissors, construction paper, and markers or crayons for each student

Processing Questions:

1. Why is breakfast called the most important meal of the day?
2. What types of foods are good to eat at breakfast?

✓ **Assessment:** Students will be able to list at least three healthy breakfast foods.

Nutrition　　　　　　　　　　　　　　Grades 3–6

Valued Outcome: Students will identify the six essential nutrients needed to maintain a healthy body and how the body benefits from each of the nutrients.

National Health Education Standard: 1

Description of Strategy: Explain to the class that today's lesson is about being able to identify the six essential nutrients needed for maintaining a healthy body and the benefits from each nutrient. Introduce the six nutrients (carbohydrates, proteins, lipids, water, vitamins, and minerals) and list them on the board. Tell the students that some foods contain many nutrients; for example, pasta contains carbohydrates, peanut butter contains protein, ice cream contains fat (lipids), and so on. Pick students to go to the board three at a time and write a food under each category for the six nutrients. Each student will have an opportunity to write a food on the board. Explain the importance of each of the dietary nutrients in relation to its function in the body. Explain that they are the substances in food needed to support life functions. For example, fats are an important part of cell membranes and tissues; and proteins build and repair body tissues, function as enzymes, antibodies, and so on. Finally, have students complete Worksheet 18.1 on page 495 to reinforce the material.

Materials Needed: overhead projector and pens or board and markers, Worksheet 18.1

Processing Question: Why is it important to consume each of the nutrients daily?

○ **Integration:** Science

✓ **Assessment:** Students will be able to name the six essential nutrients and one key function in the body for each nutrient.

Breakfast Book Grades K–5

Valued Outcome: Students will be able to explain how a healthy diet can increase the likelihood of physical and mental wellness.

National Health Education Standards: 1, 7

Description of Strategy: If your school has a breakfast program, explain to the students that these meals are nutritionally balanced to provide the fuel needed to help their bodies work. Ask the students for suggestions, and make a "Healthy Breakfast List" on large chart paper. Include food from at least three of the food groups. Some ideas are peanut butter on toast, yogurt, cereal with fruit, cold pizza, fresh or dried fruit, a glass of juice, a sandwich, and a glass of milk. Have the students write a Big Breakfast Book about the foods they like to eat for breakfast; include things such as what they like to eat, whom they eat with, how they feel when they do not eat breakfast, and so on. Have each student write or dictate his or her own words and illustrate them. Then bind all pages together into a book; let the students choose the title for their book. When the book is complete, read it to the class, let each student author read his or her own page to the class, or let the principal come in for an authors' reading. Display the book for the students to see.

Materials Needed: chart paper, pencils, markers or crayons, and paper for each student, materials to bind a student work into a book

Processing Question: Why is breakfast the most important meal?

○ **Integration:** Writing

✓ **Assessment:** Students will be able to list three of their favorite healthy breakfast foods, and explain at least two benefits of eating a healthy breakfast.

Source: Utah Education Network 1996, 1997b

Eating for Healthy Teeth Grades K–5

Valued Outcome: Students will be able to identify foods that are good for the teeth.

National Health Education Standards: 1, 7

Description of Strategy: Share the following information with the students. Unhealthy foods often stick to your teeth and/or contain a lot of sugar. Healthy foods can include those foods, like apples, that can help clean your teeth as you eat them. Other healthy foods for teeth include foods high in calcium and phosphorus. Remind students that even healthy foods can promote tooth decay if trapped food is not removed from teeth by flossing and brushing daily, since bacteria can grow in food left on and around teeth.

Have students bring in at least ten pictures—drawn or cut out of magazines and glued or taped onto paper—of healthy and unhealthy foods for our teeth. Have them label each picture healthy or unhealthy.

Write Healthy and Unhealthy on the board and provide examples for both categories. Then divide the class into groups of three or four. Say, "Please work as a group. Copy the chart and words off the board. As a group, complete the chart by listing healthy foods for teeth under the Healthy side and the unhealthy foods under the Unhealthy side." Walk around the room to monitor for understanding. Allow time for them to complete the assignment. When all groups have finished, have the class help you complete the chart on the board. Have them explain why they put certain foods under certain categories. Have students review the labels they put on their magazine pictures. Should any of these labels be changed?

Materials Needed: board and markers or overhead projector and pen; magazines, glue or tape, paper, and pencils for each student

Processing Questions:

1. What are the healthiest foods to eat for our teeth?
2. What foods will hurt our teeth?

✓ **Assessment:** Students will be able to list at least two foods that are healthy for teeth and two foods that are unhealthy for teeth.

Food Preference Grades 3–4

Valued Outcome: Students will be able to explain the difference between their own food tastes and preferences and the tastes and preferences of others.

National Health Education Standard: 2

Description of Strategy: Have the students write down their favorite ethnic food (Italian, American, Mexican, etc.), their overall favorite food, their favorite fruit, their favorite vegetable, and their favorite dessert. Explain why some of the foods are more nutritious than others, the different foods that each ethnic group cooks, and the nutritional value of those foods. Announce a category (e.g., favorite ethnic group), and have all the students with the same answer stand together. Do this until all the categories are completed. Then, as a class, talk about everyone's favorite foods.

Materials Needed: paper and pencils for each student

Processing Question: Does everyone have the same tastes and favorite foods? Why or why not?

✓ **Assessment:** Students will demonstrate the ability to recognize the differences in taste, preference, and favorite foods among different people and different cultures.

Food Labels in the Classroom   Grades 3–5

Valued Outcome: Students will be able to use food labels to determine the nutritional content of various foods.

National Health Education Standards: 1, 7

Description of Strategy: Give each student several food labels. Then have each student read thoroughly all information given on the packaging and write down all nutritional information such as grams of protein, carbohydrates, and fat per serving. Use current health references (nutrition textbooks and brochures) to go over the six essential nutrients, which are carbohydrates, protein, lipids, vitamins, minerals, and water, and look for these dietary requirements on food labels. Make a classroom list of packaging and labeling techniques meant to attract the consumer; classify these appeals into categories such as good taste, low cost, convenience, and health. Under the health category determine which health factors are being considered (low in calories, no cholesterol, fiber, and no additives). Answer any questions that the students have regarding the food labels. Finally, reinforce the material by having students complete Worksheet 18.2 on page 496.

Materials Needed: food labels brought in by students, brochures and textbooks on nutrition, overhead projector and pens or board and markers, Worksheet 18.2

Processing Questions:

1. What information can you find on a food label to determine if a food is healthy?
2. What advertising claims found on food labels might influence your decision to buy the food?
3. How important is it to read food labels carefully before buying a product?

✓ **Assessment:** Students will be able to list at least three pieces of information on the food label that can help them determine if the food is healthy.

Source: Teacher Store 1999; Roger 1994

Assess Your Food Intake   Grades 3–5

Valued Outcome: Students will be able to compare their food intake for one day to the recommendations from ChooseMyPlate.gov.

National Health Education Standards: 1, 7

Description of Strategy: The online dietary assessment at www.ChooseMyPlate.gov provides information on diet quality, related nutrition messages, and links to nutrient information. Each student will track a day's food intake. The students will then access the ChooseMyPlate.gov website to receive their own nutrient recommendations. They should create overall evaluation of their daily food intake by comparing the amounts of food and the nutrients they ate to current nutritional guidance. The students should be given the assignment at least one day in advance so they can track their food over the course of a day, rather than trying to remember what they've eaten.

Processing Questions:

1. Did your food intake meet the recommendations of the MyPlate assessment?
2. What other choices do you think you should have made to better fulfill your daily nutrient recommendations?

✓ **Assessment:** Students will print out their food intake assessment and write a one-paragraph description of their food intake. They should demonstrate an understanding of food groups and basic nutrient needs.

Source: United States Department of Agriculture 2011.

Snack Machines in the Schools Debate   Grades 3–5

Valued Outcome: Students will be able to debate whether snack machines should or should not be installed in the school cafeteria.

National Health Education Standard: 8

Description of Strategy: Should snack machines be placed in the school cafeteria? Have two debate teams argue the issue. Act as moderator and keep the debate on track. Then follow with a general class discussion.

Processing Questions:

1. Why are snack machines present in some schools?
2. Does the presence of such machines encourage poor eating habits on the part of some students?

✓ **Assessment:** Students will be able to state at least two valid reasons why snack machines should or should not be placed in schools.

Food Basket Turnover
Grades 4–5

Valued Outcome: Students will be able to demonstrate knowledge of the food groups of MyPlate.

National Health Education Standard: 1

Description of Strategy: Using masking tape, create the outline of MyPlate on the classroom floor. Designate each area by a sheet of paper affixed alongside each section (the label should contain the name of the food group and the amount of servings suggested daily). Instruct students to brainstorm different foods that fit into each category of MyPlate and write them on a piece of paper. Have them include at least one food that they have never tried and one food that they dislike in each food group and place NT beside the food he or she has never tried and DL beside the food he or she dislikes. Compile a written list of foods (grouped by category) on the overhead, while the students name the food group in which it belongs.

Explain that the class will play a game called "Food Basket Turnover" to help them learn how many servings of each food group are necessary for a healthy diet. Have each student draw one food task card from a group of prepared task cards (each containing a picture of a different type of food), take the card, and move to the appropriate location on the classroom floor. After all task cards have been chosen, visually check for accuracy and declare, "Food Basket Turnover!" On this signal, the students return to their desks. Repeat the MyPlate activity two additional times. Have students share orally with classmates one fact learned from their experience and participation in the MyPlate activity.

Materials Needed: masking tape, paper and pencils, overhead projector and pens, large MyPlate chart, food task cards (one per student, each with a picture of a specific food)

Processing Question: How is MyPlate helpful in planning our daily diets?

✓ **Assessment:** Students will demonstrate the ability to match foods to the correct category in MyPlate and accurately state the recommended daily servings for each group.

Food Journal
Grades 4–5

Valued Outcome: Students will be able to describe their eating habits.

National Health Education Standards: 4, 7

Description of Strategy: Have the students keep a journal of what they eat for one week, starting on a Sunday and ending on the following Saturday. (Provide them with charts such as the sample table below.)

Date and Time	
Foods	
Servings	
Place	
With Whom	

Have them bring this to class on the Monday after it is completed. In pairs, have students use MyPlate to decide the number of servings from each food category that were eaten each day. Students should record this information on a separate sheet of paper. After the number of servings for each category for each day has been tallied, make a class graph showing the food groups and the number of servings eaten for any one day. (Decide which day you want to use. You may want to use one weekday and one weekend day to compare.) Use the graph to talk about how many students are eating the correct number of servings. Lead a discussion on what foods they need to eat more or less of to be healthier.

Materials Needed: pencil or pen and journals for each student, chart, a copy of MyPlate, materials to compile a class graph

Processing Questions:

1. In which areas of the MyPlate did you eat enough, and in which did you not eat enough?
2. Why do we eat sometimes even when we are not hungry?

✓ **Assessment:** Students will demonstrate the ability to correctly state the number of servings they are eating from each food category in MyPlate.

Nutrition IQ
Grades 4–5

Valued Outcome: Students will be able to test their nutrition knowledge by completing the worksheet.

National Health Education Standard: 1

Description of Strategy: Have each student complete Worksheet 18.3 (page 497) containing questions related to nutrition. Have the students turn in their work or discuss the questions as a class.

Materials Needed: Worksheet 18.3 and pencils for each student

Processing Question: Why is it important to our health to have a good "nutrition IQ"?

✓ **Assessment:** Students will correctly answer at least 75 percent (nine out of twelve) of the T/F questions.

Being Healthy! Grades 4–5

Valued Outcome: Students will be able to explain the effects of a proper diet on their physical and mental health.

National Health Education Standards: 1, 7

Description of Strategy: Have the students write down four to six sentences about how they feel mentally, physically, and emotionally when they eat nutritious foods. Then, have them do the same thing about how they feel when they eat nonnutritious foods. Write the three aspects of health on the board, and discuss the answers.

Materials Needed: pencil and paper for each student, board or overhead projector and markers

Processing Question: How can food affect your ability to learn?

○ **Integration:** Writing

✓ **Assessment:** Students will be able to list one mental, physical, and emotional effect of eating healthy and unhealthy foods.

Foods from Around the World Grades 4–5

Valued Outcome: Students will be able to report on foods grown in different countries and regions.

National Health Education Standard: 2

Description of Strategy: Locate countries or regions on a world map. Have the students choose a particular country or region and research the history of a food or type of food from that country. Students will then present in oral, written, or pictorial form their information about the foods from a specific country.

Materials Needed: maps and dietary information about different countries, chart paper, and markers for students who choose the written or pictorial form

Processing Question: How does the preparation and type of food that you researched differ from American food?

○ **Integration:** Social Studies

✓ **Assessment:** Students will demonstrate the ability to research and discuss the different types of foods commonly eaten around the world.

Diet Goals Grades 4–5

Valued Outcome: Students will understand each of the seven diet goals for health.

National Health Education Standards: 1, 7

Description of Strategy: List these seven diet goals on the board:

1. Eat a variety of foods.
2. Be at a healthful weight.
3. Eat few fatty foods.
4. Eat more fiber.
5. Eat less sugar.
6. Use less salt.
7. Do not drink alcohol.

Have the students write the diet goals on a 30" × 50" index card. They should keep the index card with them and refer to it at mealtimes until they have memorized the goals. This will help them become accustomed to considering the diet goals when selecting foods. Discuss each diet goal. For example:

- *Eat a variety of foods.* Ask students to identify the food groups and give the number of servings from each group that should be eaten daily.
- *Be at a healthful weight.* Explain that your body works best when you are at the weight that is right for you. Let the students know that the doctor can tell them if they are at a healthful weight. Explain to the students that they can make wise choices to help them be at a healthful weight and how important it is to exercise and eat properly balanced meals.

Materials Needed: board and markers or overhead projector and pen, 30" × 50" index cards

Processing Questions:

1. Why is each of these goals important?
2. Which goal is easiest for you to reach? Which is most challenging for you to reach?

✓ **Assessment:** Students will be able to list the seven diet goals and explain why each is important.

School Cafeteria Menus Grades 4–5

Valued Outcome: Students will be able to write sample menus incorporating a variety of foods from the school lunch program.

National Health Education Standard: 8

Description of Strategy: Have the school dietitian bring various cafeteria menus to class and show how a variety of foods is incorporated into them. Have the students write sample menus incorporating a variety of food characteristics for the school lunch program.

Materials Needed: pen and paper, MyPlate diagram (optional for each student)

Processing Question: Does your school lunch menu have foods from each category of MyPlate?

✓ **Assessment:** Students will be able to write at least two sample school lunch menus using MyPlate.

Diet Modification Grades 4–5

Valued Outcome: Students will be able to compare diet modifications.

National Health Education Standards: 1, 3, 7

Description of Strategy: Give the students a problem such as modifying diets for athletes or planning inexpensive party menus. Have them consult at least three different sources of information. Compare the conclusions that might be reached from the information derived from the three sources.

Materials Needed: resources for diet information

Processing Questions:

1. How do professional nutritionists help us eat more healthfully?
2. Why is it important to plan the meals for events such as those listed in the Description of Strategy?

✓ **Assessment:** Students will be able to plan at least two meals for a specific special needs person or event.

Diet and Athletic Performance Grades 5–6

Valued Outcome: Students will be able to research and report on the relationship between proper diet and improved athletic performance.

National Health Education Standards: 1, 3

Description of Strategy: Have the students research the relationship between proper diet and improved athletic performance. One suggestion is to have them interview a local high school athlete or coach for his or her own eating behaviors. Report the results to the class.

Materials Needed: resource information on diet and athletic performance

Processing Questions:

1. What effect does a nutritious diet have on athletic performance?
2. What effect does a poor diet have on athletic performance?
3. What types of foods should be eaten to enhance athletic performance?

✓ **Assessment:** Students will be able to state one effect a healthy diet has on athletic performance, and one effect an unhealthy diet has on athletic performance.

Food Label Activity Grades 5–6

Valued Outcome: Students will be able to identify and report on regulations concerning labeling food.

National Health Education Standards: 1, 3, 7

Description of Strategy: Have the students research the regulations concerning labeling of packaged foods and present their reports either orally or in writing. Individualize the activity by having each student prepare a report on a specific food product. Then have the student discuss his or her findings in class, explaining what information is contained on the label of the package for his or her product. Later, put all the packages on display so that students may examine them.

Materials Needed: various packaged foods, resources and information about food labeling requirements

Processing Questions:

1. Why do packaged foods have labels?
2. How can such labels help us eat healthier?

✓ **Assessment:** Students will be able to accurately list and explain the FDA food label requirements.

Weight Management Programs Grades 6–8

Valued Outcome: Students will be able to learn healthy weight reduction methods.

National Health Education Standards: 1, 7

Description of Strategy: Invite a leader of a weight reduction group that stresses balanced nutrition in its program to discuss the effects and health implications of prolonged overeating, crash diets, and surgery for weight loss. Have students submit questions on index cards in advance to be answered by the resource person.

Materials Needed: index cards for each student

Processing Questions:

1. What are the dangers of dieting improperly?
2. Why are fad diets so popular?
3. What are the dangers of surgery for weight loss?

✓ **Assessment:** Students will be able to describe one healthy strategy for weight loss and one unhealthy strategy for weight loss.

Experiments and Demonstrations

Food and the Five Senses Grades K–3

Valued Outcome: Students will be able describe how the five senses affect food selection.

National Health Education Standard: 1

Description of Strategy: Use a food, such as an apple, to teach about the senses. Cut the apple, and ask the students how the apple looks different on the outside and inside (using sight). Give everyone a chance to smell an apple that has been cut and one that is whole. Which has more of an odor (smell)? Have the students determine if the apple is warm or cool, soft or firm, light or heavy (touch). Have students bite into an apple and describe the sound (hearing). Have the students describe whether the taste was sweet, bitter, or salty (taste). (This activity may be done with a variety of foods.)

Materials Needed: apples, knife to cut apples (for teacher only)

Processing Question: How do the various senses work together to enhance our enjoyment of foods?

✓ **Assessment:** Students will be able to list the five senses and give one way in which taste, appearance, smell, sound, or feel of a food can impact food selection.

Say Cheese   Grades K–5

Valued Outcome: Students will be able to compare and contrast the taste and texture of various cheeses. Students will be able to determine that cheeses are part of the dairy section of MyPlate.

National Health Education Standard: 1

Description of Strategy: Display a variety of cheeses such as cheddar, colby, blue, Swiss, mozzarella, Monterey Jack, etc. Have students compare and contrast the cheeses regarding the texture, taste, and smell. Give each student a handout that lists the different cheeses. Have the students fill in the three columns (texture, smell, and taste). Have students write down if the cheese is soft, hard, crumbly, or smooth to touch. Next, have the students describe the way the cheese smells. Last, have the students write down if the cheese is peppery, sharp, tangy, or buttery when they tasted it. After the students have tasted, felt, and smelled the cheeses, have them compare the results to see which cheeses are similar and which ones are different. Graph the students' results on the board. Follow the activity with a discussion about why cheese belongs in the dairy section of MyPlate.

Materials Needed: a variety of cheeses, handout for each student listing types of cheeses, pencils

Processing Questions:

1. Which type of cheese did you like the best?
2. Did you find any cheeses that tasted the same?
3. What food category of MyPlate does cheese belong to?

✓ **Assessment:** Students will understand that cheese is in the dairy food group.

Is It Healthy or Not?   Grades K–5

Valued Outcome: Students will be able to determine if a group of foods comprises a healthy meal.

National Health Education Standards: 5, 7

Description of Strategy: Set up several meals on a table. Have a highly nutritious meal, a nonnutritious meal, a somewhat nutritious meal, etc. Divide the class into groups of four. Have the groups go to each meal and look at them, but tell students they must work individually. Give them five to seven minutes at each station and have them decide whether the meal is nutritious. Tell them that they are not allowed to talk to anyone. Have them write whatever comments they want about the meal. Then have the groups get together and discuss what they wrote. Have a group discussion about every meal. Let the groups explain what they wrote and why.

Materials Needed: food (or pictures of food set on plates), plates, glasses, utensils

Processing Question: What criteria do you use to decide whether or not a meal is nutritious?

✓ **Assessment:** Students will be able to correctly state why the healthy meal is healthy and why the least healthy meal is unhealthy.

Sugar and Salt Detectives   Grades K–5

Valued Outcome: Students will be able to identify fatty foods, different kinds of sugars, and salt content of various foods and follow a plan to eat fewer of all three food types. They will be able to identify sources of fiber by reading cereal box labels and follow a plan to eat more fiber.

National Health Education Standards: 1, 7

Description of Strategy: Place a piece of bacon and a slice of an apple on a brown paper grocery bag to demonstrate how the bacon leaves a grease spot but the apple does not. Explain to the students that fats such as that which left the grease spot can collect on arterial walls. Then, using empty cereal boxes, have the students read the cereal labels to determine which cereals contain sources of fiber. Instruct the students to create a name for a cereal that tells the consumer that the cereal contains fiber.

Write the following words on the board: *glucose, sucrose, maltose, fructose, lactose, and corn syrup.* Explain that these are words for different kinds of sugar. Add the word *sodium* and explain that this word is used for salt. Have the students pretend they are sugar and salt detectives. They are to read labels at home to find what kinds of foods contain sugars and salt and should make a list of five foods that contain sugars and five foods that contain salt.

Materials Needed: slices of bacon, an apple, empty cereal boxes, board and markers or overhead projector and pen

Processing Questions:

1. Why should we eat more fiber? How does that make us healthier?
2. Why should you keep your arteries clear of fat? What else could you do to keep them clear of fat? (exercise)

3. Why should you eat less sugar?
4. Why should you use less salt?
5. Why is it important to read food labels?

✓ **Assessment:** Students will be able to correctly give three alternative names for sugar and one alternative name for salt. Students will also be able to correctly state why too much fat can be unhealthy for the body.

Differences in Milk   Grades K–5

Valued Outcome: Students will be able to compare the taste of various milk products.

National Health Education Standard: 1

Description of Strategy: Display a collection of milk products: whole, skim, evaporated, condensed, chocolate, buttermilk, etc. Compare the various milk products regarding taste, smell, feel, consistency, and appearance. Discuss what the different types of milk are used for and ask why consuming dairy products is so important.

Materials Needed: variety of milk products

Processing Questions:

1. What nutrients are found in milk?
2. Which type of milk is most nutritious for children under age two? Which is most nutritious for people over age two? Why is there a difference?
3. Which type of milk do you prefer?

✓ **Assessment:** Students will be able to state which milk products are highest and lowest in fat and sugar content.

Fats and the Heart   Grades 3–5

Valued Outcome: Students will be able to describe the effects of a poor diet on the heart.

National Health Education Standard: 1

Description of Strategy: Have a picture of the heart on the wall. Point out the different valves. Explain how the blood enters and leaves the heart. Ask a variety of questions about the heart. Show the fact that eating too much junk food that contains fat can block one of the valves. When a valve is blocked it can cause the heart to beat abnormally. If the heart doesn't beat normally, it can stop and this can cause a heart attack. Show students a section of hose or pipe that has been cut open lengthwise (to simulate a blood vessel) and has a piece of chewed gum or some putty stuck to an inside wall (to simulate a fatty deposit, or plaque). Point out that blocked blood vessels can also trigger a heart attack. Bring in pieces of fat. Try to get a pound of fat (or suet) so students can see what it looks like when you gain a pound of fat.

Materials Needed: picture of the heart (must show interior structures), hose or pipe cut lengthwise, piece of chewed gum or putty, a pound of fat (suet)

Processing Questions:

1. How do nutritious foods help the heart function better?
2. How do nonnutritious foods harm the functioning of the heart?

✓ **Assessment:** Students will be able to explain two ways that an unhealthy diet can harm the health of the heart and blood vessels.

Foods Eaten in the Cafeteria   Grades 3–5

Valued Outcome: Students will observe various foods eaten by students in the school cafeteria.

National Health Education Standard: 1

Description of Strategy: Have the students observe the kinds and amounts of foods eaten by students in the school cafeteria. Record the information by grade level, if possible, on an observation form (see the following example). This activity can be followed with the next activity, "Food Waste."

Sample Observation Form	
Servings of Meats	
Servings of Vegetables	
Servings of Fruits	
Servings of Grains	
Servings of Dairy	

Materials Needed: observation form and pencils or pens for each student

Processing Questions:

1. Do most students in your school eat healthy lunches in the cafeteria?
2. Does your school lunch program offer various alternatives for eating?

✓ **Assessment:** Students will be able to discuss the amounts and types of foods eaten in their school cafeteria.

Food Waste   Grades 3–5

Valued Outcome: Students will identify foods that are wasted by the students in the school cafeteria.

National Health Education Standard: 1

Description of Strategy: The previous activity "Foods Eaten in the Cafeteria" could be followed up with a food waste survey to determine which foods are not eaten from each food group. Have the students observe what types of food and how much are discarded into the trash cans by students. Then, using a chart like the one shown below, make a graph of the information and present arguments to increase selection of the food groups that are not chosen or eaten often.

Food Waste Observation Survey	
Meats Discarded	
Vegetables Discarded	
Fruits Discarded	
Grains Discarded	
Dairy Discarded	

Materials Needed: food waste survey, graph paper and pencils or pens for each student

Processing Questions:

1. Do you think a lot of foods are wasted in your cafeteria?
2. What types of food are wasted the most?
3. What environmentally healthy act can be done with the wasted food?

✓ **Assessment:** Students will be able to describe the amounts and types of at least three foods commonly thrown away in the cafeteria.

Our Bodies Need Water

Grades 4–5

Valued Outcome: Students will measure and physically see how much water is recommended each day. Students will estimate if their intake meets the daily requirements.

National Health Education Standards: 1, 7

Description of Strategy: Make the following statements about water and the ways it helps your body: Water in blood lets it flow through the body, carrying nutrients and oxygen. Water helps cool our bodies when we sweat. Water helps our bodies remove wastes. The body needs at least a quart of water each day to replace water that it uses.

Group the students in pairs. Each pair needs either a four-ounce glass, an eight-ounce bottle of water, a sixteen-ounce thermos, or a thirty-two-ounce pitcher of water. Each group also needs a quart container filled with water. Have the groups measure out how many of their containers equals one quart of water. Record their answers on the board. Display pictures of bottled water, watermelons, fruit juice, celery, lettuce, and tomatoes. Ask students which foods are sources of water (all of them). Have students cut out pictures of foods that are sources of water. Have each student make a collage. Show them how much a quart of water is in a clear container. Ask them if they drink that much every day.

Materials Needed: one container for each pair of students (available container sizes should be four-, eight-, sixteen-, and thirty-two-ounces), one quart of water for every two students; board and markers or overhead projector and pen; pictures of various drinks and foods for display; magazines, scissors, construction paper, glue for each student

Processing Questions:

1. Why is water important to us?
2. Do you drink enough water?

◯ **Integration:** Math

✓ **Assessment:** Students will demonstrate the ability to measure the amount of water required by the body each day.

Source: Health Strategies, Inc. 2002

Complete Proteins

Grades 4–5

Valued Outcome: Students will be able to describe complete proteins.

National Health Education Standard: 1

Description of Strategy: Explain how complete proteins contain all nine essential amino acids. Animal sources of protein (meat, fish, eggs, milk, and milk products) contain complete proteins. Plant sources of protein (dried beans, peas, nuts, breads, and cereals) contain incomplete proteins. These are low in one or more essential amino acids. Write the names of foods that provide incomplete proteins ("Beans," "Rice," "Grains") on several index cards. Take two blank cards and put them together. Label this "Complete protein." Then take one incomplete protein card and add another incomplete protein card to show how to make a complete protein, such as "Beans and Rice." Explain the fact that this method of combining foods to make a complete protein is what most vegetarians do because they don't eat meat.

Materials Needed: index cards labeled as described in Description of Strategy

Processing Questions:

1. What role does protein play in our diet?
2. What would happen to the body if we did not eat enough of the right kind of proteins?

✓ **Assessment:** Students will be able to name three foods that provide complete proteins and three foods that provide incomplete proteins.

Puzzles and Games

Food Alphabet

Grades K–3

Valued Outcome: Students will be able to list the names of foods for each letter of the alphabet.

National Health Education Standard: 1

Description of Strategy: Divide the students into teams, and assign each team a number of letters of the alphabet. For example, one team can be assigned letters *A* through *E*, the next team letters *F* through *J*, and so on. Challenge each team to write down at least one food for each letter assigned to the team.

Materials Needed: pen and paper for each team

Processing Question: What are the names of foods that start with each letter of the alphabet?

✔ **Assessment:** Students will be able to give one food for each letter assigned to their team.

MyPlate Bingo   Grades 3–6

Valued Outcome: Students will be able to place foods in the proper group by using MyPlate.

National Health Education Standard: 1

Description of Strategy: Hand out the bingo cards to the students. Each card will have six columns across it, labeled to represent the six categories of MyPlate. The spaces below the columns will be blank. Draw index cards with the names of various foods on them, and read them aloud to the students. Students will then write the name of the foods in the correct category on their cards. The student who writes in six foods in a row wins. Let the person who wins lead the next game.

Materials Needed: bingo cards (as described above); index cards with various food names on them, pencils or pens for each student

Processing Questions:

1. Which food group should you have the most of in a day?
2. Why is it important to have more of this category than any other?

✔ **Assessment:** Students will demonstrate the ability to accurately place foods in the correct MyPlate categories on their bingo cards.

Online Nutrition Games   Grades K–5

Valued Outcome: Students will be able to access the various online nutrition games through their computer or cell phone, complete the games, and report their outcome to the teacher.

National Health Education Standards: 1, 2, and 3

Description of Strategy: Direct your students to access one (or more) of the following websites with nutrition-related games. Additional nutrition-related games such as

Munch-a-day (to track daily food intake) are available for handheld devices (such as iPhones).

- National Dairy Council: *Explore the World of Nutrition with Nutrition Explorations.* Games focus on helping athletes select appropriate food before a race, making nutritious choices throughout a day, shopping smart, and tracking meals and serving sizes. Access at www.nutritionexplorations.org/kids/activities-main.asp.
- Nourish Interactive: *Game Room.* Activities are focused on the importance of nutrition and exercise. Access at www.nourishinteractive.com/kids/scrolls.htm.
- Dairy Council of California: *Kids Games.* Games focus on eating a healthy breakfast and on dairy-related concepts (calcium intake, exploring a dairy farm, etc.). Access at www.dairycouncilofca.org/Tools/KidsLearningTools.aspx.

After completing the online nutrition game(s), the student will either print out their score (if available) or write down their score, and report this in writing to the teacher. Also, the student should write a brief paragraph about what they learned about nutrition while playing the online nutrition game.

Processing Questions:

1. How did the game relate to nutrition?
2. Did the game help you learn about nutrition?

✔ **Assessment:** Students will be able to list a minimum of two concepts they learned while completing the online nutrition game(s).

Wheel of Food   Grades K–5

Valued Outcome: Students will be able to participate in a game identifying certain foods from MyPlate.

National Health Education Standard: 1

Description of Strategy: This game is set up like "Wheel of Fortune." The spinner spins the wheel indicating from which food category the secret word will be chosen. One student will act as the host; the remainder of the class will take turns being the player(s) and serving as card holders. Students serving as card holders will be given the correct cards to spell out a food name. The blank sides of these cards will be held toward the class until the card holder is instructed by the host to turn the card. Remind the students that the food they will be trying to spell out will come from the food category chosen. This first team, or student, chooses a letter; if the letter is in the word, they continue. If the first team/student is incorrect, the second team/student gets a turn and so on. The team to turn or guess all letters and spell the name of the food is the winner.

Materials Needed: wheel with the five categories from MyPlate; cards arranged in sets that spell out names of different foods; MyPlate for display

Processing Questions:

1. What are the different categories of foods within MyPlate?
2. Why is it important to know the foods within each category?

✓ **Assessment:** Students will correctly guess letters for foods that fall into the selected MyPlate category.

Alphabet Game   Grades 3–5

Valued Outcome: Students will be able to spell the names of foods and nutrients correctly.

National Health Education Standard: 1

Description of Strategy: Divide the students into three groups. Write the letters of the alphabet onto index cards (some letters may be repeated) and give a set to each group. Ask the students a question such as "This nutrient is responsible for building new cells and tissues in growing children." The group must work together to think of an answer and then spell the word correctly (protein). Each student should have only one letter in his or her hand. The group should be standing in a straight line with the word spelled correctly. The group who can do this first wins.

Materials Needed: three identical sets of index cards with letters of the alphabet written on each card, a list of questions

Processing Question: What is the function of each nutrient?

✓ **Assessment:** Students will give the correct answers to the questions.

Learning MyPlate   Grades 3–5

Valued Outcome: Students will be able to describe MyPlate.

National Health Education Standard: 1

Description of Strategy: Divide the class into groups of four to five students. On each table have some magazines, paper bags, five poster boards or pieces of construction paper, scissors, and glue. Each student should have his or her own paper bag. Have each group label one poster board for each category of MyPlate. Then have them cut out pictures of different foods from the magazines and place them in their bags. Have the students exchange bags with each other. Tell them to remove the different foods from the bag and paste each on the correct poster board according to the category of MyPlate in which it belongs. Once the students finish, have each group show their poster boards. At the end of class, hang the posters around the classroom.

Materials Needed: magazines or grocery store advertisements, scissors, glue, poster boards or construction paper for each group; paper bags for each student

Processing Questions:

1. What are the categories in MyPlate?
2. Why is it important to know the various categories in MyPlate?
3. Which foods did you have trouble placing in the proper category? Why?

✓ **Assessment:** Students will demonstrate the ability to place the foods in their bag in the correct MyPlate category.

What Kind of Food Am I?   Grades 3–5

Valued Outcome: Students will be able to guess types of food from clues.

National Health Education Standard: 1

Description of Strategy: Say "Now we are going to play the 'What kind of food am I?' game." Tape the name of a food on each student's back. "No one is allowed to tell you what your food is, and you are not to tell anyone the name of his or her food." Once everyone has become a food, start the game. Call the students up to the board one at a time. Have them turn around so their classmates can see the food. One at a time, the classmates will start describing the food—which food group the student belongs to, the shape, color, or size, or even other foods it might taste good with or be found in. After each hint, the student may guess which food she or he is. After the student guesses his or her food, write it on the board under the correct category. Allow students to keep their food tags.

Materials Needed: tape, paper for food tags for each student

Processing Question: What types of clues (characteristics) about foods will help identify those foods?

✓ **Assessment:** Students will be able to give accurate clues to describe the mystery food.

Label Scavenger Hunt   Grades 3–5

Valued Outcome: Students will be able to identify certain foods just by reading the food labels.

National Health Education Standard: 1

Description of Strategy: Clip the Nutrition Facts panel and ingredients list area from several food labels (that have been removed from the products) and give them to groups of students. Have students try to determine what food each of the ingredient labels is describing. Points can be awarded to the groups on the basis of guessing the correct food from the labels.

Materials Needed: Nutrition Facts panel and ingredients list area from several food labels

Processing Question: How can the information from food labels help us to identify foods?

✓ **Assessment:** Students will be able to correctly identify at least two foods from the Nutrition Facts panel and/or ingredients list of the food labels.

Cultural Foods Game   Grades 3–5

Valued Outcome: Students will be able to recognize food cards representing foods from different cultures and identify the country of origin.

National Health Education Standard: 2

Description of Strategy: Paste or draw pictures of different ethnic foods in the center of an index card. Write the name of the food at the top of the card. The player must name the country when he or she sees the name of the food. Suggested number of cards is thirty for two to four players, more for larger groups.

How to Play:

1. Shuffle the deck of index cards well.
2. Deal five cards to each player face down.
3. The player on the dealer's left draws one card from the deck. He or she may either keep the card or discard it right side up next to the deck. If the card is kept, the player must discard another (the player must have five cards in his or her hand at all times).
4. The opponent(s) may either take the card that is right side up or draw from the deck and then discard a card.
5. The game continues until a player has five different cultures of food represented by his or her cards.
6. The player lays down his or her hand for the opponent(s) to see and check. If correct, he or she is then declared the winner.

Variation: Players can decide to play for one culture of food, in which case six cards should be made for each of five cultures. When a player sees the first five cards he or she is dealt, he or she can decide which country is best represented (by the most cards) in his or her hand. This will determine which country he or she plays for, and he or she will try to get a "set" of five cards for that country. The first player to get a set is the winner.

Materials Needed: one package of 30" × 50" index cards, pictures of at least six different foods from cultures studied (foods from Mexico, France, China, Germany, Italy, and Hawaii are especially interesting)

Processing Questions:

1. What are some foods from other countries that are different from ours?
2. Why is it important to know about other cultures' foods?

✓ **Assessment:** Students will be able to correctly identify the cultures for foods listed on at least five index cards.

Balanced Meals   Grades 4–5

Valued Outcome: Students will be able to name the five food categories, and select and construct a balanced meal.

National Health Education Standards: 1, 7

Description of Strategy: This game has two parts. In the first part—"The Balance Game"—students identify whether a meal is balanced or not. Then in the second part—"Meals on Wheels"—the students identify whether the balanced meal provides the daily amounts needed in a healthy diet.

Show the students six plates, each containing a different meal (construct the food from paper or cut out pictures from magazines). Have students decide if each meal is balanced. Instruct them to clap if it is or to rub their head if it is not. The game is played with a makeshift balance. If the meal is balanced, do not move the balance, but if the meal is not balanced, adjust the balance so that it is uneven. This is designed to visually show the students what a *balanced* meal is.

After completing "The Balance Game," use an interactive bulletin board titled "Meals on Wheels" to decide if each meal contains the proper daily amounts of nutrients. Write the names of the food groups in a different color on a wheel (refer to MyPlate). Give the students colored stickers that correspond to the colors of the food groups. Have them break down each meal into individual food groups. For every item in the meal, place a colored sticker on the wheel in the appropriate food group. Then have the students add up the number of stickers in each category to see if they had the daily amounts that they needed in order to have healthy meals that day.

Materials Needed: paper food to represent six meals, poster-board balance scale that can be tipped, wheel with names of the five MyPlate categories written in different colors and stickers in corresponding colors

Processing Question: What does it mean for a meal to be balanced?

✓ **Assessment:** Students will be able to accurately list foods that construct a balanced meal.

Other Ideas

Field Trips   Grades 3–5

Valued Outcome: Students will be able to participate in a field trip relating to food or dairy products.

National Health Education Standards: 1, 7

Description of Strategy: Arrange to take the class on a field trip to a dairy, bakery, food processing plant, or other nutrition-related operation. Be sure to prepare your class thoroughly for the trip before they go. Discuss the nature of the operation that they will see. Explain the processes they will observe, and have the students prepare a list of questions they will want to ask.

Processing Question: How do the processes of food preparation vary for different foods?

✔ **Assessment:** Students will demonstrate knowledge on the nutritional quality of the food made or sold at the field trip destination.

Poster Contest   Grades 3–5

Valued Outcome: Students will be able to construct a poster using topics concerning all aspects of food.

National Health Education Standards: 1, 7

Description of Strategy: Each week assign a theme for individual posters, using such topics as the MyPlate, table manners, essential nutrients, and so on. Post the completed art in the classroom or in the school cafeteria.

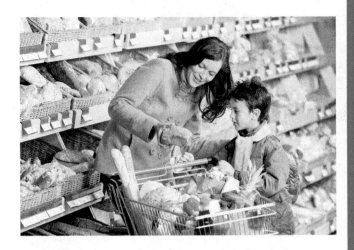

A field trip to the grocery store is an excellent strategy for teaching nutrition.

Materials Needed: poster board, art supplies to construct posters

Processing Questions:

1. How do such signs serve as reminders for good food-related behavior?
2. What are some essential messages that should be related through such signs?

○ **Integration:** Art

✔ **Assessment:** Students will be able to draw or clip at least three appropriate pictures for the assigned poster topic.

Access more material online at www.pearsonhighered.com/anspaugh. At this companion website for *Teaching Today's Health*, you'll find chapter quizzes, web links, flashcards, a glossary, additional Worksheets, and more to help you succeed.

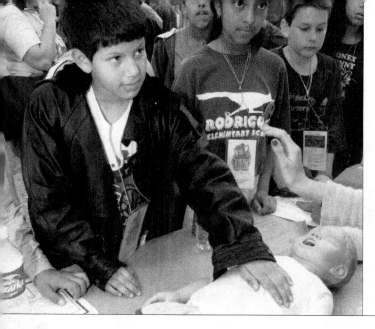

Injuries: Accident and Violence Prevention

Many of us remember a time when walking and bicycling to school was a part of everyday life. In 1969, about half of all students walked or bicycled to school. Today, however, the story is very different. Fewer than 15 percent of all school trips are made by walking or bicycling, one-quarter are made on a school bus, and over half of all children arrive at school in private automobiles.

—*U.S. Department of Transportation (2011)*

NATIONAL HEALTH EDUCATION STANDARDS

1. Students will comprehend concepts related to health promotion and disease prevention to enhance health.

4. Students will demonstrate the ability to use interpersonal communication skills to enhance health and avoid or reduce health risks.

5. Students will demonstrate the ability to use decision-making skills to enhance health.

7. Students will demonstrate the ability to practice health-enhancing behaviors and avoid or reduce risks.

Valued Outcomes

After completion of this chapter, you should be able to:

- Discuss the difference between intentional and unintentional injuries.

- Discuss the major human and environmental causes of accidents.

- Describe the characteristics of an accident-prone person.

- Discuss young people's attitudes toward violence.

- List the ways for a child to protect himself or herself against violence.

- List the ways for a child to protect himself or herself against adult and stranger abuse.

- Describe why risk taking is a necessary evil.

- Discuss the major parts of a school safety program.

- Contrast a positive approach to safety education with a negative approach.

- Discuss the growing violence problem in U.S. society.

Reflections

As you read through this chapter, reflect upon the dangers to personal safety found in your environment—including the possibilities of both intentionally and unintentionally inflicted injuries. As you reflect upon these dangers, you will become more aware of strategies that can be employed to protect your personal safety and that of the people around you.

Children, Accidents, and Violence

Injuries and violence affect us all, but three quarters of all deaths among young people are the result of injuries and violence (CDC 2011). Children are especially susceptible to unintentional injuries, mainly because they are unaware of dangers. Among persons aged one through thirty-four

> **TEACHING TIP**
>
> Integrate lessons about safety and injury prevention into reading lessons. If a character in a reading assignment acts unsafely or gets injured, start a discussion about how the injury might have been prevented.

years, unintentional injuries alone claim more lives than any other cause. For those ages five through thirty-four in the United States, motor vehicle crashes are the leading cause of death, claiming the lives of 18,266 Americans each year (CDC 2011).

According to the most recent data available, homicide is ranked as the third leading cause of death among children ages one through four and ten through fourteen, and the fourth leading cause of death among children ages five through nine (CDC 2007).

▪ The Crime and Violence Epidemic

We want our schools to be safe places for teaching and learning and free of crime and violence. Students are less likely to be victims of a violent crime at school than they are away from school, but any crime or violence at school not only affects the individuals involved but also may disrupt the educational process, the school itself, and the surrounding community. Schools should be safe havens for teaching and learning, free of crime and violence. In addition to affecting the individuals directly involved, crime and violence at school may also disrupt the educational process. It has been established that victimized children are more prone to truancy, poor academic performance, dropping out of school, and violent behaviors. Incidents of victimization can also affect teachers as well, leading to professional disenchantment or departure from the profession (National Center for Education Statistics [NCES] 2010). If a teacher is a victim of crime and/or violence, he or she is more likely to be disenchanted with teaching and will be more likely to leave teaching altogether.

It is difficult to measure the magnitude of crime and violence in schools because of the large amount of attention devoted to isolated incidents of extreme school violence; however, parents, school staff, and policymakers need an accurate understanding of the extent and nature of the problem to effectively address school crime. Establishing and monitoring indicators of the current state of school safety across the nation helps ensure safer schools locally (NCES 2010).

The Need for Safety Education

Fortunately, most accidents that happen to children are not serious or fatal. Unfortunately, accidents occur often enough to make safety an extremely important part of elementary health instruction. As a teacher, your involvement in safety education is imperative because of the number of accidents that occur while the child is at school. Your efforts, combined with those of the school administration, can make a difference. It is very important for teachers to comply with and periodically review school district policies concerning safety and first-aid procedures.

The number of accidents among children is unnecessarily high. Although accidents will always occur, given the nature of children, accidents don't just happen. In most instances, they are caused by human error or carelessness, and these factors can be positively influenced by safety education. Children do not have to learn safe behavior through trial and error; they do not have to continue having accidents in order to recognize the importance of safety. They can be taught the elements of safety in a positive way that will result in fewer accidents of all types, both at school and away from school. As a teacher of health education, this should be one of your major goals.

This chapter presents an overview of the elements of safety education and violence prevention. Topics include risk taking and safety procedures, positive characteristics of safety, accident prevention, violence and violence prevention, types of accidents, violence in schools, and the school safety program.

Safety and Risk Taking

We take risks in almost any of our activities, from going to school or work in the morning, to cooking or eating a meal, to engaging in daily tasks and recreational activities. If safety were our only concern, logically many of these efforts would have to be curtailed: One could be hit by a truck while crossing the street, choke on a piece of food, or suffer a fatal injury while at work or at play. What is an acceptable degree of risk depends on the needs and desires of the individual and the activity. Some adults, for instance, make their living by engaging in highly risky activities—as race drivers, deep sea divers, law enforcement officers, and so forth. Such individuals are often held in high esteem and even glamorized by the rest of the population, demonstrating that risk taking is viewed positively in our society.

▪ Fostering Safety Behavior

Children develop an unrealistic view of risk taking from viewing the glamorous aspects, and this attitude may tempt them to enter into situations that are potentially very

Injuries are the leading cause of death for Americans ages one to forty-four, and a leading cause of disability for all ages. More than 180,000 people die from injuries each year, and approximately one in ten sustains a nonfatal injury serious enough to be treated in a hospital emergency department. Most events resulting in injury, disability, or death are predictable and preventable.

Overall Goal: Prevent unintentional injuries and violence, and reduce their consequences
Selected Objectives for 2020:

Injury Prevention

- Reduce fatal and nonfatal injuries.
- Reduce emergency department visits and hospitalization for nonfatal injuries.
- Improve tracking of injury-related data.
- Increase access to trauma care.
- Reduce fatal and nonfatal motor vehicle crash-related injuries.
- Reduce pedestrian deaths and injuries on public roads.
- Increase the proportion of motorcycle operators and passengers using helmets.

Violence Prevention

- Reduce homicides.
- Reduce nonfatal physical assault injuries.
- Reduce physical fighting among adolescents.
- Reduce bullying among adolescents.
- Reduce child maltreatment deaths.

Source: U.S. Department of Health and Human Services 2011. *2020 Topics and Objectives: Injury and Violence Prevention.* (Available at www.healthypeople.gov/2020/topicsobjectives2020/overview.aspx?topicid=24.)

hazardous. This, combined with natural curiosity and energy, can greatly increase the chance of serious accidents. Part of your job in teaching safety education is to make children aware that unnecessary risk taking is not socially endorsed behavior, and that it is important to safely prepare for necessary activities in which there are some risks involved. This cannot be accomplished, however, by simply providing your students with a list of safety don'ts. Children, especially younger children, should be emphatically warned of dangers in the environment. However, the "don't" approach to safety education, when used exclusively, is negative and not likely to influence behavior permanently.

A Positive Approach to Safety

You are more likely to influence children's behavior toward safer personal practices when you take a positive approach. Emphasize that safety is largely a matter of individual choice and responsibility. Although an acceptance of risk is a part of living, embracing risk without recognizing and accepting the possible consequences is not wise. In considering role models, point out that even adults who make their living in the most hazardous of ways do all they can to minimize the risk involved.

As in all areas of health education, stress the importance of personal decision-making skills. Accidents happen not because of chance or fate, but because of the inherent risk involved in the activity combined with the possibility of human error. When children understand and internalize this concept, they will be in a better position to enhance their own personal safety. By recognizing their own choices and responsibility, they will begin to be better able to assess the risk involved in a given activity and to take steps to minimize the possibility of making errors when engaged in that activity.

To become mindful of safety, a person must become analytical. What are the risks involved in the activity contemplated? What can be done to lessen those risks? After determining the probable answers to these questions, the individual can then act accordingly. The process of becoming analytical about decision making begins in childhood. You can do much to help children develop analytical decision-making skills by providing a variety of learning opportunities that require them to think before they act.

Of course, you cannot expect a child to have the analytical skills of a competent adult, and therefore you must also supervise children's activities to prevent needless accidents. This supervision should take place in the classroom, gymnasium, cafeteria, hallways, and playground. As much as possible, however, relate your supervision to individual decision-making skills. Always keep a positive approach to safety.

Accident Proneness

The term *accident prone* was first coined in 1918 when researchers were studying the relationship between certain personality traits and risk for injury. Studies have led to several conclusions regarding the increased chances of a person having more accidents than others. In particular, when motor vehicle accidents are examined, those people who appear accident prone are emotionally less mature and responsible, more antisocial, have had more involvement with criminal justice and social service agencies, and show lower academic achievements (U.S. Department of Justice 2011). Also, according to the U.S. Department of Justice (2011), "most of the traditional correlates of criminality—early dating, working, and smoking; less stable marital relations; and low skill occupations—have also been associated with accident proneness. The factor common to accidents, crime, and social deviance appears to be a high willingness to engage in risky behaviors with little regard for long-term consequences."

Certain people are more prone to accidents than others. Statistics indicate that people who have had one accident are more likely to have another one than those who have not had any previous accidents. The accident-prone person may be impulsive, drawn to adventure and excitement, or always in search of immediate pleasures. This type of individual does not like to plan ahead and may harbor resentment against authority figures. The rebellion may be a response to a strict upbringing in childhood. He or she usually cannot tolerate discipline, including the self-discipline caution requires.

Characteristics of an accident-prone person may include aggression and overactivity. Although statistically boys are three times more likely than girls to have an injury-prone personality, studies show that other possible factors include:

- **Economic status**—Over a three-year period, a group of economically deprived children at a summer camp had a disproportionately high number of accidents.
- **Personal characteristics**—Cognitive abilities and personality traits may play a role; extroverts, for example, have more accidents than introverts.

Accidents

▪ Types of Accidents

Accidents involving schoolchildren can be classified into six categories: school, traffic, recreational, home, personal, or disaster. Disaster situations include floods, hurricanes, tornadoes, and earthquakes. Because these are general emergencies involving a large segment of the population, disaster situations will not be detailed here.

School Accidents. Most school accidents occur in physical education classes, during playground activities, and in sports contests. These activities expose the students to greater levels of risk. Emergency departments in the United States treat more than 200,000 children ages fourteen and younger for playground-related injuries. Children ages five to nine visit emergency departments for playground injuries more than any other age group does. A higher percentage of girls (55 percent) than boys (45 percent) are injured in this age group. On public playgrounds, more injuries occur on climbers than on any other equipment or at home playgrounds.

Plan carefully to ensure maximum safety. First of all, the teacher in charge should make sure that sports and playground equipment are in good condition and suitable for the activity. Work closely with school administrators, other faculty members, and the school custodians. Equipment that is not in use should be stored so that it does not interfere with the ongoing activity. Swings and other play equipment should be inspected regularly. The playground should also be routinely inspected for hazards, such as broken glass and damaged fencing, before children are allowed to play. Metal playground equipment that is standing in the sun should be checked before children use it in order to avoid potential burns.

Next, be sure that all physical activities are properly supervised by an adequate number of faculty members. Some schools now require teachers supervising playground activities during school to stand and watch children carefully rather than completing paperwork or other distracting activities. Teachers should confine all activities to designated areas and make sure that the activity of one group of children does not interfere with that of another group. Keep any activity you are supervising well ordered, and watch for signs of fatigue. When a child becomes tired, the chances for an accident increase. Finally, when your students have finished the activity, make sure that equipment is properly stored. Lock all equipment cabinets to prevent unauthorized, unsupervised use.

Safety in the hallways, stairways, cafeteria, and other parts of the school outside the actual classroom should be maximized by teacher supervision. Stress the importance of polite, considerate behavior rather than simply demanding that students follow rules. Hall monitors should not function as prison guards. Work with school administrators and custodians to keep the school environment free of potential hazards. Stairways should have banisters and adequate lighting. Water fountains should have the appropriate amount of water pressure—not too low to cause children to bump their teeth and not too much to cause water to spill on the floor. Spills of any sort should be wiped up promptly, and litter should be removed. Doors to maintenance areas should be locked.

In the classroom itself, make sure that you also maintain a safe environment. Keep equipment and supplies stored until they are needed. Supervise all activities closely. If you prepare any experiment or classroom demonstration that could be hazardous, do not take unnecessary risks. For example, if a demonstration involves the use of a sharp object or a chemical, do not have students help you. Also, be especially careful with any electrical apparatus.

Asbestos. Asbestos was widely used as an insulating material in schools for many years and in other commonly occurring items, such as brake linings in cars. Asbestos is considered a danger to health only if the insulation is disturbed regularly through contact. If this happens, fibers that can block breathing passages will be released into the air.

People who are exposed to asbestos through their occupations (such as construction work) have developed several types of life-threatening diseases, including lung cancer. Continuing use of asbestos and asbestos products has decreased, but they are still found in many settings and continue to pose a health risk to workers and others

(National Institute for Occupational Safety and Health 2011). Many school systems are replacing asbestos with safer types of insulation.

Traffic Accidents.
Going to and from school accounts for few school accidents. This is surprising when one considers the potential dangers that children face as pedestrians, bicyclists, and bus and auto passengers. The low accident rate speaks well for school safety patrols and pedestrian and bicycle safety programs. Nonetheless, traffic accidents do occur, and they are often serious. Help your students recognize the importance of following established safety procedures when they are pedestrians, bicyclists, and vehicle passengers.

As pedestrians, children should understand how to interact with motor vehicles. Traffic laws are designed not only for operators of motor vehicles, but also for pedestrians. Each has an obligation to the other, a point you should stress. Help younger children learn the meaning of traffic signs and signals, and explain the reasons behind traffic regulations. Youngsters usually do not appreciate the physical principles involved in the operation of a motor vehicle and do not understand that a car cannot stop immediately or that the child can see the car much better than the driver can see him or her. Further, children often become so engrossed in their own activities that they simply do not consider the vehicular traffic around them. They may dart into the street after a ball without thinking.

Bicycle safety should also be emphasized. Children often assume that traffic laws and regulations apply only to motorized vehicles. They see themselves not as operators of vehicles—which they are—but rather as mounted pedestrians. To some degree, this is a values-related issue and must be approached as such because children do not see themselves as being irresponsible when they fail to heed traffic regulations.

Most children are regular passengers on school buses and in family vehicles. Because of the large numbers of children being transported to and from schools in buses and cars, children need to become aware of proper safety practices in buses and cars. Drivers of school buses are responsible for supervising students during their ride. Cooperate with drivers in establishing firm guidelines for safe student behavior while loading, riding, and unloading the buses. Unruly students can easily distract a driver so that an accident results. Make clear the possible consequences of unruly behavior, and point out that the well-being of many people can be affected by poor behavior. Also provide instructions for safe behavior. Children should enter the bus in an orderly manner and move to their seats quickly and carefully. They should remain seated during the ride. Books, lunch boxes, and other objects should be kept out of the aisles. Windows should remain closed unless the driver opens them. If windows are opened, children should not stick their arms or heads out or throw objects out the windows. Finally, students should remain well clear of the bus when it is approaching the bus stop and after they have been dropped off.

Motor vehicle injuries are the leading cause of death among children in the U.S. During 2005 in the United States, 1,335 children ages fourteen and younger died as occupants in motor vehicle crashes, and approximately 184,000 were injured (CDC 2011). That's an average of four deaths and 504 injuries each day. Many motor vehicle-related deaths can be prevented through habitual use of passenger safety devices. Placing children in age- and size-appropriate car seats and booster seats reduces serious and fatal injuries by more than half (CDC 2011).

It should be emphasized to children that even though it may look easy, driving a car requires the full attention of the driver. Children should not distract the driver and should not lean out of windows. Stress the importance of wearing safety belts and using child safety or booster seats, even if the parents of some children do not regularly use them.

In the United States, many states now require the use of safety belts by passengers. Many other states are considering such legislation. Not wearing a safety belt is essentially irrational behavior. Excuses given for not using safety belts are varied. Some drivers find them constricting or uncomfortable. Others say that they are not needed for short trips. A few claim to fear being trapped inside the vehicle in case of an accident. None of these reasons hold up. The truth is that people refuse to wear safety belts either because of laziness or because of a belief that somehow preparing for an accident by wearing a belt will actually allow an accident to take place. This type of reasoning for not wearing a belt is a psychological device called *denial*.

Recreational Accidents.
A large portion of recreational accidents happen to children in and around water. Thus, water safety should be an important component of the instruction that you provide. All children should be taught to swim at an early age. This is something that you can encourage by getting parents and students involved in organized recreational programs.

Even if children know how to swim, however, the danger of accidental drowning always exists. Most drownings happen to people who are not dressed for swimming, which implies that they were not planning to be in the water. Victims usually fall into the water, whether in a home pool, from a boat, or by a river or lake. Emphasize to your students that any body of water should be treated with respect and caution, including a flooded drainage ditch. In

> **Creativity in the Classroom**
>
> Bring a wheelchair or a walker to class to help children understand the physical limitations that can be a consequence of a serious physical injury. Students can experiment with the restricted mobility imposed by relying on a mobility aid in day-to-day activities.

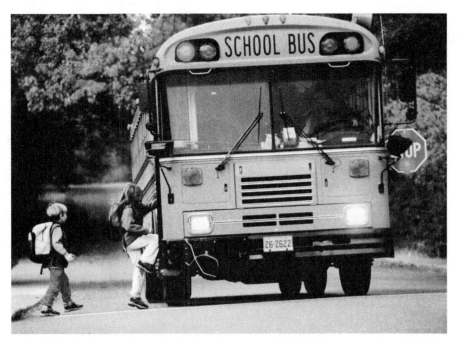

Being safe in and around the school bus is an important part of a student's life.

your discussion of water safety, include the rules for boating safety, such as always wearing a life vest.

Camping and hiking activities contribute to many recreational accidents. Falls from cliffs and other high places result in hundreds of fatalities and injuries each year. Stress the importance of being cautious in unfamiliar terrain.

Skateboards also cause many recreational accidents among children. The popularity of skateboards is high, as is the number of resulting accidents. Emphasize the need to wear proper protective equipment. Also note that skateboards should not be used on streets. A collision between a car and a child on a skateboard can be fatal for the child. See the Health Highlight box on page 342 for examples of precautions students should take during skateboarding.

Your treatment of recreational safety should also include any forms of recreation popular in your area.

Home Accidents. "There's no place like home" implies that home is a pleasant place to be. Unfortunately, there's also no place like home for accidents. More accidents happen in the home than in any other place, partly because most people spend a great deal of time at home.

The leading cause of death in the home is fire. Most home fires occur in the kitchen and bedroom. For the latter, smoking in bed is often the cause. Home safety, including fire safety, is primarily a parental responsibility, but you can help by making your students aware of possible hazards. Work with parents and children to ensure that every family has a fire safety and fire evacuation plan.

For younger children, emphasize the danger of playing with matches or with the kitchen stove. Encourage parents to install smoke detectors and to keep cookware handles turned toward the back of the stove. Teach children what to do if a fire breaks out in the home, especially at night. Too often, frightened children seek shelter in a closet or other enclosed area rather than fleeing, and some will be frightened by the sight of a firefighter dressed in turnout gear. Follow each fire drill in school with a discussion of home fire drills. Every member of the family should know the evacuation route and an alternative route if the primary one is blocked by smoke or flames.

Poisoning is another common home accident, especially among younger children. Explain the dangers of ingesting any substance, such as medicines, food that may have gone bad, and household chemicals. Make sure that parents understand the dangers of accidental poisoning from such substances as aspirin, and encourage them to keep a list of emergency procedures on hand and the telephone number of the local poison control center.

Electrical appliances are a common source of home accidents. Make sure that children understand the danger of playing with any electrical device. Also discuss how electrical overloads can lead to home fires and how electrical appliances can electrocute someone if they are knocked into water.

Your instruction in home safety techniques should include specific recommendations, such as not leaving toys or other objects on stairs or sidewalks, and wearing protective eye equipment when using power tools or lawn equipment. Encourage parents to do all they can to keep the home a safe environment for themselves and their children. For example, you may wish to prepare a checklist

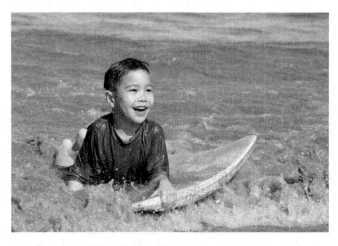

Teach about forms of recreation that are popular in your area, such as snowmobiling, skiing, hunting, and fishing.

HEALTH HIGHLIGHT | Skateboarding Safety Tips

Skateboarding is a popular activity enjoyed by many people, but it is also an activity that causes many unintentional injuries. According to the U.S. Consumer Product Safety Commission (CPSC), in 2006 there were 65,000 skateboard injuries, including fractures, to children younger than fifteen years old. Deaths as a result of collisions with motor vehicles and from falls (often due to irregular riding surfaces) are also reported. The National Safety Council offers these skateboarding tips to avoid injury:

Equipment

- Select a board that fits the intended type of riding (i.e., slalom, freestyle, or speed) and that is rated for the weight of the intended user.
- Wearing protective equipment (such as closed, slip-resistant shoes, helmets, and specially designed padding) can reduce the number and severity of cuts and scrapes.

- Padded jackets and shorts, wrist braces, and special skateboarding gloves can help absorb the impact of a fall.
- Protective equipment currently on the market is not subject to government performance standards; careful selection is necessary.
- Select a helmet that fits properly, allows free movement, and that does not block vision and hearing.

How to fall

Learning how to fall may help reduce the chances of a serious injury:

- If you are losing your balance, crouch down on the skateboard so that you will not have as far to fall.
- Try to land on the fleshy parts of your body and try to roll rather than absorb the force with your arms.
- Try to relax your body, rather than go stiff.

Using a skateboard

Provide young skateboarders with the following tips for using the skateboard:

- Give your board a safety check each time before you ride.
- Always wear safety gear.
- Never ride in the street.
- Obey the city laws. Observe traffic and areas where you can and cannot skate.
- Don't skate in crowds of non-skaters.
- Only one person per skateboard.
- Never hitch a ride from a car, bicycle, etc.
- Don't take chances; complicated tricks require careful practice.

Source: From National Safety Council, http://downloads.nsc.org/pdf/factsheets/Skateboarding_Safety_Tips.pdf, © 2011. Used by permission.

---

for students to take home to their parents. Discussion of items on the checklist can provide a valuable learning experience for all involved.

Just as a family should have a home evacuation plan in case of fire, it should also have a general disaster plan. Encourage students and their parents to work out a plan for any disaster that might hit their community. Depending on the locale, disasters might include earthquakes, floods, tornadoes, or blizzards. Each family member should know what to do in case a disaster strikes, including knowing the name and phone number of someone who does not live in the immediate vicinity and who may act as a contact person in the event of a major disaster.

School Violence: An Overview

Schools should be safe and secure for all students, faculty, and staff so teaching and learning can occur. Contrary to the image of pervasive violence in schools that is projected by the popular media, more violence occurs against children and youth away from rather than at school.

The National Center for Educational Statistics (NCES) conducts a survey on school violence annually (NCES 2011). In the 2009–10 school year, selected data from the NCES show that:

- The rate of violent incidents per 1,000 students was higher in middle schools (forty incidents) than in primary schools or high schools.
- Some 46 percent of schools reported at least one student threat of physical attack without a weapon, and 8 percent of schools reported such a threat with a weapon.
- Some 25 percent of schools reported at least one incident of the distribution, possession, or use of illegal drugs, a higher percentage than that of the distribution, possession, or use of alcohol (14 percent of schools) or prescription drugs (12 percent of schools).
- Some 10 percent of city schools reported at least one gang-related crime, a higher percentage than that reported by suburban (5 percent), town (4 percent), or rural schools (2 percent).
- A higher percentage of middle schools reported that student bullying occurred at school daily or at least once a week (39 percent) than did high schools or primary schools (20 percent each).
- A lower percentage of schools with 50 percent or less white student enrollment reported that cyberbullying among students occurred daily or at least once a week (5 percent) than did schools with higher percentages of white student enrollment (7 to 13 percent).

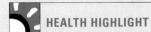

HEALTH HIGHLIGHT | **Home Alone!**

Every parent must eventually leave their child home alone for the first time. The trust involved in allowing a child to stay home alone (even if the parent is just running to the grocery store!) can be a positive experience for a mature child, but even well-prepared children can face risks when left unsupervised. It is important for a parent or guardian to review the local laws and child protective policies in determining when to leave a child alone. If a child appears to be neglected or inadequately supervised, a local child protective services (CPS) agency or the Childhelp® National Child Abuse Hotline (800.4.A.CHILD or www.childhelp.org) should be contacted.

The following are recommendations from the Administration for Children and Families (2007):

- Consider the child's physical, mental, and emotional well-being, as well as laws and policies in the State regarding this issue; States that do not have laws may still offer guidelines for parents.
- There is no agreed-upon age when all children are able to stay home alone

safely. Because children mature at different rates, the decision should not be based on age alone. Consider:

Is the child physically and mentally able to care for him- or herself?

Does the child obey rules and make good decisions?

Does the child feel comfortable or fearful about being home alone?

- When and how a child is left home alone can make a difference to his or her safety and success. Consider:

How long will the child be left home alone at one time? Will it be during the day, evening, or night? Will the child need to fix a meal?

How often will the child be expected to care for him- or herself?

How many children are being left home alone?

Is the home safe and free of hazards?

How safe is the neighborhood?

- The child needs to know what to do and whom to contact in an emergen-

cy situation. Knowledge of basic first aid is also useful. Consider:

Is there a safety plan for emergencies? Can the child follow this plan?

Does the child know his or her full name, address, and phone number?

Does the child know where the parent is and the relevant contact information?

Does the child know the full names and contact information of other trusted adults, in case of emergency?

- There should be a trial period when the child is left home alone for a short time while the parent stays close to home.
- Establish rules. Make sure the child knows what is (and is not) allowed when home alone.
- Check in.
- Don't overdo it. Even a mature, responsible child shouldn't be home alone too much.

Source: U.S. Department of Health and Human Services. Administration for Children and Families 2007. *Leaving Your Child Home Alone.* (Full text available at www.childwelfare.gov/pubs/factsheets/homealone.cfm.)

- For students involved in the use or possession of a weapon other than a firearm or explosive device at school, 40 percent of students received out-of-school suspensions lasting five or more days, 36 percent of students received other disciplinary actions (e.g., suspensions for fewer than five days, detention, etc.), 19 percent of students received transfers to specialized schools, and 6 percent of students received removals with no continuing services for at least the remainder of the school year.

- A lower percentage of schools with 1,000 or more students reported that more than 75 percent of students had a parent or guardian who attended regularly scheduled parent-teacher conferences (23 percent) than did schools with lower enrollments (53 to 56 percent).

▪ Children's Exposure to Violence

The debate about the connection between children's exposure to violence and the number of violent crimes committed by children is heated, ongoing, and currently inconclusive.

It is undeniable, however, that many of America's children consume a steady diet of verbal and physical violence that begins early in life with cartoons and video games, and continues throughout life with movies, other popular media, and even the evening news. (Numerous reports state that children in the United States spend more time watching television than attending school.)

Exposure to violence when young, such as child abuse, can have emotional, psychological, and/or physical effects that can last a lifetime. A child who has been abused may go through life with a poor self-image and be unable to love and trust other people. Children who are abused often grow up to demonstrate criminal or antisocial violent behavior (Los Angeles County Department of Children and Family Services 2011).

Sometimes, simply engaging parents to take an interest in their child's behavior and welfare is more than half the battle in stopping school violence. But more and more parents work outside the home, which makes them less accessible to school officials. Some parents are tired of dealing with their child's problems and simply give up trying. Unfortunately, these attitudes cross all socioeconomic strata. But parents who abuse their children or who fail to provide guidance and discipline can be assured that they are likely contributing to the spread of school violence.

In generating statistics on school violence, researchers generally survey students and teachers regarding several key areas, including:

- violence at school as opposed to away from school
- prevalence of threats or intentional injury
- physical fighting
- bullying
- violent acts involving teachers

The NCES provides an extensive breakdown of such statistics by student characteristics (gender, age, race/ethnicity, and so on) and by type of crime. Following are some statistical highlights from students and teachers surveyed in recent years. You may find it interesting to compare the NCES statistics to those in your local area.

▪ Bullying

Although we don't typically think of bullying as an act of violence, it can contribute as much as does violent crime to a climate of fear and intimidation. In 2007, about 32 percent of twelve- to eighteen-year-old students reported having been bullied at school during the school year and 4 percent reported having been cyberbullied (NCES 2011). Additional data from the 2007 survey include:

- Students who were bullied at school during the school year reported that bullying consisted of being made fun of; being the subject of rumors; being pushed, shoved, tripped, or spit on; being threatened with harm; being excluded from activities on purpose; and in some cases students reported someone tried to make them do things they did not want to do and that their property was destroyed on purpose.
- Of those students who reported being bullied, 79 percent said that they were bullied inside the school, 23 percent said that they were bullied outside on school grounds, 8 percent said they were bullied on the school bus, and 4 percent said they were bullied somewhere else.
- Of these students who had been bullied, 63 percent said that they had been bullied once or twice during the school year, 21 percent had experienced bullying once or twice a month, 10 percent reported being bullied once or twice a week, and 7 percent said that they had been bullied almost daily.
- Thirty-six percent of students who were bullied notified a teacher or another adult at school about the event(s).
- Thirty-three percent of female students reported being bullied at school compared to 30 percent of male students.

Of those who were cyber-bullied:

- About 4 percent of students reported having been cyberbullied anywhere (on or off school property) during the school year.
- Two percent of students said that they had experienced cyberbullying that consisted of another student posting hurtful information about them on the Internet; and 2 percent of students reported unwanted contact, including being threatened or insulted, via instant messaging by another student during the school year.
- Seventy-three percent said it had occurred once or twice during that period, 21 percent said it had occurred once or twice a month, and 5 percent said it had occurred once or twice a week.
- Thirty percent of students who were cyberbullied notified a teacher or another adult at school about the event(s).
- Five percent of female students reported being cyberbullied anywhere, compared to 2 percent of male students.

▪ Violence against Teachers

Most teachers feel safe in their schools during the day, but after-school hours they may not (especially in urban areas). Strict teachers who insist students adhere to rigorous standards are most at risk of being victimized. During the 2007–08 school year (NCES 2011):

- Seven percent of teachers were threatened with injury by a student from their school
- A greater percentage of teachers in city schools than teachers in suburban, town, or rural schools reported being threatened with injury and being physically attacked.
- A greater percentage of public than private school teachers reported being threatened with injury and being physically attacked.
- A greater percentage of secondary school teachers than elementary school teachers reported being threatened with injury by a student, and this pattern held for teachers in suburban schools as well as for teachers in rural schools.
- A greater percentage of male teachers reported having been threatened with injury than female teachers.

▪ Strategies to Prevent School Violence

The most common school security measure used requires school staff, in particular teachers and security staff, to monitor students' movements in and around the school. Equally effective, and less costly than guards, is the use of students' parents as monitors and teachers' aides. Youths are less likely to misbehave or engage in violent acts if parents from their neighborhood are highly visible.

The following measures should also be considered when establishing strategies to prevent school violence.

1. **Institutionalization of discipline and dress codes.** These codes should be developed collaboratively by administrators, teachers, parents, and students. Schools must be sure that the rules created have a purpose and that they explicitly tell students what kinds of behavior are acceptable and how the school will deal with students who break the rules.

2. **Some school communities seek to counter lack of effective parenting by establishing tutoring programs and providing mentors for students.** The mentors are community volunteers from business, service organizations, colleges and universities, churches, and retiree organizations. Some schools have established counseling programs for students; however, most elementary schools do not have them, and most high school counselors have 350 to 400 students each.

3. **Use of conflict resolution strategies to defuse potentially violent situations by persuading those involved to use nonviolent means to resolve their differences.** Schools that have adopted conflict resolution strategies are trying to teach young people new ways of channeling their anger into constructive, nonviolent responses to conflict. Some schools use students as a conflict resolution team to help maintain order in the school by counseling their peers and intervening in disputes among students. Conflict resolution teams also help by encouraging peers to talk through their problems and by training other students to use conflict resolution strategies.

4. **Schools should strongly consider the establishment of crisis centers for students who commit violent acts or threaten violence.** Crisis centers should not be used for long-term interventions, but rather as in-school areas where students can be sent to "cool off" and to receive on-the-spot counseling.

5. **Reduce the number of property crimes by providing part-time employment for students during the school year and full-time employment during the summer months.** The goals of these work programs include building self-esteem and a sense of responsibility, learning the value of money and the importance of getting a good education, and staying in school until graduation.

6. **Extend the number of hours that the school is open.** Students can participate in organized activities such as sports, gymnastics, crafts, art, music, and tutorial programs.

7. **Several urban school districts have organized youth collaboratives.** These collaboratives focus on school dropout prevention and the preparation of youth for the workforce. These groups promote the need to provide coordinated services for youth and families. With the business community, school districts seek to address the needs of students at risk of educational failure through the combined efforts of the city government, health, law enforcement, education, social service agencies, and the religious community.

8. **Efforts to prevent violence in schools must involve teachers at every step of the process.** Whether or not through formal communications channels, all teachers should be aware of the discipline problems that occur in their school. Strategies designed to eliminate or reduce such problems will not work unless teachers are involved in the design and implementation of programs to establish a safe, orderly environment in the school. Faculty members who are aware of what is going on in the school and of strategies to address problems are apt to become actively involved in supporting schoolwide efforts to correct the problem. It is also important for teachers to be able to discuss any major discipline problems they are having with students in their classrooms. These discussions can be part of regular monthly faculty meetings or special sessions.

9. **Critical to the elimination of violent acts in schools is support for teachers' efforts to address discipline problems.** Since teachers are the front line, it is paramount that they receive support from their administration. Administrators must provide teachers and other school staff with the assurance that violent students will be dealt with swiftly and firmly, and that teachers will receive support in their efforts to maintain an orderly classroom.

10. **A teacher must set forth both academic and behavioral expectations for the classroom.** It is very important for them to establish control on the first day of school and maintain it steadily thereafter. Students are perceptive: They quickly become aware of teachers who are not in control of their classrooms. Being in control does not mean being rigid or being a tyrant; it means asserting authority and demanding and getting respect. Teachers also must ensure that the behavior standards are followed— and they must do so in a manner that is fair but firm and consistent. Students who fail to comply with the discipline standards must be dealt with quickly and firmly.

11. **Equally important, and often a factor ignored in discussions about discipline and violence in schools, is the academic side of the issue.**

Classrooms where the academic objectives are unclear are fertile for disruptive student behavior and perhaps violence. This does not mean that every student should be seated quietly at a desk with a book open or busy filling in the blanks on a form. It does mean that the lessons have been carefully planned to elicit maximum teaching and learning. It means students are actively engaged in learning activities—sometimes in groups. It means using strategies to ensure that students comprehend what is being taught and are able to demonstrate their learning. It means insisting that all students strive to meet the academic as well as behavioral standards for the class and assisting those who have difficulty doing so.

Disruptive or violent behavior in the classroom is a way for some students to mask their frustration and anger over their academic deficiencies. The fact that all students do not acquire knowledge the same way must be reflected in the teacher's instruction. Applied strategies of effective teaching, along with lesson plans that respond to students' cultural diversity and learning styles, can significantly reduce instances of potentially disruptive or violent behavior in our nation's schools.

▪ Personal Safety

Becoming a victim of violent behavior or sustaining an unintentional injury can harm your health as much as any of your own unhealthy behavior. Intentional injuries reflect violence committed by one person acting against another person.

Unfortunately, many children suffer from injuries inflicted on them by adults, sometimes parents or relatives of the children and sometimes by strangers. Children need to be taught to trust their feelings when they do not feel right about a person or a situation. For example, if being touched by an adult, and the touch feels uncomfortable, the child needs to know to inform another adult. Emphasize to children that they have a right and a responsibility to determine when and how they wish to be touched. Teach them to assert their own personal space, or privacy. They need to be taught to keep their distance from people who make them feel most uncomfortable.

Each child should be taught to be more aware of his or her surroundings—that is, be aware if someone is following him or her. Walk in the middle of the sidewalk, and try to walk with someone else. Stay away from dark places when alone. Tell them it is all right to scream if they are approached by someone intending to do them harm.

▪ The School Safety Program

Instruction in safety education should be only one part of your school safety program. The total program should consist of these components:

- providing instruction by and for faculty, staff, and students

- planning and implementing safety procedures
- providing safe transportation, including bus travel, walking, and bicycle safety
- establishing accident reporting and recordkeeping procedures
- making sure there is liability insurance protection for staff
- providing emergency health care for all people attending or employed by the school
- creating a safe environment

The responsibilities of each person involved in the safety program should be defined by the school. Additionally, the school should instruct each person regarding specific duties or responsibilities. Supervision should be provided for all school activities, including travel to and from school, physical education, playground time, and after-school gatherings.

Some schools have established school safety councils to develop rules, policies, and procedures for safe living within the school and for school activities. Safety councils provide excellent learning opportunities and allow for student involvement. For example, a school safety council could do a needs assessment or accident survey for the school. This procedure makes the students and others involved aware of the accident situations in their school environment, thus helping to prevent future accidents.

Generally, any accident that causes a student to miss school or go home from school, or that involves property damage should be reported. Some schools have specific forms for reporting any type of accident in or around the school. Accident reports can provide data for studying accident trends in the school environment. They are also valuable in the event of lawsuits filed against the school.

First-Aid Skills

First aid means just that: providing aid before more qualified medical help can be obtained. Adults and children alike should have some knowledge of first-aid procedures so they can help an accident victim in an emergency. Often such knowledge can make the difference between life and death in extreme cases. However, first aid should never be dispensed casually—and not at all if more qualified help can be obtained quickly. As a classroom teacher, you should learn basic first-aid procedures and instruct your students in them. Most often, first-aid procedures are used in common incidents involving cuts, nosebleeds, sprains, and so on.

Begin your own preparation by checking with the school administration and medical personnel to determine established procedures for handling medical problems and emergencies. This is extremely important as far as liability is concerned and cannot be stressed too strongly. In most instances, you will probably be told not to offer any medical assistance except under clearly life-threatening circumstances or when there is no possibility of obtaining more qualified assistance. In some instances, however, administering first aid may be acceptable and provided for in the school safety program.

Keep in mind that first aid is not treatment; instead, it is protection of the victim until treatment can be given. The purpose of first aid is to offer emergency care, prevent further injury, lessen the victim's pain, and ward off unnecessary complications, such as shock. While this is being done, help should also be sought. (Links to more information about first aid can be found on the book website at www.pearsonhighered.com/anspaugh.)

▪ Emergency Situations

The best way to prepare yourself to handle an emergency medical or accident situation is to become qualified to handle emergencies. If you are not qualified, you should become qualified by taking a first-aid and CPR (cardiopulmonary resuscitation) class through the American Red Cross, National Safety Council, and/or American Heart Association. You will gain hands-on experience in dealing with a variety of situations and will have a chance to practice basic first-aid skills before you actually have to use them.

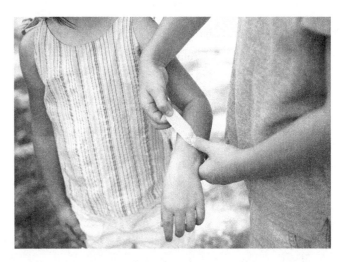

Children should have some knowledge of first-aid procedures to be of help in emergency situations.

Chapter In Review

Summary

- Elementary school children are subject to many injuries, some intentional and some unintentional.

- Accidental deaths are the leading cause of death for this age group, but deaths and injuries from violence are on the rise.

- Children are becoming involved in violent behavior in increasing numbers, both as perpetrators and victims.

- Safety education that covers both safety and violence prevention should be a vital part of health instruction.

- Safety education will help students to increase their awareness of the potential for and cause of accidents; provide them with factual knowledge about safety; help them adjust to new, unfamiliar environments; and heighten their potential for living full, productive lives.

- Positive, safe behavior should be seen by the students as an important part of living.

- The emphasis in safety education should be on positive attitudes and values.

- Learning opportunities in safety should be designed to help students recognize potentially hazardous situations, develop a sense of responsibility for their own safety and others', and make wise decisions regarding their behavior.

- Do not provide safety instruction that is limited to accident statistics, safety rules, or scare tactics. Instead, stress that living is much more enjoyable when a person is safe.

- Teach the students how to prevent violence in their own lives and how to respond if they are faced with violence.

- As the teacher, you should set a good safety model for your students.

- The classroom and other parts of the school environment should be examples of safe, efficient places to work and live.

- Be aware of your responsibility as a teacher regarding liability in various school situations.

- Students should learn how they can be of help in emergency situations.

- Because so many accidents happen to children while they are attending school, you should learn basic first-aid skills and CPR to treat injuries resulting from accidents.

Discussion Questions

1. Describe the factors that lead to a disproportionate number of accidental deaths among children.

2. Discuss the reasons for some people taking risks in our society.

3. How can we teach children to assume a positive approach to safety?

4. Describe the emotional makeup of an accident-prone individual.

5. Discuss the ways to make a playground safer for children.

6. Describe the proper behavior for a child while riding on a school bus.

7. Discuss the steps to take when confronted by someone who is threatening to attack you.

8. Enumerate the rules for children to follow to ensure their personal safety from strangers.

9. Discuss the first-aid procedures to follow in a breathing emergency.

10. Discuss the types of educational programs designed to prevent violent behavior.

Critical Thinking Questions

1. Consider the case of an automobile accident in which a driver runs into the back of another automobile when the roads are wet and visibility is low. How much of this type of unintentional accident would you attribute to human factors and how much to environmental factors?

2. Explain your willingness to take the risk to perform daily tasks, such as driving or riding to work and school, crossing a busy street, and walking through a parking lot.

3. Compare the response of students who are taught safe behavior from a positive point of view versus a negative point of view.

4. Do you think that some individuals have more accidents than others because of coincidence? Or, do you think that each of those individuals' inordinate amount of accidents can be explained by emotional factors (e.g., accident proneness)?

5. Considering your own personal beliefs, character, and past experience, what do you think would be the best approach for you to take if someone is threatening to attack you? What preventive steps would you be willing to take to prepare yourself for such an event?

6. Despite having training in first-aid and crisis procedures (such as hurricanes, etc.), some people are concerned that they would panic in such a situation. Detail some steps to take to prevent such a panic reaction.

7. Design what you would consider a feasible school safety plan to prevent intentional and unintentional injuries.

Access more material online at www.pearsonhighered.com/anspaugh. At this companion website for *Teaching Today's Health*, you'll find chapter quizzes, web links, flashcards, a glossary, additional Worksheets, and more to help you succeed.

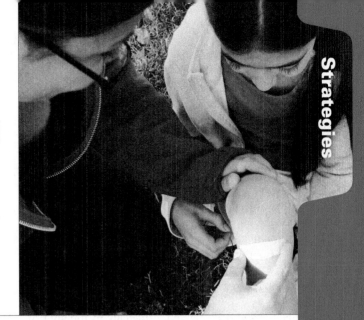

20 Strategies for Teaching Injuries: Accident and Violence Prevention

Valued Outcomes

After completion of this chapter, you should be able to convey the following to your students:

- Each person is to a large degree responsible for his or her own personal safety.
- Peers exert a tremendous influence over safety practices.
- Obedience to safety rules enhances the quality of life.
- Risk taking is a part of living, but unnecessary risk taking greatly increases the risk of harm to oneself and to others.
- The degree of risk in any particular activity can often be determined by analytical thinking.
- Rules and procedures for safe behavior help prevent accidents in the home, school, and community.
- Hazardous conditions should be corrected whenever possible.
- There are many people and community agencies that can help when accidents occur.
- Elementary school children have more fatal accidents than any other age group.
- More than half of all accidents involving children happen at school.
- Playground rules are important for safe activities.
- Elementary students need to practice safe behavior in traffic.
- Home and school fire escape routes should be practiced frequently.
- Acting without thinking often results in an accident.
- Basic first-aid skills are important for everyone.
- Improper first aid can do more harm than good.
- Safety is not just a matter of luck. Safe behavior must be learned.

Reflections

As you use the strategies in this chapter, reflect on how you can emphasize assuming personal responsibility in one's safety and risk-taking behavior. Also, consider how each of these strategies can emphasize taking a positive approach to safety behavior as opposed to using scare tactics.

We have a wealth of information about accidents, causes of accidents, and methods for teaching safe behavior. School safety programs work; however, administrators and teachers need to use the resources they have available to present a coordinated safety program and to provide a safe learning environment for students.

NATIONAL HEALTH EDUCATION STANDARDS

1. Students will comprehend concepts related to health promotion and disease prevention to enhance health.

2. Students will analyze the influence of family, peers, culture, media, technology, and other factors on health behaviors.

3. Students will demonstrate the ability to access valid information and products and services to enhance health.

5. Students will demonstrate the ability to use decision-making skills to enhance health.

7. Students will demonstrate the ability to practice health-enhancing behaviors and avoid or reduce risks.

8. Students will demonstrate the ability to advocate for personal, family, and community health.

Fostering Safety Behavior

Progress has been made in virtually every area of health education in the previous century, including disease prevention, environmental sanitation, and nutritional habits. If there is one area in which health education has lagged behind, however, it is safety and accident prevention. Safety education has lagged behind partially because many teachers and organizations tend to teach safety education in a negative way, emphasizing rules and a list of "don'ts" for the students to follow. Also, some educators and organizations use scare tactics in safety, but these tactics have very little long-term value in changing behavior.

Many laws have been passed, especially in the area of traffic safety. Some states are passing mandatory safety belt and stiffer drunk-driving laws. These laws should help save more lives on the road; however, despite these and other legislative safety efforts, thousands of Americans die or are injured each year because of needless accidents. The situation will not change significantly until Americans reject an attitude of apathy toward safety and adopt a lifestyle of safe behavior.

Shown to the right of each activity title in this chapter is the suggested grade level(s) for which the activity might be appropriate. However, many of the suggested activities could be modified for use at various grade levels.

Information Assessment Activities

Stranger Safety   Grades K–3

Valued Outcome: Students will be able to make safe decisions about interactions with strangers.

National Health Education Standard: 7

Description of Strategy: Pose a series of statements to the students and have them respond by giving thumbs up for "OK to do" and thumbs down for "not OK to do." Show a picture card of each situation as you make each statement. Some example statements you might use are:

- I would accept candy or gifts from someone I did not know.
- I would accept a ride from someone I did not know.
- I would talk to my mother's friend.
- I would let someone I did not know into my house.
- I would help someone find his or her puppy, even if I did not know that person.
- I would talk to my school counselor.
- I would tell someone I have met on the Internet where I go to school.

Alternately, you can give students Worksheet 20.1 on page 498 to complete.

Materials Needed: large cards with pictures of people correlated with the statements, Worksheet 20.1, pencils

Processing Questions:

1. Why are some of these behaviors dangerous and other behaviors safe?
2. What should you do if a stranger approaches you?

✓ **Assessment:** Student will be able to describe individuals who may threaten their safety.

Safety Habits Beliefs   Grades K–5

Valued Outcome: Students will define their knowledge of safety habits.

National Health Education Standard: 1

Description of Strategy: Before spending time discussing safety rules and habits, have the students complete a series of statements that show how they feel when it comes to safety (Worksheet 20.2 on page 499). On a volunteer basis, discuss the values implicit in the statements on the handout.

Materials Needed: Worksheet 20.2 and pencils for each student

Processing Questions:

1. Why do we need safety rules and regulations?
2. If we don't follow rules, what might happen?
3. Why did you select what you did for the most important thing you can do to try to remain safe?
4. How can your attitude toward safety improve your safety?

✓ **Assessment:** Students will be able to explain why specific safety behaviors, such as fastening a safety belt or using a crosswalk, will lessen their chances of injury.

Safety Values   Grades K–3

Valued Outcome: Students will be able to respond to safety-related statements based on their values.

National Health Education Standard: 7

Description of Strategy: Have your students raise their hands to agree or disagree with the following statements:

- Some accidents are caused by people showing off.
- All the medicines in my house are stored in a safe place.
- Some medicines can be taken without parents' permission.
- I know the number of the local poison control center.
- I read labels on all medications before I take them.
- It is important to wear a safety belt even on short trips.

Lesson Title: First-Aid Kits

Date: April 2, 2012   **Time:** 9:00 A.M.   **Grade:** Three   **Teacher:** Lavender

I. National Health Education Standards

Health Education Standard 5: Students will demonstrate the ability to use decision-making skills to enhance health.

II. National Health Education Standards Performance Indicator

5.5.1 identify health-related situations that might require a thoughtful decision.

III. Valued Outcomes

- Students will identify basic components of a first-aid kit.
- Students will identify situations when a first-aid kit might be used.
- Students will react more confidently when accidents occur in the classroom.

IV. Description of Strategy

1. Explain that you think a first-aid kit should be assembled. Explain what a first-aid kit is and what it can be used for. Discuss why it is important to have first-aid kits in the classroom.
2. Divide the class into groups of three to four students. Have each group make a list of things that they think should go into the first-aid kit and why.
3. After students are finished, have each group explain what they put on their list and why. Write all items on the board. After the first group speaks, each consecutive group should mention only items that have not already been said. Then, discuss any items that might be missing.
4. Show students first-aid supplies and ask them what should go into the first-aid kit and why.
5. Demonstrate how each item in a first-aid kit is used and for what it is used. Make sure students know where the kit will be located so they can get it if needed.

V. Materials Needed

- paper/pencils
- board/markers
- first-aid supplies

VI. Formative Evaluation

Benchmarks

- Level 1: Student was able to identify some items in a first-aid kit.
- Level 2: Student was able to identify all items in a first-aid kit and describe what some are used for.
- Level 3: Student was able to list all items in a first-aid kit and describe what all are used for.
- Level 4: Student was able to list all items in a first-aid kit and explain what all are used for. Student was able to choose appropriate supplies for a given situation.

VII. Points of Emphasis

1. Make sure students know what everything in a first-aid kit is used for.
2. Explain to students appropriate times for a first-aid kit to be used.
3. Explain that a teacher must always be notified when a first-aid kit is used.

Teacher Evaluation

1. Keep the lesson as taught?   yes _____   no _____

2. What I need to improve _____

3. Next time make sure _____

4. Strengths of lesson _____

Lesson Title: Basic Water Safety/Reaching Assists

Date: April 9, 2012   **Time:** 10:00 A.M.   **Grade:** Five   **Teacher:** Maya

I. National Health Education Standards

Health Education Standard 5: Students will demonstrate the ability to use decision-making skills to enhance health.

II. National Health Education Standards Performance Indicator

5.5.2 analyze when assistance is needed when making a health-related decision.

III. Valued Outcomes

- Students will discuss basic safety rules for swimming.
- Students will identify when help is needed for a distressed swimmer.
- Students will demonstrate reaching assists for distressed swimmers.

IV. Description of Strategy

1. Get information about water safety from the American Red Cross or a local pool.
2. Have students describe water safety rules that they already know. Write the rules on the board and explain why each should be followed. Go over any rules that students did not mention.
3. Describe a distressed swimmer and have students give ideas about what to do if they see a swimmer in trouble. Emphasize that students should get help in this situation.
4. Explain reaching assists, describe when one would be used, and demonstrate the proper technique. Have students give examples of things that could be used for reaching assists.
5. Use masking tape to outline a "swimming pool" in your classroom. Demonstrate a reaching assist and have pairs of students practice reaching assists.
6. Review reaching assists and safety rules. Finish with a summary of safety rules and explain that if rules are followed, it is less likely someone will become a distressed swimmer.

V. Materials Needed

- masking tape
- rescue equipment

VI. Formative Evaluation

Benchmarks

- Level 1: Student was able to describe some basic water safety rules.
- Level 2: Student was able to describe basic water safety rules and explain why they are needed.
- Level 3: Student was able to describe basic water safety rules and explain why they are needed. Student was able to identify a distressed swimmer.
- Level 4: Student was able to describe basic water safety rules and explain why they are needed. Student was able to identify a distressed swimmer and demonstrate a reaching assist.

VII. Points of Emphasis

1. Describe specific water safety rules for lakes, pools, and beaches.
2. Explain why it is important for people to be able to recognize distressed swimmers.
3. Explain why a child should never jump in the water to try to save a distressed swimmer.

Teacher Evaluation

1. Keep the lesson as taught?   yes _____   no _____

2. What I need to improve _____

3. Next time make sure _____

4. Strengths of lesson _____

Processing Question: What variables help you determine your values about safety practices?

✓ **Assessment:** Students will be able to answer all statements and explain their answers.

Escaping a Home Fire   Grades K–1

Valued Outcome: Students will be able to describe the importance of a fire escape plan.

National Health Education Standards: 5, 7

Description of Strategy: Ask the students the following questions related to fire safety and to escaping a fire:

Question: What happens in a fire drill at school?

Sample Answer: *The fire alarm sounds and then we all go outside to our meeting place.*

Note: If they don't say the meeting place, tell them where it is.

Question: How do you know when to leave during a fire drill?

Sample Answer: *The fire bell rings or the smoke alarm sounds.*

Question: A fire can also happen in our houses or apartments where we live. How will you know if a fire happens in your home?

Sample Answer: *There may be something on the ceiling or wall that looks like this* (show a smoke alarm). *It's called a smoke alarm. Fires make a lot of smoke, and this smoke alarm is always sniffing the air to check for any smoke. If it finds a lot of smoke, then it beeps very loudly to let you know that there is a fire. It's on the ceiling or high on the wall to smell the smoke.* (Show photo of alarm on wall/ceiling.)

Question: Have you ever seen a smoke alarm in your home? Have you heard what it sounds like? (Take answers of several children.) I'll push this button so you can hear the sound it makes if a fire happens in your house or apartment. Cover your ears because it will be very loud! (Push button to demonstrate sound of smoke alarm.) If you hear that sound in your home, what do you think you should do?

Sample Answer: *You should go outside as quickly as you can. Even if you are scared, you should never hide in a closet or under the bed. And don't stop to get any toys. Get outside!* (Show photo of family leaving house.)

Note: Emphasize this point because many children have been known to hide in a fire, and it can make it difficult for firefighters to find them.

Question: Do you know why the smoke alarm beep is so loud?

Sample Answer: *Because if you are asleep, you want it to be able to wake you up.*

Note: You may hear children talk about the smoke alarm beeping and their parent fanning it or pushing a button so the smoke alarm goes off, or taking the battery out of the alarm. You can explain that sometimes normal cooking can make the smoke alarm go off, but that they should always expect the beep to mean that there might be a fire and to ask their parent/guardian to check if there is a fire.

Materials Needed: a smoke alarm, a sample home escape plan, photo of a smoke alarm in a residence, photo of people leaving a home (as though they are evacuating during a fire alarm)

Processing Questions:

1. How does a smoke alarm work?
2. What should you do if you hear a smoke alarm at home?

✓ **Assessment:** Students will write their answers to the questions you ask and turn in their completed sheet at the end of the lesson.

Source: SafeKids.org 2011. *Escaping a Home Fire.* (www.safekids.org/assets/docs/for-educators/lesson-plan-pedestrian-safety-lesson-plan.pdf.)

Learning about Personal Safety and Strangers   Grades 2–3

Valued Outcome: Students will be able to explain how to deal with potentially dangerous strangers in order to maintain personal safety at home, in their yard, at school, at the park or playground, etc.

National Health Education Standards: 1, 2, 5

Description of Strategy: The teacher will read *Once Upon a Dragon: Stranger Safety for Kids (and Dragons)*, discussing ideas in the book either during or after the reading. The teacher will then help the group brainstorm how to determine who, for safety purposes, is and is not considered a stranger; all criteria should be covered. Next, each student should write and/or illustrate one way to identify a stranger. Papers will be collected to make up the classroom's Safety Book.

Materials Needed: *Once Upon a Dragon: Stranger Safety for Kids (and Dragons)* by Jean E. Pendziwol (Kids Can Press, 2006); paper, pencils, markers, etc.; a binder to create the Safety Book

Processing Question: Describe several ways you can distinguish the people you trust from strangers.

○ **Integration:** Art

✓ **Assessment:** Students will demonstrate understanding of personal safety guidelines through writing and illustration.

How to Stay Safe Online
Grades 3–5

Valued Outcome: Students will be able to explain how to protect their safety when using the Internet.

National Health Education Standard: 2

Description of Strategy: This lesson teaches students how to use the Internet, how to interact with websites, and mostly, how to keep themselves safe online. Direct students to access the website www.teachingideas.co.uk/welcome/3711.htm. They should then click on "What Do You Need" to access the worksheet for this lesson. With the worksheet accessible, the students then click on "How do you start?" and follow the lesson while completing the worksheet.

Materials Needed: computer with Internet access and speakers, printer access

Processing Question: What threats to personal safety may you be exposed to when using the Internet?

✔ **Assessment:** Students will turn in completed worksheets after all parts of lesson have been completed.

Source: Teaching Ideas 2011. *Staying Safe.* Available at www.teachingideas.co.uk. Used by permission.

Field Trip Documentaries
Grades 3–5

Valued Outcome: Students will be able to make and deliver to their classmates an audio/video documentary of a safety field trip.

National Health Education Standard: 3

Description of Strategy: Plan a field trip related to some aspect of personal safety. Prepare students for their projects by introducing them to video cameras, video editing software, and audio recording. Divide the students into groups of four to five. Give them specific responsibilities on the aspects of the field trip they are to report on. During the field trip, each group is responsible for videotaping their assigned aspect of the field trip. During the next few days in class, the groups will add the audio portion to the video, and then the groups will deliver their field trip safety-related presentation to the class.

Materials Needed: video camera, access to computer video editing/recording programs (e.g., Garage Band or GoldWave)

Processing Question: How can technology be used to deliver "safe behavior" messages to students?

○ **Integration:** Social Studies

✔ **Assessment:** Students will be evaluated on each phase of the documentary: 1) video, 2) recording the audio portion, and 3) presentation of the documentary to the class.

School Safety Newspaper
Grades 4–5

Valued Outcome: Students will be able to utilize their Internet skills to research information about safe behavior in and around the school, and complete a student-oriented School Safety newspaper.

National Health Education Standards: 2, 3

Description of Strategy: Set up the students in groups of three or four. Each group of students will research information about a specific area of the school in which safe behaviors are important (classroom, playground, etc.). The students will access appropriate Internet sites (such as .gov sources) to research safety standards and recommendations related to their assigned area. They will organize their information so they can keep their information and source documentation on file. Each group will write a brief (100-word) newspaper article using the information they found through research and observation of their assigned area. Groups should format the information and upload it onto the class webpage (intranet) or publish it in a printed newspaper.

Materials Needed: supervised access to areas for safety observation and research, computer with Internet access, word processing program, article layout program, school intranet or newspaper

Processing Questions:

1. How can the media/newspaper articles affect safe behavior at school?
2. Is the assigned area up to safety standards? If not, what could be done to improve it?

○ **Integration:** Language Arts

✔ **Assessment:** Students will be evaluated on their ability to write the articles as well as successfully uploading the articles in newspaper format on the intranet server at their school.

Pool Safety
Grades 3–5

Valued Outcome: After a class discussion about water safety, the students will be able to categorize the listed behaviors as safe or unsafe and write two of their own water safety rules.

National Health Education Standard: 7

Description of Strategy: Lead the class in a discussion about water safety. To begin, ask the students "How many of you like to swim?" Then, "Do any of you swim at a pool or a lake where there are lifeguards? Who can tell me one thing a lifeguard does?" Answers will vary.

Next, lead a class discussion using prompts: "Why does a lifeguard sit on such a high chair/stand?" (so he or she can see the whole pool area), "Why would a lifeguard need to be able to see everyone?" (to keep everyone safe and make sure everyone is following the rules), "What should you do if you hear the lifeguard blow his or her whistle?" (stop what you are doing and give the lifeguard full attention), "What are some of the pool rules?" (do not run on deck, no pushing each other in or under water, no diving in the shallow end of the pool, get out of the pool when the lifeguard tells you to), "Why do they have these rules?" Go through each one: No running because someone could fall and get hurt on the deck or fall into the water; it is dangerous to horseplay in water because someone could drown; no diving in shallow water because the diver could hit his or her head on the bottom of a pool and be injured or drown; and get out as soon as the lifeguard gives the instruction because there is most likely a danger such as lightning, or the pool water has been contaminated (with vomit, feces, etc.).

Explain to the students that following pool rules keeps them, others, and the lifeguards safe. Wrap up this part of the discussion by having the student recall some fun things they can do at a pool (swim, float, talk to their friends, play a water sport, go down a water slide, etc.).

After the discussion, do the following activity. Give each student the following items: two paper plates, one with a sad face and one with a happy face, two blank slips of paper, and slips of paper with the following statements written on them (each slip should contain one statement):

- Play tag on the pool deck. (unsafe)
- Play with a beach ball in shallow water. (safe)
- Take turns with a friend holding each other under the water. (unsafe)
- Ignore the lifeguard's whistle if I am sure it is not directed at me. (unsafe)
- Cannonball into the deep end if the area is clear. (safe)
- Dive off a diving board after checking that the area is clear. (safe)

At the front of the room, place an additional set of plates and a master set of statements to sort later. At their desks, have the students sort the slips of paper into safe (happy) and unsafe (sad) piles. Then have the class sort the master slips together by reading each statement aloud and asking the students which plate it should go on. Then, have the students write their own safe or unsafe behaviors on the blank slips of paper. Have each student read his or her statement aloud before placing it on the appropriate plate. Be sure to have them write their names on the back so you will be able to evaluate what they have learned.

Materials Needed: two paper plates per student and one teacher set (one with a happy face and one with a sad face), pencils and slips of paper with statements for each student

Processing Questions:

1. What are two safe and two unsafe behaviors?
2. What is the most important rule to remember when at the pool?

✓**Assessment:** Students will be able to describe safe and unsafe swimming behaviors.

Decision Stories

The teacher and students will follow the procedures outlined in Chapter 4, pages 60–62, for decision stories.

For each of the decision stories, write a list on the board of ideas generated by the class for how each situation should be dealt with. Ask the students to discuss the merits of the methods suggested.

Assessment for Decision Stories: Students can identify health-enhancing behaviors and exhibit positive decision-making skills.

Show and Tell   Grades K–2

Valerie and Davina are in the same second grade class. One day during lunch, Davina tells Valerie she has something to show her when they are back in the classroom. After lunch, while the teacher is busy talking to another student and they are putting away their lunch boxes, Davina pulls out a gun from her backpack to show Valerie and says, "I found this in my dad's room. Isn't it cool?" Valerie knows guns are dangerous because their teacher had a police officer talk to the class about gun safety. Valerie knows that she should not touch guns and that guns are not allowed at school.

Focus Questions:

1. What should Valerie do?
2. Why are guns dangerous?

National Health Education Standards: 2, 5, 7

Around the Neighborhood   Grades K–3

Joseph and Eli are best friends in the same third grade class. Sometimes Eli plays at Joseph's house, and Joseph often plays at Eli's house after school. Many times they like to ride their bikes around Eli's neighborhood. There is a lot of traffic on Eli's street, and Joseph and Eli know they should always wear their helmets. In class, they have learned about bike safety and what they should do to be safe. Joseph always wears his helmet, but Eli does not. Eli says, "Helmets are for babies, and I don't play with babies." Joseph doesn't want to argue with Eli or lose his friendship.

Focus Questions:

1. What should Joseph do?
2. What could Joseph say to Eli to convince him to wear his helmet?

National Health Education Standards: 2, 5, 7

Fire! Grades K–5

Marilyn is alone in her house. She goes into the hallway on the second floor and sees flames coming from the room down the hall. The flames are between Marilyn and the only staircase to the downstairs part of the house.

Focus Question: What should Marilyn do?

National Health Education Standards: 5, 7

The Hill Grades K–5

George and Mario like to ride their bikes to school. There is a hill on the way to school. Near the top of the hill, there is a stop sign, but if they stop, getting over the hill is difficult. George usually stops, but Mario never does. George has to get off his bike and start again. Mario kids him about this and calls him a chicken. George does not want to seem a coward to his friend, but he knows that he should stop for traffic signs.

Focus Question: What should George do?

National Health Education Standards: 2, 5, 7

Cyberbullying Grades K–5

Valued Outcome: Students will be able to apply the instructions in order to prevent cyberbullying.

National Health Education Standard: 2

Description of Strategy: Have the students access the website http://learninglab.org. Students should watch the first video (Garfield cartoon), then try and apply the cyberbullying lessons taught through writing and illustrating a cyberbullying scenario.

Materials Needed: computer with Internet access and speakers, pencils and markers, drawing paper

Processing Questions:

1. What are the different ways that one can be "cyberbullied" online?
2. What are strategies that can be used to avoid being cyberbullied?

✔ **Assessment:** Students will draw and color their own sheet illustrating how to avoid cyberbullying.

Source: Virginia Department of Education 2011. (http://learninglab.org.)

Safety Belts Grades K–5

Jaime's friend, Warren, and Warren's parents came to Jaime's house to take Jaime and Warren to a party. When Jaime got into their car, he noticed Warren and his parents were not wearing their safety belts, and the one at his seat was hard to find. Jaime had been taught always to wear his safety belt, but he was afraid he would embarrass Warren and his parents if he were the only one in the car to wear his safety belt.

Focus Question: What should Jaime do?

National Health Education Standards: 5, 7

The Stranger Grades K–5

Beth and her sister Harriet are walking home from school. Just then a car pulls up by the curb. The driver is a man Beth and her sister have never seen. He asks them their names, and they tell him. Then the man says that he is a good friend of their father. He says that their father has asked him to pick them up and take them for a ride. The stranger offers to buy the girls some ice cream, too.

Focus Question: What should Beth and her sister do?

National Health Education Standards: 5, 7

Emergency Care Grades 3–5

Mary came home from school and found her grandmother lying at the foot of the stairway unconscious. She could not wake her.

Focus Questions:

1. Who should Mary call?
2. What else should she do for her grandmother?

National Health Education Standards: 5, 7

Violence Prevention Presentation Grades 3–5

Valued Outcome: Students will be able to use information from a violence prevention-related Decision Story and produce and deliver a PowerPoint presentation to their classmates.

National Health Education Standards: 2, 3

Description of Strategy: After teaching a decision story to the class, tell students to use Microsoft PowerPoint to develop each aspect of the decision story and the decision they reached. Each slide will be illustrated by an appropriate picture related to that aspect of the decision story. The PowerPoint presentations can be narrated live or recorded beforehand.

Materials Needed: access to a computer and PowerPoint software, pictures

Processing Question: How can technology be used to deliver violence prevention messages to students?

✔ **Assessment:** Students will be evaluated on setting up the PowerPoint presentation and delivery of the PowerPoint presentation to the class.

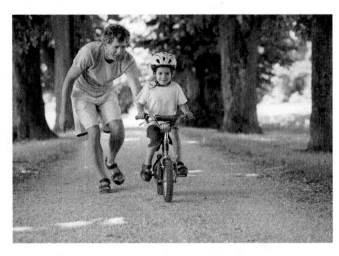

Learning to be safe while riding a bicycle can prevent many accidents.

Dramatizations

Safety Puppet Show
Grades K–2

Valued Outcome: Students will be able to demonstrate their ability to react in emergency situations.

National Health Education Standards: 5, 7, 8

Description of Strategy: Have students make or use puppets (such as "Safe Susan" and "Hazardous Harry") to perform safety-related skits. Topics could include disaster situations, handling medical emergencies, fire safety, recreational safety, and safety in the home.

Materials Needed: paper bag or cloth for making puppets and markers for each student

Processing Questions:

1. Why is it important to plan ahead for disaster situations?
2. How can you help your family during a disaster?

○ **Integration:** Art

✓ **Assessment:** Students will have their puppets react appropriately in an emergency situation.

School Bus Behavior
Grades K–5

Valued Outcome: Students will be able to identify proper conduct on a bus.

National Health Education Standards: 1, 2, 5, 7

Description of Strategy: Divide the class into groups. Give each group a situation that has happened on the bus. Have students decide what should be done.

• Case 1: Two students are fighting.

• Case 2: Two students are sitting on the same seat; one student wants the window up, the other student wants the window down.
• Case 3: A student is holding his arms and head out of the window.

Processing Question: Why is it important to behave well on the school bus?

✓ **Assessment:** Students will be able to describe safe and unsafe bus behavior.

Looking for Hazards
Grades K–5

Valued Outcome: Students will be able to identify hazardous areas in the school setting.

National Health Education Standards: 1, 7

Description of Strategy: Assign students to visit various classrooms, such as the gym, looking for hazards. Have them report the findings to the class and then return to the same classroom in one week to see if the hazard still exists.

Materials Needed: form for each student that lists classrooms in the school

Processing Questions:

1. What safety hazards are typically found in schools?
2. What can students do to help eliminate these hazards?

✓ **Assessment:** Students will demonstrate that they can identify hazards in school classrooms.

Phoning for Help
Grades K–5

Valued Outcome: Students will be able to learn the proper technique for using the phone during an emergency situation.

National Health Education Standards: 1, 7

Description of Strategy: In many emergency situations, assistance can be obtained by calling 911, or telephoning the proper authority or agency. Stress the importance of knowing what to say on the telephone. Have the students prepare a list of emergency telephone numbers for their area, including those of the fire department, the poison control center, and so on. Then have them role-play emergency situations. One student plays the part of the telephone operator or official. Another student then phones for help. Point out that information given over the telephone should be stated clearly and accurately. Let each student role-play the part of an emergency caller at least once. Follow the activity with general discussion of proper use of the telephone.

Materials Needed: telephone book, pencils and paper for each student

Processing Questions:

1. What's the first phone number you should dial in an emergency? What other phone numbers should you have on hand in case of an emergency?
2. What information should you give over the phone in case of an emergency?

✓ **Assessment:** Students will be able to state the correct phone number to call in an emergency, and the information that should be given.

Disaster Drama
Grades 3–5

Valued Outcome: Students will be able to learn first-aid procedures to use during a disaster.

National Health Education Standards: 1, 7

Description of Strategy: Have the students enact a mock disaster. Set up the classroom as if a tornado or hurricane had hit the area, and the students are the only trained first-aiders who can help. Assign some students to be victims with a variety of injuries (provide descriptions of injuries and symptoms on index cards), and the other students will play the parts of emergency care personnel who will perform first aid for the victims.

Materials Needed: first-aid kits, bandages, cards with descriptions of injuries and symptoms

Processing Questions:

1. How can you help during a disaster?
2. What first-aid skills would you need to know?

✓ **Assessment:** Students will demonstrate knowledge of which first-aid procedures to use in specific emergency scenarios.

Safety Attitudes
Grades 3–5

Valued Outcome: Students will be able to role-play positive and negative attitudes concerning safety.

National Health Education Standards: 1, 7

Description of Strategy: Attitudes play a large part in safety behavior. Have students role-play people with positive and negative attitudes while participating in several activities (such as bicycling or playing ball). Positive attitudes include consideration, maturity, courtesy, and honesty; negative attitudes include selfishness, impatience, childishness, competitiveness, showing off, daydreaming, and unnecessary risk taking.

Processing Questions:

1. How can one's attitude about safety cause or prevent an accident?

2. What are examples of positive safety attitudes? of negative safety attitudes?

✓ **Assessment:** Students will be able to describe positive and negative safety attitudes.

Discussion and Report Techniques

Home-Alone Safety
Grades K–5

Valued Outcome: Students will be able to write from memory two safe or unsafe behaviors associated with home-alone safety.

National Health Education Standards: 1, 7

Description of Strategy: As an introduction to the lesson, have students indicate whether the following statements are true or false. After students answer the statements, give the correct answers and ask a student who answered correctly to explain why his or her answer is correct. (This will give you an idea of focus areas for subsequent lessons and expose the class to home-alone safety awareness.)

True or False

T/F 1. If the door is open or unlocked when I arrive home alone, I should go in and check things out.

T/F 2. It is okay to give out information to adults on the phone.

T/F 3. I can watch television or talk on the phone with my friends.

T/F 4. If someone knocks on my door, I should open it.

T/F 5. I should shut and lock the doors to my house.

T/F 6. I can play outside as long as I stay near the house or in my yard.

After the class discussion, have each student write about two safe or unsafe home-alone safety behaviors.

Materials Needed: paper and pencils for each student, master list of quiz questions

Processing Questions:

1. Why would you not answer the door when you are home alone?
2. What if the person knows your name and your parents' names or says your mom or dad asked him or her to come?
3. What should you do if your door is already open and unlocked when you arrive home?

✓ **Assessment:** Students will understand the differences between safe and unsafe behaviors when home alone.

Accidents around the Home
Grade 1

Valued Outcome: Students will be able to explain how to remove common household dangers and make their homes safer, create a family escape plan known by all family members, and have an emergency phone number sheet posted in their homes.

National Health Education Standards: 1, 3, 5, 7

Description of Strategy: The teacher will show students a skeleton drawing of a two-story house that includes a kitchen, bathroom, two bedrooms, a staircase, an exterior deck, a yard, and a garage. The teacher will go room by room, asking students to brainstorm typical safety hazards that can be found in each room (electrical outlets, cleaning supplies, gasoline, paint cans, decks without childproof railings, etc.), filling in any hazards that students don't mention. As homework, each student will pair up with a parent to seek out and list any such dangers in their own homes. On the day homework is turned in, teacher will ask students to describe safety hazards they discovered in their homes and what they plan to do to reduce or remove them.

Students will also be sent home with a fill-in-the-blank Family Escape Plan and an Emergency Telephone Numbers sheet. After returning completed sheets to school for credit, students will take them home to post in a visible place.

Materials Needed: drawing of house, Family Escape Plan sheet, Emergency Telephone Numbers sheet

Processing Questions:

1. What steps can you take to make your home safer?
2. Does everyone in your family know your emergency escape plan?
3. Does everyone in your family know where the emergency phone number sheet can be found?

✓ **Assessment:** Students will share safety hazards uncovered at home. Students will complete both the family escape plan and the emergency phone numbers sheet.

Bike Safety Laws
Grade 3

Valued Outcome: Students will be able to name important bike safety laws and discuss why each should be followed.

National Health Education Standards: 1, 2, 3

Description of Strategy: Students will be led through the process of creating posters about bike safety laws to display in the classroom and/or around the school. First, the class will brainstorm known bike safety laws, writing them down on the board. Once student knowledge is exhausted, teacher will fill in any missing laws. The teacher will explain the difference between safety laws and best practices. Each student will then choose a law to make a poster for, and use a piece of paper to sketch ideas for their concept. Students may focus on images, language, or both. Once initial concept sketches are completed, the teacher will present them to the class, with students offering feedback on ideas and execution. Students will then design full-sized posters incorporating class feedback; they may choose to work alone, or partner with others to combine the best images and ideas.

Materials Needed: 8.5 × 11 drawing paper, pencils, markers, poster board

Processing Questions:

1. What is the difference between bike safety laws and bike safety best practices?
2. Why is it important to follow bike safety laws?

○ **Integration:** Art

✓ **Assessment:** Posters will be displayed to conclude lesson.

Resiliency Skills Blog
Grades 4–5

Valued Outcome: Students will be able to set up, make entries into, and implement a blog on the Internet.

National Health Education Standard: 2

Description of Strategy: After studying a unit on bus safety, familiarize students with blogging. The students will set up a blog on the school's or district's intranet where they will blog about their thoughts on waiting at the bus stop, boarding the bus, riding on the bus, and departing the bus safely. They can brainstorm about ways to encourage other students to practice safety in all those areas of behavior and write about real-life situations they have experienced or might experience. The students can have one class blog or their own individual blogs. When students visit each other's blogs, they can brainstorm with them, provide feedback, and offer suggestions.

Materials Needed: computers, school intranet (This would be much more secure than an Internet blog, where the entries would be visible to others outside the school network.)

Processing Question: How can safe behavior reduce accidents on the bus?

✓ **Assessment:** Students will be graded on their ability to set up, make entries, and publish their blog on the school intranet.

Disaster Demonstration
Grades K–5

Valued Outcome: Students will be able to demonstrate proper behaviors during various disasters.

National Health Education Standards: 1, 7

Description of Strategy: Assign groups of students to demonstrate the proper behaviors during various emergency situations, such as a tornado, hurricane, earthquake, or an armed intruder. (Be sure to include whatever types of disasters are more likely to occur in your geographic area.) Have them give instructions to the other students, and actually carry out the drill.

Processing Questions:

1. What types of disasters could occur in your area?
2. Does your family have a plan to follow if such a disaster occurs?

✓ **Assessment:** Students will be able to name natural (and other) disasters that might occur in their area, and describe the appropriate action to take if such an event occurred.

Holiday Safety Diary   Grades K–5

Valued Outcome: Students will be able to list hazards that occur during holidays.

National Health Education Standards: 1, 7

Description of Strategy: As a class, identify major holidays, and list them on the board or on an overhead transparency. Have students make a list of accidents or safety hazards that occur more often during each holiday and ways in which those accidents could be reduced or prevented.

Materials Needed: overhead projector and pen or board and markers, pencils and paper for each student

Processing Questions:

1. Which holidays are most likely to have disasters associated with them?
2. How can holiday disasters be prevented?
3. If such a disaster cannot be prevented, how can we plan in order to reduce the number and severity of accidents?

✓ **Assessment:** Students will be able to name some possible emergencies associated with various holidays, and ways to prevent them.

School Safety Books   Grades 3–5

Valued Outcome: Students will be able to list school safety rules.

National Health Education Standards: 1, 7

Description of Strategy: Have students work in groups of three. Have students list safety rules they should follow at school. Examples include no running in the halls, put supplies away when finished, share, wait your turn in lines and on playground equipment, follow all school bus safety rules, and follow the teacher's instructions. Have the

groups share their answers with the rest of the class, and write the responses on the board or on an overhead transparency.

Have each student write and illustrate a short book on school safety. Have them go through the writing process of prewriting, drafting, editing, revising, rewriting, and publishing. After their story has been through the writing process, have them write their story on the pages in a booklet or type it into the computer and then illustrate it. Display the books in the classroom or, if possible, the library. (Since the students will take their stories through the writing process, this activity will take several days to complete.)

Materials Needed: computer or sheets of white paper folded into a booklet for each student; crayons, pencils, notebook pages, colored pencils or markers for each student; overhead projector and pen

Processing Question: How do school safety rules benefit you as an individual?

○ **Integration:** Writing

✓ **Assessment:** Students will be able to write out and explain school safety rules.

Don't Touch That!   Grades 3–5

Valued Outcome: Students will be able to determine the difference between safe and unsafe items and situations found at home.

National Health Education Standards: 1, 7

Description of Strategy: Discuss the safety hazards that are found in and around a house. Explain that many accidents occur at home. Have each student make a page with newspaper and magazine clippings of accidents that have occurred in people's homes. Then have students write a sentence explaining how the accident happened and how it could have been avoided. Put all the papers together to construct a class scrapbook.

Materials Needed: scrapbook; newspapers, magazines, pictures, glue or tape, pencils or pens for each student

Processing Question: What steps can you take to prevent home accidents?

✓ **Assessment:** Students will be able to list common accidents that occur in the home and explain how they can be avoided.

Emergency!   Grades 3–5

Valued Outcome: Students will be able to identify the correct action to take in emergency situations.

National Health Education Standards: 1, 5, 7

Description of Strategy: Each of the following items describes an emergency that was handled incorrectly. Read each item. Identify the incorrect action, and tell why it was incorrect. Explain what you would do in the situation.

- Leroy was hit in the head by a moving swing and was knocked unconscious. Since it was a very hot day, his friend Eddie moved him into the shade before going for help.
- While Liz was babysitting for the Jacksons, two-year-old Timmy drank some liquid from an unlabeled bottle. When Liz found him, Timmy was pale and sweaty, with stains from whatever he drank around his mouth. Liz immediately gave him some syrup of ipecac to make him vomit. Then she called the poison control center.
- While José and Ben were sledding, José was thrown from his sled, hitting his head on a rock. Although conscious, he felt nauseated and too dizzy to walk. Before going for help, Ben covered José with his coat and gave him some hot chocolate from their thermos to keep him warm.
- Nancy and Kayla were in the park, eating hamburgers and talking. Kayla, who had been lying on her back while she ate, suddenly jumped up and made strange wheezing sounds as if she couldn't breathe or speak. Nancy saw that Kayla was probably choking and ran to get some water for her.

Processing Question: Why is it important to know the correct action to take in emergency situations?

✓ **Assessment:** Students will identify the incorrect actions taken in each scenario and explain why they were incorrect.

Safety Belt Discussion   Grades 4–5

Valued Outcome: Students will be able to explain why safety belts should be worn.

National Health Education Standards: 1, 7

Description of Strategy: Choose two teams of students to research the use of safety belts in automobiles. One team should explain why wearing safety belts, even for short trips, can save lives and prevent needless injuries in case of an automobile accident. The other team should present reasons why many people don't bother or refuse to wear safety belts. Have the class discuss why safety belts are important.

Materials Needed: resources for students to research their topic

Processing Question: Why is it important to wear a safety belt every time you ride in a car?

✓ **Assessment:** Students will be able to explain why wearing a safety belt is important.

Natural Disasters   Grades K–1

Valued Outcome: Students will know what to expect in, and how to respond to the immediate threat of, natural disasters including earthquakes, wildfires, severe storms, tornadoes, floods, tsunamis, mudslides, and volcanic eruptions.

National Health Education Standards: 1, 3, 7

Description of Strategy: The teacher will present a high-level overview of common natural disasters, using images when appropriate; he or she will then narrow the focus to natural disasters most likely to occur in the local area, showing photos from the area's most recent occurrences. Next, the teacher will divide students into small groups and assign each group a type of disaster. Each group will be given a sheet with the headings "What to Expect" and "How to Respond", with bulleted points under each heading. After reviewing (and, if age-appropriate, researching) the topic, each group will present its guidelines to the rest of the class, with each student reading at least one bullet point. At the conclusion, all students will be provided with sheets for every type of disaster covered. Students may also be quizzed on their basic knowledge of each type of disaster.

Materials Needed: Sheets describing "What to Expect" and "How to Respond" for each type of natural disaster that normally occurs in the local area; testing sheet/s based on the same material.

Processing Question:

1. What can you expect when (x-type of natural disaster) strikes?
2. How will you respond when (x-type of natural disaster) strikes?

✓ **Assessment:** Students will present the information about their assigned natural disaster and listen to the presentations of others. Students will then be tested on retention of this information.

Fire Safety   Grades K–1

Valued Outcomes: Students will be able to identify fire hazards in a home. They will know what to expect if a fire occurs; how to Stop, Drop, and Roll; and how to dial 911.

National Health Education Standards: 1, 3, 5, 7

Description of Strategy: Teacher will play clips from the Firefighter George series of videos, demonstrating (1) Stop, Drop, and Roll, (2) home fire safety tips, and (3) when and how to dial 911. Teacher will pretend the classroom is a home and lead students through the proper responses to a fire. Teacher will then take students outside the classroom and lead them through proper responses to a fire when outside. While outside, all students will practice the Stop, Drop, and Roll maneuver.

Materials Needed: Firefighter George and Fire Trucks: Volumes 1 & 2 DVDs (from Start Smarter Videos), equipment to play DVDs

Processing Questions:

1. What can you do to make your home safer from fire?
2. What do you do if there is a fire in your home while you're outside?
3. What do you do if there's a fire in your home while you're inside? Asleep?

✓ **Assessment:** Each student's ability to demonstrate the proper actions (Stop, Drop, and Roll; crawling low; dialing 911, etc.) will be assessed.

Pedestrian Safety Lesson Plan   Grades K–5

Valued Outcome: Students will be able to demonstrate knowledge of pedestrian safety techniques.

National Health Education Standards: 1, 4, 7

Description of Strategy: The teacher begins discussion by asking students what the following terms mean: *pedestrian, yield, right-of-way.* Ask the students who taught them how to walk in traffic and cross streets and discuss what they know. Ask the students what they learned and what they know already about pedestrian safety and make a list of their responses on the board. Discuss why signs, signals, and laws are needed to keep pedestrians safe while they are walking. Ask the students if they have ever observed any of the signs during their walk to school or any other time they walk. Discuss dangerous and safe things the students have seen pedestrians do while walking, and then discuss what steps students can take to make them more safe as pedestrians.

Processing Question: Why is it important for pedestrians to know about traffic laws and pedestrian safety?

✓ **Assessment:** Students will be assessed by how they respond to the various scenarios and relate knowledge of pedestrian safety issues during discussion.

Source: SafeKids.org © 2011. Used by permission.

Safe Crossing Demonstration   Grades K–5

Valued Outcome: Students will be able to demonstrate knowledge of road safety/traffic signs and safe crossing techniques.

National Health Education Standards: 1, 4, 7

Description of Strategy: Using signs and mock cars provided, have students role play different situations they may experience as a pedestrian. Have students take on the role of a driver or a pedestrian and simulate the scenarios using the signs and cars, and create a crosswalk using masking tape (if indoors) or sidewalk chalk (if outside).

Students should have an opportunity to hold the signs, be a driver, or be a pedestrian. Sample scenarios:

- Use a traffic light sign (red, yellow, or green) and Walk or Don't Walk signs. Have students demonstrate crossing the street with these signals present. Try with and without a crosswalk.
- Use the Stop sign and/or the Yield to Pedestrian sign and simulate a car and pedestrians. Try with and without a crosswalk.
- Use all of the signs (Stop sign, traffic lights, Yield to Pedestrian, Don't Walk and Walk) and have the students come up with three possible scenarios of what they have seen or might see while walking. Incorporate the cars and try with and without a crosswalk.
- Have students demonstrate looking left, right, and left again at a crosswalk when cars are approaching.
- Demonstrate behaviors of a driver that follows rules (stopping at a crosswalk or the Stop sign) and one that doesn't (not stopping at a Stop sign or not obeying the Yield to Pedestrian sign)

Materials Needed: signs/props (Stop sign, traffic lights, Walk sign, Don't Walk sign, Yield to Pedestrian sign, cars, crosswalk)

Processing Question: Why is it important for pedestrians to know all the traffic signs?

✓ **Assessment:** During the activity, the students will be assessed by how they respond to the various scenarios and signs.

Fire Safety at Home   Grades K–5

Valued Outcome: Students will be able to evaluate a situation involving fire and smoke and decide the best way to exit a building.

National Health Education Standards: 1, 7

Description of Strategy: Have the students discuss what they already know to do when a fire happens in school and at home. Most students only practice the school drill twice a year and never at home, so it will be important to go through the school procedure before the actual drill occurs so that they know what to do. Have the students help you make a fire plan using a school map and procedures just for your classroom. After the discussion and plans are made, have students quietly practice entering and exiting the building. When outside, find your special spot to meet and tell the students as they walk outside to make a chain and do not let go until all are in the meeting spot and class roll has been taken. Practice this several times until the students feel comfortable.

After the students have practiced entering and exiting the building, have them help you set up two houses (a one story and a two story) in the classroom. Assign some students to the houses and others to the audience. Students will describe their plan for escape from their home and then demonstrate it for the audience. If the students want, they can set up special situations such as fire in the hallway on the first floor or other obstacles. Once each group has practiced escaping out of the homes, ask the students to practice stopping, dropping, and rolling in the event their hair or clothing catches on fire.

Some points of which to remind students include:

- Using the back of your hand, feel the surface of any closed door you must open during your escape. If the door is hot, find a different way out.
- Toxic gases may be low across the room, and smoke may be up higher. Crouch down or crawl on hands and knees in smoke-filled rooms.
- *Do not hide* inside the building.
- Take the easiest and fastest exit out of a building if it is not blocked. Try the door first (instead of the windows).

Materials Needed: blankets, mats/small pieces of carpet, chairs or sturdy tables to make the homes

Processing Questions:

1. What is the best measure of protection when there is a lot of smoke in the house or classroom?
2. Why is it important to have a special meeting place?
3. Why is it important to have plans at home and at school?

✓ **Assessment:** Students will demonstrate their ability to find the best way to exit a building that contains fire and/or smoke.

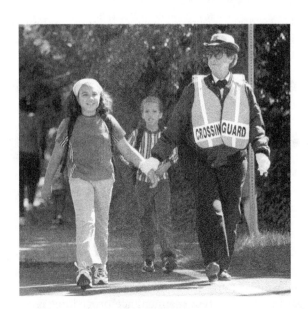

Students need to be safe pedestrians.

Cuts, Scratches, and Abrasions   Grades 3–5

Valued Outcome: Students will demonstrate a basic knowledge of cuts, scratches, and abrasions and what to do if they get one.

National Health Education Standards: 1, 5, 7

Description of Strategy: Begin the class by walking into the room with a bandage on your arm. Ask the students what they think is wrong with your arm. Explain to the students that you cut your arm, and you had to try to make it better.

Explain to the students what a cut, scratch, and abrasion is and how they might happen. Cuts are deeper and caused by sharp objects like knives, scratches are shallow and caused by sharp objects like a fingernail or thorn, and abrasions are caused when large areas of skin are rubbed away. Tell the students the steps to follow to help your cut heal: Apply pressure to stop the bleeding, clean the cut with soap and water, apply antibacterial cream (if approved by school and if needed), and put a bandage on the cut. Show the students a picture of someone with stitches and explain that stitches may be needed if a cut is very deep. Review these steps with the students a few times, and make sure they all understand what they are doing.

Tell students to find a partner and practice cleaning and putting an adhesive bandage on the cut. Have plenty of bandages available for the students to practice with. While the students are practicing, walk around the room and make sure students are doing it properly. Have the students come up one at a time and perform the techniques for you while all the other students continue to practice.

Materials Needed: soft cloths, antibacterial cream, different types of bandages, picture of a cut with stitches

Processing Questions:

1. What is the difference between a cut, a scratch, and an abrasion?
2. What is the proper technique for cleaning and bandaging a cut?
3. What materials are needed to treat a cut?

✓ **Assessment:** Students will demonstrate how to properly clean a cut or abrasion and apply a bandage.

Strains and Sprains   Grades 3–5

Valued Outcome: Students will demonstrate the basic knowledge of sprains and strains and what to do if they have one.

National Health Education Standards: 1, 3, 7

Description of Strategy: Begin the class by walking into the room with a splint or air cast on your ankle. Ask the students what they think is wrong with your ankle. Tell them that it is sprained (but not really). Explain to the students how you get a sprain or strain. Sprains are caused when the ligaments that reinforce a joint are stretched or torn. Strains, also called "pulled muscles," occur when a muscle is overstretched or torn by overuse or abuse; the injured muscle may become inflamed, and adjacent joints are usually immobilized. Tell the students what to do if they think they have hurt their ankle: They should not move it and should tell an adult what has happened. They may have to go to the doctor. If you have a sprain or strain, you may have to wear a splint or temporary cast.

Explain to the students that RICE is a mnemonic that stands for Rest, Ice, Compression, and Elevation. Explain to the students why each of these steps is important. Have the students draw and color a picture of them following the RICE method. While they are doing that, call them up individually and have them tell you what RICE stands for.

Materials Needed: a splint or temporary cast, paper and crayons for each student

Processing Questions:

1. What is the difference between a sprain and a strain?
2. What is the proper technique for taking care of the sprain or strain?

✓ **Assessment:** Students will be able to describe how to correctly give first aid (RICE) for an ankle strain or sprain.

Backpack Safety
Grades 3–5

Valued Outcome: Students will demonstrate basic knowledge of backpacks and how to use them safely.

National Health Education Standards: 1, 7

Description of Strategy: Begin the class by having the students pack their backpacks as if they would be going home for the day. Walk around to make sure that the students pack everything that they normally take home in their backpack. Ask them if they think that their backpacks are too heavy. Tell the class that a backpack should weigh only 10 percent of their own body weight. Let the class take turns measuring how much they weigh and how much their backpack weighs, and then tell them if their backpack is too heavy. Explain to the students that a heavy backpack can cause your back, shoulders, and neck to ache. The weight can cause damage to the disks that are between the vertebrae in your back and can also do damage to your nervous and circulatory systems. You may have problems for the rest of your life if you do not follow the safety tips for using a backpack.

Tell the students that there are many ways to make sure that their backpacks are safe. They can make sure they get a backpack with two shoulder straps and a waist strap, put the heaviest things closer to their back, and do not carry anything that is not necessary. Backpacks should

not be carried over just one shoulder; use both shoulder straps. They could also get a backpack that has wheels or one with a lot of pockets that can spread out the weight. Have the students draw a picture of themselves with their backpack using one of the safety tips. Call the students up while they are working on their picture and have them explain why the improper use of backpacks can be bad for your health.

Materials Needed: a scale, paper and markers for each student

Processing Questions:

1. How can backpacks cause back pain?
2. What are some ways to prevent backaches from backpacks?

✓ **Assessment:** Students will be able to describe two ways they can help keep their backpacks from harming their health.

Resuscitation Annie
Grades 5–8

Valued Outcome: Students will learn mouth-to-mouth resuscitation.

National Health Education Standards: 1, 3

Description of Strategy: If you have a CPR (cardiopulmonary resuscitation) mannequin available, demonstrate the proper technique for mouth-to-mouth resuscitation. Contact your local chapter of the American Heart Association or American Red Cross for assistance in presenting this demonstration. Students must weigh enough to do proper chest compressions.

Materials Needed: CPR mannequin

Processing Questions:

1. How does resuscitation help a victim with a breathing problem?
2. Can you perform these procedures?

✓ **Assessment:** Students will correctly demonstrate mouth-to-mouth resuscitation on a CPR mannequin.

Fire Extinguishers
Grades 3–5

Valued Outcome: Students will learn the proper techniques of using a fire extinguisher and be able to identify the classes of extinguishers.

National Health Education Standard: 1

Description of Strategy: Show the students how to operate the extinguisher. Identify the different classes of extinguishers. (You may wish to contact your local fire department on current maintenance procedures required for fire extinguishers.)

- **Class A:** used for wood, paper, or textile fires
- **Class B:** used for oil, grease, or paint fires
- **Class C:** used on electrical equipment

Materials Needed: fire extinguishers from each class

Processing Questions:

1. Does your family have a working fire extinguisher in your home?
2. Do you know how to use the extinguisher?

✓**Assessment:** Students can name the three types of extinguishers and demonstrate how to properly use a fire extinguisher.

The Hug of Life   Grades 7–8

Valued Outcome: Students will be able to demonstrate the Heimlich maneuver.

National Health Education Standards: 1, 7

Description of Strategy: Have a trained representative from the American Heart Association or American Red Cross demonstrate the proper use of the Heimlich maneuver. Emphasize that this is only a mock demonstration, and be careful not to apply too much pressure.

Processing Questions:

1. How does the Heimlich maneuver work to help a person who is choking?
2. How is this procedure conducted differently for children and adults?

✓**Assessment:** Students will be able to describe how the Heimlich maneuver works and demonstrate the proper technique.

Puzzles and Games

Safe Route Home   Grades K–5

Valued Outcome: Students will be able to determine the safest route home from school.

National Health Education Standard: 7

Description of Strategy: Have students map out a safe route to their home from their school. Students should have their parents or guardians provide input to help chart the safest route. Ask them to identify an alternative route to use in the event of a problem with the safest route.

Materials Needed: pencils and paper for each student

Processing Questions:

1. How do you travel from school to home?

2. If you walk or ride your bicycle, do you have a safe route planned?
3. If you walk from the school bus stop to your home, do you have a safe route planned?

✓**Assessment:** Students will be able to describe the safest route from their house to the school and explain why this route is the safest.

Other Ideas

Traffic Safety Obstacle Course   Grades 2–5

Valued Outcome: Students will learn the importance of traffic signs.

National Health Education Standard: 1

Description of Strategy: Set up a simulated obstacle course on the playground (or in a parking area that has been blocked off to traffic) illustrating such traffic hazards as busy intersections, unmarked intersections, and so on. Mark each potentially hazardous part of the course with traffic safety signs, including speed limit signs, yield signs, and pedestrian signals. Have some students wear appropriate bicycle safety gear and go through the course on bicycles, while others play the part of pedestrians. (You may wish to review bicycle safety rules at this time. If bicycle helmets are to be shared, provide plastic liners for the helmets.) Discuss the importance of following traffic safety signs, signals, and regulations.

Materials Needed: poster board, markers, scissors, construction paper, bicycles and bicycle safety gear, plastic sheets or bags to line bicycle helmets that will be shared

Processing Questions:

1. Why is it important to practice negotiating traffic obstacles?
2. What dangerous activities by students cause accidents in traffic situations?
3. How can you help eliminate some of these dangerous activities?
4. How do traffic signs prevent accidents?

✓**Assessment:** Students will be able to identify the meaning of various traffic signs and describe how the signs improve street safety.

Field Trips   Grades K–5

Valued Outcome: Students will be able to inspect a fire station or other safety-related agency or equipment and learn how it operates.

National Health Education Standard: 1

Description of Strategy: If feasible, take the class on a field trip to the local fire station or other safety agency outlet (ambulance or police car might visit the school, etc.). Prepare the class thoroughly for what they will see, and have them write down a list of questions they wish to ask those in charge.

Materials Needed: pencils and paper for each student

Processing Questions:

1. What items are available to help deal with specific emergencies?
2. How does each safety agency help the public prevent accidents?

✓ **Assessment:** Students will be able to list and describe the various safety agencies available for emergency situations.

21 Consumer Health

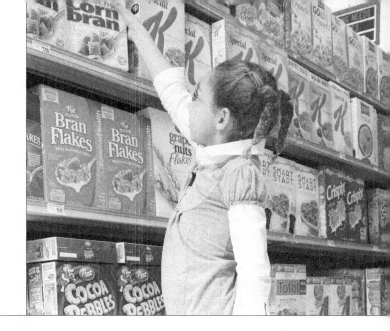

Valued Outcomes

After completion of this chapter, you should be able to:

- Analyze the role of advertising in consumer purchases.
- List various advertising approaches.
- Discuss how quackery affects health care.
- State criteria for selecting a health care professional.
- State criteria for selecting a health care facility.
- List the rights of the consumer.
- Discuss private and governmental agencies that help protect the consumer.

Reflections

Over the past decade people have become increasingly concerned about their quality of health care. Health consumers are asking questions of their health care providers, seeking second opinions, and sometimes choosing to forgo treatments. As you reflect upon this chapter, see if you can identify several guidelines or principles that health care consumers might keep in mind when selecting products or services.

The most violent element in society is ignorance.

—Emma Goldman

> **NATIONAL HEALTH EDUCATION STANDARDS**
>
> 1. Students will comprehend concepts related to health promotion and disease prevention to enhance health.
>
> 2. Students will analyze the influence of family, peers, culture, media, technology, and other factors on health behaviors.
>
> 3. Students will demonstrate the ability to access valid information and products and services to enhance health.

A Nation of Consumers

We are all consumers. A consumer is anyone who selects and uses products to fulfill personal needs and desires. Consumer products range from the clothes we wear, to the foods we eat, to the over-the-counter (OTC) drugs we buy for self-medication. Consumer services include those provided by physicians, dentists, and other medical professionals. In this chapter, we examine the area of **consumer health**, which is defined as the intelligent purchase and use of products and services that will directly affect one's health. At first, this may seem only a small percentage of consumer goods and services, but in fact many more are health related than may be supposed. For example, buying a car may not seem to be a health-related matter, but it is, at least in part. One car might be safer than another vehicle because it is equipped with dual airbags, antilock brakes, and side-impact protection, all of which are not in another model.

This chapter cannot discuss all aspects of consumer health, only the more directly health-related issues. We also look at consumer psychology and how various forces attempt to manipulate consumer attitudes and behavior. In addition, we discuss consumer rights, consumer-oriented legislation and government agencies, and the role of the teacher in consumer health education. Some of the information may seem to be very adult oriented, but if children are going to be wise consumers as adults, the process must begin in the elementary school years.

Advertising and Consumer Behavior

Everyone has consumer needs and desires. From childhood, we are barraged with advertising that attempts to foster these needs and desires so that one blurs into the other. A need becomes a desire, and a desire is perceived as a need. Our economic system is built on supply and demand, and producers do all that they can to nurture a growing demand.

This manipulation of consumer psychology and behavior begins in early childhood, often by means of television commercials aimed specifically at young children. Typical products promoted are toys, candy, and breakfast cereals. As children grow older, the products change, but the message is still one of persuasion. In fact, the methods used to advertise the products are quite sophisticated. By law, advertising of any kind may not be false or misleading. The advertising agencies do an excellent job of stimulating desire and creating a belief about need.

Businesses spend billions of dollars each year on advertising; more money is spent on advertising health products than on any other category of items. Prescription drug manufacturers now spend more than $4.3 billion per year to advertise in magazines, newspapers, and on television. This is in addition to the several billion dollars spent each year promoting prescription drugs to physicians (Howard 2009). A great deal of psychological research goes into advertising so that the target group—whether children, teenagers, homemakers, young adults, or older adults—can be effectively reached. The entire point of this endeavor is to get consumers to buy a particular product or engage in a specific activity. Advertising seeks not to inform, but to persuade.

There are dozens of different brands of products from which to choose. In many ways, the U.S. consumer is fortunate to have so many choices. Competition for the consumer dollar also stimulates the development of better and more efficient products and services. Consider the level of quality that would be available if only one brand of each type of product or service were offered. By providing us with so much choice, however, our economic system also makes it more difficult to make informed decisions about purchases. Many of the products on the market are virtually indistinguishable from one another as far as quality and effectiveness are concerned. Price may be the only difference, and even that may not be much of a factor. For example, all brands of aspirin are basically the same in quality and effectiveness, regardless of advertising claims to the contrary (Barrett, Jarvis, Kroger, and London 2002).

Because the purpose of advertising is to persuade, most advertising contains little informational content. Even that which appears to be informational is carefully selected so that the product being advertised will appear to be uniquely better in some way. Certainly, no manufacturer could be expected to state, "Our product is no different from our competitors' products, but please buy ours anyway."

> **TEACHING TIP**
>
> Make consumer issues relevant to students by asking them to bring in recordings of commercials or copies of print advertisements for products they are interested in. Ask the students to analyze the approaches used in each ad and lead a class discussion about how consumers can avoid being manipulated.

Advertising Approaches

Advertising is a sophisticated kind of manipulation. Advertising experts understand that, despite the lack of information conveyed about the actual merits of a product, consumers can be convinced that one particular brand should be sought out from among the dozens of very similar products on the market. The reason for this is that advertising seeks to appeal to the irrational, not the rational, aspects of human psychology. By making a particular product sound more appealing, *for any reason*, an advertiser can increase the market share of the product. This can be done in a variety of ways, almost all of them noninformational in nature. It is important to remember

Table 21.1 Common Advertising Techniques		
Techniques	**Appeals**	**Questions to Ask**
Bandwagon	Typical phrases: *everyone uses, nation's leading, used by millions, preferred by most, used for more than twenty years*	Is it really true? Who says?
Costs	Typical phrases: *cost-effective, costs less than the competition*	Is the cost really less? What is the quality?
Effectiveness	Typical phrases: *most effective, relieves pain, relieves itch, protects, easy to use*	What is the evidence? How long is it effective? Does it really work?
Endorsements and testimonials	Use of actors, athletes, dentists, physicians to promote	What are the spokesperson's qualifications to endorse the product?
Scientific appeal	Typical phrases: *many doctors recommend, hospital tested*	Is the information accurate? What is the evidence? Where did the information come from?
Slogans and humor	Use of humorous lyrics, cartoon characters, phrases such as *Morning Mouth*	Does the product really work?
Snob appeal and superiority	Use of famous person or use of phrases such as *people who know*; use of words *long-lasting, natural, extra strength*; claims to contain some ingredient from Europe, etc.	Does the person really know? What is the real implication of the words used? Does it work as claimed?
Social	Claims to make you more attractive, better smelling, more socially acceptable	Does the product really work?

that the same appeals are used on children as on adults. Table 21.1 lists some of the most common advertising techniques.

Many advertisers combine the approaches mentioned in Table 21.1 with visual and/or emotional imagery. Whether in a magazine advertisement or television commercial, the visual aspects of the advertisement are just as important as the written or spoken message. If the visual message of the commercial is pleasant, the reader or viewer will more likely associate positive thoughts with the product. Students should be made aware of the powerful stimuli provided by advertisements. Consumers must learn to recognize that there is a great deal of puffery in almost any commercial or advertisement, regardless of the approach used to convey the message. Often there is little difference in effectiveness between one health product and another, and price is not a big factor either. We are all manipulated by advertising, and even if a person actually feels better about using one product over another, usually there is no difference in health consequences whether Brand X or Brand Y is selected. For children and adults, what is important to their consumer health is to develop

an understanding of how advertising seeks to manipulate them so that when more serious health problems arise, they will not be deceived by advertising claims. Perhaps

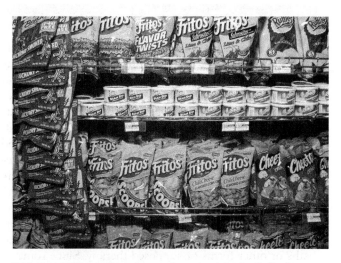

Packages and advertisements can be powerful stimuli. Students should be made aware of this.

most important, the limited effectiveness of OTC drugs and self-medication must be recognized.

Other Influences on Product and Service Choices

Consumer decisions are influenced not only by advertising, but also by an individual's level of education, family beliefs, religion, socioeconomic status, community, and personal goals. A host of other factors may be involved, including one's physical and emotional needs, motives, and personality. People may model their buying patterns and selections after those of family members, friends, or peers. The more status or importance that the person being modeled has, the greater his or her influence.

With all these influences, it might seem that a person can hardly be blamed for sometimes making poor choices about consumer health products and services. But this denies personal responsibility. Not everything can be blamed on advertising or outside influences—people often make harmful health decisions quite independently of either. They may use advertising claims to shore up these decisions, for example, by relying on OTC products in an attempt to cure ill health when they actually know that they should be seeking more effective medical treatment. Such individuals are only too willing to create a false sense of security or relief by accepting advertising claims uncritically or by enlarging on such claims themselves in order to find easy answers where no such answers exist. In the final analysis, consumers can make informed choices if they want to do so. As with other aspects of wellness, each individual must accept self-responsibility. Consumers can then seek out information on products and services, analyze each on its own merits, and make better decisions accordingly.

Consumer Myths and Misconceptions

Some consumer health myths might be classified as folk beliefs. Although not based on any scientific facts, many of these myths are widely believed. In some instances, belief in certain of these myths can lead to unwise consumer health decisions. For example, a belief that organic or natural foods are always better than regular produce available in stores can lead to wasteful spending on overpriced specialty products. Some consumer health myths are believed because the person is desperate for relief. Sufferers of arthritis, which is an incurable condition at present, may wear a copper bracelet in the hope that perhaps the myth about the curative properties of copper really has some truth to it. They may also spend money on mud baths or other forms of supposed therapy. Since some of these treatments do provide relaxation, leading to a feeling of temporary relief, they are not entirely without value.

But consumers who place their faith in them are deluding themselves as to long-term benefits.

Consumer misconceptions also lead to wasteful spending and, occasionally, to actual harm to health status. Perhaps the most common misconception is that producers manufacture only products that are needed; therefore, if a product is on the market, it must be fulfilling a need. In fact, many products are marketed to create a need that does not actually exist. For example, many mouthwashes, tonics, and other nostrums provide few health benefits. However, most consumers believe that any product that continues to be sold must be meeting a real need. Constant advertising reinforces this misconception through sheer repetition. Even better-educated individuals are often ignorant about consumer health information and hold many misconceptions.

Clearly, consumers must become better informed if they are to make wise consumer health decisions. They must recognize the negative impact that myths and misconceptions can have on personal health. They must also become more aware of how advertising seeks to manipulate consumer behavior and learn to reject appeals to emotion in favor of facts and accurate information. Obtaining factual information about health products and services is not always easy. By law, advertisers must tell the truth about their products, prove the claims they make, be specific about any guarantee or warranty, and avoid making misleading statements. In addition, the advertising code subscribed to by most business advertisers puts forth similar guidelines. However, most products are still made to sound more effective than they really are. It is ultimately the consumer's responsibility to see through this misleading advertising and make wise decisions accordingly. To accomplish this, children and adults must strive to become intelligent health consumers. Cornacchia and Barrett (1993, 10–11) offer six guidelines for intelligent consumers:

1. The intelligent consumer is well informed and knows how to make sound decisions.
2. The intelligent consumer seeks reliable sources of information.
3. The intelligent consumer is appropriately skeptical about health information and does not accept statements appearing in the news media or advertising at face value.
4. The intelligent consumer is wary of inept practitioners, pseudopractitioners, and pitchmen in the business and medical worlds and can identify quacks and quackery.
5. The intelligent consumer selects practitioners with great care and questions fees, diagnoses, treatments, and alternative treatments.
6. The intelligent consumer willingly speaks out by reporting frauds, quackery, and wrongdoing to appropriate agencies and law enforcement officials.

Quackery

There are many models of medical treatment. Some of them are valid and time tested; some are new and their advocates are working to gain acceptance. Others, however, do not seek scientific validation and, in fact, avoid scientific inquiry. The first category of medical models includes conventional medicine practiced by physicians who are licensed and certified in their fields. The second category includes such approaches to health care as biofeedback and holistic health, which may be of value in treating certain health conditions. The third category is quackery, the use of worthless approaches that often promise miraculous results.

Quacks usually try very hard to appear scientific. Their offices may closely resemble conventional physicians' offices, even to the framed degrees (but often from diploma mills) on the walls. They may dress as physicians, in a white laboratory coat or with a stethoscope around their neck, employ scientific-looking gadgets, and use scientific-sounding language to explain their supposed treatments. But it is all a sham, and a quack will always find an excuse for not permitting the form of quackery to be subject to independent scientific scrutiny. Although some quacks may sincerely believe in the efficacy of their treatments, most are simply out to victimize the consumer to make money.

Quackery flourishes in the United States for a variety of reasons. The primary reason is ignorance. Many Americans do not know the difference between legitimate and illegitimate medical practitioners. Anyone who claims to be a doctor or a healer is taken at face value. Another reason quackery exists is that quacks often promise cures or relief that legitimate medical practitioners cannot offer. For those suffering from incurable diseases, the false hope that quacks hold out may seem irresistible. Since nothing else can help them, they turn to quacks in desperation. People also sometimes consult quacks because they hope to get around the high cost of legitimate medical attention; the quack promises a quick and inexpensive cure. In other instances, people turn to quacks because they wish to avoid surgery or other involved legitimate medical treatment. Some individuals may not realize the difference between scientifically proven methodologies and legitimately trained professionals versus those who are trained in treatments that are outside this body of knowledge. Still, of course, many people actually believe the deceptive claims made by quacks (Payne and Hahn 2006).

If quacks cannot effect cures, why do so many people continue to have faith in them? In some instances, quacks do seem to provide relief or cures. In such cases, the patient may be a hypochondriac who has no actual physical problem. If the person believes that help is being provided, the problem disappears. In cases where an actual problem does exist, the natural healing powers of the body may be responsible for a cure attributed to a quack. Finally, temporary relief or remission may be mistaken for a cure.

Not only is the consumer's pocketbook shortchanged in quackery treatments, medications, and devices, but people's health can be undermined. Quackery delays proper treatment and increases the possibility of a more serious outcome. Using good sense and seeking information from physicians or some reputable agency is a good start to finding proper information (Butler 2012). Some nonprofit agencies that may be able to help provide reliable information and referrals include the Consumer's Union, American Cancer Society, Arthritis Foundation, American Heart Association, American Lung Association, American Medical Association, American Dental Association, and the Better Business Bureau.

Health Care

The U.S. health care delivery system continues to evolve. Rising medical care costs, as well as the ever-increasing number of uninsured or underinsured individuals, are significant factors contributing to many of the proposed changes. The reasons for increasing health care costs include current reimbursement practices, increasing technology, and rising physicians' fees and other health care salaries (which are in part due to increasing litigation and litigation insurance costs). Another factor in high health care costs, particularly in hospitals, is the cost of care for the poor, uninsured, and underinsured. The poor and the elderly are the people who suffer most from the current health care delivery system. Government programs such as Medicare and Medicaid help, but for many individuals the portion of the bills not paid by these programs is still financially overwhelming.

The vast majority of Americans cannot afford the costs of medical care without some form of health insurance. Health insurance is a contract between an insurance company and either an individual or a group for the payment of medical costs. Health insurance usually requires the individual or group to pay a premium to the insurance company each month. The insurance company then pays for all or part of the health care costs, depending on the type of coverage provided.

▪ Medical Insurance

As fees for medical and health care services continue to climb, it is more important than ever to have adequate medical insurance. A typical plan may pay 80 percent of medical costs, and the individual is responsible for the remaining 20 percent. Premiums for this coverage are paid by employer contributions and employee pay deductions. Group insurance plans typically have a deductible that the insured is responsible for paying before costs are covered by the insurance company.

Basic health insurance includes benefits for hospital, surgical, and medical expenses. Some plans will include provisions for dental and vision coverage. The extent of benefits differs from contract to contract. Individual employees (self-employed) may purchase insurance that covers these areas, but today most workers are covered by a group plan at their place of employment.

In addition, most insurance plans will offer what is called comprehensive coverage that is designed to offset large medical expenses resulting from serious illness or injury. These programs are designed to take over where basic insurance plans stop coverage. Comprehensive insurance coverage usually covers every type of medical situation prescribed by a physician for both in and out of the hospital. Examples of potential services covered include office visits, nursing care, physical therapy, emergency ambulance service, prescription drugs, prosthetic appliances, and psychiatric care.

Government Health Insurance

Two examples of government insurance plans are **Medicare** and **Medicaid**. Medicare is financed by Social Security taxes and is designed to provide health insurance for people sixty-five years and older, the blind, the severely disabled, and those requiring specialized treatments, such as kidney dialysis. Medicaid is underwritten by federal and state taxes. It provides limited health benefits for people who are eligible for assistance from two programs: Aid to Families with Dependent Children and Supplementary Security Income. Like Medicare, Medicaid is directed to people age sixty-five or older and for younger people who have disabilities.

When to Seek Health Care

Sometimes it is difficult to determine when to seek health care attention. Some people tend to wait too long before seeking health care, while others may seek help unnecessarily. For many, the ability to tolerate discomfort determines whether or not they seek help. Health care decisions are largely personal and based on the perceived severity of the symptoms. Being in tune with one's body and having knowledge of the signs and symptoms of illness can help someone make the decision to seek or wait to get medical attention.

Several symptoms indicate the need for medical attention. Blood present in urine, feces, vomit, sputum, or other body fluids indicates the need for medical advice. Pain in the abdomen, especially when accompanied by nausea, may indicate a wide range of conditions, ranging from appendicitis to pelvic inflammatory disease—all of which need a physician's attention. A stiff neck accompanied by fever may indicate meningitis, which may be lethal if left unattended. And obviously, any disabling injury requires prompt medical assistance (Anspaugh, Hamrick, and Rosato 2011).

Presence of fever is another area of concern when someone is deciding to seek medical care. A fever is an indication that the immune system is working to fight an infection. If left untreated, a fever may damage various body organs and structures. Self-treatment in the form of aspirin, acetaminophen, or ibuprofen usually lowers temperature. However, if there is no improvement in twenty-four to thirty-six hours, or if a low-grade temperature continues over an extended period, a physician should be consulted. Fever in children should always be discussed with a physician.

Selecting a Health Care Professional

Nearly everyone should have a primary care physician. If a medical emergency arises, a person can seek help immediately from a trusted health care professional who knows the patient's history. Just as important, by having a personal physician or other health care professional, a person can better maintain good health by means of regular checkups or consultations with the provider about health concerns. A health care professional should be selected carefully. Some suggestions for doing so are listed here.

1. Choose your physician while you are in good health. If you wait until a medical crisis arises, you will have to rely on whomever you can find. Having a physician you trust and feel comfortable with *before* a crisis will lessen anxiety in a crisis.

2. To locate physicians who are accepting new patients, telephone the physician's office or call the local county medical society. (You can find the number in the telephone book yellow pages.) If you are not sure what kind of physician you need, such as a specialist or a general practitioner, the medical society can also offer some initial advice. Generally you will be given the names of two or three physicians you can call. A local hospital can also be a good source of information about physicians who are accepting new patients.

3. Select a board-certified family practitioner for a family physician, a pediatrician for children, and a gynecologist for females (see Table 21.2 for other types of specialists).

4. Check the credentials of physicians you are considering. Don't be afraid to ask questions about how the person is keeping current in the field.

5. Get details about office hours, emergency care, whether house calls will be made, and so forth. Also try to determine how long a patient usually has to wait before seeing the doctor.

6. Determine the fee schedule for checkups and different types of treatment. Doctors often base their fees on recommended prices recorded in a fee schedule book produced by the American Medical Association. The fees are recommended ranges, not fixed prices, and a physician may charge on the high or low end. Keep in mind that the most expensive physician is not necessarily the best.

Table 21.2   Health Care Specialists

Name of Specialist	Field of Specialty
Medical Specialists	
Allergist	Allergic conditions
Cardiologist	Coronary artery disease; heart disease
Dermatologist	Skin conditions
Family practice physician primary came physician	General care physician
Gastroenterologist	Stomach, intestines, digestive system
Geriatrician	Diseases and conditions of the aged
Gynecologist	Female reproductive system
Hematologist	Study of blood
Internist	Treatment of diseases in adults
Neurosurgeon	Surgery of the brain and nervous system
Obstetrician	Pregnancy, labor, childbirth
Oncologist	Cancer, tumors
Ophthalmologist	Eye disease and treatment
Orthopedist	Skeletal system
Otolaryngologist	Head, neck, ears, nose, throat
Pathologist	Study of tissues and the essential nature of disease
Pediatrician	Childhood diseases and conditions
Psychiatrist	Mental illnesses
Radiologist	Use of X-rays
Dental Specialists	
Dentist	General care of teeth and oral cavity
Orthodontist	Teeth alignment, malocclusion
Pedodontist	Dental care of children
Other Specialists	
Chiropractor	Emphasizes the use of manipulation and adjustment of body structures to treat disease
Optometrist	Examines and tests eyes for visual defects and prescribes vision correction lenses
Osteopath	Emphasizes structural integrity of the body; uses manipulation along with medical therapies
Psychologist	Study of human behavior

7. Choose a physician who is able to communicate with you in terms you can understand. You have a right to know what is going on during any treatment, and the doctor has an obligation to keep you informed. Regardless of their medical skills, however, some physicians are better communicators than others.

8. Choose a physician with whom you feel comfortable. The doctor's age, sex, and personal manner may all be factors that make you more comfortable or less comfortable. Set up an appointment to talk with the professional to see whether he or she is willing to communicate openly and honestly.

9. Choose a physician in whom you can have confidence. Even if the person is highly qualified and well thought of in the profession, you may be put off by some personal quality.

10. Change physicians if you are not satisfied with the way you are being treated. Find a doctor with whom you feel comfortable.

Ask questions! The more questions you ask, the fewer mistakes will occur, and the more power you have in the doctor–patient relationship (Devita 1995).

■ Choosing a Health Care Facility

If given a choice, few people would select the use of an emergency room (ER) or hospital. Unfortunately, most people will need the services of these facilities at some time. Consequently, knowing what to consider when choosing a health care facility should be weighed long before it is needed.

ERs should be used only in an absolute emergency; most ERs are understaffed, overcrowded, and harried. If the ER personnel view a particular situation as less serious, the patient will probably have a longer wait than someone in an acute state will. Tests that may be needed are more difficult to arrange, and the cost for an ER visit is higher than the cost of a visit to a physician's office.

When there is time to select a hospital, it is wise to discuss with your physician the options that are available. Many times, physicians hold admitting privileges at more than one hospital. Every attempt should be made to find out as much as possible about the hospital. Some possible questions to consider include the following.

1. Why does your physician use this hospital?
2. What is the patient-to-nurse ratio?
3. What are the room rates?
4. What are the costs of laboratory services, X-rays, and so on?
5. How frequently does the hospital perform the procedure you require?
6. What is the history of malpractice charges against the hospital?

7. Can you tour the hospital?
8. What are your rights as a patient?

Choosing a hospital is serious business. Don't be afraid to ask questions.

Health-Related Products

Americans spend billions of dollars each year on health care products ranging from OTC drugs to cosmetics. Many of these products are used to help relieve symptoms, to aid in curing illnesses, and to provide cosmetic effects. Unfortunately many products are not needed, don't provide the advertised effect, and may have the potential to harm health.

■ Over-the-Counter Drugs

There are more than 500,000 OTC health care products. These vary widely from mouthwashes to pain relievers. In fact, some of the most beneficial OTC drugs can also create problems. For example, pain relievers such as aspirin and ibuprofen (a nonsteroid anti-inflammatory drug) can damage the lining of the stomach, which can lead to ulcers and other problems. Large doses have been associated with kidney damage. Another pain reliever, acetaminophen, also relieves pain and reduces fever and is the drug of choice for relieving pain in children. However, with heavy doses, the drug can cause bleeding and liver damage. All three of the above-mentioned pain relievers should be taken with food and a full glass of water to reduce irritation to the lining of the stomach.

Two other frequently used OTC products also provide good examples of potentially hazardous use. Nasal sprays relieve congestion by shrinking the blood vessels in the nose. If used for too long, more and more spray is required to maintain effectiveness and the vessels begin to swell, which worsens the congestion. This is called the rebound effect. Prolonged use can result in bleeding and partial or complete loss of the sense of smell. Another product that holds potential misuse problems is laxatives. Many people, especially the elderly, consider a daily bowel movement necessary. Chronic use of laxatives destroys much of the flora in the intestinal tract, making constipation even worse. Bulk laxatives are better than regular laxatives, but exercise and a high-fiber diet are much safer alternatives for promoting normal defecation.

■ Cosmetic Products

Many health care products are intended to be used externally. Some of these have little effect but, due to massive advertising campaigns and misconceptions about their effectiveness, are extensively used.

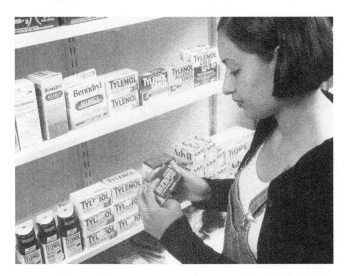

All OTC products must be checked carefully for potentially harmful ingredients.

Skin Products. Some products are designed to prevent or cure acne, rejuvenate skin, prevent body odor, or protect against excessive sun exposure. Acne products, in conjunction with washing the face with a mild soap, may help control the condition. OTC skin rejuvenators have not been shown to be effective at actually changing skin properties, regardless of the claims that are made. A moisturizer can help with the dry skin associated with aging, although it does not actually change the skin. Retin A, a prescription drug, does seem to help treat acne, delay skin deterioration, and restore a more youthful appearance for those individuals who can use it, but it irritates the skin and may result in peeling, blotching, or other undesirable side effects. Deodorants and antiperspirants can help control body odor, but no product can prevent sweating in extremely hot weather or during exercise (nor is this desirable because sweating is the body's primary means of cooling itself). Regular washing is essential if the bacteria and other odor-causing substances are to be removed.

Hair Products. Hair products run the gamut from removing hair to restoring, cleaning, and coloring the hair. Several products are designed to remove hair. Shaving can be used in almost all circumstances and is a safe method of hair removal except for the risk of cutting oneself. Tweezers can be used to pluck unwanted hair but present some danger of infection because the adjacent skin may not be clean. Chemicals can be used to soften and remove hair at the root; wax can be warmed and used to tear hair from the roots as it hardens on the skin; and a fine pumice stone can be used to prevent hair from growing above the skin. Although these products are usually safe, if sometimes painful, there is always the possibility of skin reactions, irritations, and infections. A dermatologist should be consulted if any symptoms appear.

Most hair-restoring products do not work—many products advertised in the media have not been proven to be effective. A drug invented by the Upjohn Company, minoxidil (Rogaine), does seem to grow limited amounts of hair in some people. Rogaine can now be purchased over-the-counter; however, it has never been shown to totally restore hair (Propecia 1998, 26). Surgery can replace lost hair, but it is extremely expensive, painful, and may take a year or two to complete. Certainly, before considering surgery, the person should consider multiple medical opinions.

Hair-cleaning products are generally safe. A wide variety of products are available, and personal preference is usually the primary criterion for selecting a particular product. Some people may have allergic reactions to hair products, but this tends to be atypical. Most people consider dandruff a hair problem, but it is actually a scalp problem in which the scalp sloughs off dead skin cells. If hair is washed daily, dandruff is not usually a problem, so it is unnecessary to purchase a special hair product to help fight dandruff—any hair-cleaning product will serve to remove the flakes. People who have a severe problem may wish to use an antidandruff shampoo, however. The Food and Drug Administration (FDA) considers antidandruff shampoos to be a drug. These products can help control dandruff but cannot cure it. Dandruff may be the result of a social or psychological problem but usually poses no medical or health threat unless it is a symptom of psoriasis, seborrhea, or dermatitis, all of which require a physician's attention.

Hair-coloring products should be used with caution since many of these products can cause skin irritation or harm the eyes upon direct contact. These products are used for cosmetic reasons only. Consequently, care should be used by testing the product on a small area of the hair prior to covering all the hair with the product.

Oral Products. Oral products include toothpaste, mouthwashes, and gargles. There are many toothpaste products that, when used with dental flossing, serve to protect against tooth decay. Living in an area where the water supply contains fluoride also helps prevent dental cavities. Toothpaste that has fluoride should be used. It is unwise to purchase toothpastes that have whiteners since they contain abrasives that can damage the teeth.

Mouthwashes and gargles do little to eliminate unpleasant odors or treat a sore throat. Because unpleasant odors do not develop in the mouth but are carried from the intestines to the lungs and exhaled, these products can only mask smells. Bad breath also may be a symptom of other conditions such as infections, tumors, or diabetes. In fact, excessive use of mouthwash can actually dry the mucous membranes, making a sore throat even more irritated.

HEALTH HIGHLIGHT | **Your Medical Rights**

The following is a brief list of some of your rights as a consumer in the health care system. It is the responsibility of each of us to make sure we are not denied these rights.

- We have the right as a parent to stay with our children during tests and treatments, provided there is no interference with the medical treatment or child abuse is not suspected.

- We have the right to request that a relative or friend accompany us during a test, treatment, or hospitalization.

- We have the right to see our medical records if the state in which we live so allows. State laws vary on this issue.

- We have the right to emergency care whether or not we have insurance.

- We have the right to refuse to sign any form. The provider can also refuse to provide treatment in the absence of your signed authorization.

- We have the right to a second opinion, but our doctor can also stop treating us for challenging him or her.

- We have the right to leave the hospital at any time, even against medical advice or without paying the bill.

- We have the right to refuse or stop any treatment.

- We have the right to an itemized, detailed bill for all medical services.

- We have the right to know the results of all tests unless the doctor has reason to believe that the information will be harmful.

Consumer Rights and Protection

One of the basic premises of wellness or high-level health is that individuals should be responsible for their own health behavior. This is certainly true for consumer health. With so much competition for every dollar spent and with so much available to buy, consumers need to guard against wasteful spending on products and services of dubious value. For the most part, consumers do not protect themselves properly through informed consumer health behavior. Fortunately, government agencies and private organizations have stepped in to establish consumer rights and offer some protection. On March 15, 1962, President John Kennedy sent to Congress his "Special Message on Protecting the Consumer Interest." The message stated that additional legislative and administrative actions were required to assist consumers in the exercise of their rights. Kennedy outlined these rights:

- *Right to safety*—to be protected against the marketing of goods that are hazardous to health or life

- *Right to be informed*—to be protected against fraudulent, deceitful, or misleading information or advertising

- *Right to choose*—to be assured that consumer interests will receive full and sympathetic consideration in the formulation of government policy on consumer matters

Additionally, as outlined by Woolley and Peters (1999–2011), basic consumer rights have been expanded to include: the right to be heard, the right to satisfaction of basic needs, the right to redress, the right to consumer education, and the right to a healthy environment.

These consumer rights, of course, are meaningless unless they are backed up with the power of legislation. Over the years, hundreds of federal, state, and local laws have been passed to ensure the rights of consumers and to protect consumers from fraudulent or harmful products and services.

Consumer Protection Agencies

Many federal agencies work to protect the consumer. One of the most active of these agencies is the FDA. Responsibilities of the FDA include periodic inspection of foods, drugs, devices, and cosmetics. The agency demands proof of the safety and effectiveness of any new drug before it is marketed and has the power to recall possibly unsafe drugs or other substances from the market. The FDA also enforces the laws against illegal sales of prescription drugs, investigates therapeutic devices for safety and truthfulness of labeling claims, and checks importation of foods, drugs, devices, and cosmetics to ensure that they comply with U.S. laws.

Another government agency, the Federal Trade Commission (FTC), is responsible for eliminating unfair or deceptive practices in commerce that curtail competition. In other words, this agency prevents the free enterprise system from being suppressed by fraudulent trade techniques or by a company creating a monopoly on a product or service. The FTC has the authority to stop the dissemination of advertisements of foods, drugs, devices, or cosmetics when such action is in the best interest of the consumer. Also, if a label on a product is misleading, the FTC can order the withdrawal of that product from the shelves.

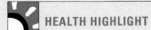

HEALTH HIGHLIGHT | Patients' Bill of Rights

As a patient at a health care facility the consumer has the following rights and expectations.

1. **Information Disclosure.** You have the right to receive accurate and easily understood information about your health plan, health care professionals, and health care facilities. If you speak another language, have a physical or mental disability, or just don't understand something, assistance will be provided.

2. **Choice of Providers and Plans.** You have the right to a choice of health care providers that is sufficient to provide you with access to appropriate high-quality health care.

3. **Access to Emergency Services.** If you have severe pain, an injury, or sudden illness that convinces you that your health is in serious jeopardy, you have the right to receive screening and stabilization emergency services.

4. **Participation in Treatment Decisions.** You have the right to know all your treatment options and to participate in decisions about your care. Parents, guardians, family members, or other individuals that you designate can represent you if you cannot make your own decision.

5. **Respect and Nondiscrimination.** You have a right to considerate, respectful, and nondiscriminatory care from your doctors, health plan representatives, and other health care providers.

6. **Confidentiality of Health Information.** You have the right to talk in confidence with health care providers and to have your health care information protected. You also have the right to review and copy your own medical record and request that your physician amend your record if it is not accurate, relevant, or complete.

7. **Complaints and Appeals.** You have the right to a fair, fast, and objective review of any complaint you have against your health plan, doctors, hospitals, or other health care personnel. This includes complaints about waiting times, operating hours, the conduct of health care personnel, and the adequacy of health care facilities.

Source: FirstGov for Consumers 2006

The Consumer Product Safety Commission, established by the federal government in 1973, protects the public against unreasonable risks of injury from products. This commission oversees the enforcement of the Flammable Fabrics Act, the Federal Hazardous Substances Act, and the Poison Prevention Packaging Act, among many others. Under these acts, the Consumer Product Safety Commission is responsible for regulating the manufacture for sale of all highly flammable wearing apparel and fabrics. This is especially helpful for the consumer, because the majority of fabrics used in today's clothing burn quite easily.

In January 1964, President Lyndon Johnson established the President's Committee on Consumer Interests. This committee was replaced by the Office of Consumer Affairs in 1971. The main purpose of this office is to act as a consumer voice in the presidential administration, but it also coordinates all governmental activities in the field of consumerism; conducts investigations on consumer problems; handles consumer complaints; facilitates communication on consumer affairs between the government, business, and the consumer; and helps disseminate helpful information to the consumer.

Various department-level organizations within the federal government also aid the consumer. The U.S. Department of Commerce encourages industry to avoid packaging proliferation that can lead to consumer confusion in shopping. This department can request mandatory packaging standards. The Department of Labor provides the consumer price index, the measure of changes in the nation's economy and currency, and also surveys employment trends and studies prices of various commodities. The U.S. Department of Agriculture (USDA) inspects meat and food animals before slaughter to prevent any diseased meat from reaching the stores. The USDA establishes grades of meat to help the consumer in identifying the different levels of quality. The U.S. Postal Service investigates any incidence of mail fraud and regulates attempts to sell worthless or harmful merchandise or medicines through the mails. There are also many trustworthy websites that seek to protect the consumer (see Health Highlight box, "Can a Website Be Trusted?").

Private Agencies

Many private agencies also assist the consumer by providing accurate, unbiased information about products or by attempting to eliminate fraud and deception by businesses. For example, Consumer's Union publishes *Consumer Reports*, a magazine that provides impartial information about products; it informs the consumer about the best buys and the most reliable products. *Consumer Reports* also helps the consumer by interpreting advertising on many products.

Better Business Bureaus are private, nonprofit, business-supported groups that help the consumer mediate misunderstandings between customers and businesses. These groups provide information about a company, help resolve complaints against companies, foster ethical advertising and selling practices, alert consumers to bad business practices, and provide

HEALTH HIGHLIGHT | Can a Website Be Trusted?

With the explosion of information on the World Wide Web, the question arises whether the information found at a website can be trusted to be scientifically accurate and truthful. It is important to remember that the Internet is filled with good/bad, true/false, complete/incomplete, and even dangerous information.

To help determine if the information can be trusted, ask the following questions:

- **Where does the information come from?** Reputation counts. Information from established medical institutions or government agencies can usually be trusted.
- **Does the website reflect more than one opinion?** Quality sites will often feature a variety of perspectives.
- **How often is the information updated?** Good websites update at least monthly, sometimes weekly.

- **Does the website promote products or procedures?** Do not trust websites that rely on anecdotal records and testimonials to promote their products. Be suspicious of websites that dwell on the shortcomings of mainstream medical practice.

the media with informational materials on consumer subjects. Better Business Bureaus have no legal powers, but they can arbitrate between consumers and businesses. When illegal practices are discovered and a business refuses to cooperate, the matter is turned over to the appropriate law enforcement agency. These bureaus are one of the more important sources of help to which consumers may turn when they need assistance, especially with regard to health products and devices (Cornacchia and Barrett 2006).

Many cities have chambers of commerce that are supported by businesses in that community. These organizations publish a business consumer relations code of ethics. Their work is quite similar to a Better Business Bureau in that they act as liaisons between the consumer and business. They also protect the consumer by attempting to eliminate fraudulent business practices.

Even with all these government and private agencies working to protect the consumer, however, it remains the individual's responsibility to be informed about products and services in order to increase the probability of satisfaction when purchasing a product.

Common Health Fraud Targets

The FTC and FDA indicate that health fraud is most common in areas in which people have special needs or feel helpless and overwhelmed by their conditions. Fraud promoters target those who are overweight or who are afflicted with serious conditions such as cancer, diabetes, arthritis, HIV/AIDS, multiple sclerosis, or Alzheimer's disease. Many of these people become convinced that devices, products, or treatments offer a "cure-all" for these conditions. Unfortunately, these people are bilked out of their money, their time, and maybe even their lives because of delay in seeking legitimate treatment or stopping treatment to begin a fraudulent treatment or procedure. The FTC

has provided guidelines for awareness of potential false claims. Some signs of a fraudulent claim include:

1. Statements that the product is a quick and effective cure-all or diagnostic tool for a wide variety of ailments. For example, "beneficial in the treatment of rheumatism, arthritis, infections, prostate problems, cancer, heart disease, and more."
2. Statements that suggest the product can treat or cure diseases; for example, "shrinks tumors" or "cures impotence."
3. Promotions that use words such as "scientific breakthrough," "miraculous cure," "exclusive product," "secret ingredient," or "ancient remedy."
4. Promotions that use impressive sounding terms; for example, for a weight-loss product: "hunger stimulation point" and "thermogenesis."
5. Undocumented case histories or personal testimonials by consumers or doctors claiming amazing results. For example, "After taking Product X my husband now leads a normal life and we enjoy everything again as we once did."
6. Limited availability and advance payment requirements. For example, "Hurry, this offer will not last!" or "Send us a check to reserve your supply."
7. Promises of a no-risk money-back guarantee. For example, "If after thirty days you are not satisfied, we will return your money and you keep the remaining product."

Teaching Consumer Health Education

Consumer health education teaches students to learn to make wise decisions about buying and using products and services, especially in health-related areas. Children need to become knowledgeable about consumer rights and consumer responsibilities. They (like their adult counterparts) have rights as outlined earlier in the chapter, but rights are balanced with responsibilities. These responsibilities include seeking out accurate information about products and services, being skeptical of advertising claims, recognizing the differences between needs and desires, and making wise consumer choices. This process must begin early in life and be fostered throughout the elementary school years. Even though the information presented in this chapter may seem more appropriate for adults, the concepts that lead to becoming an effective consumer as an adult are instilled in each child early in life.

The most effective way that all consumers, regardless of age, can protect themselves in the area of consumer health is through preventive health care. By learning about proper nutrition, exercise, and health care, students can avoid feeling the need for many consumer health products such as tonics, diet products, or some other worthless health product or service.

When it comes to teaching consumer health education, the importance of critical thinking cannot be overemphasized. Children must recognize that, just because a product is advertised on television or in a newspaper, it is not necessarily worthwhile or useful. They should learn to see how wants can be fostered artificially. In addition, they should learn not to accept advertising claims or promises without thinking about them critically. Children need to understand that much of what is said in a commercial or print advertisement is meaningless. For example, a product may be touted as new or improved. Is new necessarily better? Improved in what way? If a product is advertised as being "25 percent more effective," students should ask, "More effective than what?" Generally, no answer to these questions can be found.

The intent of consumer education is not to teach students *what* to buy, but rather *how* to buy. Students should be encouraged to get the facts, comparison-shop, consider the consequences of all purchases, and budget their money the same as any wise adult would do. By learning the importance of wise consumer behavior, students can incorporate the concepts taught into their own value system. Finally, students should be informed of their rights as consumers and what recourse they have if they are victimized in the marketplace. All consumers have legal rights. Exercising these rights can help put an end to deceitful health care practices and services as well as worthless health care products.

Chapter In Review

Summary

- A consumer is anyone who selects and uses goods and services.
- Consumer health education is concerned with those products that directly or indirectly affect personal health.
- Consumers become aware of available products primarily through advertising.
- Advertising seeks to influence consumer psychology and behavior by confusing wants with needs and by fostering desires.
- Many advertisements for health products seek to give the impression that the products are more effective than they actually are.
- Consumers are persuaded to buy a product because of a variety of appeals.
- Quackery is widespread in the United States despite legal measures designed to prevent it.
- Resorting to a quack can prevent a person from getting proper or even life-saving treatment.
- Many people today are not insured or are underinsured.
- A physician and health care facility must be selected with care.
- Private and government agencies help protect consume rights, evaluate the quality and effectiveness of health-related products, and police business practices.

- The primary responsibility of each consumer is to become knowledgeable when making health-related consumer decisions.
- Helping students learn to become informed, wise consumers is a vital part of teaching consumer education.

Discussion Questions

1. How does advertising manipulate consumer psychology and behavior?
2. Discuss the most typical advertising approaches.
3. Describe the influences, other than advertising, that affect consumer behavior.
4. List and discuss some common health-related consumer myths.
5. Discuss the teacher's role in combating consumer misconceptions.
6. Discuss the role of Better Business Bureaus in protecting consumers' rights.
7. What are some considerations that should be made when selecting a physician?
8. What are some of the agencies that help protect the health consumer?

Critical Thinking Questions

1. What types of myths and misinformation develop concerning consumer health issues? Why?

2. Discuss the preparations you would make before a doctor's appointment.

3. How much help do you think you get from government consumer protection agencies? What responsibilities do you have in protecting yourself against quackery or fraud?

4. What guidelines would you develop for acceptable advertisement of health-related OTC products?

Access more material online at www.pearsonhighered.com/anspaugh. At this companion website for *Teaching Today's Health,* **you'll find chapter quizzes, web links, flashcards, a glossary, additional Worksheets, and more to help you succeed.**

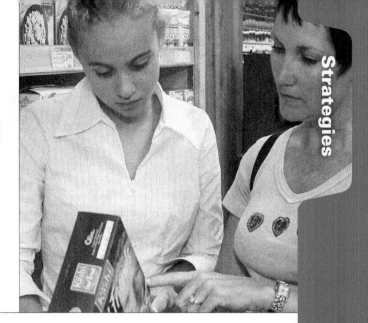

22 Strategies for Teaching Consumer Health

Valued Outcomes

After completion of this chapter, you should be able to convey the following to your students:

- Discuss why it is important to obtain accurate information concerning health care information.

- Describe why not all products and services are worthwhile or necessary.

- List ways that advertising seeks to persuade or induce use of a product.

- Describe why many advertising claims are inflated or misleading.

- Discuss why all labels on health care products should be read carefully.

- List ways in which quackery in health care products can be identified.

- Understand that many health care products are not useful and are even dangerous.

- Discuss why medical treatment should be obtained only from qualified professionals.

- List the governmental and private agencies that work to protect the consumer.

- Realize that making wise consumer decisions concerning health care products and services is a personal responsibility.

Reflections

As you read through the activities found in this chapter, reflect on the many choices students must make as consumers. What concepts should be emphasized in helping students become aware of their options and how to make informed decisions? Select one concept and describe the types of activities at each grade level that would best illustrate the concept.

One human frailty is to believe what we are told by others.

—*Warren E. Schaller and Charles R. Carroll*

NATIONAL HEALTH EDUCATION STANDARDS

1. Students will comprehend concepts related to health promotion and disease prevention to enhance health.

2. Students will analyze the influence of family, peers, culture, media, technology, and other factors on health behaviors.

3. Students will demonstrate the ability to access valid information and products and services to enhance health.

4. Students will demonstrate the ability to use interpersonal communication skills to enhance health and avoid or reduce health risks.

5. Students will demonstrate the ability to use decision-making skills to enhance health.

7. Students will demonstrate the ability to practice health-enhancing behaviors and avoid or reduce risks.

8. Students will demonstrate the ability to advocate for personal, family, and community health.

Establishing Consumer Behavior Patterns

The patterns established in childhood of appraising, selecting, and using consumer products and services can influence a person's physical, psychological, and social well-being for a lifetime. To choose wisely requires accumulating knowledge and formulating attitudes about different kinds of products and services. Students must learn that products and services differ in quality, cost, and intrinsic value. They must also recognize how advertising and social forces influence ideas about needs and desires. Above all, they must understand that the responsibility for making wise consumer decisions ultimately is a personal one.

Consumer health pertains to products and services that either directly or indirectly relate to personal health. Most directly related health products and services include over-the-counter (OTC) medications, cosmetics, and medical and dental treatment. Broadly speaking, however, almost any product or service purchased can in some way be health related. For example, choice of foods has a bearing on nutrition. Choice of clothing relates not only to physical needs, but also to psychological expression of personality. Choice of discretionary purchases, ranging from toys to jewelry to stereo equipment, affects income available for necessities.

In this chapter, both the rights and the responsibilities of the consumer are emphasized. A variety of suggestions for learning activities will assist you in helping students establish responsible consumer behavior patterns.

Shown at the right of each activity title in this chapter is the suggested grade level(s) for which the activity might be appropriate. However, many of the suggested activities could be modified for use at various grade levels.

Information Assessment Activities

Why Do I Buy? Grades 4–6

Valued Outcome: Students will be able to identify the reasons they purchase various products.

National Health Education Standard: 2

Description of Strategy: Each student should think of a product that he or she buys from time to time. It can be any sort of product, not necessarily a health-related one. Ask the students the questions below. Have them explain and discuss the answers they give. How do they relate their decisions to their values?

- How does advertising convince consumers to buy a product?
- If your friends use a certain product, would you use it also?

- Does cost affect what you buy?
- If you didn't like a product, but it was the only kind available, would you buy it?
- If you had your choice of two products, one in a bright, colorful box and one in a plain box, which would you buy?
- Would you buy a product because your family likes it?
- Does the quality of a product matter?
- Would you try several brands to find one you like?
- Do you tell other people about products you like/buy?
- What kind of products would you buy because of an associated name; in other words, because of who wears them or whom they represent?

Processing Questions:

1. What factors do you think influence your buying decisions?
2. What types of ads are most likely to get you to buy the product?

✔ **Assessment:** Students will be able to state two factors that influence their purchasing decisions.

Assessing Attitudes Grades 4–6

Valued Outcome: Students will be able to analyze why they purchase products.

National Health Eucation Standards: 2, 3

Description of Strategy: Give each student a copy of Worksheet 22.1 (page 500). Have students assess their own attitudes about each statement. By doing so, the students will become more aware of why they make choices.

Materials Needed: Worksheet 22.1 for each student, pencils

Processing Questions:

1. What seems to be most important in determining why you buy a product?
2. Are there products you buy that perhaps you could do without?
3. Are any of the products you buy potentially harmful to you?
4. Do all the products you buy seem to be as good as you thought they would be?

✔ **Assessment:** Students will be able to state two factors to consider before buying a health-related product.

I'm a Wise Consumer Because... Grades 4–6

Valued Outcome: Students will be able to identify their positive purchasing habits.

| **Daily Lesson Plan**

Lesson Title: Consumer Reports

Date: April 16, 2012   **Time:** 11:00 A.M.   **Grade:** Five   **Teacher:** David

I. National Health Education Standards

Health Education Standard 3: Students will demonstrate the ability to access valid information and products and services to enhance health.

II. National Health Education Standards Performance Indicator

3.5.2 locate resources from home, school, and community that provide valid health information.

III. Valued Outcomes

- Students will learn about comparison shopping.
- Students will learn where to obtain reliable product information.
- Students will identify product validity.

IV. Description of Strategy

1. Use a typical thirty-minute television program and 200-page magazine to describe the ratio between advertisements and content.
2. Explain that when purchasing something, people should look for reliable information on the quality of the product. A good source is *Consumer Reports* magazine.
3. Get back issues of *Consumer Reports* from the school library or a public library, and discuss some of the products tested. Point out that the magazine has no advertisements. Ask students what the lack of advertisements indicates. Give other examples of places to find reliable product information.
4. Ask students to choose a brand-name product. Have them research the item and compare it to similar products. Have students write about whether they still want the product and why.
5. Close the lesson with a discussion about the advantages of being an informed consumer.

V. Materials Needed

- copies of *Consumer Reports*

VI. Formative Evaluation

Benchmarks

- Level 1: Student was able to identify techniques of comparison shopping.
- Level 2: Student was able to identify techniques of comparison shopping and describe advantages of comparison shopping.
- Level 3: Student was able to identify techniques of comparison shopping and describe advantages of comparison shopping. Student was able to list places to find reliable product information.
- Level 4: Student was able to identify techniques of comparison shopping and describe advantages of comparison shopping. Student was able to list places to find reliable product information and explain how to determine product validity.

VII. Points of Emphasis

1. Explain marketing techniques and how much research goes into targeting a market.
2. Remind students that just because someone says it on TV that does not mean it is true.
3. Explain advantages of having the best product, not just the most attractive product.

Teacher Evaluation

1. Keep the lesson as taught?   yes _____ no _____

2. What I need to improve _____

3. Next time make sure _____

4. Strengths of lesson _____

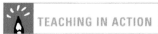 TEACHING IN ACTION | **Daily Lesson Plan**

Lesson Title: Dr. I. M. A. Quack

Date: April 23, 2012   **Time:** 1:00 P.M.   **Grade:** Seven   **Teacher:** Barrett

I. National Health Education Standards

Health Education Standard 3: Students will demonstrate the ability to access valid information and products and services to enhance health.

II. National Health Education Standards Performance Indicator

3.8.1 analyze the validity of health information, products, and services.

III. Valued Outcomes

- Students will recognize phony health claims.
- Students will recognize phony medical treatment claims.
- Students will have a better understanding of product validity.

IV. Description of Strategy

1. Begin class by showing students infomercials, commercials, and ads that make questionable claims. Discuss with students how each advertisement makes us want to buy the product. Discuss what makes the claims believable and how ad companies stretch the truth.
2. List things that students can keep in mind when selecting health care products or services. Describe key words or phrases that are used to convince the consumer a particular product is effective. Remind students that if it seems too good to be true, then it probably is.
3. Divide the class into groups, and have each group come up with a quack product or service. Each group will make a presentation to the class and try to convince the other students that the product or service is actually of value. Encourage students to use their imaginations.
4. The class should listen to the presentations and then identify any fallacies of the product or service. Have the class list exaggerated truths in each presentation. After the presentations, have the class list products other than health care products that have phony claims.

V. Materials Needed

- video and magazine ads

VI. Formative Evaluation

Benchmarks

- Level 1: Student was able to describe false claims in advertising.
- Level 2: Student was able to describe and recognize false claims in advertising.
- Level 3: Student was able to describe, recognize, and identify false claims in advertising.
- Level 4: Student was able to describe, recognize, and identify false claims in advertising. Student was able to identify exaggerated claims that make us desire a product.

VII. Points of Emphasis

1. Explain that a marketer's job is to make us think we cannot live without certain products.
2. Describe words or phrases commonly used to mislead consumers.
3. List ways to differentiate valid time-tested products from quack products.

Teacher Evaluation

1. Keep the lesson as taught?   yes _____ no _____

2. What I need to improve _____

3. Next time make sure _____

4. Strengths of lesson _____

HEALTH HIGHLIGHT | **A Thought on Generic Drugs**

Substantial savings to consumers can be obtained through the use of generic drugs. Generic drug sales have increased dramatically since 1984 when the U.S. Congress passed the Drug Price Competition and Patent Term Restoration Act. The Food and Drug Administration (FDA) issues guidelines to ensure that generic drugs retain the same quality and potency as brand-name drugs. Almost 80 percent of generic drugs are produced by brand-name firms in their manufacturing plants. The FDA's Office of Generic Drugs conducts reviews and approves generic drugs for marketing. What does this suggest to you concerning generic drug use?

National Health Education Standards: 2, 7

Description of Strategy: Ask each student to complete the following statement in a written paragraph of twenty-five words or less: "I'm a wise consumer because…" Each answer should be based on actual behavior or attitudes. Discuss each student's response in a general class discussion. Ask students to explain on what values their statements are based.

Processing Questions:

1. What makes you a wise consumer?
2. What do you consider before buying a product?
3. What consumer tips did you learn from others in your class?
4. How can these tips help you in the future?

○ **Integration:** Writing

✓ **Assessment:** Students will be able to state two positive habits they regularly employ when purchasing products.

Health Fact or Fiction   Grades 4–6

Valued Outcome: Students will be able to identify factual health-related information.

National Health Education Standard: 3

Description of Strategy: Create a handout from the following questions and give a copy to each student. Ask him or her to place a checkmark in the blank under the appropriate answer.

	Agree	Disagree	Not Sure
1. Raw eggs are more nutritious than cooked eggs.	—	—	—
2. Eating an egg a day is harmful.	—	—	—
3. Fish and celery are brain foods.	—	—	—

	Agree	Disagree	Not Sure
4. Frozen orange juice is less nutritious than fresh juice.	—	—	—
5. All fruits and vegetables should be eaten raw.	—	—	—
6. It is dangerous to leave food in a can that has been opened.	—	—	—
7. Drinking too much water will make you retain fluid.	—	—	—
8. Drinking ice water causes heart trouble.	—	—	—
9. If one vitamin pill a day is good, two are better.	—	—	—
10. Meat is fattening.	—	—	—
11. Toast has fewer calories than bread.	—	—	—
12. Special diets help people with arthritis.	—	—	—
13. Acupuncture is a reliable method of treating illness.	—	—	—
14. Cooking with an iron skillet increases the amount of iron in the food cooked.	—	—	—
15. Cooking with aluminum pots and pans may increase the likelihood of getting Alzheimer's disease.	—	—	—

Materials Needed: handout for each student

Processing Questions:

1. What are some additional statements you have heard concerning health fact or fiction?

2. Why is misinformation about health issues
   a problem?
3. How does misinformation concerning health issues
   begin?
4. How is misinformation concerning health issues
   disseminated?

✓ **Assessment:** Students will be able to state two factual and two mythical pieces of health information and explain why the statements are true or false.

Use Technology to Make Wise Consumer Decisions
Grades 5–8

Valued Outcome: Students will be able to describe various factors that influence consumer decisions.

National Health Education Standards: 1, 2, 3

Description of Strategy: Working in groups of three to four, students will investigate 1) factors that influence online consumer decisions (peer pressure, desire for status) and 2) online advertising techniques (facts and figures, glittering generalities, endorsement and testimonial). Each group should identify the importance of the factors and techniques they find. Once these factors have been investigated, a PowerPoint or poster board presentation outlining in what way the students think each factor influences consumer decisions should be developed and presented to the class. After these presentations, each group should then select a type of health care product (toothpaste, wrinkle cream, sun screen, etc.) and analyze it using the factors identified during the group presentation. A report should be prepared by eat group reporting on what they have learned about the influences affecting purchases of the product they selected.

Materials Needed: computer, Internet, and PowerPoint program or poster board and markers.

Processing Questions:

1. What social factors and economic principles impact consumer decisions?
2. What criteria do you think are important in comparing and evaluating health care products and services based on major factors?
3. What strategies will you use when buying health products?
4. How do price, appearance, features, and quality affect consumer decisions?
5. How can technology be utilized to access consumer information (e.g., products, services, and resources)?

✓ **Assessment:** Students will be able to identify a variety of print and electronic resources that are available to assess consumer health products and select criteria that are important for consideration when selecting health care products.

Where Is the Help?
Grades 5–8

Valued Outcome: Students will be able to discuss agencies that can help protect consumers.

National Health Education Standard: 3

Description of Strategy: Ask the students to investigate the following agencies to determine the types of services/protection they can offer the consumer:

> Better Business Bureau (BBB)
> Small Claims Court
> Consumer Product Safety Commission (CPSC)
> Food and Drug Administration (FDA)
> Federal Trade Commission (FTC)

Have them list the types of services offered by each. Prepare a handout from the following information and have each student complete the form.

Where Is the Help?
Directions: Indicate which agency(ies) could provide help with the problems listed below:

a. BBB
b. Small Claims Court
c. CPSC
d. FDA
e. FTC

Agency

___ 1. Your new toy truck has small pieces that your younger sister might swallow.
___ 2. Food purchased at your local store was found to have worms and was spoiled.
___ 3. You are looking for information on a new drug.
___ 4. Your mom has purchased a product that is labeled as hamburger, but it does not look or smell like hamburger—your mom suspects it was mislabeled.
___ 5. Your new CD player gives you a slight shock every time you turn it on.
___ 6. Your dad takes his car to the serviceman for repair. But the car still does not work, and the serviceman says it is not his fault.
___ 7. Your deodorant has caused you to break out.
___ 8. Your family wants to check out a local company before doing business with it.
___ 9. You see an advertisement that is false or misleading.

Materials Needed: copy of worksheet for each student

Processing Questions:

1. Do some of the agencies cover a variety of complaints and issues?
2. Which agencies can respond most quickly to a consumer complaint?

3. What are the responsibilities of the consumer before purchasing a product or service?

✓ **Assessment:** Students will be able to state the purpose and roles of at least two of the listed agencies.

What Is Best? Grades 5–8

Valued Outcome: Students will be able to identify the major OTC pain relievers and discuss differences among them.

National Health Education Standards: 1, 3, 7

Description of Strategy: Introduce the concept that there are several types of OTC pain relievers. Ask the students to identify by brand name products that they know help to relieve pain, fever, and headaches. Write their responses on the board or on an overhead. Introduce the notion that each of these products has an active ingredient (drugs such as acetaminophen, acetylsalicylic acid, ibuprofen, naproxen). Have the students research which of the products they identified are in each of the four categories of active ingredients. Ask them to identify similarities, differences, and potential dangers associated with each type of product and record them on a chart similar to the one here.

Drug Chart

Name of Product	Main Ingredient	Purpose of Drug

Materials Needed: chart listing the various pain relievers, drug books or computer access to Internet, overhead projector and pen or board and markers

Processing Questions:

1. Have you taken any of these drugs for pain relief? Does the drug that you normally take have any potential side effects?
2. Do some of the drugs require a higher dose than others? Did all the drugs provide pain relief for the same amount of time?
3. Were all the medications safe for children to take?
4. Did any of the products offer different benefits or advantages?

✓ **Assessment:** Students will demonstrate knowledge of the name brands of types of pain relievers and be able to discuss potential side effects.

Budget Diary Grades 6–8

Valued Outcome: Students will develop insight into the reasons they purchase products.

National Health Education Standard: 2

Description of Strategy: Have each student keep a notebook diary of all purchases made for a week or longer. Every purchase should be recorded in the diary, along with the reasons for that purchase. Money spent on food, snacks, toys, video games, school supplies, transportation, books and magazines, pet supplies, hobbies, and health care products should all be recorded. Explain to the class that the amount of money each student spends is not as relevant as how the money is spent. After the diaries have been completed for the assigned time period, have each student analyze his or her purchases and answer the processing questions below. Answers to these questions should be written out so that students can clarify their thoughts better and come to personal conclusions about their patterns of consumer behavior. On a volunteer basis, have students explain to the class what they learned from this activity. Follow this with a general discussion.

Materials Needed: notebook diary for each student

Processing Questions:

1. What items did you buy that brought you a great amount of pleasure?
2. What items did you buy that disappointed you?
3. Do you think that you spent any money unwisely? Why?
4. Does this diary suggest ways that you could budget your spending money better? How?
5. What does this diary tell you about your consumer habits? Are there patterns in the way you spend your money?

○ **Integration:** Writing

✓ **Assessment:** Students will be able to list the items on which they spend the most money and discuss whether these are wise purchases. Students will also be able to discuss ways to improve their purchasing decisions.

What Is Really Happening? Grades 4–6

Valued Outcome: Students will be able to identify the amount of time companies spend in attempting to influence consumer spending and habits.

National Health Education Standards: 2, 3

Description of Strategy: Assign the students to watch television for one hour. Ask them to keep track of the amount of time spent in advertisements during the hour. Provide a chart such as the one shown below for their recordkeeping.

Television Viewing Form

Name of Program	Number of Minutes of Program	Type of Commercial	Number of Seconds/ Minutes
1.			
2.			
3.			
4.			

Total Minutes of Programs ____
Total Seconds/Minutes for Commercials ____

Materials Needed: stopwatch, calculator, viewing form for each student

Processing Questions:

1. How much time was devoted to advertising?
2. To whom did the advertising appeal: children, young adults, and/or grown-ups?
3. What type of product was on most of the commercials you saw?
4. What message was each commercial trying to get across?
5. Did you think all the commercials were truthful?

✓ **Assessment:** Students will be able to describe the amount and nature of advertising shown during a typical one-hour block of television programming.

Techniques that Sell
Grades 6–8

Valued Outcome: Students will identify the strategy used to sell a particular product.

National Health Education Standard: 2

Description of Strategy: After reviewing the various strategies used to sell products, divide the class into groups of three to five students. Assign each group a different selling strategy. Have them review media such as magazines, newspapers, radio, and television to find examples of their strategy. If possible, have them record or provide examples of their technique.

Materials Needed: magazines, newspapers, radio, television, and audio or video recorder for each group

Processing Questions:

1. Were you able to find all the techniques discussed?
2. Why are there so many different techniques?
3. What technique(s) were used most often?
4. What type of technique appeals to you?
5. Why does that particular technique appeal to you?

✓ **Assessment:** Students will be able to state at least two commonly used advertising techniques and give examples of ads that use them.

What Is in There?
Grades 6–8

Valued Outcome: Students will realize the many drugs that they have in their household.

National Health Education Standard: 1

Description of Strategy: Ask the students to request a parent to review the different drugs found in their household. With adult supervision, each student should list the drug and the main ingredient of each drug and its intended purpose. Students can then research any ingredient they don't understand or research that drug on the Internet. Provide a chart such as the one shown below to list the different drugs.

Drug Chart

Name of Product	Main Ingredient	Purpose of Drug

Materials Needed: copy of drug chart for each student, computer(s) with Internet access

Processing Questions:

1. What types of drugs are kept on hand in your house? What is the purpose of each drug?
2. Do some of the drugs serve the same purpose?
3. How many of the ingredients did you not know the effect of?
4. Did any of the ingredients of the various products have the potential to interact with one another?

✓ **Assessment:** Students will be able to state at least three drugs kept on hand in their home, and the primary purpose of each.

Decision Stories

Follow the procedures outlined in Chapter 4, pages 60–62, for presenting decision stories such as these. For each of the decision stories, write a list on the board of ideas generated by the class for how each situation should be dealt with. Ask the students to discuss the merits of the methods suggested.

Assessment for Decision Stories: Students can identify health-enhancing behaviors and exhibit positive decision-making skills.

Broken Promises
Grades 1–3

Ricardo saw a model car advertised on television. It looked like a fun toy. He saved up his money and bought the model. But when he opened the package, the car didn't look as well made as it did on television. He started playing with it, and the car broke. He was angry and disappointed. He felt like throwing the car away, but it had cost a lot of money.

Focus Question: Was it Ricardo's fault that the car broke?

National Health Education Standard: 2

Vitamins for Vera? Grades 2–4

In her health class, Vera has been learning about the importance of vitamins for good health and growth. She wonders if she is getting enough vitamins because sometimes she feels tired and worn out. One day, Vera's mother asks her to go to the grocery store to buy some milk. While at the store, Vera sees a shelf with many different kinds of vitamin pills on it. She has some money of her own with her. Maybe she should buy some vitamins so she might feel healthier.

Focus Question: What should Vera do?

National Health Education Standards: 3, 5

Munch or Lunch Grades 4–6

Miguel likes to play video games at the arcade. He spends a lot of his money playing Munchman, his favorite video game. He is getting better and better at it, but playing Munchman often leaves him without any money for other things. His parents give him lunch money every day. Up to now, he hasn't spent this money on anything except lunch. But maybe he could cut a few corners. Maybe he could buy less for lunch and use the rest of the money to play video games.

Focus Question: What should Miguel do?

National Health Education Standards: 2, 5

Shampoo of the Stars Grades 4–6

Ling's friends have been telling her about a new shampoo called Hairdoyoudo. They say that it makes their hair feel soft and look pretty. Ling has also seen the product advertised on television. A famous young model with beautiful hair says that she uses it. Ling would like to use Hairdoyoudo, also, but her mother buys another brand of shampoo that is less expensive and seems to work fine. Ling asks her mother to buy Hairdoyoudo, but her mother refuses, saying it is overpriced. Ling is very upset because she wants her hair to look as nice as her friends' hair. But how can that be if she has to use another shampoo?

Focus Question: What should Ling do?

National Health Education Standards: 2, 3

Spots and Shaun Grades 6–8

Shaun has acne. He is very embarrassed about his spots and blemishes. One day he sees an advertisement for a new acne medication in a magazine. The advertisement promises a miracle cure within thirty days. The product has a money-back guarantee, but it can only be purchased by mail. The advertisement also says that the product has a secret ingredient that no other product has. It sounds like just what Shaun has been looking for, even if the product costs $19.95 a tube.

Focus Question: Should Shaun order the product?

National Health Education Standards: 2, 3, 5

Dramatizations

Finding a Doctor Grades 2–4

Valued Outcome: Students will be able to identify criteria for selection of a physician or a dentist.

National Health Education Standards: 3, 7

Description of Strategy: After discussing the procedures that can be used for locating a qualified physician, have students role-play the techniques. For example, one student plays the part of a representative from the county medical society who recommends physicians who are accepting new patients. Another student calls on the telephone and asks for the names of such physicians, or one student can play the part of a doctor while the other plays the part of a prospective client. The latter should ask questions about availability of services, fees, qualifications of the doctor, and so forth.

Materials Needed: two telephones (optional)

Processing Questions:

1. Where would you look to find a physician or dentist?
2. How would you contact a physician or dentist?
3. What questions would you ask before using the services of a health care professional?

✓ **Assessment:** Students will be able to accurately describe how to find a health care provider and state two questions to ask the provider before using his or her services.

Medicine Safety Rules Grades 2–4

Valued Outcome: Students will be able to list the rules for safely taking medicine.

National Health Education Standards: 1, 7

Description of Strategy: After discussing the medicine safety rules detailed in the following list, divide the class into seven groups, and let each group develop a brief skit—two to five minutes—dramatizing each rule. The rest of the class will try to determine which rule is being acted out by each group.

- Don't take any medicine without asking an adult about it first.
- Only take medicines that you really need.
- Take only the medicine prescribed by your doctor especially for you.
- Never take more than one medicine at a time, unless your doctor tells you to do so. Different medicines may interact in a way that can be dangerous or even fatal.
- Don't take any medicine unless you are sure you know what it is.
- Throw away medicine that doesn't have a label or that has passed the expiration date.
- Keep all medicines out of the reach of younger children.

Materials Needed: medicine safety rules listed on poster board

Processing Questions:

1. Why are medicine safety rules so important?
2. Are there other medicine safety rules you could think of to help protect us?

✓ **Assessment:** Students will be able to give two safety rules to follow when taking a prescription medication and will be able to explain why the rules are important.

Now for This Commercial Message
Grades 5–8

Valued Outcome: Students will be able to analyze commercials to determine misleading or overstated claims concerning health care products.

National Health Education Standards: 2, 7

Description of Strategy: Ask the students to work together in pairs or small groups to reenact commercials they have seen on television for health care products or services. Let each group decide on the commercial they wish to reenact. Draw up a master list to avoid duplication. Have the students closely study the commercial of their choice at home. Then let them work together, rehearsing their reenactment. Each student should play a different role. For example, one student can recommend the product, and another student can act out trying the product, as in many aspirin commercials. When the students are ready, have each commercial reenacted in front of the class. After the reenactment, the students who played the roles should explain what might have been misleading or overpromising about what they said or did. Video recording will allow reuse of some of the commercials at a later time.

Materials Needed: video recording equipment (optional)

Processing Questions:

1. What types of commercials seem to be the most misleading?
2. How do these commercials seem to overstate the effectiveness of the product?
3. What is misleading about the commercials you have just seen?

✓ **Assessment:** Students will demonstrate that they can critically evaluate television commercials and describe what aspects of commercials may be misleading.

Complaints
Grades 6–8

Valued Outcome: Students will practice appropriate ways to complain about defective or ineffective health care products.

National Health Education Standards: 4, 7, 8

Description of Strategy: Have small groups of students role-play how they would act when complaining about a defective or ineffective health care product or service. One student should act the part of the disgruntled consumer, another the part of the seller, and a third the part of a consumer advocate or representative of a local Better Business Bureau or other consumer-oriented group.

Processing Questions:

1. What agencies can help consumers with defective products?
2. Where do you begin when filing a consumer complaint?
3. Who is ultimately responsible for protecting us in consumer issues?

✓ **Assessment:** Students will be able to describe the appropriate process for filing a complaint about a defective product.

Discussion and Report Techniques

Health Myths
Grades 4–6

Valued Outcome: Students will make a collection of health myths and state why they are accurate or inaccurate.

National Health Education Standards: 3, 7

Description of Strategy: Students can research and collect health myths such as "Feed a cold and starve a fever," "Toads cause warts," and "An apple a day keeps the doctor away." Develop a bulletin board or scrapbook listing and illustrating the adages as well as whether they are true or false. Discuss the scientific accuracy for the sayings that may have relevance and why people continue to subscribe to such beliefs today.

Materials Needed: list of myths, construction paper, markers, glue

Processing Questions:

1. Are all health myths completely false?
2. Why do you think people first developed these myths?
3. Why do people continue to believe these myths today?

✓ **Assessment:** Students will be able to list two health myths and explain where they came from and why they are false.

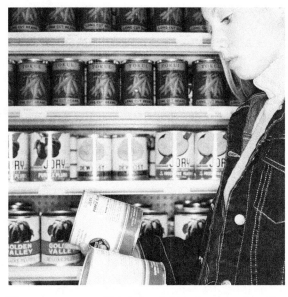

Wise consumers read labels carefully and compare brands before purchasing products.

Do Only Ducks Quack? Grades 4–6

Valued Outcomes: Students will be able to describe quacks and quackery.

National Health Education Standards: 3, 7

Description of Strategy: Develop a class discussion around the topic of quacks and quackery. Questions that can be used include:

- What is quackery? What are some examples that you've seen?
- Why does quackery continue to flourish?
- Who are the people most likely to believe what quacks say?
- How can consumers be protected from quackery?
- What can be done if you think a legitimate physician is in error?
- Why would people give testimonials about products that have no proven value?
- In what areas of health concern would it be easiest to get people to buy products?

After the discussion, divide the class into groups. Each group is to develop and build a pretend fraudulent medical device and/or medicine to present to the class. Have the students formulate advertisements to stimulate interest in their phony product. After completion, projects can be displayed in the classroom. Presentations can be videotaped.

Materials Needed: materials to build devices or to present medicines, poster board and markers for each group, video recording equipment (optional)

Processing Questions:

1. Do you think fraudulent medicines and cures are very prevalent?
2. Should there be strong laws against people advertising phony remedies? Why or why not?

✓ **Assessment:** Students will demonstrate knowledge of what quackery is and give at least two examples that they have seen.

Advertising: Don't Buy It Hook, Line, and Sinker Grades 4–8

Valued Outcome: Students will be able to understand the role of advertising in product purchases.

National Health Education Standards: 2, 7

Description of Strategy: Create a handout from the questionnaire below and distribute it to the students. Ask students to bring various advertisements to class. Help them determine the types of appeal used in each advertisement and list them on the board. Then have students circle the appropriate letter to best complete the statement or question.

1. When a product's package says, "Free coupon inside," the advertising appeal being used is
   a. cost and rewards.
   b. scientific appeal.
   c. snob appeal.
   d. testimonial or authority figure.

2. People who purchase and use goods and services are called
   a. advertisers.
   b. consumers.
   c. researchers.
   d. shopkeepers.

3. Advertising is designed to do all of the following except
   a. entertain.
   b. dissuade.
   c. persuade.
   d. promote.

4. In evaluating an advertisement that features an endorsement by a famous person, the most important question should be
   a. How is this person qualified to judge the product?
   b. How much money is this person being paid?
   c. Does this person really like the product?
   d. Does this person use the product regularly?

Answers: 1. a, 2. b, 3. b, 4. a

Materials Needed: copy of questionnaire for each student, board and markers or overhead projector and pen

Processing Questions:

1. What is the most important role advertising serves?
2. Why do famous people serve as spokespersons for various products?
3. Do any health products have potentially dangerous consequences?

✓ **Assessment:** Students will be able to identify the technique used in at least one advertisement and state factors that consumers should consider when thinking about purchasing that product.

Health News   Grades 5–8

Valued Outcome: Students will gather current health information and present it in newspaper form.

National Health Education Standard: 3

Description of Strategy: Have students research, develop, and publish a copy of a newspaper dealing with health issues. Included in the paper should be articles, cartoons, editorials, advertisements, and human interest stories written by the students. If students are using the Internet to research health information, remind them to consider the source of the information and to rely only on reputable sources, such as the Centers for Disease Control and Prevention, the American Heart Association, etc.

Materials Needed: sources containing health information such as magazines and newspapers, computers with Internet access

Processing Question: What did you learn about health that you did not know before?

○ **Integration:** Writing

✓ **Assessment:** Students will be able to list and describe credible sources of health information.

The Laws of Advertising   Grades 5–8

Valued Outcome: Students will be able to list at least three laws that protect consumers.

National Health Education Standards: 1, 3

Description of Strategy: Have students research the laws that protect consumers against fraud or useless products and services. They can begin by looking up "consumer protection" on the Internet, or in the catalog system, at the library. They can also visit the laws and regulations sections of government websites such as www.fda.gov and www.usda.gov. Have students write the laws on the poster board and discuss the laws with the class.

Materials Needed: poster board, computer with Internet access

Processing Questions:

1. Why was it necessary to pass laws to protect us against fraud?
2. Do you think most consumers know about these laws?
3. What is the key to consumers being protected against fraud?

○ **Integration:** Social Studies

✓ **Assessment:** Students will be able to name and describe at least two laws that help protect consumers.

Labels Are Important   Grades 5–8

Valued Outcome: Students will learn how to read and interpret OTC drug labels correctly.

National Health Education Standards: 1, 7

Description of Strategy: With the cooperation of parents, have each student analyze the information given on the package of an OTC drug. Use the processing questions below for the analyses. Students should prepare individual reports about what they find.

Materials Needed: labels from OTC drugs

Processing Questions:

1. What information did you find on the label?
2. Are any drugs safe for everyone to take?
3. Why do you think the warnings were placed on the label?

4. The labels of OTC drugs caution against using the product if you have certain allergies or medical conditions. What do you think would happen if you had an allergy or condition that might cause a reaction, but you took the drug anyway?

✓ **Assessment:** Students will be able to describe the information found on the labels of OTC drugs.

How Are Your Health Habits? Grades 6–8

Valued Outcome: Students will be able to evaluate their health to determine what lifestyle changes they might make.

National Health Education Standards: 2, 3, 7

Description of Strategy: Have students develop and conduct a survey of health habits at their school. Answers should be either yes or no and should include questions dealing with superstitions and personal health habits. For example: "Have you ever bought a product just because you saw it advertised on television or in a magazine?" "Have you ever ordered anything online and been disappointed with the merchandise?" "Do you take vitamins?" Tally the results and post them on a bulletin board. Also, post the medically correct answers so students can assess their own knowledge, or lack of knowledge, concerning health issues.

Materials Needed: a list of possible questions to be asked in the survey (enough questions should be provided to help students start the project)

Processing Questions:

1. What did you discover from the survey?
2. How should you change any negative lifestyle habits you identified?
3. What positive health habits did you identify?

✓ **Assessment:** Students will be able to state two trends they were able to identify from the health survey.

Health Promotion Agencies Grades 6–8

Valued Outcome: Students will learn what health promotion agencies are responsible for specific activities.

National Health Education Standard: 3

Description of Strategy: Hand out Worksheet 22.2 (on page 501). The handout has a list of agencies involved in health promotion programs and the description of each agency's function.

Materials Needed: worksheet for each student, pencils

Processing Questions:

1. What agencies can you name?
2. What agencies do you think are most important to our personal protection?

✓ **Assessment:** Students will be able to name at least two health promotion agencies and describe what they do.

Health Options? Grades 6–8

Valued Outcome: Students will identify forms of treatment other than traditional medicine.

National Health Education Standards: 1, 3

Description of Strategy: After dividing the class into small groups, have the students investigate complementary and alternative health care choices. The following could be included: acupuncture, chiropractic, faith healing, holistic health, homeopathy, visualization, laughter therapy, or positive self-talk. Reports are then given to the class. Students should discuss the scientific basis of each, the feasibility of trying alternative kinds of medical care, under what circumstances they might try an alternative form, and the intrinsic value of each method. A master list of alternative treatments may be given to the class to help the students choose their topics. Presentations can be videotaped.

Materials Needed: list of alternative health care choices to hand out to students, video recording equipment (optional)

Processing Questions:

1. Would you try any of these alternative forms of treatment?
2. Do you think some or all of these alternative forms of treatment are useful?
3. What are some guidelines we should keep in mind when deciding if we might try an alternative treatment?

✓ **Assessment:** Students will be able to list and describe at least three forms of complementary or alternative medicine.

Where Can I Go for Help? Grades 6–8

Valued Outcome: Students will learn about health care services offered in their community.

National Health Education Standards: 1, 3

Description of Strategy: Have students research legitimate health care services available in the community and write reports on their findings. Community health care resources include private physicians, dentists, therapists, hospitals, clinics, health maintenance organizations

(HMOs), telephone referral services, and so on. Keep a list of the type of services each student chooses, so that not too many will have the same topic. Have students discuss their resource in class. Students should seek information concerning eligibility for services, types of services, where the facility is located, the types of staff employed, and the duties of the staff.

Materials Needed: list of the health care services offered in the community with headings for categories of services, phone numbers, and descriptions of services to be filled in by the student

Processing Questions:

1. Are there many health organizations in your community?
2. What services does your organization provide?
3. How do the various health services differ?

✔ **Assessment:** Students will be able to list and describe at least three health care facilities in their community.

Experiments and Demonstrations

Is There Any Difference? Grades 3–6

Valued Outcome: Students will taste different unlabeled cola drinks and try to determine what each one is.

National Health Education Standards: 1, 7

Description of Strategy: Many products are indistinguishable once removed from their packaging. To demonstrate this, bring in some different brands of cola drinks. Pour small amounts of three or four different brands into paper cups, and have the students do taste comparisons. Let them try to guess which cup contains a particular brand.

Materials Needed: liters of several different colas, small cups

Processing Questions:

1. Do you have a favorite cola drink? Could you tell which one it was?
2. How much do you think advertising affects what you buy?

✔ **Assessment:** Students will demonstrate understanding that different brands of the same product may be nearly identical.

Comparison Shopping Grades 4–6

Valued Outcome: Students will learn to compare similar products from a cost perspective.

National Health Education Standards: 1, 7

Description of Strategy: Have the students develop a list of five or six health care products, such as toothpaste, deodorant, soap, eye drops, dental floss, and antiseptic cream. Let each student comparison-shop for these items and report on which stores in the community sell each brand of product for the best price. This can be done either by visiting stores or by checking prices in newspaper advertisements. You may wish to have the students comparison-shop for specific brands that they normally use, or you may suggest that the students look for the cheapest and most expensive brand of each type of product. Compare the results in a class discussion.

Materials Needed: sheet for each student for listing products, price, and comments

Processing Questions:

1. Do the same products cost the same at various stores?
2. What is the difference in cost between the most expensive and the least expensive version of a certain item?
3. Is the most expensive product always the best? Is the least expensive product always the worst?
4. On what criteria should you base your purchases?

✔ **Assessment:** Students will be able to describe the cost differences between different brands of similar items and discuss why similar items are not priced the same.

Listen Carefully Grades 4–6

Valued Outcome: Students will increase their awareness of meaningless phrases used in advertising.

National Health Education Standards: 2, 3, 7

Description of Strategy: Record some radio or TV commercials and play them back for the class. First, play the commercial in its entirety, asking students to listen or watch for any misleading statements. Play the commercial again, this time stopping the recording to discuss statements such as "Now more improved than ever" or "America's number one choice!" Explain that these types of statements are especially meaningless since the comparison is not specifically stated. List these statements so the students can review them.

Materials Needed: audio or video of commercials, tape player or video recorder and television, poster board, board and markers or overhead projector and pens

Processing Questions:

1. What types of statements do you find used most often?
2. How are certain statements misleading?
3. What are examples of other commercials on television or radio that are also uninformative or misleading?

✓ **Assessment:** Students will be able to state at least three phrases often used in commercials and explain what the phrases mean.

Which Is Better?   Grades 5–8

Valued Outcome: Students will exchange consumer products such as shampoo or soap to determine if there are actual differences between them.

National Health Education Standards: 2, 3

Description of Strategy: Ask students to bring a particular brand of shampoo or soap to school, making sure that the brands are not all the same. Then have students trade the products they now use with someone using another brand of shampoo or soap. Let each volunteer use the alternate product for a week or two and then report on the results.

Materials Needed: index cards or paper for each student for recording comments

Processing Questions:

1. Did the alternate shampoo or soap do just as effective of a job, or were differences noted?
2. Were any differences a matter of individual preference?
3. Are different products perhaps more or less effective for different individuals?

✓ **Assessment** Students will be able to compare and contrast the alternate brand of product with the brand that they normally use.

Puzzles and Games

Consumer Health Tic-Tac-Toe   Grades 3–5

Valued Outcome: Students will develop health-related questions and use them to beat an opposing team at tic-tac-toe.

National Health Education Standard: 1

Description of Strategy: This game can be played either by two players or by the whole class divided into two teams. Have each team come up with a health-related question for one of the tic-tac-toe squares. The opposing side or player tries to answer and to mark a particular square. The correct answer must be given. If an incorrect answer is given, no mark on the tic-tac-toe board is to be made. Each side plays in turn until there is a winner.

Materials Needed: health-related questions, poster board with tic-tac-toe grid for each group, two different colors of counters for each group

Processing Questions:

1. Can you correct all the answers that were missed?
2. What are some additional questions?

✓ **Assessment:** Students will be able to answer at least three of the health-related questions correctly.

Consumer Riddles   Grades K–3

Valued Outcome: Students will solve these riddles about consumerism.

National Health Education Standard: 1

Description of Strategy: Use the following riddles on consumerism to assess student knowledge of consumerism.

- I am a fraud, but I sound like a duck. What am I? (a quack)
- An inflated advertising claim is a huff and a. (puff)
- My initials are BBB. I can help you if you have a consumer problem. What am I? (Better Business Bureau)

Materials Needed: riddles

Processing Questions:

1. What other riddles can you identify that illustrate an aspect of consumerism?
2. Can you think of an example for each of the riddles?

✓ **Assessment:** Students will be able to answer at least one riddle correctly.

Scrambled-Up Health   Grades 4–6

Valued Outcome: Students will learn discretion when using health care products or services.

National Health Education Standards: 2, 3, 7

Description of Strategy: Through various media, people are constantly being bombarded with ads about goods and services that supposedly improve health or appearance. Give students a worksheet that has scrambled words that name some items that should be considered with caution and discretion. Have students unscramble the words and write them in the blanks.

Materials Needed: worksheet of scrambled words for each student

Processing Questions:

1. Have you heard or read health claims that might not be truthful?
2. How can you determine if a health claim is accurate and truthful?

✓ **Assessment:** Students will be able to unscramble at least six of the nine words.

Shopping Game   Grades 4–8

Valued Outcome: Students will participate in a game to increase their knowledge of consumer spending.

National Health Education Standards: 2, 7

Description of Strategy: Prepare a shopping game board as shown in Worksheet 22.3 on page 502. The game can be played by two to six players. Each player is given $200 in play money at the start. A "bank" is given $100 in play money; this is where students place or remove money for their purchases or refunds. Participants roll dice in turn to determine the number of moves. The winner is the player with the most money at the end of the game. Play can continue until only one player has money left. Let each player decide to what extent he or she won or lost by the consumer decisions the game dictated. Follow with a discussion of options in buying products and services.

Materials Needed: Worksheet 22.3 of shopping game board for each group of students, dice (one per group), play money ($200 per student and $100 in assorted denominations in the central store), game pieces such as buttons (one per student)

✓ **Assessment:** Students will understand the costs associated with the various activities listed on the game board.

Other Ideas

Packaging   Grades 4–6

Valued Outcome: Students will recognize the importance of attractive packaging in influencing the purchase of a product and will design a package for a product of their own.

National Health Education Standard: 2

Description of Strategy: Some of the appeal of a product results from the way it is packaged. Have the students bring in empty packages from various health care products. Discuss the visual appeal of each one, then have the students design packages of their own for the products. First, they should try to design a package they think would be very appealing to consumers. Then they should design a package that would not appeal to consumers. These can be shown to other students for feedback.

Materials Needed: construction paper, glue, markers, empty health care product packages

Processing Questions:

1. Was it difficult to design a package that would help sell your product?
2. What did you find the most attractive—certain colors or designs or wording?
3. How much do you think packaging influences what you and your family buy?

○ **Integration:** Art

✓ **Assessment:** Students will be able to explain what is appealing and unappealing in a product's packaging.

The Pharmacist and You   Grades 4–6

Valued Outcome: Students will learn what a pharmacist does.

National Health Education Standards: 1, 3

Description of Strategy: Have students visit a pharmacy, or invite a pharmacist to class to discuss his or her training and educational level and exactly what he or she does as a pharmacist. Students can work together to make a list of questions to ask the pharmacist about the job, how he or she likes it, his or her income level, the industry's view of the use of generic medications, and the decisions he or she makes in collaboration with both doctors and pharmaceutical salespeople. Questions can also be asked, or research done, into the history of pharmacy and how modern technology has enabled it to evolve into an exacting science today. Perhaps brainstorming with the students can help them generate questions of interest to the group.

Materials Needed: list of questions to be asked at interview

Processing Questions:

1. Would you be interested in a career in pharmacy?
2. What kinds of questions could a pharmacist help you answer about drugs and medications?
3. What is the most important thing a pharmacist does?

✓ **Assessment:** Students will be able to explain what a pharmacist does.

Slogans—Do They Sell?   Grades 5–8

Valued Outcome: Students will discuss the impact of slogans on the health care products they purchase.

National Health Education Standards: 2, 3, 7

Description of Strategy: Create a handout that offers options of matching slogans with product names, and provide each student with a copy. You may wish to use slogans that are popular in your area. Or, students can develop their own lists using magazines, videos, and television.

Materials Needed: handout for each student with slogans for various products, pencils or pens

Processing Questions:

1. What other slogans you can think of?
2. Why do slogans influence what we buy?
3. Do any of the slogans provide you with actual information about the product?

4. Do you find that you purchase products more if you like and remember the slogan associated with it?

✓**Assessment:** Students will be able to define the term *slogan* and discuss why a slogan might help an advertiser sell a product.

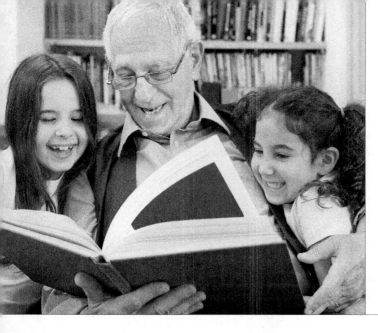

Aging, Dying, and Death

Our country is at a critical juncture in its history where the numbers of people over age 65 are expected to double in the next 30 years. The good news is that older adults are living longer, healthier, and more productive lives. As a Nation, we must do everything we can to support their independence and provide opportunities for them to make meaningful contributions to our society.

—*U.S. Department of Health and Human Services, 2008*

Valued Outcomes

After completion of this chapter, you should be able to:

- Discuss aging as a normal part of the life cycle.
- Describe how ageism affects the elderly in our society.
- Describe the current demographic aspects of the elderly in the United States.
- Explain the factors that can help delay or retard the physiological changes that occur in aging.
- List the reasons why elderly people have problems with nutrition.
- Describe Alzheimer's disease.
- Suggest intergenerational contact programs for school-age students and the elderly.
- Discuss the factors that will lead to better quality lives for the elderly in the future.
- Discuss the fears of a dying person.
- Describe the relationship of personal beliefs in facing dying and death.
- List ways in which family members cope with and help in times of a relative's death.
- Describe healthy ways to grieve.
- Discuss the purposes of funerals, hospice care, and living wills.
- Describe the warning signs for suicide in children.
- Describe effective methods of teaching death education.

Reflections

Aging. Consider your own relationships with elderly people—your grandparents and relatives or other elderly individuals around you. Reflect on how you can increase the quality of these relationships.

Death and Dying. As you read through this chapter, consider the ways that you and those around you practice and observe the denial of death and dying—in behavior, in common phrases, on television, and so on.

The Normalcy of Aging

Aging is a normal developmental process, not a pathological phenomenon, as it is often viewed. When we speak of aging, we must avoid the misconception that the process affects only those over 65; each of us is aging every day. We generally consider the changes taking place in the body as "development" until postadolescence and refer to the changes as "aging" after that. Many people view growth as positive and aging as negative—but, in fact, both are part of one process. The process of aging is a continuous experience that begins at birth and ends at death.

Exactly how we age is not clearly understood. Many theories have been advanced, but some aspects of the aging process are still mysteries. In any case, the number of elderly in the United States has risen sharply in the past two decades, and this trend will continue. Because of advances in medical technology, improved health care delivery, reduced infant mortality, and control of diseases, more people are living longer. In this chapter, we examine the ramifications of this fact and consider the ways in which aging is viewed in our society.

The Significance of Aging Education

Aging education is relatively new compared to other health topics. Because the number and proportion of elders are expanding rapidly in the United States, education about aging and the aged is becoming increasingly important. Myths and misconceptions about the elderly and the aging process can have serious consequences, such as ageism and discrimination against the elderly. It is important that health educators counteract these myths and misconceptions with the truth and realities about the aging process and the elderly. Elders have a tremendous impact on our society through their talents, wisdom, and psychological support for younger age groups.

People face many changes and challenges in life as they age. The problems of the elderly are problems that affect all of us. Major challenges facing the elderly include income, fitness, acute illness, nutrition, housing, sexuality, mandatory retirement, and the changing character of society.

U.S. society places a great deal of emphasis on youth and productivity; the elderly person's role is considered less significant. Also, because of financial reasons (sharing housing costs) and social factors (desiring to live with or near peers and living nearer service-oriented agencies), some elderly people have opted to move into housing and communities for the aged. This further segregates them from the remainder of society and makes them less visible.

Children today are less likely to have significant contact with the older generations than in the past. Many of today's children have little regular contact with grandparents. Children today experience many changes in their lives and in their families. Further, they are more likely to

live greater distances from their grandparents than were children in previous generations. As a result, children may feel isolated and separated from their grandparents. Just a generation ago, it was common for family members of different generations to talk with each other and spend time together. This interaction does not occur as often today. This lack of meaningful contact with the elderly, coupled with any misleading stories children read and hear, often leads to fears and misconceptions. Students need to be taught about the elderly and aging early in their lives. They need to understand that they themselves will one day be old and that the elderly were once young like themselves.

Intergenerational Contact

Intergenerational contact programs can be one of the most effective ways for secondary teachers to implement an aging education program. Such an experiential approach to intergenerational contact has been implemented in programs throughout the country. Notable examples are the Foster Grandparent Program and the Retired Seniors Volunteer Program. Volunteers and paid aide programs, tutoring projects, free lunches, and guest speaker days have all served to involve the elderly with the schools. Only as students are given the opportunity to understand aging and the aged will many false beliefs be dispelled. The positive attitudes gained from aging education can help students realize their full potential throughout their lives as they themselves age. By studying aging, students will be better able to understand and interact with their parents and grandparents.

There are several things for young adults to consider when planning for later life. For example, the better educated elderly may be better able to cope with the challenges of later life; therefore, younger adults should place an emphasis on continuing their education. A related factor that will help a young adult prepare for later life is the development of hobbies; therefore, continuing education does not have to include a program that results in a formal degree. Some courses can be taken to investigate various interests and hobbies. Young adults should become active in organizations and/or movements, such as environmental issues, women's rights, and charitable organizations, in which they have concerns or interests. This activity contributes to one's self-concept by providing a purpose in life and can enhance the quality of life in later years. Finally, young adults should carefully consider financial planning for later years. It is difficult for a young

> **TEACHING TIP**
>
> Today's children are limited in their involvement with elderly people and, therefore, hold many myths and misconceptions about the elderly and aging. As often as possible, invite elderly persons (maybe students' grandparents) to interact with the students.

adult to contemplate financial needs that are thirty to forty years away—especially in a society that promotes instant gratification. Financial concerns usually top the list of problems for elderly people in our society, and this trend is likely to continue; therefore, it is vital for young adults to develop a sound financial plan in order to ensure quality health care, housing, and living standards for themselves in later life.

Population Demographics

According to the U.S. Administration on Aging, the U.S. population of persons sixty-five years or older numbered 39.6 million in 2009. This number represents 12.9 percent of the U.S. population, over one in every eight Americans. In 2009, there was a sex ratio of 135 older women for every 100 older men. The percentage of Americans sixty-five and older has more than tripled since 1900 (from 4.1 percent to 12.9 percent in 2009), and the older population itself is increasingly older; in 2008, the eighty-five and older group was forty-six times larger (U.S. Department of Health and Human Services 2011).

The older population itself is getting older. People are expected to live longer, thanks to medical advances and improvements in health-related care, reducing the death rates among children, young adults, and the elderly, especially males. Americans today have a greater life expectancy than at any time in history, according to the latest U.S. mortality statistics released by the CDC's National Center for Health Statistics.

Women are expected to live longer than men. However, the gap between male and female life expectancy closed from five years in 2008 to 4.9 in 2009; this is a small change, but the gap is significantly smaller than the peak of 7.8 years in 1979 (CDC 2011). Americans are living longer than ever before, and life expectancies at older ages have increased. Men and women who live to age sixty-five can expect to survive an average of 18.5 more years, which is about four years longer than people age sixty-five in 1960. The life expectancy of people who survive to age eighty-five today is 6.8 years for women and 5.7 years for men (U.S. Department of Health and Human Services 2011).

Race has played a significant role in life expectancy in the past, and the racial and ethnic diversity among the elderly population is expected to increase into the future. Based on the 2011 Population Profile of the United States from the U.S. Census Bureau, from 1990 to 2050, the proportion of elderly is expected to increase from 13 to 23 percent for Whites; 8 to 14 percent for Blacks; 6 to 13 percent for American Indians, Eskimos, and Aleuts; 6 to 15 percent for Asians and Pacific Islanders; and 5 to 14 percent for Hispanics (U.S. Census Bureau 2011). According to data tracked by the National Vital Statistics Reports, white females have the highest life expectancy followed by, in order, black females, white males, and

black males. This pattern has not changed from 1975 through 2009 (CDC 2011).

The higher the socioeconomic group an individual is born into, the better the chances are that the person will be better educated, get a better or higher paying job, and will be aware of the importance of healthy habits as they contribute to longer life expectancy. The gap in life expectancy at birth for those born to a higher socioeconomic status versus those born in the lowest socioeconomic group has grown from 2.8 years in 1980 to 4.5 years in 2000 (U.S. Congressional Budget Office 2008). It is not completely understood why the differences in life expectancy occur among socioeconomic groups, but it is assumed that some basic factors contribute to the disparity. These include smoking, obesity, self-management of disease, healthy lifestyles and use of health care, and insurance coverage (U.S. Congressional Budget Office 2008).

The Aging Process

Aging is a complex process influenced by physiological, psychological, and sociological factors. Before the specific changes associated with the aging process are discussed, it should be emphasized that the changes occur to different people at different times. Most of these changes are gradual, and adjustments can often be made to offset them. Many changes can be slowed through proper exercise, nutrition, and other preventive health maintenance.

▪ Biological Aspects of Aging

Gender, genetics (a person's hereditary predisposition toward or resistance to certain diseases and conditions), and general environment (exposure to various hazards or special benefits that affect health and well-being) are all factors that affect how long people live and how healthy they will be over their life span.

Many physical changes, only some of which are affected by lifestyle choices, occur with the passage of time (National Institutes of Health 2010). These include:

- The amount and distribution of lean tissue (muscles and organs), bones, water, and other substances in the body.
- An increase of fat tissue toward the center of the body, including around the abdominal organs.
- Bones become more brittle and may break more easily as they lose some of their minerals and become less dense (osteoporosis).
- A loss in height due to changes in the bones, muscles, and joints. People typically lose about 0.4 inches every ten years after age forty.
- Changes in the muscles, joints, and bones affect the posture and gait, and lead to weakness and slowed movement.
- The joints become stiffer and less flexible.

- Inflammation, pain, stiffness, and deformity may result from breakdown of the joint structures.

- The risk of injury increases because gait changes, instability, and loss of balance may lead to falls.

Some physical changes can often be slowed or reduced through regular exercise; avoiding smoking, alcohol, and illicit drugs; and by following a healthy diet. For example, osteoporosis in women can be addressed by consuming adequate amounts of calcium and vitamin D throughout the lifespan. Other changes are simply a result of the body changing as it ages.

Dementia and Alzheimer's Disease.

The majority of people over the age of eighty retain normal brain function, but various biological phenomena involving progressive degeneration of mental functions may occur as people age. **Dementia** is a general term for the progressive loss of cognitive and intellectual function and is caused by a variety of factors, the most common of which is a structural brain disease. According to the National Institutes of Health (2011), at the most basic level, those with dementia "have significantly impaired intellectual functioning that interferes with normal activities and relationships." The impaired functioning can include a loss in the ability to solve problems, less emotional control, personality changes, behavioral problems, memory loss, impaired language skills, and hallucinations. Dementia is not a normal part of the aging process, and is instead often a symptom of Alzheimer's disease, Huntington's disease, and Creutzfelt-Jakob disease. There is no drug available to halt or reverse brain damage as a result of these diseases, but some drugs are available to improve symptoms and slow progression of the dementia. Symptoms of dementia have also been seen in reactions to medications, nutritional deficiencies, infections, poisoning, brain tumors, and heart and lung problems, so a diagnosis of dementia is made only after a thorough examination by a health care professional to rule out other possible causes of symptoms of dementia (National Institutes of Health 2011).

The majority of cases of dementia, however, are due to **Alzheimer's disease**, a progressive and irreversible disease involving the death of nerve cells and deposition of plaques of amyloid (a protein) in the brain. The causes of Alzheimer's disease are not entirely known, but it is posited that genetic, environmental, and lifestyle factors each play a part. More than 90 percent of cases are seen in people age sixty-five and older; there are cases of "early onset" Alzheimer's disease seen in individuals in their thirties and older who have a mutation in an inherited gene. The initial symptoms of Alzheimer's disease are memory loss and confusion that then slowly develop into other symptoms of dementia. Ultimately, there is a severe loss of mental function in patients with the disease. As mentioned above, there are currently no medications that can slow the progression of the disease (National Institutes of Health 2011).

■ Psychological and Sociological Aspects of Aging

The psychological and sociological changes that accompany the aging process affect some elderly individuals more than others. Each individual will respond to aging in a way that reflects his or her personality, philosophy of life, and the way that he or she is treated by society as a whole. Better treatment of and more positive attitudes toward the elderly would do much to limit many of these detrimental attitudes and behaviors.

Ageism. Many psychological changes are the result of negative attitudes and behavior toward the elderly, who often are treated as sickly and unproductive by the younger generation regardless of their actual health and abilities. Phrases and images in our language and media reflect these stereotypes. The term for discriminating against someone based on his or her age is **ageism**. This form of prejudice is different from other forms (e.g., sexism, racism) because a person's age changes throughout a lifetime, and older age (and thereby discrimination due to older age) is something that the majority of adults will eventually experience, especially in U.S. society, which stresses the importance of being young, healthy, and economically prosperous.

Coping with Changes. In helping individuals cope with changes that do occur with aging, it must be recognized that the elderly face many losses, including peers, jobs, spouses, and physical senses. Problems with making adjustments to these losses overwhelm some elderly people, whereas others are able to face the challenges and find satisfaction. Changes may include:

- loss of the child-rearing function (the empty nest syndrome)

- loss of a spouse

- mandatory retirement (or a change in role if retirement is voluntary)

- problems with transportation

- lack of community involvement

- lack of knowledge of community resources

- inadequate medical services

- financial problems

- a need for leisure activities and ways to use their time

- loneliness

- loss of role identification

- victimization through crime or abuse

Again, it should be noted that some of these sociological aspects of aging are the result of discrimination and inappropriate treatment from younger people. With proper education and attitudinal changes in the general population, many of these detrimental changes could be alleviated among some of the elderly in America. The validity of this premise can be demonstrated by contrasting the role of the

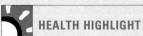

The number of adults in the U.S. aged sixty-five or older is expected to surpass 71 million by the year 2030. This number will place large demands and expectations on available health care and other age-related services. Steps can be taken to prevent some future demands, such as addressing potential chronic diseases before symptoms manifest. This is particularly important as about 80 percent of older adults have one chronic condition, and 50 percent have at least two. Focusing on prevention or reduction of risk of infectious diseases (like influenza) can also remove some future anticipated burdens on the system. The CDC is focusing on some specific areas of prevention (2011). These include:

- **Promoting healthy lifestyle behaviors to improve the health of older adults through environmental and policy approaches.** This can include programs to encourage regular physical activity and nonsmoking to reduce incidence of future chronic diseases.

- **Increasing the use of clinical preventive services.** Only about 25 percent of adults aged fifty through sixty-five years are current on recommended immunizations and cancer screenings.

- **Addressing cognitive impairment that affects health and long-term care needs.** Assessing and monitoring the perceived burden of future cognitive impairment should help states and communities develop policies and strategies to address this issue.

- **Addressing issues related to mental health.** Public health efforts focus on ways to better assess mental health among older adults.

- **Providing education on planning for health care in case of serious or terminal illness.**

Source: Centers for Disease Control and Prevention 2011. More information available from www.cdc.gov/chronicdisease/resources/publications/AAG/aging.htm.

---

elderly in the United States with that of the elderly in some other cultures, such as Japan. In Japan, individuals enjoy higher social status and prestige as they grow older—almost the opposite of what happens in the United States.

Major Challenges Facing the Elderly

Income and Employment

Chief among the challenges facing the American elderly is the lack of financial resources. The primary source of income for older persons in 2007, as reported by the Social Security Administration, were Social Security earnings, income from assets, and public and private pensions. Lack of sufficient income is the result of inflation that has eroded the savings many elderly acquired during their working years. Retirement benefits from Social Security are not sufficient to meet all their needs.

Poverty level impacts a person's longevity, overall health, and general lifestyle. Although income among the elderly increased between 1972 and 1992, wide disparities in income exist between men and women and among race and Hispanic-origin groups, and the poverty rate of 9.4 percent (in 2006) among the elderly is an issue of concern (Center for American Progress 2008). In 2008, 3.4 million people age sixty-five and older lived below the poverty line.

Housing and Living Arrangements

Housing continues to be a major issue for the elderly. Nearly two-thirds of the elderly in the United States own their own homes. However, even if the house is paid for, the owners are still responsible for taxes and insurance costs, and older homes can have higher maintenance costs. Some elderly have to make a decision between drastic improvements in their current home and moving, but they are sometimes limited financially as to where they can move. Some government housing is available based on current income—the lower the income, the lower the monthly payment. Some elderly share housing to reduce the monthly costs. For many elderly, however, there are few housing options. Some housing alternatives are apartments for the aged that are sponsored by private, public, and nonprofit church-related groups. Also, for older persons requiring assistance, boarding homes and nursing homes that provide both intermediate and skilled care are available.

More than half of older noninstitutionalized people (55 percent of men and 41 percent of women) lived with their spouse in the year 2009, but this proportion decreases with age. Because men tend to die younger than women do, women are more likely to be living without their spouse or others as they advance in age. In 2009, about 716,000 grandparents aged sixty-five or over maintained households with grandchildren present and another 942,000 grandparents aged over sixty-five years lived in family households that included their grandchildren. Only of a small percentage of the older population of the United States (1.6 million or 4.1 percent of older individuals) lived in institutional settings such as nursing homes. As individuals age, they are increasingly likely to be living in a nursing home (USDHHS 2011).

Health

Maintaining good health is a major challenge of growing old. An individual's health affects every aspect of life—relationships to spouse, family, and community; income-producing ability; and leisure pursuits. The health problems that beset the elderly are usually associated with the aging process, in addition to those related to environmental causes and trauma. Chronic ailments, such as heart disease, are the most common affliction of the elderly.

Escalating medical and health-related expenditures are a major concern for the older population. Of economic necessity, the health care of many elderly people is crisis oriented. Because they cannot afford to visit a physician every time they are ill, many do not seek help until they feel it is absolutely necessary—and their more advanced illnesses may be more difficult to treat. At the same time, there are many areas in which the elderly needlessly spend money on health remedies or could spend their money more wisely for greater health benefits. Federal programs such as Medicare and Medicaid have helped in some ways, but even these programs do not pay enough of the health care bills of some elderly because of the ever-increasing costs of health care delivery.

Medicare and Medicaid. The U.S. government provides financial assistance for medical care through two major programs authorized through the Social Security Act and administered by the Centers for Medicare and Medicaid Services (CMS). **Medicare** is the nation's largest health insurance program, providing coverage for nearly 40 million individuals who are either age sixty-five and older or who are qualifying younger but medically disabled individuals. Generally, older individuals or their spouses must have worked for at least ten years in a Medicare-covered job (i.e., they are entitled to Social Security or railroad retirement benefits) and must be a citizen or permanent resident of the United States in order to receive Medicare benefits. Most of these individuals are covered by Medicare Part A, which helps pay for care in a hospital or skilled nursing facility, home health care, and hospice care, and they will not need to pay additional costs to participate in the program. Additional coverage may be obtained by qualified individuals through a subscription (i.e., at additional cost) to Medicare Part B, which is a supplemental medical insurance to help pay for doctors' fees, outpatient hospital care, and other medical services.

Medicaid is a federal subsidy program for state programs that finance health care for qualified (usually low-income) individuals. Each state makes its own health care regulations, has its own program administration, and determines its own benefits and rates of payment, but these must remain within limits set by federal regulations. A large portion of Medicaid spending is used as reimbursement for nursing facilities.

Nutrition. Some of the health problems faced by the elderly result from improper nutrition. Nutrition is as important for the elderly as it is for other age groups. Because of limited finances, loneliness, various disease states, and a reduction in the senses of smell and taste, many elderly skip meals or do not otherwise eat well.

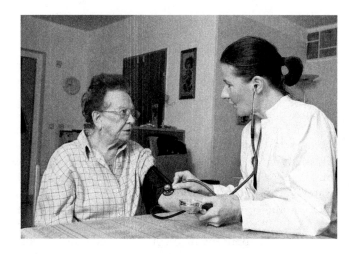

One factor that will determine the quality of life in the elderly is access to medical services.

Sometimes emotional problems, such as depression, keep elderly people from eating.

Because an elderly person's basal metabolism is reduced, the person's caloric requirements are also reduced. For this reason, better planning is required to ensure proper nutrition. Less food is required, but the quality must remain high. Programs such as Meals on Wheels, which delivers meals to homebound elderly, and the federal government's Food Stamp Program and Nutrition Program for the Elderly (Title VII of the Older Americans Act of 1965, which is updated every three years) help defray the cost and improve the nutrition of the poor elderly.

Medications. Older people take more medications than any other segment of the population does. Because the older population has the highest rate of chronic or long-term illnesses, this group also tends to take more than one drug at the same time. Drug use in older adults may cause greater problems than in younger people because of slower metabolic rates and more illnesses. Polypharmacy (taking more than one medication at a time) and prescription drug misuse and abuse are prevalent among older adults (SAMHSA 2006).

According to the Center for Substance Abuse Prevention, an increasing number of seniors may be abusing drugs, prescription medication (taken for a variety of illnesses that tend to accompany senior citizenship), and alcohol.

Some otherwise harmless over-the-counter (OTC) drugs can be dangerous if taken in conjunction with certain prescription medications. Prescription drugs may interact with each other. Many drugs react poorly with alcohol. It is critical to check with a pharmacist before taking any medication or allowing anyone in your care to take medication. Also, the pharmacist must be aware of *all* medications (OTC, prescription, and even vitamin supplements) the person is taking so that such interactions can be avoided.

Prescription medications can pose further risks when in the homes of seniors who have young grandchildren. Accidental poisonings can happen when children explore the medicine cabinets and nightstands of their grandparents. The danger of accidental poisoning increases when an elderly person moves in with family members who have young children.

The responsibility for overseeing and safekeeping seniors' medication often falls to a caretaker or family member. Regardless of who ultimately dispenses the medication, there are some key recommendations for safety precautions. The USDA recommends that the patient and/or caretaker talk to health care professionals about all conditions, medicines, and dietary supplements; learn about the medicines and keep track of side effects or possible drug interactions; use an aid (calendar, pill box) to track what medication should be taken, when, and for what purpose; purge the medicine cabinet of old or expired medicines yearly; and keep all medicines out of the sight and reach of children (USDA 2010).

Crimes against the Elderly. Medical quackery also affects the elderly. Arthritis sufferers, mostly older individuals, spend $300 million yearly on quack remedies. Other types of crime against the elderly range from muggings and theft to financial exploitation and physical abuse by members of their own family.

Transportation. Transportation is a major challenge for some older individuals, many of whom do not drive or have not adjusted to today's complicated traffic patterns. Those who drive with failing eyesight and hearing are more likely to be involved in accidents. The cost of automobile maintenance and gasoline prohibits some older people from operating a car. Nondrivers must seek other means of transportation. Taxis can be expensive, but public transportation, although cheaper, is much less convenient because it requires more walking and takes more time. Often it is not designed with the elderly in mind. For these reasons, many elderly are restricted to their homes and apartments except for going out to get health care, groceries, and other necessities.

Caregiving for the Elderly How to care for elderly parents is a concern for many future caregivers. Some of the major issues are how to ensure good health care, how to find the right living situation, and how to handle legal questions. While it can be difficult to discuss the issues of aging, the family who has discussed the options and agreed on plans will be better able to handle whatever happens. Ideally, older adults can make plans and decisions before an emergency happens. Individuals who will soon be reaching their older years should investigate their options and decide which is most appropriate for retirement and for life-sustaining medical care, and make sure documents, instructions, and powers of attorney are available to those who are designated to take responsibility of their care in an emergency. All plans and elder care instructions should be discussed with the potential caregiver to make wishes clear. The caregiver should ask questions and ensure instructions are clearly understood. Advance planning can also help in a financial sense; medications and care services are not always covered by existing insurance plans and should be discussed at length.

Talking with the elderly about their living situations and the possible need for change is not always easy, even if plans were made for future care. A successful conversation depends partially on the existing relationship between the caregiver and the elderly person, and also on the elderly person's mental, emotional, and physical conditions. The designated caregiver should understand that certain signs (sudden weight loss, deterioration of personal habits, general forgetfulness, increased accidents, and consistent disorientation) may be signals that elder care is necessary. When it comes time to address a change of living situation, it is important to help the elderly person retain all possible control of their own decisions and be certain both the caregiver and the elderly person are clear on legal, financial, and medical matters (U.S. Department of State 2011).

The options for elder care have grown in past years as the numbers of elderly have increased. The resources to help with in-home care (emergency aid buttons, modified bathroom fixtures, lightweight wheelchairs) can delay or ease a transition to a retirement community or nursing home. Home care and meal delivery services are also available in many communities, allowing an elderly person to remain at home for a longer period of time.

A caregiver should understand that they are taking on significant responsibilities emotionally, legally, and even financially. It is necessary for caregivers to have support systems to help if an elder care situation becomes overwhelming.

Considering Death

Death is a vital part of the life cycle for every creature on earth. Death is included in the natural order of birth, growth, aging, and dying. Death is a certainty—it will come to every person. These seem like elementary statements, but many people in contemporary society believe that life and death are mutually exclusive phenomena.

The contemplation of death can be trying. The various aspects of dying and death are extremely complex and confusing because there is so much about death we do not comprehend. Many questions regarding death, such as "If we are born to die, then why do we live?" and "If death is natural, why do so many people regard it as bad?" have still not been answered satisfactorily. None of the numerous attempts to come up with answers to such questions have been able to satisfy everyone. The unknowns have caused much confusion and put an aura of mystery around death, but they have also been the source of many interesting attitudes and philosophies on the subject.

Death is as much a part of human existence, of human growth and development, as birth is. Death sets a limit on our time in this world, and life culminates in death. Recognizing that death is a natural end to life can have a profound influence on our lives. Our lifestyles can depend on our attitudes toward death. Much information on death and dying is now available, but many misconceptions and problems concerning issues of death and dying still exist. For example, medical and nursing schools do not do enough to prepare their students to handle end-stage care issues related to dying and death.

Another problem with death and dying concerns students of secondary school age. Parents often protect their children from the trauma of death-related events, thinking they are doing the best thing for the child. However, this treatment tends to propagate fears and misconceptions. For example, children tend to regard death as happening only to the old. This is a result of parents telling them not to worry about death until they are older.

In the remainder of this chapter, we examine these and other death-related issues. We also look at attitudes toward death, the needs of dying people and their families, the grief experience, funerals and related rituals, death education for students, personal beliefs about death, and other issues surrounding death.

Common Attitudes toward Death and Dying

The current attitude of Americans toward death is contradictory. We are both intimidated and fascinated by death. We enjoy living, but we take risks by driving dangerously and taking part in high-risk sports. We want safety and happiness, but we behave in self-destructive ways, for instance by abusing drugs. We consider the subject of death to be a social taboo but insist on reading and talking more about it now than we did in the past. We say we need weapons for war, but at the same time we are concerned about spiritual rebirth.

Our typical response to death is denial. This results from our resistance to imagining death and is predicated on our fears of death. We deny death by not planning for it (e.g., by not making out a will) and by participating in high-risk activities as if we were impervious to dying. Students often feel they are impervious to death and will live forever; but death is inevitable, and students need to learn to live with and accept this fact of life. Some of the many reasons students may fear death include the following.

- Fear of the unknown.
- Fear of what comes after death.

- Concern about what would happen to their parents, siblings, or other family members or friends after their death.
- Fear of change.

Many people display an outright hatred of death. They hate death because they think people die too young or because they are afraid of what comes after death. The hate and fear might not result so much from the unknown factor as from the hopelessness regarding what is beyond death.

Open, honest discussions of dying and death are often denied because of the belief that death should be considered a taboo topic for discussion. Death also may be a taboo topic because of the mystery and danger associated with it, an attitude that is influenced by society's emphasis on youth and secularism. Attitudes toward death are influenced by past experiences with death, by early parental messages, cultural influences, life experiences, religious beliefs, level of education, and maturity. Attitudes are formed largely by childhood experiences and carried into adulthood.

It is interesting that many people today who would rather not discuss death in an open and frank manner actually talk about death in other ways. For example, "You'll be the death of me" or "My shoes are killing me" or "That loud noise scared me to death!" In other cases, death is the subject of humor, such as jokes about Saint Peter at the "Pearly Gates." Often, people who talk about death in these ways show both an aversion to death as a topic of conversation and a fascination with death. They may be subconsciously trying to show themselves and others that death really doesn't bother them, even though serious contemplation of the subject makes them extremely uncomfortable.

We also treat death in a very special way. We set aside special places for death—the funeral home, cemeteries, hospices, and hospitals. We set aside special times for remembering deaths—Memorial Day, Day of the Dead in Mexico, and Good Friday, a day celebrated by Christians for remembering the death of Jesus. The deaths of other celebrated and martyred persons are remembered with special days. We have special symbols for death, such as black armbands worn by athletes when a teammate has died or a flag flown at half-mast in memory of someone who has died.

Several factors have contributed to our very narrow and stereotyped attitudes toward death and dying. Because many people encounter death so infrequently, we fail to accurately contemplate its nature. We blindly believe in modern medicine to the point that we subconsciously feel we may never die. Many never come to realize that death is a fact of life with which all people must cope and reason out for themselves. Most Americans say they want to die quickly or in their sleep. This response reflects reluctance to accept the possibility of a painful or slow death in which one is conscious of what is going on.

Our attitudes toward death and dying are confusing and contradictory. We normally detest the taking of another person's life, as in homicide, yet we train soldiers to do just that in war. In fact, we make heroes of soldiers who tempt death and kill the enemy. In every state in the nation there is serious debate regarding capital punishment. Is it right to kill people because they have committed heinous crimes, such as murder? Is the use of capital punishment a statement that we condone the killing of a criminal and that killing under these circumstances will solve the problem? Another controversial issue involving death is abortion. Such groups as the Right to Life organization say that abortion is murder, akin to genocide. Yet abortion is legal if certain guidelines are followed—for example, if it is performed in the first trimester of pregnancy or if the mother's life is at risk.

Some Americans have very negative attitudes toward death, primarily because they are uncomfortable with their own mortality. Many people associate death only with loss, pain, suffering, frustrated desires, and uncompleted goals. They see death as a separation from people they love, from places or objects they treasure, and from a part of their own self-identity, and they fail to see anything positive in death.

Otherwise mature individuals often find themselves unable to cope with the thought of death. These people generally choose to try to ignore death, to pretend on a subconscious level that they are immortal. This attitude is assumed primarily out of a fear of death. Furthermore, other people's deaths remind us of our own vulnerability, causing us to feel totally helpless, as if nothing we can say or do can change a thing.

Many people try to avoid even mentioning death. When the subject of personal death or the death of someone close comes up, there are often looks of dismay and discomfort until someone changes the subject. When people refer to death, they often use euphemisms that do not imply the finality, totality, and complete separation from life that death is. These euphemisms include "passed away," "departed," "gone to his rest," and "gone to her great reward." Such phrases make it easier to talk about and think about death because they soothe the harshness of its reality. The use of euphemisms is an extension of the denial attitude that many Americans take toward death.

These attitudes can have a profound influence on people's lives. If death is nothing but fear, and if fear prevents people from thinking and acting, they then risk becoming less than human. Also, if the fear of death does limit an individual's view of the future, this negative attitude can hinder the person's ability to plan ahead, to anticipate both hazards and opportunities in life.

■ Positive Approaches to Death

Death should not be considered taboo. It should be seen as a natural part of our existence. The more absolute death becomes, the more meaningful life can become. Death is as much a part of human existence and the life cycle as birth. It is not an enemy to be conquered, but an integral part of life that gives meaning to human existence. Death sets a limit on our time in this life, urging us to do something meaningful with that time as long as it is ours to use. Dying is the final chance to grow, to become more truly who you are. Those who truly are reconciled to their own

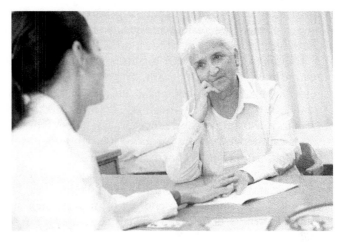

Recognizing that death is a natural end to our lives can have a profound influence on our lives.

mortal existence are the ones who get the most out of life. Such a positive approach to death frees one to focus on the daily tasks of living life more fully.

A normal and healthy fear of death is considered essential to the preservation of life because this fear leads us to take certain precautions. But we should not allow this fear to affect our emotional health in a negative way. We must find ways to cope effectively with death and dying, and it is not enough to intellectualize. The quality of our life depends on our ability to acknowledge reality and to deal appropriately with death and dying. The first step in overcoming a fear of death is to face it openly and resolve any unrealistic fears by looking into the causes of those fears. Frank and open discussion about death can help a person to diminish fear, anxiety, aggression, and other conflicts associated with death and to develop a positive attitude.

Various studies show that those who have religious beliefs generally have a decreased anxiety tevel about dying and death (U.S. National Library of Medicine 2010). Most religions believe that death comes only to the physical self and that one's spirit (or soul) will survive.

Furthermore, people who have shared in the death of someone who understood death's meaning tend to develop a more positive attitude toward dying and death. Those who have a healthy attitude toward death and who consider it truly one phase of existence have profited from this frame of mind. Positive attitudes toward dying can enhance the meaningfulness and richness of life for many, even for the terminally ill.

Needs of a Dying Person

Fear is the most typical psychological response that a dying person experiences. Dying people often fear humiliation, a sense of failure, a loss of self-worth, and anxiety about the future. Other common fears of the dying are:

- Fear of unknown
- Fear of loneliness

- Fear of loss of family and friends
- Fear of loss of self-control
- Fear of loss of body parts and disability
- Fear of suffering and pain
- Fear of sorrow
- Fear of loss of identity
- Fear of regression
- Fear of mutilation, decomposition, and premature burial (Endlink 2006)

In a sense, dying people have no model to follow. They feel like strangers to healthy and living individuals because no one understands what they are going through. Most dying people want to talk about death and their own illness; unfortunately, sometimes they cannot find anyone willing to discuss these matters.

▪ Adjusting to Dying

Adjusting to dying during the grief process consists of a number of phases, such as shock and numbness, denial, intense grief (which consists of yearning, anger, guilt, and disorganization), and finally reorganization or resolution. This adjustment period occurs differently in each individual and does not necessarily happen in sequential process. Understanding these stages of adjustment to impending death is critical in understanding the needs of the dying person. These phases occur in the person who learns that he or she is going to die as well as in the bereaved person grieving the loss of the deceased.

Shock and numbness are the most immediate reactions to death—the dying person cannot accept the fact that he or she is going to die, and the bereaved cannot consciously believe that the death just occurred. They are typically followed by a period of denial. This is the mind's normal reaction to protect the person from something he or she may not be able to handle emotionally at that time.

Intense grief includes a collection of fears (as discussed earlier in this chapter) on the part of the dying person and a subconscious searching for the deceased by those still living because the thoughts and behavior of the bereaved are focused on the deceased. Hallucinations are not uncommon because of the intense desire for the return of the deceased. Anger is manifested by irritability directed at anyone who comes in contact with the dying person or the bereaved, and it is sometimes even directed at God. The anger may be directed at oneself because of thoughts such as "If I had only done this with my life" or "If I had only done this while he or she was alive." During this intense grief, the dying person and the bereaved often experience despair. Apathy, aimlessness, futility, emptiness, and disorganization are all manifested during this time.

Resolution occurs when a person realizes cognitively and emotionally that death is inevitable. People at this stage of grief accept the fact that they are dying but do not necessarily give up trying to live while they are alive. A dying person and those who are grieving the inevitable death are able to accurately express their feelings. They are then able to deal with logistical matters surrounding the death and deal with relationships as well.

It should be noted that each person is as unique in death as in life, and everyone responds differently. Some may progress naturally through these phases, whereas others might reach one of the latter phases of adjustment, then regress. Further, not all dying people will reach the phase of resolution before they die.

The Family of a Dying Person

Impending death affects family members of the dying person in various ways. Sometimes there is a strong prohibition in the family against talk of death because family members feel this may bring about death more quickly. Some family members think that a discussion of death would make the others in the family more uncomfortable, and any discussion may seem to be related to an undue interest in the estate of the dying person. The loss of an important family member, such as the head of a household, can threaten certain social and psychological arrangements. This can lead to enormous stresses and cause tension among all remaining members.

Besides grief, emotional reactions to the death of a family member may range from guilt and anger to fear, anxiety, and money worries. Sometimes the anger is directed toward the person who died: "He died and left me with all these debts" or "She deserted us during a crucial time in our lives." Further, death is a reminder of the survivors' own vulnerability, which evokes fear in itself. If the dying person lives in the home before death, tension and resentment can develop. When family members have to sacrifice their own friends and activities to provide care, feelings of hostility and anger toward the dying person can develop. Then the anger turns to guilt, which has been described as anger turned inward. Some family members tend to feel inadequate when confronted with this overwhelming situation. They tend to want to protect themselves and the dying relative by not speaking to the person. This is wrong because it leads to emotional abandonment, making the situation all the more difficult for the dying person. Compassion, not isolation, should be given.

When circumstances permit, the family can help the most by maintaining an emotional and social environment consistent with the person's past life. This means keeping the person at home or in a hospice rather than in a hospital or nursing home, if possible. The family should include the dying relative as a participant in every discussion, especially those that involve decisions about that person's care and welfare. The family should do all they can to show their love and concern without doing it in ways that make the person feel guilty for being a burden to them. Family members should not allow their inability to face death to hinder the dying person's adjustment. When the person is

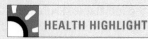

HEALTH HIGHLIGHT | **Emotional and Psychological Responses to Life-Threatening Illness**

The task-based approach is the most common model used to account for how individuals cope with a life-threatening illness. Several significant limiting factors have been ascribed to the older model, a stage theory based on the original work of Elizabeth Kubler-Ross, including whether the stages used in the Kubler-Ross model (denial, anger, bargaining, depression, and acceptance) actually exist. There is no evidence that all individuals experience these stages, or that movement exists from one stage to another in a sequential pattern. Further, individuals may regress in their mourning experience.

The task-based model does not imply any order or sequence and is therefore viewed as a more flexible model than the stage-based model, and it helps the patient and his or her family as they grieve. Four phases, or segments, of a life-threatening illness have been

identified and a task-based concept has been applied to understand how individuals confront each phase: prediagnostic, acute, chronic, and recovery or death.

The prediagnostic phase of a life-threatening illness is the period of time prior to the diagnosis of illness, when an individual recognizes symptoms or risk factors that make him or her prone to illness and during which diagnostic studies are performed. This does not necessarily happen in a single moment; rather, this phase may culminate in one moment when the diagnosis is first spoken.

The acute phase centers on the time in which a person is forced to understand the diagnosis and make decisions regarding his or her medical care.

The chronic phase of an illness is the period of time between the diagnosis and outcome. Individuals attempt

to cope with the demands of life while simultaneously striving to maintain and comply with treatments and side effects. Until recently, the period between a cancer diagnosis and death was typically measured in months, most of which were spent in the hospital; however, today people can live for years after the diagnosis of cancer.

During the recovery or death phase, persons may experience recovery from their disease and thus have to deal with the psychological, social, physical, spiritual, and financial after-effects of cancer. Other individuals encounter a final, or terminal phase of illness when death is no longer just possible, but inevitable. At this time medical goals change from curing illness or prolonging life to providing comfort and focusing on palliative care.

Source: National Cancer Institute 2005

---

ready to accept the reality of dying, the family should share that acceptance. An absence of support at this crucial time will mean that the person will die without dignity.

The Grief Experience

Grief is usually described as sorrow, mental distress, emotional agitation, sadness, suffering, and related feelings caused by a death. **Bereavement** refers to a state of experiencing grief. **Mourning** is composed of culturally defined acts that are usually performed when death occurs.

The closer the relationship of the bereaved to the deceased, the stronger the emotional response. Among these emotions and patterns of behavior are sadness, anger, fear, anxiety, guilt, loneliness, tension, loss of appetite, weight loss, loss of interest in things once interesting, a decrease in socialization, and disrupted sleep. These responses are usually greater when the death is unexpected.

Studies of mourning show that it is therapeutic for survivors to talk about the deceased and work through their death-related problems in counseling sessions (Davis 2004). Another form of therapy involves going to work, going to school, or participating in organizational activities. Americans seem in need of much more elaborate death ceremonies than some other cultures. This may explain

why many in our society place a strong emphasis on the rituals of funerals and burials.

Funerals and Related Rituals

The **funeral** is an organized, group-centered response to death. It involves rituals and ceremonies during which the

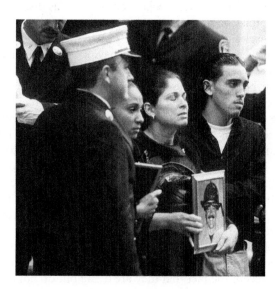

Funerals meet many emotional needs of the survivors.

body of the deceased is usually present. The traditional funeral includes speaking to the needs of the mourners. Some religions include a eulogy of the deceased, and some include an open casket that survivors view as part of the ceremony.

An alternative to the traditional funeral is a memorial service. Memorial services are sometimes held in conjunction with a cremation (with the urn present or absent) or when the body is not present for some reason (such as being donated to a medical school immediately on death or the family preferring not to have the body present). This service is held in a church, chapel, home, or whatever place is considered appropriate by the family. The service is not a eulogy but a chance to show thankfulness for having known the person. It also gives an opportunity for the expression of grief and sharing with family members. Generally, individuals who hold a memorial service are using this time to celebrate the life of the deceased while on earth, as opposed to mourning. Memorial services are most common among families who have strong religious convictions and the belief in life after death. Memorial services are becoming more common even among the nonreligious.

A primary purpose of the funeral is to dispose of the body. It also meets many emotional needs, such as grief and mourning, of the survivors. The visitation part of the funeral ceremony is important for friends to show their respect for the deceased and support for the survivors. Also, viewing the casket, which is part of some funeral home visits, is important to some for realization (seeing and thus believing that the person is dead) and recall (providing an acceptable image for recalling the deceased). For these reasons, the funeral home visitation can be therapeutic for friends as well as family.

Cemeteries, with markers for each grave, formerly were thought of as very sacred places where relatives and friends could go in quiet and peace to show their respect to the dead. Now, however, many cemeteries are crowded, congested, and impersonal. The relatives and friends of the deceased may also live many miles from the burial site. For these reasons, cemetery visits are less common than they once were. This ritual is not used as often as it once was for working out grief and mourning among the survivors.

Issues Surrounding Death

Some topics related to death have become the focal point of controversy in recent years. These issues include the definition of death, organ transplants and donations, the right to die, wills, and suicide.

▪ Definitions of Death

For thousands of years, the time of death was clearly defined as the time of cessation of life functions. Now, however, with advanced medical technology, life can be sustained beyond when death formerly would have occurred. The problem of defining it is much more complex—for example, not just knowing when a person is dead, but being able to determine the exact moment of death. This is important in the case of potential organ transplants, when every second is critical. Some say that a person is brain dead when the entire brain is dead, even if respiration and circulation could be maintained artificially. Others argue that a person is dead when the outer surface of the cerebrum of the brain has ceased to function. This individual may still breathe spontaneously via control of the brain stem, but thinking and reasoning ability would have ceased.

Definitions of death center around "brain," "heart," or "physiological" death, when various organs cease to function, and around "clinical" death, when there is a total lack of response to any external or internal stimuli, lack of spontaneous respiration, fixed and dilated pupils, lack of brain stem reflexes, and a flat electrocardiogram (i.e., no heartbeat). The significance of the definition of death is not just for the purpose of organ transplants. It also indicates which human lives can be saved, possibly with life-support systems such as heart–lung machines.

▪ Organ Donation and Transplants

Some people wish to donate their organs or their entire body for scientific and medical uses. This sometimes involves an urgent decision at the time of the donor's death. Biological, medical, and legal ethics are all involved in this issue. For those who wish to donate an organ, the Uniform Anatomical Gift Act of 1978 sets guidelines underlying the donor laws of each state. Some individuals donate their entire bodies to medical schools for dissection. Other parts of the body that can be donated include eyes for corneal transplants, ear bones to temporal bone banks for use in research into ear diseases, kidneys for kidney transplants, pituitary glands for use in producing growth hormone for those who lack this vital substance, and hearts for heart transplants.

Medical advances now enable an average of seventy-five people each day to receive organ transplants to save or enhance their quality of life. Due to a shortage of donated organs, about eighteen people die each day while waiting for a donation (U.S. Department of Health and Human Services 2011). In 2011, more than 86 million people were signed up to be an organ and/or tissue donor; it is believed that each person could help as many as fifty people by being an organ and tissue donor. The number of people in need of a transplant far exceeds the number of donors: approximately 4,100 people are added as candidates each month to the national waiting list (U.S. Department of Health and Human Services 2011). The donor must die in a hospital because surgery must be performed within hours if the organ(s) is to be used. For example, the heart is suitable for transplantation for only four to five hours after death. For this reason, surgeries are usually begun simultaneously for the donor and the recipient. The liver must also be transplanted within four to five hours, but the kidneys are suitable for transplantation for thirty-six to forty-eight hours after death.

It is not always known for sure who will receive the transplant, nor is such information as the donor's name or hometown usually given. General information is provided, though. An example of this would be the information that the kidney of a thirteen-year-old who died in an automobile accident was used. Anyone eighteen years or older and of sound mind may donate by signing a donor card. Anyone under eighteen years may become a donor if either a parent or the legal guardian gives permission. Most body parts from a person who is over fifty-five are not accepted for donation.

Although much of transplant surgery is still classified as experimental, the future is encouraging. Medical knowledge and technology are improving every day. Today two-thirds of the patients receiving liver transplants live beyond the first year. Even when a transplant patient lives only a few months, most families consider the operation worthwhile, because the patient's quality of life was probably vastly improved.

■ The Right to Die and Euthanasia

Euthanasia, the act of ending a life a permitting a death (often referred to as "death with dignity"), is not just a medical problem; it also involves legal, ethical, social, personal, and financial considerations. For this reason, the debate over euthanasia involves many professionals and paraprofessionals, as well as the patients and their families. The arguments now have to do with the dignity of the patients, the quality of their lives, their mental state, and sometimes their usefulness to society. For example, the patient who is in a vegetative state is considered dead by some but not by others, and this case presents substantial ethical and logistical problems. Some people say that to intervene in any way is to "play God," while others maintain that the rights of the patient are violated if the medical staff does not allow the patient to die. Such procedures as using a life-support machine to sustain life are sometimes seen as heroic acts, but some people think this only prolongs the suffering of the patient. Therefore, the line between heroic procedures (or unnecessary care) and giving up (or neglecting the patient) is difficult to draw. This distinction would be simple if we could just ask patients which treatment they wanted, but this is not possible in a majority of such cases.

Today we are being forced to rethink our ideas and choices about life, dying, and death. The issue of euthanasia is an excellent example of this. Currently, there is a change in emphasis in the euthanasia debate. The focus is less on allowing people to die a natural and painless death and more on allowing death to occur by withholding medical treatment. Typically, patients involved in a case of euthanasia are severely deformed or severely diseased infants or the terminally ill. Often the decision to practice euthanasia is more of a decision between letting the person die now or later, rather than a choice between life and death. Some argue that the movement in favor of euthanasia may be rooted in our fear of facing death, and that euthanasia is used to hasten death so that we will not have to cope with the consequences associated with the actual process of dying. A related issue that intensifies the problem is that many times the life, living, dying, or death decision is made by medical staffs or families about someone else's life or death.

Active euthanasia, which implies an individual deliberately ends the life of a person who is terminally ill or injured to prevent further suffering, is also described by some as *mercy killing*. When performed by a physician who supplies the materials needed for a patient to end his or her life this practice is termed *physician assisted suicide*. Active euthanasia is generally illegal in the United States (this is discussed again later in the chapter).

In the early 1990s, Dr. Jack Kevorkian intensified the debate over assisted suicide. He created a suicide machine that delivered an anesthetic and a lethal injection of potassium chloride through an intravenous line. Though he was not convicted for providing such assistance with this machine, Kevorkian was convicted of second-degree murder for actively administering lethal drugs to an incurably ill person, even though that person had requested his assistance. Kevorkian's actions provoked discussion of the thin line separating passive euthanasia, which is legal in this country, and active euthanasia. Opponents of Kevorkian's actions state that he is practicing assisted suicide, which is illegal. Proponents of Kevorkian's actions argue that the patient's right to control his or her medical treatment is sufficient justification for assisted suicide.

In the United States and Canada, a physician is permitted legally to accede to a mentally competent patient's desire to refuse medical treatment, even if the refusal will result in death. These laws do not permit physicians to assist a patient to die—this is considered a form of murder or manslaughter. Today the majority of states have legislation defining suicide assistance as a felony punishable by several years in prison. The Criminal Code of Canada also prohibits suicide assistance.

In the last several years, those who favor legalizing assisted suicide in the United States and Canada have challenged the constitutionality of these laws. The Supreme Court of the United States allows each state to determine whether or not to prohibit or permit assisted suicide (Beauchamp 1997–2003). Recently, the Supreme Court blocked the Bush administration's attempt to punish doctors who help terminally ill patients die. Assissted suicide is legal in the three American States of Oregon, Washington, and Montana.

Rapid advances in medical technology have given the medical profession the ability to sustain or prolong life through extraordinary methods, so that those who might have died quickly now have a chance of survival with life-sustaining artificial support mechanisms. An adult in this country is considered to have the right to determine whether this type of medical technology should be employed. The person has the right to expressly prohibit life-saving surgery or other medical treatments. In other words, the right to die with dignity is inherent for every individual, as much as the right to live. Some individuals fear the indignity and humiliation of existing merely as a vegetable, with others making decisions for them and caring for their every need. These people would rather die a "good death" than exist in this manner. The proponents of euthanasia state that saving a life is not always the same as saving people, as some do not wish to go on living or be revived. They argue that further extension of life should not be forced on the person just so life itself is preserved. This places an emphasis on the quality of life rather than just the literal existence of life.

Some families are using Health Care Advance Directives to handle this situation. Such a directive allows a person who is unable to speak for himself or herself to designate a person to make health care decisions (such as the kind of health care desired in such a situation) for him or her.

One example of a Health Care Advance Directive is a *living will*. In this type of document, a person is allowed to state his or her desires about life-sustaining medical treatments in case it becomes impossible to state those wishes later. Another document, a Health Care Power of Attorney, allows a person to appoint a designated person to make medical treatment decisions for him or her. If you do not wish to name such a person, you may state very specific wishes, such as the desire to donate certain organs.

A Health Care Advance Directive is intended to be used when a person cannot make or communicate decisions because of a temporary or permanent illness or injury. Such a document allows a person to keep control over important health care decisions through a designated agent. The person chosen as an agent for an advance directive will be making decisions on your behalf. If you do not appoint a person, the health care provider or a court-appointed guardian will have this responsibility; this person may not be aware of your wishes and beliefs. While it is not necessary to have a lawyer for many advance directive documents, many people do seek legal counsel. It is advisable to fully discuss advanced directives with the appointed person and clearly communicate decisions about the following (from the American Association of Retired Persons 2010):

- *Living will.* This will alert medical professionals and your family to the medical treatments you want to receive or refuse, and under what conditions. This will only go into effect if you meet specific medical criteria and are unable to make decisions.
- *Health care power of attorney.* This will delegate a trusted person to make health care decisions for you if you are unable to do so.
- *Letter of instruction.* This outlines any special requests, such as plans for a funeral and names of people to contact. It also should include important contact

information, such as an employer or insurance agent. Some people also include a list of meaningful possessions they'd like to give to certain loved ones. This is not a substitute for a will, but it helps clarify intentions.

The health care agent should have a copy of these documents in case they are needed, and a copy should be placed in your permanent medical record. These documents should be reviewed every few years or as living situations change.

Wills

The *last will and testament* is a legal instrument declaring a person's intentions concerning the disposition of property, the guardianship of children, or the administration of the estate after a person's death. A will is a legal document in which a person states how he or she wants property and possessions to be distributed after his or her death. By making such a document, people can ensure how their property will be distributed, the cost and time of settling the estate can be reduced, consequences of estate and inheritance taxes may be avoided, an executor can be named, family quarrels can be averted, a guardian can be appointed, and a testamentary trust can be created. For most people, ensuring the desired distribution of their property and possessions is sufficient reason for writing a will. Further, a person can enact a living trust that entrusts an estate to another person while the owner of the estate is still alive. A living trust keeps the estate private instead of public, even when the owner of the estate dies. A living trust can avoid probate, attorney fees, and some taxation when the owner of the estate dies.

Perhaps because ours is a society that denies death, most people delay writing a will. It is not surprising that most Americans, even many with sizable estates, do not have a will because writing a will reminds people of their own mortality. For individuals who die without wills, property passes according to state law. In other words, the state will decide which relatives get which part of the estate, even if the deceased person may have wished otherwise.

Near-Death Experiences

The near-death experiences that have been reported are remarkably similar to each other, whether they occur in young people or old, whether the result of an accident or illness, and whether the person is actually near death or just thinks he or she is. This has led many to believe that these experiences are not merely dreams, as was thought initially. Some physicians report not only that their patients have similar experiences, but also that the events occur in much the same sequence. Some report being able to watch events transpiring from several feet in the air (including resuscitation attempts on themselves) or feeling a sense of passing into another dimension or foreign region. Some see light, often as if at the end of a tunnel, with their vision clearer and their hearing sharper. Some recall seeing scenes from their earlier life and/or seeing loved ones who have died.

Many people who have near-death experiences as hospital patients undergoing surgery can recall procedures used on them and remember what each person in the room said. One patient, a nurse in a coma, had total recall of the exact procedures used. These patients also reported an instant replay of their own lives. Some patients have multiple experiences during a prolonged illness—some of these experiences are bad (usually the first ones), while others are very good. The patients themselves interpret whether the experience is good or bad.

▪ Hospices

A hospice is a program, type of care, or facility that cares for the terminally ill and their families. Sometimes hospice care is given in the patient's home and at other times in a separate wing of a hospital. Generally the goal of hospice care is to enhance the quality of a dying person's life during the last days and to allow the person to live as comfortably and inexpensively as possible.

▪ Suicide

For youths between the ages of ten and twenty-four, suicide is the third leading cause of death in the United States, resulting in approximately 4,500 deaths each year. Of the total number of these suicides in 2008, 83 percent of the deaths were males and 17 percent were females. More people in this age group survive attempts at suicide than actually die; in fact, each year about 149,000 people ages ten to twenty-four in the U.S. are given emergency medical care for self-inflicted injuries (CDC 2008).

There is more guilt associated with suicide than with any other type of death. Parents or relatives often feel they are somehow to blame. Some feel that a suicide reflects badly on the parents and family, but this is not always the case. Some hold a religious view that suicide is morally wrong or that one who commits suicide cannot enter heaven.

Any suicidal threat, however subtle, must be taken seriously. Most individuals who commit suicide provide significant clues to their contemplated action. These include obvious changes in mood or behavior, excessive use of drugs, changes in any set of habits, preoccupation with personal health, decreased academic performance, and insomnia.

There are four commonly recommended steps for helping someone who seems in danger of suicide. First, one should talk to the person who threatens suicide and determine how deeply troubled the individual really is. Second, one should not challenge the individual to act on the threat. Such a challenge may force the person to act to prove the validity of the threat. Third, someone can help the person postpone the decision and offer other options to consider. Fourth, one should be knowledgeable about resources that can provide aid. The person threatening suicide might have exhausted all personally known avenues of assistance and might need professional help.

Suicide prevention is a community responsibility, and everyone can play an important part in its resolution. However, many people have misconceptions about suicide. For example, they think a person who talks about suicide will not commit suicide, that a person talking about suicide just wants attention, or that a person who is suicidal at one point in his or her life is suicidal forever.

Young People and Death

Many young people in the United States no longer experience many aspects of the formerly traditional American life cycle. Most do not live with grandparents or on farms, so they do not observe aging and death in their immediate environment. Death education is necessary for the proper development of children. Death education should be viewed as a natural topic for inclusion in education because students are not immune to experiencing the death of a loved one, a pet, or a classmate.

Youths in our country continue to commit suicide. As stated earlier, suicide is the third leading cause of death for youths ages fifteen to twenty-four, and it is also the sixth leading cause of death for youths ages five to fourteen. For younger children, the causes for increasing numbers of suicides are stress, confusion, pressure to succeed, and financial uncertainty. For older youths, causes include divorce, problems in adjusting to a blended family, or difficulty making new friends in a new school or community.

Many of these stated reasons are treatable through counseling, especially if the problems are recognized and diagnosed appropriately. However, some parents fail to recognize the warning signs for suicide in their own children.

According to the American Association of Suicidology (2011), parents and teachers should watch for warning signs of acute risk, including a person:

- Threatening to hurt or kill him or herself
- Talking about wanting to hurt or kill him/herself
- Looking for ways to kill him/herself by seeking access to firearms, available pills, or other means
- Talking or writing about death, dying, or suicide (when these actions are out of the ordinary)
- Increasing substance (alcohol or drug) use
- Experiencing anxiety, agitation, an inability to sleep, or desire to sleep all the time
- Who expresses feeling trapped or hopeless
- Who withdraws from friends, family, and society

- Who displays rage, uncontrolled anger, or seeks revenge
- Who acts reckless or engages in risky activities, seemingly without thinking
- Who displays dramatic mood changes

If anyone makes a statement indicating a desire to take his or her own life, the statement should be taken seriously, and the person should be referred to a psychiatrist or psychologist. Though most people refrain from talking about death, a person making such a statement should be asked if he or she is depressed or thinking about suicide. This will let the young person know that you care and that you are willing to listen to his or her problems. With support from family and professional treatment, children and teenagers who are suicidal can heal and return to a healthier path of development (Youth Suicide Prevention 2001).

Education about death is much more open than in the past, allowing for more candid discussions between parents or teachers and youths. Talking about death and dying in a classroom can help students indentify thoughts, feelings, and beliefs about death, and understand better what happens at the end of life (Iowa Department on Aging 2011).

■ Death Education

Positive attitudes toward death can help prepare succeeding generations to face death more realistically. We can help young people accept the reality of death by preparing them properly for funerals and by allowing them to mourn, cry, recover from the loss of a pet or a relative, and express grief as part of the healing process. We should talk to them about death in terms they can understand. This discussion can be either from a religious or a factual point of view, depending on the preference of the parents and of the student.

We should explain the cause of death in order to eliminate any fear or guilt the young person might develop as a result of experiencing a death. Do not deceive them by using euphemisms or half-truths. One way to teach young people about death is to allow—but not force—them to attend a funeral or burial service. A recommended method is to take them first to the funeral of a neighbor or distant relative. Because the parents would not be as physically or emotionally involved in such a situation, they could devote time and energy to their children. Make the funeral a learning experience. Prepare the children before the funeral, ask them to watch for certain things during the funeral, and encourage their questions afterward. Education through attendance at a funeral will help young people gain a more complete understanding of death and make it more likely that they will develop a healthy attitude about death.

Finally, young people should be encouraged to talk openly about their fears and feelings. This will help eliminate any misgivings they have and help the parents to respond more appropriately to the emotions expressed. Of course, this assumes that the parents know how to respond and that they will share their own emotions with their children.

Fortunately, people today are more willing than before to discuss death and dying. The many books available on the subject, the courses being taught in schools and universities, the increased number of bereavement societies and hospice groups, and the increasing number of documentaries, specials, and films are evidence of this. This openness about death is refreshing—a challenge to the previous treatment of death as a taboo topic for conversation, research, and writing. Communication about death can improve the quality of our lives and help us grow as individuals. Even if we fumble through a discussion on death, as a friend or parent, our effort is very helpful.

Death is a universal part of living, even though it is often a taboo topic in our society. Young people are interested in knowing more about the subject of death, but they are generally shielded from such exposure. Many parents are reluctant to talk with their children about death because they wish to protect their children (and themselves) from the pain of loss. Young people are often prohibited from some hospital wards, health care institutions, and other places where people are dying. Such apparent secretiveness may result in fear or curiosity, and as a result of their lack of firsthand knowledge, young people tend to learn about death through the media, which can be confusing and misleading.

Sooner or later, students must confront death to understand the needs of the dying, to have some preparation for the experience, and to deal with their own feelings. Education about death is a legitimate subject for students. It is an important topic worthy of open, informed, and sensitive discussion. Death education can guide students toward greater understanding about death and dying, and, even though it might be painful for them and for the teacher, gaining such understanding can be essential for sound mental health.

In death education, the teacher should come to terms with his or her own feelings about death and not just learn the material. He or she needs to be aware of the students' willingness to express their feelings on this sensitive topic and be ready to let them discuss the subject openly and frankly. Never tell students they need to wait until they are older to talk about death. Many adults use this ploy as an excuse to avoid their own insecurities about death. Teachers need to answer any question at the students' level of understanding. The students' feelings and emotions related to death should also be allowed to be expressed in the classroom, even encouraged. Teachers can use experiences in the classroom, such as the death of a flower, a pet, or a classmate, to teach students about death feelings and rituals.

Chapter In Review

Summary

- Aging is a normal part of the life cycle, not a pathological condition. We are all aging every day.

- The number of elderly has risen sharply in the past two decades, and this trend is predicted to continue.

- The life expectancy for all Americans is increasing.

- The majority of older Americans still own their own homes, and fewer than 5 percent are institutionalized.

- Both intrinsic and extrinsic factors affect the aging process for each individual.

- Many biological, psychological, and sociological changes occur as a person ages. Some of these changes present unavoidable problems for the elderly, but successful adjustments can be made to other changes.

- Elderly Americans face many challenges in life, but these issues affect all members of society, not just the aged. Among these challenges are income, retirement, housing, health problems, nutrition, crime, and transportation.

- Some of the problems facing the elderly are the result of discrimination and misconceptions.

- Stereotypes about the elderly largely result from lack of knowledge and insufficient contact with the elderly.

- Intergenerational contact programs in schools can be one of the most effective ways to help students understand aging and the elderly, helping dissolve some of the many myths about aging.

- The elderly of the future will generally enjoy a better standard of living.

- Death is the natural end to life, yet many in our society try to deny its existence.

- Death is mysterious because we do not know what is beyond death.

- Many people fear death and refuse to discuss the topic openly and frankly.

- Everyone has personal beliefs about death. Some of these beliefs are helpful in facing death because they help demystify it.

- Facing death is a traumatic experience for both the dying person and survivors.

- The dying person has many emotional needs that often go unmet by relatives and the medical profession. This may leave the dying person feeling lonely and abandoned.

- An individual goes through various stages of adjustment to impending death. If we understand these stages, we can better help the dying person.

- Controversies and issues surround death, including the definition of death, the person's right to die, organ donation and transplants, wills, and suicide.

- Most young people in our society are not exposed to the dying process and lose relatively few individuals with whom they are close.

- Young people go through definite stages in their understanding of death.

- Young people are interested in knowing more about the subject of death. Thus, death education is a legitimate, worthy topic in schools.

Discussion Questions

1. Discuss the significance of aging education and death education in the school curriculum.

2. Describe the benefits of intergenerational contact.

3. Discuss the current demographics of the elderly in the United States.

4. Predict the lifestyle of the elderly in the United States in the year 2020.

5. Why do most people fear death?

6. How can the family help in the adjustment of a dying person?

7. Differentiate between grief, bereavement, and mourning.

8. Why is there more guilt associated with a death by suicide than with other types of deaths?

Critical Thinking Questions

1. Rate your personal health in relation to the aging process. In other words, what health skills and behaviors do you possess that will help you age in a healthy way?

2. What are three things that you consider most positive about getting older? What are three concerns you have about aging?

3. It is likely that you will be the primary caregiver for your parent or grandparent. What steps can you take now to prepare for this event?

4. Consider a situation in which you or a close relative have received a diagnosis of a terminal illness. What activities or tasks would you accomplish? What type of circumstances would you desire for your impending death?

5. Contemplate your own attitude toward death—is it negative or positive? What factors in your own life experiences have affected your attitude toward dying and death?

6. Some argue that without proper legislative controls, passive euthanasia may lead to active euthanasia. Propose several controls to prevent this from occurring.

7. Think about the most recent funeral you attended. How would you want your own funeral to be similar or different?

8. How would you design a suicide prevention program specifically for the age of the students you desire to teach?

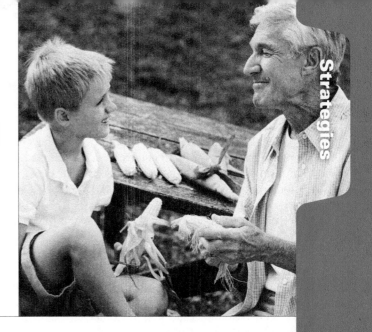

24 Strategies for Teaching about Aging, Dying, and Death

Valued Outcomes: Aging

After completion of this chapter, you should be able to convey the following to your students:

- Aging is a natural part of the life cycle.
- Exercise and proper diet can slow down the aging process to some degree.
- Most elderly people are healthy and alert.
- People use their retirement years for different activities from those done in preretirement times.
- Elderly people make positive contributions to society.
- Nutritional needs change as one ages.
- The elderly in the United States are often discriminated against.
- Many social agencies provide services for the elderly.

Valued Outcomes: Dying and Death

- Death is a natural end to the life cycle.
- Our society generally avoids the topics of death and dying in discussion and conscious thought.
- Dying people and the family of a dying person have special needs.
- Grief and bereavement naturally follow the death of a close friend or relative.
- Funeral and burial rituals have significant meaning in our society.
- There are ways to help a friend who is contemplating suicide to reconsider the action.
- Organ donation can be considered an "ultimate gift of life."

Reflections

Aging. As you teach about aging, have the students reflect upon the positive aspects (e.g., more experience, more confidence, more wisdom) of getting older.

   Death and Dying. As you teach about the rituals and customs of death and dying, consider how to use these strategies to help your students express their feelings about the customs. Ask them to reflect on how a positive attitude about the concepts of death and dying can enable them to add to the quality of their life and how they can help their friends and family develop positive feelings about these issues.

We need to present realistic and accurate information to students about aging, the aged, and death. Both the positive and the negative aspects of each should be examined.

NATIONAL HEALTH EDUCATION STANDARDS

1. Students will comprehend concepts related to health promotion and disease prevention to enhance health.

4. Students will demonstrate the ability to use interpersonal communication skills to enhance health and avoid or reduce health risks.

5. Students will demonstrate the ability to use decision-making skills to enhance health.

7. Students will demonstrate the ability to practice health-enhancing behaviors and avoid or reduce risks.

8. Students will demonstrate the ability to advocate for personal, family, and community health.

Introduction: Aging

The percentage of elderly adults in our population is growing extremely fast; therefore, the study of aging is becoming important to everyone. Our culture typically propagates ageism through inaccurate portrayals of elderly people in television, movies, and literature. These stereotypes are shared by young people in this country, primarily because of a lack of opportunity to learn about aging and the aged and through a lack of contact with older people. Young people often fear older people and the aging process.

We need to present realistic and accurate information to students about aging and the aged. This will allow students to decide for themselves what aging and the elderly are really like. When students are able to understand and develop healthy attitudes toward aging (including their own aging process), they will be able to live a higher-quality life as they grow older.

Introduction: Dying and Death

The death of a relative, close friend, or even a pet can be traumatic to people of all ages, including children. For this reason, some parents approach the problem by trying to shield their children from experiences related to dying

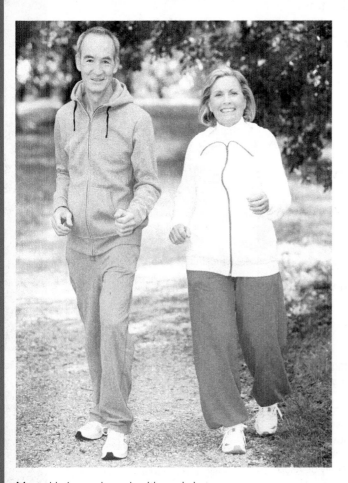

Most elderly people are healthy and alert.

and death. Rather than solving the problem, this avoidance leaves the child unprepared to face a natural part of the life cycle. Many children, though they may not have an accurate concept of death, want to know about the many aspects of life related to dying and death, such as funerals and cemeteries. Death education in the elementary schools can help meet this need. Its objectives are to allow students to clarify their values about death and dying, to provide factual information about the subject, and to encourage students to discuss openly the vital issues concerning the natural end of the life cycle.

Shown to the right of each activity title in this chapter is the suggested grade level(s) for which the activity might be appropriate. However, many of the suggested activities could be modified for use at various grade levels.

Information Assessment Activities: Aging

How Does It Feel to Be Old?   Grades K–3

Valued Outcome: Students will understand thoughts we associate with the word *old* and how they affect everyone around them (including themselves).

National Health Education Standard: 4

Description of Strategy: Draw a big circle on the board with the word *kids* in the center. Then draw lines coming from the outside of the circle in toward the word at the center. Ask the class what words they think of when they hear, see, or think the word *kids*. Write the words on the lines of the board. After about three minutes, ask the class how people think of young people their age. Ask how negative and positive attitudes have made them feel. Introduce ageism, a form of discrimination that places people in a limited position because of their age. Draw a second large circle with radiating lines on the board, and put the word *old* instead of *kids* in the center. After three minutes, ask the students how people think of old people and how they think negative and positive attitudes make older people feel.

Materials Needed: board and markers or overhead projector and pen

Processing Question: How do you feel about growing old?

✔ **Assessment:** Students will be able to state one positive and one negative attitude often felt toward kids and older adults.

Aging Voting   Grades K–5

Valued Outcome: Students will be able to determine for themselves if they agree with aging-related statements.

National Health Education Standard: 4

TEACHING IN ACTION | **Daily Lesson Plan**

Lesson Title: Physical Activity in Older Age

Date: April 30, 2012   **Time:** 1:00 P.M.   **Grade:** Three   **Teacher:** Kaplan

I. National Health Education Standards

Health Education Standard 1: Students will comprehend concepts related to health promotion and disease prevention to enhance health.

II. National Health Education Standards Performance Indicator

1.5.2 identify examples of emotional, intellectual, physical, and social health.

III. Valued Outcomes

- Students will describe feelings about exercise in older age.
- Students will witness seniors who are active and enjoy exercise.
- Students will see how achieving health is a lifelong process.

IV. Description of Strategy

1. With permission, go to a YMCA, senior center, or retirement community and film exercise classes for older adults. Choose several classes (e.g., water, weight training, or tai-chi), and then interview some seniors. Ask for their thoughts on exercise.
2. Ask students to write down their thoughts about exercise and the elderly. Ask students to describe how they envision senior exercise classes. Have students discuss what they wrote.
3. Show students the video of seniors exercising.
4. Ask students to write about the video and how it was similar to or different from what they imagined. Have students discuss their responses, feelings, and perceptions after seeing seniors exercise.
5. Explain that while some seniors have a hard time getting around, many seniors are still involved in exercise programs. Discuss how exercise in old age can improve quality of life.

V. Materials Needed

- video of seniors exercising
- paper/pencils

VI. Formative Evaluation

Benchmarks
- Level 1: Student was able to describe negative perceptions about senior exercise.
- Level 2: Student was able to describe negative perceptions about senior exercise and explain contradictions to this stereotype.
- Level 3: Student was able to describe negative perceptions about senior exercise and explain contradictions to this stereotype. Student listed reasons why some seniors still enjoy exercise.
- Level 4: Student was able to describe negative perceptions about senior exercise and explain contradictions to this stereotype. Student listed reasons why some seniors still enjoy exercise and discussed how exercise can improve quality of life.

VII. Points of Emphasis

1. Explain that there is a spectrum of activity levels among seniors.
2. Explain that because of better medicines and longer life spans, active seniors are becoming more common.
3. List other nonmedical things that seniors do to keep healthy.

Teacher Evaluation

1. Keep the lesson as taught?   yes _____ no _____

2. What I need to improve _____

3. Next time make sure _____

4. Strengths of lesson Strategies _____

TEACHING IN ACTION | **Daily Lesson Plan**

Lesson Title: Determining Causes of Death

Date: May 7, 2012   **Time:** 9:00 A.M.   **Grade:** Five   **Teacher:** Ali

I. National Health Education Standards

Health Education Standard 1: Students will comprehend concepts related to health promotion and disease prevention to enhance health.

II. National Health Education Standards Performance Indicator

1.5.1 describe the relationship between healthy behaviors and personal health.

III. Valued Outcomes

- Students will identify common diseases.
- Students will identify common death-causing diseases.
- Students will compare common causes of death in 2000 and 1900.

IV. Description of Strategy

1. Have students identify ten to fifteen diseases that may result in death. Write the causes on the board.
2. Describe the difference between infectious and degenerative diseases. Ask students to identify which diseases on the list are infectious and which are degenerative.
3. Show students a list of the most common causes of death in the United States in 2000 (available on the National Center for Health Statistics website). Now show students a similar list for the causes of death in the United States in 1900 and worldwide in 2000.
4. Compare causes of death in the United States between 1900 and 2000. Are any causes on both lists? Discuss why death causes have changed so much in only 100 years. Ask students if they see a shift in the infectious/degenerative disease ratio. If so, ask students to explain the change. Also ask why the U.S. list differs from the worldwide list in 2000.

V. Materials Needed

- board/marker
- lists of common causes of death from United States in 2000 and 1900 and worldwide in 2000

VI. Formative Evaluation

Benchmarks

- Level 1: Student was able to list some common causes of death.
- Level 2: Student was able to list and compare common causes of death in 2000 and 1900.
- Level 3: Student was able to list and compare common causes of death in 2000 and 1900. Student was able to describe the difference between infectious and degenerative diseases.
- Level 4: Student was able to list and compare common causes of death in 2000 and 1900. Student was able to describe the difference between infectious and degenerative diseases and explain how causes of death have changed over time.

VII. Points of Emphasis

1. Explain some of the risk factors for potentially fatal diseases.
2. Explain how some of the diseases could be prevented by healthier lifestyles.
3. Explain how some nonfatal health problems can accumulate to become fatal diseases.

Teacher Evaluation

1. Keep the lesson as taught?   yes _____ no _____

2. What I need to improve _____

3. Next time make sure _____

4. Strengths of lesson _____

Description of Strategy: Have students vote by raising their hands if they agree or disagree with the following statements about aging:

- Good health habits may affect the length of your life.
- Having good health habits always means that you are going to live longer than people with bad health habits.
- Bad health habits can shorten the life span.
- It is important to develop good health habits in order to be able to enjoy more years of life.
- Retirement is the worst part about growing old.
- Grandparents are fun to be around.
- Growing old makes a person wiser.
- Growing old is a normal part of life.
- Old people are not very bright.

Materials Needed: list of statements

Processing Question: What factors determine your attitudes about growing old?

✓ **Assessment:** Students will be able to state at least two true statements about how health behavior can affect aging.

Rank-Ordering
Grades 3–5

Valued Outcome: Students will be able to decide which qualities associated with aging they most desire.

National Health Education Standard: 4

Description of Strategy: Prepare a list of positive qualities often associated with aging. After discussing these qualities, have students individually rank each in order of importance. Follow with a discussion of why some students feel certain qualities are more desirable than others. Note the importance of individual preferences. Tell students to number each of the following items from 1 to 5. Have them use 1 to show the quality or condition about becoming older that appeals to them the most, 2 for the second most appealing quality or condition, and so on.

__ retirement
__ wisdom
__ grandchildren
__ leisure time
__ satisfaction

Materials Needed: overhead or handout for each student with list of positive aspects of aging

Processing Question: Why are some qualities associated with aging more desired than others?

✓ **Assessment:** Students will be able to state the top three most appealing aspects of older adulthood and explain why they are appealing.

Sentence Completion
Grades 3–5

Valued Outcome: Students will be able to complete statements related to aging.

National Health Education Standard: 4

Description of Strategy: Create a handout from the sentences shown below. Instruct students to complete each sentence on the handout by writing down their immediate reaction to the statement. Point out that statements should be honest, even if some are negative. After the exercise, discuss the responses on a volunteer basis. Note varying points of view and discuss possible reasons for these opinions. After the discussion, pass out another copy of the handout for students to fill out and see how their answers may be different.

1. Aging is _____.
2. Growing old is _____.
3. My grandparents are _____.
4. Retirement from full-time work is _____.
5. I think that old people are _____.

Materials Needed: handouts with sentences and pencils for each student

Processing Question: Are your immediate responses the same as they were after you thought about the statement for awhile?

✓ **Assessment:** Students will be able to state one positive and one negative attitude they have about aging.

Aging Collage
Grades 3–5

Valued Outcomes: The students will be able to communicate the changes they have gone through as they have grown, and to use software to make and illustrate a collage.

National Health Education Standards: 2, 3

Description of Strategy: After the introduction of an information session on how everyone ages, assign students homework: Each should gather pictures of themselves at different ages since birth. (Note: Their parents or guardians may prefer to provide scans or copies instead of original photos.) Students should use a computer program (such as KidPix) to create a collage of their lives, showing how they have changed as they have grown. For example, students can divide a page into several blocks, with a picture of themselves at a different age in each block; they can then type in labels or captions in each box to describe themselves at that particular age. Descriptions could include physical differences (taller? different haircut?) or changes in their interests or friend groups. Print the collages and discuss again how everyone ages. Use the collages for display in class.

Materials Needed: group of photos of each student, access to a computer and presentation software, access to Internet or software program with pictures, access to a scanner (to scan photos) and a color printer

Processing Question: How can technology be used to illustrate a health concept?

✓ **Assessment:** The students will be evaluated on their understanding of changes that occur during aging, and on setting up and illustrating the collage.

Source: Adapted from Wacona Elementary School 2003. www.wacona.com/kidpix/kidpix.html.

Value Voting   Grades 4–5

Valued Outcome: Students will be able to verbalize their bioethical values regarding death-related issues.

National Health Education Standard: 4

Description of Strategy: Present a series of controversial statements such as those shown below to your class. Explain that each statement represents the way some people feel about death-related issues, then ask students to raise their hands if they basically agree with the stance or to keep their hands down if they disagree. After each show of hands, allow students who wish to comment on the statement to do so. Follow the activity with a general discussion of issues that came up.

- Euthanasia is murder.
- Euthanasia is a peaceful way to die.
- Euthanasia is murder only if the patient is conscious.

Materials Needed: list of statements

Processing Question: Why is euthanasia (or other topic discussed in class) such a controversial issue?

✓ **Assessment:** Students will be able to state their position on the controversial issue and give two supporting reasons why they feel the way they do.

Information Assessment Activities: Dying and Death

Values Statements   Grades K–5

Valued Outcome: Students will be able to clarify their values regarding death.

National Health Education Standard: 4

Description of Strategy: Have the students complete each of the statements about death on Worksheet 24.1 (page 503) with their immediate reaction to the statement. Point out that statements should be honest, even if some are negative. Afterward, discuss how different individuals react and feel about each issue raised in the statements.

Materials Needed: Worksheet 24.1 and pencils for all students

Processing Question: What events in your life have determined your attitudes about death?

✓ **Assessment:** Students will be able to explain how they feel about death.

Personal Views on Suicide   Grades 4–5

Valued Outcome: Students will be able to clarify their values regarding suicide.

National Health Education Standard: 4

Description of Strategy: Have students answer and discuss these questions in class or give them a handout of the questions:

1. Do you feel that an individual has the right to make the ultimate decision as to whether he or she should live or die?
2. What would you do if a friend said to you, "I think I might commit suicide—would you help me?"
   a. call the police
   b. do nothing
   c. ask why
   d. call a doctor
   e. send my friend away with the statement "Sorry, but I can't help you."
   f. try to help by talking to him or her
3. What do you feel might be one possible answer to suicide prevention?

Materials Needed: list of questions or handout

Processing Question: Why do some people feel more strongly about suicide as opposed to other types of deaths?

✓ **Assessment:** Students will be able to state how they would respond to a friend or family member who threatened to commit suicide.

On Living and Dying   Grades 4–5

Valued Outcome: Students will be able to decide if death-related ideas are acceptable to them.

National Health Education Standard: 4

Description of Strategy: Have students look over the various statements on a handout created from the following list. Have the students ask themselves, "Would this idea be acceptable or unacceptable to me?"

Rating Scale: Death, Dying, and Living
1 = very acceptable   2 = acceptable   3 = unsure
4 = unacceptable   5 = not acceptable at all

__ being killed in an auto accident
__ living forever

__ dying slowly
__ dying of cancer
__ being saved through medical help but unable to walk again
__ being able to choose when you will die
__ living to age 110
__ dying before your spouse
__ dying after your spouse dies
__ choosing how you will die

Materials Needed: handouts with statements and pencils for each student

Processing Question: Why should we consider our own deaths?

✓ **Assessment:** Students will be able to list two death-related statements that make them uncomfortable, and discuss why this is the case.

Decision Story: Aging

(Follow the procedures outlined in Chapter 4 on pages 60–62 for presenting decision stories.)

For each of the decision stories, write a list on the board of ideas generated by the class for how each situation should be dealt with. Ask the students to discuss the merits of the methods suggested.

✓ **Assessment for Decision Stories:** Students can identify health-enhancing behaviors and exhibit positive decision-making skills.

Going for a Visit   Grades K–5

Maya's grandparents live in a retirement village in another state. Her family is going to fly there for a visit next month, but Maya doesn't want to go. She visited her grandparents a few years ago, when she was younger. She remembers that there was nothing for her to do at her grandparents' home. There were no other kids around, and her grandparents made such a fuss over her. They were nice, but they treated her like a baby. Maya doesn't like that, and she wishes her grandparents would realize that she is growing up.

Focus Question: What should Maya do?

National Health Education Standard: 5

Decision Stories: Dying and Death

A Gift of Life   Grades 3–5

Loretta is dying of kidney disease. She knows it and has accepted her coming death. Now her doctors would like to use her heart in a transplant operation. They tell her that her heart could be used to help another person live. Loretta isn't sure about the matter.

Focus Question: What should Loretta do?

National Health Education Standard: 5

Sally's Grief   Grades 3–5

Valued Outcome: The students will be able to use information from the following decision story and produce and deliver a PowerPoint presentation to their classmates.

National Health Education Standards: 2, 3

Description of Strategy: After the introduction of the following decision story to the class, the students (singly or in assigned groups of two to three students) will use Microsoft PowerPoint or a similar presentation program to develop each aspect of the decision story and the decision they reached. Each slide should be illustrated by an appropriate picture related to that aspect of the decision story. The presentations can be narrated live or recorded beforehand.

"Sally's Grief"

The mother of Maki's best friend, Sally, died in an automobile accident. Sally had not called Maki yet, but Maki knew that she needed to talk to Sally. She had heard that Sally was not coping with her mother's death very well. Maki also wanted to see Sally, but she was unsure of what to say or do once she saw Sally.

Focus questions:

1. How long should Maki wait before she calls Sally?
2. What should she say when she calls Sally?

Materials Needed: a computer with Internet access, presentation software and a source for pictures, in-class projector or other method of viewing completed presentations

Processing Question: How can technology be used to convey methods for dealing with grief to students?

✓ **Additional Assessment:** The students will be evaluated on thoughtful creation of the presentation and delivery of the presentation to the class.

Dramatizations: Aging

Elderly Puppet Show   Grades K–2

Valued Outcome: Students will be able to describe physical attributes of the elderly.

National Health Education Standard: 1

Description of Strategy: Have three students enact the following: A young boy and girl set out on a hike in the morning and come to a bridge. An old troll there is angered by their presence and casts a spell on them to make them "old for a day." They examine themselves and find the following traits, which they discuss with each other: wrinkled skin with age spots, gray hair (boy becomes bald), inability to move quickly, lack of strength, and shortness of breath on their hike.

Materials Needed: five puppets (young boy, young girl, old troll, old man, old woman), puppet bridge

Processing Question: What physical effects occur during the aging process?

✓ **Assessment:** Students will be able to list three physical changes that occur with aging.

Grandparents and Grandchildren   Grades K–5

Valued Outcome: Students will be able to discuss relationships with grandparents.

National Health Education Standard: 4

Description of Strategy: Assign several students to role-play a situation involving grandchildren and grandparents. The roles will be grandfather, grandmother, mother, father, sister, and brother. The scene is a visit from the grandparents. The dad will ask the children to remain at home for the day and visit with the grandparents. One child will be instructed to play the role with a lot of enthusiasm, while the other child will resent being made to stay home because of missing the afternoon playing with friends.

Processing Questions:

1. How should a child relate to grandparents—with enthusiasm or resentment?
2. Do you have any meaningful relationships with an older or elderly person?

✓ **Assessment:** Students will be able to explain at least three benefits of spending time with grandparents.

Now I Am Old   Grades 3–5

Valued Outcome: Students will be able to differentiate between an active and an inactive retirement lifestyle.

National Health Education Standards: 1, 7

Description of Strategy: Have two volunteers role-play situations in which two elderly retirees are planning the day's activities. One situation could include two retirees who are very active, and another could involve two retirees who are inactive. Follow up the activity by asking the students with which of the characters they most identified.

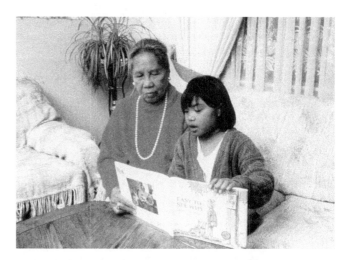

Good relationships with grandparents can enhance a child's life.

Processing Questions:

1. What activities might an active older adult include in his or her day?
2. What activities might an inactive older adult include in his or her day?
3. Which lifestyle do you think is healthier? Why?

○ **Integration:** Physical Activity (students can act out the active activities they list in the role-play)

✓ **Assessment:** Students will be able to list at least two activities that active older adults might participate in and explain why an active lifestyle is healthier than an inactive lifestyle.

Dramatizations: Dying and Death

Suicide   Grades 4–5

Valued Outcome: Students will be able to discuss ways to help a suicidal friend.

National Health Education Standard: 8

Description of Strategy: Have two students role-play that one friend is calling the other to tell him or her that their best friend just attempted suicide by taking an overdose of pills. Let the students bring the role-play to closure by discussing ways they can help their mutual friend.

Processing Question: How can a person untrained in suicide prevention help a suicidal friend?

✓ **Assessment:** Students will able to describe what they would say or do to help a suicidal friend.

Talk Can Help   Grades 4–5

Valued Outcome: Students will be able to describe how to visit a friend who is dying in the hospital.

National Health Education Standard: 4

Description of Strategy: Have one student play the role of a dying patient in a hospital. Have another play the role of a close friend who comes to visit. Role-play the situation for five minutes per pair of students. Ask each student to play the part in the way that seems most comfortable and natural. Have the students switch roles so all will have the opportunity to play the dying patient. Discuss the different approaches used in acting out this situation.

Materials Needed: bed for "dying" patient

Processing Question: What should one say when visiting a dying friend in the hospital?

✓ **Assessment:** Students will demonstrate how they would respond to a friend or family member in the hospital and explain their feelings about the situation.

Only One Week to Live   Grades 4–5

Valued Outcome: Students will be able to discuss what they would consider most important in their lives if they were facing death.

National Health Education Standard: 4

Description of Strategy: Have volunteers act out their responses when asked what they would do if they had only one week to live. This activity could be spontaneous, or you could allow the volunteers some time to think about the activities and list them.

Processing Questions:

1. What activities would you want to spend time doing if you knew you had only a week to live?
2. What would you worry less about if you knew you had a week to live?
3. How does facing death affect our outlook on life?

✓ **Assessment:** Students will be able to explain how imminent death would change their priorities.

Discussion and Report Techniques: Aging

Age, Dying, and Death   Grades K–2

Valued Outcome: Students will be able to identify and list physical characteristics of aging.

National Health Education Standard: 1

Description of Strategy: Introduce the lesson by talking to students about people they know who are older. Let them raise their hands and tell about the person they know. Ask questions such as: "Do the people you just talked about look different from you? Of course, they do because they are older. But how can we tell someone is older just by looking at them?" Let them respond. Give each student a piece of paper and markers or crayons. Have students divide the paper into four sections. In the corner of each square, write 10, 20, 40, and 60.

Example of table:

10	20
40	60

In each square, have the students draw a picture of themselves and how they think they will look at each age.

Point out that aging is not something that happens only to elderly people, but rather something that happens to everyone all the time, beginning at birth. Go over some factors related to aging, including sex, race, personality, genetics, and education. Let students share which attribute of aging they would least want (e.g., wrinkles, gray hair, etc.). Say in closing: "Today we learned that many factors cause us to age in different ways. Whether it is our personality or our genetics or other attributes, we all will age and all end up looking different from the way we do now. However, aging is a normal process, and we can learn a lot from it." Tell students to try and ask a few people older than them to show them a picture of themselves when they were younger and compare how they looked then to how they look now.

Materials Needed: markers or crayons and paper for each student

Processing Questions:

1. What factors can affect how we age?
2. What are some things that will change about our bodies as we age?

○ **Integration:** Art

✓ **Assessment:** Students will be able to state at least two physical changes of aging and one factor that affects how we age.

Life Collage   Grades K–5

Valued Outcome: Students will create and present a visual representation of their lives from birth to present.

National Health Education Standard: 4

Description of Strategy: Have students bring in items from home that are special to them and that they feel help explain who they are. Encourage them to bring things from their early childhood as well as newer things. Stress that items should be small enough to be glued or taped to poster board. (Students may also bring items to display with their poster if they don't want to tape or glue them.) Distribute magazines, and have students cut out anything that relates to their life up to the present (toys they have or had, baby for sibling). Remind them only to cut out things that already apply to them, not things they hope for in the future. Have students glue or tape items to their poster board. When they have finished, have students explain how the things they chose are significant to their life.

Materials Needed: magazines, personal items, poster board, glue, tape, and scissors for each student

Processing Questions:

1. Why is it important to include items from your early childhood?
2. What part of your collage best represents who you are? Why?

○ **Integration:** Art

✓ **Assessment:** Students will be able to explain the significance to their lives of at least five items.

Quality Time with Elderly Friends or Relatives
Grades 2–5

Valued Outcome: Students will be able to relate a positive experience with an elderly person.

National Health Education Standard: 4

Description of Strategy: Have students write a paragraph on the best time they have spent with a grandparent or elderly friend. Have volunteers share the essay with the class.

Materials Needed: paper and pens or pencils for each student

Processing Question: What type of positive experiences can a young person have with an elderly person?

○ **Integration:** Writing

✓ **Assessment:** Students will be able to state three benefits of having a close relationship with an older adult.

Challenges Facing the Elderly
Grades 4–5

Valued Outcome: Students will be able to discuss the social and emotional problems faced by elderly people.

National Health Education Standard: 1

Description of Strategy: Divide the class into small groups, and have each group research a problem area for elderly Americans. These areas should include health problems, financial problems, problems due to stereotypes and misconceptions, forced retirement, crime, and loneliness. After research is complete, have each group present a panel discussion of their findings. Group

members should be prepared to answer questions from the class about the problem area that they have researched. Finally, have students complete Worksheet 24.2 on page 504.

Materials Needed: research books, computers with Internet access, worksheet for each student

Processing Questions:

1. What health problems do elderly people face?
2. What social problems do elderly people face?
3. What financial problems do elderly people face?

✓ **Assessment:** Students will be able to state three reasons why the problem they research exists and three possible solutions to the problem.

Services for the Elderly
Grades 6–8

Valued Outcome: Students will be able to explain how the Social Security program benefits the elderly.

National Health Education Standard: 1

Description of Strategy: Ask a member of a local Social Security office to come to class and explain the Social Security system provided to elderly people, or have students research the Social Security program and present a lecture on it.

Materials Needed: materials on the Social Security system (if students do research in lieu of a presenter)

Processing Questions:

1. How does the Social Security program benefit elderly people?
2. How does an elderly person become involved in this program?
3. What was the original intent of the Social Security system? Has it accomplished its goal?
4. What potential problems does the system face in the future?

○ **Integration:** Social Studies

✓ **Assessment:** Students will be able to accurately describe the purpose of the Social Security system and how older adults can participate.

Fountain of Youth
Grades 4–5

Valued Outcome: Students will be able to discuss the implications of having a population that never grew old and died.

National Health Education Standards: 1, 4

Description of Strategy: Have students debate whether a fountain of youth would be good or bad for humans.

Processing Questions:

1. What if everyone stayed young and did not die?
2. What implications for overpopulation would there be if no one died?

✓ **Assessment:** Students will be able to state and explain three potential problems of overpopulation.

The Elderly in the Media   Grades 4–5

Valued Outcome: Students will be able to compare the media's view of the elderly with their own view.

National Health Education Standard: 4

Description of Strategy: Have students watch television programs, newscasts, and commercials and look through magazines and newspapers. Have them write comments about whether the media's portrayal of older people is consistent with their own view of the elderly.

Materials Needed: television, magazines, newspapers, paper and pencils

Processing Questions:

1. What are the similarities between the media's portrayal of the elderly and yours?
2. What are the differences between the media's portrayal of the elderly and your perceptions?
3. Do you think your perception of the elderly has been influenced by the media?

✓ **Assessment:** Students will be able to compare and contrast their perceptions of older adults with how older adults are portrayed in the media.

The Science of Aging   Grades 6–8

Valued Outcome: Students learn how scientists study aging by reviewing experiments on the effect of caloric reduction.

National Health Education Standard: 1

Description of Strategy: Ask the following questions to stimulate discussion from the class:

- Why do you think people have always been so fascinated with trying to stay young?
- Do you think you can have any control over how you age?
- What factors do you think may have an effect on how long people live? (Remember to consider both emotional as well as physical factors. Factors may include nutrition, economic conditions, environmental conditions, a positive attitude, and genetics.)

- What types of studies do you think scientists would use to determine if there was a relationship between these factors and aging? (Cross-sectional and longitudinal studies of populations of humans and of animals may be used. Cross-sectional studies compare different subgroups within a large group of humans or animals at one point in time, and longitudinal studies compare a group to itself at different points in time.)
- How might nutrition affect aging? How might scientists study the effects of nutrition on aging?

Have students write an answer to the following questions:

- What can we learn about the aging process by studying humans directly?
- What can we learn from studying the aging processes of other animals?
- How might that apply to humans?

Materials Needed: pencils or pens and paper for each student

Processing Question: What health behaviors affect how you age?

○ **Integration:** Science

✓ **Assessment:** Students will be able to accurately describe how scientific experiments on humans and animals can impact our understanding of the aging process.

Source: Science NetLinks 2002

Caloric Comparison   Grades 4–5

Valued Outcome: Students will be able to describe the different nutritional needs and caloric requirements of a person their age and an elderly person.

National Health Education Standard: 1

Description of Strategy: Discuss and show in graphic form the caloric needs of a person your students' age. Then, do the same for an elderly person. Have the students compare the differences and brainstorm why the differences exist.

Materials Needed: charts on caloric needs for elementary students and for elderly persons

Processing Questions:

1. How will your caloric needs differ as you age?
2. How will you need to modify your habits to accommodate this change and still remain healthy?

✓ **Assessment:** Students will be able to give three reasons why older adults have lower caloric needs than elementary school students.

Discussion and Report Techniques: Dying and Death

Dying: True/False
Grades K–5

Valued Outcome: Students will better understand dying.

National Health Education Standard: 1

Description of Strategy: Write on the board the following facts and have students determine whether they are true or false.

- Mature individuals often find themselves unable to cope with the thought of death.
- Individuals generally choose to ignore death.
- When death is brought up in conversation, it is usually in the form of a joke.

Engage the class in a round-robin to discuss the responses.

Materials Needed: board and markers or overhead projector and pen

Processing Question: Why is our society considered a death-denying society?

✔ **Assessment:** Students will demonstrate the ability to discuss reasons why the topic of death makes people uncomfortable.

My Pet Died
Grades K–5

Valued Outcome: Students will be able to describe the experience of having a pet die.

National Health Education Standard: 4

Description of Strategy: Most students have had pets that died—dogs, cats, hamsters, fish, or other small animals. Ask students who have had the experience of having a pet die to draw a picture or write a short report about the event. The reports should emphasize the things about the pet that the child liked most. Explain that we can remember those qualities and talk about the pleasure or companionship of a past pet, even though the pet will never return to us. Note the comfort that such fond memories can bring.

Materials Needed: paper, pens or pencils, markers or crayons for each student

Processing Question: Why should we recall qualities of pets that have died?

○ **Integration:** Art, Writing

✔ **Assessment:** Students will be able to discuss how losing a pet made them feel.

How It Felt to Go to a Funeral
Grades 3–5

Valued Outcome: Students will demonstrate, through artistic expression, what they think a funeral is.

National Health Education Standard: 4

Description of Strategy: Allow students to tell stories about a funeral they have attended or what they think a funeral involves, using felt boards with felt cutout figures and objects that represent things associated with funerals (such as flowers, religious symbols, cemeteries, coffins, and so on). Offer each child an opportunity to create a story about being at the funeral home, the funeral or memorial service, the cemetery, or the family gathering after the funeral.

Materials Needed: felt board and cutouts

Processing Questions:

1. What do you associate with funeral experiences?
2. Are they positive or negative things? Why?

✔ **Assessment:** Students will be able to describe what happens at a funeral.

The Five Stages of Grief
Grades 5–8

Valued Outcome: Students will see that adjusting to dying and understanding the five stages of grief are critical to understanding the needs of a dying person.

National Health Education Standard: 1

Description of Strategy: Create a handout from the list below. Give the following directions to the students: "There are five stages of grief, and they are listed on your handout out of order. Please put the stages in order by placing the number of the stage beside the sentence where it belongs."

____ **Depression**—the patient is saddened by the fact that death is approaching and then starts the grief process for the losses death will entail.

____ **Denial and isolation**—learning of the diagnosis of a terminal condition, the patient reacts with disbelief.

____ **Bargaining**—the patient is accepting the inevitability of death and begins to bargain (with God or others) for more time.

____ **Anger**—the reality of impending death begins to seep into the patient's consciousness, and anger is the reaction.

____ **Acceptance or resolution**—the patient resolves the issue of death.

Materials Needed: handouts with descriptions of stages and pencils for each student

Processing Question: Why is it important for each of us to understand the stages of grief?

✔ **Assessment:** Students will be able to correctly list and describe the five stages of grief.

Mourning and Funerals Grades 4–5

Valued Outcome: Students will be able to describe ways of dealing with the grief process. They will write about their experiences with funerals.

National Health Education Standards: 1, 4

Description of Strategy: Introduce the topics of death and grieving by asking students about their feelings when something bad happens. Discuss the words *grief* and *mourning*. Ask students to help figure out these words. (Grief is sorrow, mental distress, emotional agitation, sadness, suffering, and related feelings caused by death. Mourning involves culturally defined acts that are usually performed when death occurs.)

Talk about ways to deal with grief. Students may tell how they deal with grief (reading, talking about it, etc.). Talk about mourning rituals (funerals, memorial services, etc.). Allow students to act out a funeral. Close by saying that grief is acceptable and can be coped with using a variety of techniques. You may wish to repeat coping strategies that the students identified during the discussion.

Processing Questions:

1. What is the difference between grief and mourning?
2. What is the purpose of a funeral?

✔ **Assessment:** Students will be able to describe at least two different mourning rituals and explain how these rituals help people grieve.

Why Should I Have a Will? Grades 4–5

Valued Outcome: Students will be able to explain why every adult should have a will.

National Health Education Standard: 8

Description of Strategy: Discuss with the class the reasons for having a will. Describe the format of the will. Have the students prepare wills for themselves, with two classmates acting as witnesses to sign the document. Have students list their important possessions and the people to whom they would like to bequeath these things.

Materials Needed: paper and pencils for each student

Processing Questions:

1. What is the purpose of a will?
2. Who should have a will?
3. How can a will be beneficial when someone dies?

✔ **Assessment:** Students will be able to accurately describe the purpose of a will and give examples of what a will might say.

Organ and Tissue Donation Grades 4–5

Valued Outcome: Students will be able to identify organs or tissues that can be transplanted after death and will write out their feelings on transplantation.

National Health Education Standard: 1

Description of Strategy: Introduce the topic of organ and tissue donation by saying: "We have talked about death and many issues surrounding it. We know death can be very sad. However, today we are going to discuss a way that it can be very positive. Even when people die, they can help others. They can do this by organ donation." Ask the students if they know what organ donation is, and give them time to answer or figure it out. Then explain organ donation. If someone dies, everything in his or her body doesn't immediately stop working. Therefore, doctors can perform surgery to remove certain parts and give them to other people. "The doctor takes one thing from someone and gives it to someone else. We call this transplantation." Explain why we need organ donations for research and dissection in medical schools, and for sick people who can be cured with a new organ. Their body may accept the organ as their own, and they will be able to function normally, at least for a while. Discuss the following organs and tissues and their purposes:

eyes (corneas)
kidneys
pituitary glands
heart
liver
skin
pancreas
cartilage
bone marrow
lungs
bones (including ear bones, or ossicles)

Talk about the circumstances of an organ or tissue transplant. Tell the students that a potential donor usually must die in a hospital, and the organ removal surgery is performed soon afterward (e.g., a heart must be transplanted within four to five hours of the donor's death). Sometimes living people can donate organs or tissues, such as a kidney (everyone has two), a lobe of their liver (what is left of the liver will regrow), and bone marrow or blood (both of which are replaced by the body). Also, the donor must be eighteen years old or older (anyone under eighteen must have a parent's or guardian's signature). The donor and the recipient do not usually know each other, since the organ or tissue typically goes to someone on a transplant waiting list.

Finally, close by saying: "Today we learned about organ and tissue donation and how it can help people. We learned about organs and tissues that can be donated. We can now see how much medical technology is important." Give students an outline of the body with cutouts of each organ and have them glue onto the body which organs they would donate.

Materials Needed: handout with outline of the body and cutouts of each organ and glue for each student

Processing Questions:

1. How has technology in the medical field helped many people?
2. How can a person die and still help people?

✓ **Assessment:** Students will be able to list three organs or tissues that can be donated and explain why organ and tissue donation is important.

Why People Die   Grades 5–8

Valued Outcome: Students will be able to discuss why people die and how they can express themselves in a healthy fashion when a relative or someone close to them dies.

National Health Education Standard: 4

Description of Strategy: Begin by asking students why people die and in what ways people can live longer today. Divide the class into groups and talk about why people get older and what types of people live the longest. Have the students share their responses with their group, and then, as a group, have them make a poster with the best answers from their group (or any other answer their group comes up with). Have them include a written description and a picture on the poster to help give a mental image of their answers. Hang up their posters around the room, and then have each group look at the other group posters to see how their poster differed from those of other groups.

Make a class poster and have the students come up with different responses and explain them to the class. Hang the class poster outside the room in the hallway for others to see. Tell students that people who are good to their bodies, who eat right, exercise, and don't drink and smoke are likely to live longer. People who die at an early age often do so because they did not take care of their body. This includes drinking while driving, smoking, eating nonnutritious snacks and fatty foods, and not exercising. Have students share any stories that they may have about people they know who have died, and why they have died. (This has to been done very carefully without upsetting anyone, so let the students know that they don't have to share their story if they don't want to do so.)

Materials Needed: poster board, markers, tape, and pens or pencils for each student

Processing Questions:

1. Why do people die?
2. What makes a person live longer?

○ **Integration:** Art

✓ **Assessment:** Students will be able to name at least three lifestyle behaviors that can increase the risk of earlier death and explain three behaviors that can help increase life expectancy.

Experiments and Demonstrations: Aging

Last Year's Clothing   Grades K–5

Valued Outcome: Students will be able to discuss how they are aging and the implications of the aging process for them.

National Health Education Standards: 1, 4

Description of Strategy: Have students bring in articles of clothing that they wore a year earlier and try them on. Use this activity as a springboard for a discussion of growth and aging. Note that the process is a continuum and a normal part of the life cycle.

Materials Needed: clothing (brought in by students)

Processing Questions:

1. Why do we grow as we age?
2. Is aging a positive part of the life cycle?

✓ **Assessment:** Students will be able to discuss the concept of physical growth and explain why it occurs.

Aging in Humans   Grades K–5

Valued Outcome: Students will be able to describe how the aging process affects a person's facial features.

National Health Education Standards: 1, 4

Description of Strategy: Bring in photographs of a well-known person taken over a period of many years. Have the students note the aging process in the person's features from year to year.

Materials Needed: photographs of a person taken at several stages of his or her life

Processing Question: How do a person's features change as he or she ages?

✓ **Assessment:** Students will be able to identify and describe at least two facial features that change with age.

Life Cycle of a Frog   Grades 3–5

Valued Outcome: Students will observe and record the stages in the life cycle of a frog.

National Health Education Standard: 1

Description of Strategy: Order tadpoles for the classroom, and place them in a shallow, clear container. Explain the different stages of a frog's life (growing back legs, growing front legs, losing tail). When the tadpoles start to go through the first noticeable change, have students observe and record these changes in their journals. They may either write the information or draw a picture. Have students repeat this procedure for each stage in the life cycle until the tadpoles have all lost their tails.

Materials Needed: tadpoles, container, and journals and pencils for each student

Processing Questions:

1. How long did it take for the tadpoles to start growing their back legs?
2. What is the very first stage in a frog's life?

○ **Integration:** Science

✓ **Assessment:** Students will be able to describe at least three changes that occur in the frog's body as it ages.

Puzzles and Games: Aging

Aging Word Search   Grades 4–5

Valued Outcome: Students will be able to find specific aging-related words in a word search.

National Health Education Standard: 1

Description of Strategy: Provide students with a word search activity handout. Instruct the students to find the aging-related words in the puzzle.

Materials Needed: worksheet for each student, pencils

Processing Question: How many social issues facing the elderly can you find in the word search?

✓ **Assessment:** Students will be able to define at least ten of the words they find in the word search.

Other Ideas: Aging

Adopt a Grandparent   Grades K–5

Valued Outcome: Students will be able to develop a meaningful, positive relationship with an elderly friend.

National Health Education Standards: 4, 7

Description of Strategy: Have the class choose (possibly with the cooperation of the local senior citizens' group) an elderly person(s) as an adoptive grandparent. The class could invite the elderly person to class for special occasions, such as birthdays, art projects, storytime, and so forth.

Processing Question: How can a positive relationship with an elderly person enhance the quality of a child's life?

✓ **Assessment:** Students will be able to state two ways that a friendship with an older adult would be beneficial.

Elderly Health Fair   Grades 4–5

Valued Outcome: The student will be able to discuss the talents of elderly people.

National Health Education Standard: 4

Description of Strategy: Have the students plan a health fair designed for the elderly. Provide health screening services and information about health services in the community. Present arts and crafts made by the elderly. This is a great opportunity for the students to interact with the elderly and acquire an appreciation for the talents of another generation.

Materials Needed: arts and crafts made by elderly people, brochures and pamphlets about health services available in the community for the elderly

Processing Question: How can younger people appreciate the talents of the elderly?

✓ **Assessment:** Students will be able to contribute at least two ideas for items to exhibit at the health fair and discuss why these items would be useful.

What Was It Like Then?   Grades K–4

Valued Outcome: Students will be able to explain how society during an elderly person's childhood was different from today's society.

National Health Education Standards: 1, 4

Description of Strategy: Present a living American heritage lesson to your students. Have an older person in the community report on past lifestyles and historic moments for your community. Individuals might speak about their memories of the moon landing, the women's liberation movement, the civil rights movement, the Vietnam War, the rise of technology, their first exposure to the Internet, or what the world was like before cell phones and computers.

Processing Question: How was the world different when today's older people were young?

✓ **Assessment:** Students will be able to describe one thing they learned about what the world was like before they were born.

Other Ideas: Dying and Death

Poetry
Grades 4–5

Valued Outcome: Students will be able to compose a poem about dying and death.

National Health Education Standard: 4

Description of Strategy: Some of the greatest works of poetry in literature concern death and dying. Find short poems about death that are appropriate to the level of your class, and read them aloud. Discuss the meaning of each poem. Have the students write poems of their own on aspects of death and dying. The students could use a computer program to assemble their poetry into a pamphlet or book that can be reproduced for each member of the class. Various computer programs (such as KidPix) could be used to include illustrations or to add visual embellishments to their poems.

Materials Needed: poems about death and dying

Processing Question: Why do so many poems have dying and death as a central message?

○ **Integration:** Writing

✓ **Assessment:** Students will be able to say what they like about a poem they heard and describe how it made them feel.

Field Trip to a Nursing Home
Grades 3–5

Valued Outcomes: The students will (1) begin to understand the concept of a nursing home and the limitations that aging can put on elderly people and (2) be able to make and deliver to their classmates an audio/video documentary of a field trip to a nursing home.

National Health Education Standard: 3

Description of Strategy: Set up a field trip to a nursing home; be certain to communicate that you want the students to videotape during the visit. Divide the students into groups of four to five; each group will need to have access to and learn how to use a video camera and a computer-related recording program prior to the trip. Assign students specific responsibilities on the aspects of the field trip they are to report on. Documentary topics could include a focus on the assistance elderly people need to do everyday activities; the different jobs of the staff who work there; the safety precautions present in the nursing home; or the stories told by elderly people the students meet. During the field trip, each group is responsible for videotaping their assigned aspect of the field trip. During the next few days in class, the groups will add the audio portion to the video, and then the groups will deliver their field trip-related presentation to the class.

Materials Needed: video camera available to each group; access to computer recording program (e.g., Garage Band or GoldWave)

Processing Question: How can technology be used to deliver messages to students about aging and the elderly?

✓ **Assessment:** Students will be evaluated on each phase of the project: 1) video, 2) audio, and 3) presentation of the documentary to the class; they will also be evaluated on their behavior during the field trip and understanding of their documentary topic.

What Does a Funeral Director Do?
Grades 4–5

Valued Outcome: Students will be able to discuss the funeral arrangements that need to be made when a family member dies.

National Health Education Standards: 1, 4

Description of Strategy: Invite a funeral director to speak to the class about how funeral arrangements are made. Ask your guest to explain what is done, how costs are determined, and how family members are involved. The funeral director should explain any special considerations that must be taken into account for religious, cultural, or family reasons. Allow time for a question-and-answer session after the presentation.

Processing Questions:

1. What funeral arrangements have to be made when a family member or relative dies?
2. What is the significance of funeral rituals?

✓ **Assessment:** Students will be able to accurately describe the steps involved in the process of making funeral arrangements.

Obituary
Grades 6–8

Valued Outcome: Students will write their own obituaries as they would appear in the newspaper.

National Health Education Standards: 1, 4

Description of Strategy: Read several obituaries from the newspaper aloud to the class. Have students write their own obituaries modeled after the ones that they heard. Require students to include the date and cause of death and a list of survivors. Any other information provided is the student's choice (such as occupation, achievements, residence, and so on). Have students type and print out their obituaries on the computer. Display the obituaries on the class bulletin board.

Materials Needed: several obituary notices from newspapers, paper and pencils for each student, computer and printer

Processing Questions:

1. What is the purpose of an obituary?
2. What are the two main things you want people to remember about you after you die?

3. What accomplishments do you want to be able to include in your obituary?

○ **Integration:** Writing

✓ **Assessment:** Students will be able to write a two-paragraph obituary about their life and accomplishments.

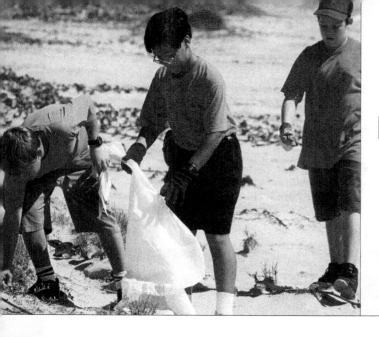

Environmental Health

Let us be good stewards of the Earth we inherited. All of us have to share the Earth's fragile ecosystems and precious resources, and each of us has a role to play in preserving them. If we are to go on living together on this Earth, we must all be responsible for it.

—*Kofi Annan (2006)*

NATIONAL HEALTH EDUCATION STANDARDS

1. Students will comprehend concepts related to health promotion and disease prevention to enhance health.

7. Students will demonstrate the ability to practice health-enhancing behaviors and avoid or reduce risks.

8. Students will demonstrate the ability to advocate for personal, family, and community health.

Valued Outcomes

After completion of this chapter, you should be able to:

- Describe the responsibilities of people in caring for the environment.

- Describe an ecosystem.

- Discuss the impact of pollution on all aspects of the ecosystem.

- Understand the connection between overpopulation and environmental pollution.

- Explain the impact of air pollution on the environment.

- State the conditions that lead to water pollution.

- Discuss what individuals can do to remedy the different types of environment pollution.

- List the sources of indoor pollution.

- Discuss the Environmental Protection Agency's (EPA) Superfund attempt to control and clean up solid waste.

- Discuss how to live a greener lifestyle.

Reflections

As you read through this chapter, consider the major hazards to the survival of the planet that you face daily, the ways you can protect yourself from these hazards, and the steps you can take personally to reduce these hazards or improve your personal environment and your community's environment.

Living in a Healthy Environment

Maintaining personal health is largely an individual responsibility. Yet, none of us lives in a vacuum. We are all subject to the influences of our environment. Thus, a person may attempt to exercise the most positive personal health behavior and still be subjected to health hazards in the form of contaminated drinking water, polluted air, and urban stress factors, such as noise and overcrowded living conditions. Clearly, our environment has an impact on our health.

Humans are the dominant species on Earth because of our power to control, manipulate, and alter our surroundings. To a large extent, we have learned to use the natural resources of the planet for our own benefit. But in doing so, we have also created a host of environmental problems. For a long time, many of these problems went unrecognized. However, with the growth of technology and industry, the problems became more and more obvious. Even then, many preferred to ignore what was happening to our environment, attributing it to the price of progress. In any case, there seemed to be no way of correcting many of the problems.

Today, more and more people are becoming aware of the negative impact human activity has had on the environment. Many of the negative changes that have occurred did not have to happen. Certainly, most do not have to keep getting worse. We can no longer plead ignorance about the effect of many of our activities on the world in which we live. We also are increasingly recognizing our responsibility toward protecting the environment and preserving our natural resources for future generations.

Ecology is the study of interactions in the environment. From this study, three principles have been determined:

1. Every system within nature is connected to every other system.
2. Matter is never destroyed but is recycled in one way or another.
3. Natural resources are finite, and nature's capacity to absorb the by-products of human technology is limited.

The implications of these three principles, separately and together, have great bearing on the health of all people and the state of the environment. At first, it may seem that these principles are beyond the control of the individual, but this is not so. Each of us has a responsibility both to understand the principles of ecology and to realize that as individuals what we do affects the operation of these principles. This is the single most important concept in the teaching of environmental health education.

Students must be taught that humans are part of the overall ecosystem of our planet, and as intelligent members of that ecosystem humans have both rights and responsibilities concerning the environment. This is a vital concept that must be stressed.

Ecosystems and Ecology

Each living thing, whether plant or animal, is part of an immediate **ecosystem**, or habitat, in which living and nonliving components interact. For example, all the organisms in a particular field or pond form an ecosystem. By interacting in a balanced fashion with all other parts of the ecosystem, a given species can generally continue to thrive while perpetuating its population. This interrelationship and interdependence with other animals and plants in the environment results in the sharing of most natural resources, including air, water, territorial space, sunlight, and soil minerals. Nonliving natural resources are usually referred to as the **abiotic factors** of the given ecosystem, while living organisms are referred to as the **biotic factors** of the ecosystem.

Each component of an ecosystem influences the other components. When the abiotic factors are altered significantly, the biotic factors will be correspondingly altered, and vice versa. As a result, ecosystems are governed by and operate through an interwoven natural organization of cycles between groups within the system. These cycles ensure that balance and stabilization of the community are sustained. Yet, balance and stability are dynamic processes, always changing in response to the alterations in these cycles as they themselves are changed by the varying interactions between the residents of the neighborhood and their use of natural resources. Thus, because ecosystems are inherently unstable, an input of energy is required in order to maintain equilibrium, or homeostasis. This input of energy produces a closed and self-sustaining cycle wherein chains of interconnections arise. For example, life is nurtured by decomposition within the system, one species feeds off another, and so forth. All resources are recycled and continually reused in one form or another because energy always remains constant. In addition, ecosystems are in continuous interaction with one another and are joined by the actions of the various abiotic and biotic factors to form a total worldwide ecosystem called the **ecosphere**, or **biosphere**.

The human species, unlike any other species, can extensively manipulate both the physical and biotic factors of ecosystems, indirectly affecting the ecosphere as a whole. Although many of these alterations are not inherently damaging, the cumulative impact on the ecosphere has taken its toll, and the natural recycling mechanisms have sometimes been overwhelmed. Ecologists have pleaded for all of us to develop a greater understanding of the scientific principles that govern ecosystems so that an increased awareness about our impact on the ecosphere will result. Then more of our decisions regarding the ways in which we choose to interact with the environment will be based on knowledge and logic rather than on ignorance or greed. Ecologists have also warned of the grave danger facing our entire planet from depletion or pollution of its rich natural resources, which are finite and must be preserved for future generations.

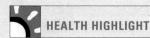

HEALTH HIGHLIGHT | **Global Warming and Climate**

According to the National Academy of Sciences, the Earth's surface temperature has risen by about 1 degree Fahrenheit in the past century, with accelerated warming during the past two decades. Evidence points to the conclusion that most of the warming over the last fifty years is attributable to human activities, which have altered the chemical composition of the atmosphere by causing the buildup of greenhouse gases—primarily carbon dioxide, methane, and nitrous oxide.

Since the beginning of the Industrial Revolution, the following changes have occurred:

- Atmospheric concentrations of carbon dioxide have increased nearly 30 percent, mostly due to human activities.
- Methane concentrations have more than doubled.
- Nitrous oxide concentrations have risen by about 15 percent.
- The twentieth century's ten warmest years all occurred in the last fifteen years of the century.
- Globally, sea level has risen 4 to 8 inches over the past century, due to thawing of glaciers.

Scientists expect that the average global surface temperature will likely rise by an additional 2°F to 11.5°F by 2100. Evaporation will increase as the climate warms, which will increase average global precipitation. Soil moisture is likely to decline in many regions, and intense rainstorms are likely to become more frequent. Global sea level is likely to rise between .59 and 1.94 feet.

Source: National Academy of Sciences 2008

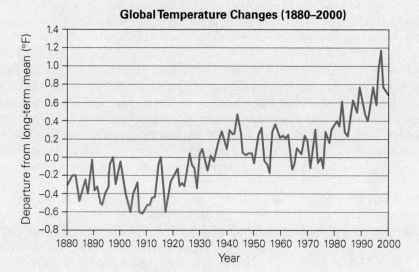

Global Temperature Changes (1880–2000)

Source: U.S. National Climatic Data Center 2008

Human Impact and Health

Human activity can have detrimental effects on the environment. For example, a growing number of diseases in children are linked to the unsafe environments in which they live, play, learn, and grow. Because they are still growing and their immune system and detoxification mechanisms are not fully developed, children are especially vulnerable to chemical, physical, and biological hazards in air, water, and soil. In both industrialized and developing countries, the development, health, and well-being of children are threatened by unsafe food and chemicals in household products and in consumer goods, and children are threatened by the overuse of antibiotics and antibacterial products (which increases the number of antibiotic-resistant strains of bacteria). Air pollution causes adverse health effects, such as asthma, leukemia, and respiratory cancer. Further, there are pathogens in our water that are resistant to standard water treatment methods. During 2005–2006, a total of seventy-eight water-related outbreaks associated with recreational water were reported by thirty-one states. Illness occurred in 4,412 persons, resulting in 116 hospitalizations and five deaths (CDC 2011).

The physical, social, and intellectual development of children from conception to the end of adolescence requires an environment that is both protected and protective of their health.

▪ Overpopulation

Many environmental health problems arise not so much from misuse of technology, but from the sheer number of

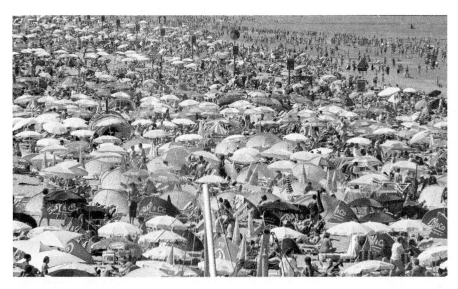

Many environmental problems arise from overpopulation.

The problems resulting from overpopulation are well recognized in countries such as China and India, where governmental incentives have been established to limit childbearing. Before condoms and diaphragms became available in the nineteenth century, birth control methods were generally unsafe and unreliable and were not widely used. However, with the introduction to the general public of the birth control pill and the intrauterine device (IUD) in the 1960s, as well as improved female sterilization and male vasectomy techniques introduced in the 1970s, birth control has become more accepted throughout the world. New contraceptive methods, such as hormone implants and male birth control pills, are being introduced.

Dissemination of information about contraceptive methods (and protection against sexually transmitted infections) has been increased to include preteens, teenagers, young adults, and older adults alike. Although some individuals and groups believe instruction about birth control is ill advised in a school setting, many school systems nevertheless have incorporated such instruction into the curriculum. The establishment of various kinds of family planning services throughout the United States and in many other nations has also aided in increasing contraceptive education.

In the United States, population growth has stabilized. The average age for marriage has increased, and many young couples delay parenthood in order to advance educationally or professionally. In developing nations, where population control is more of a problem, efforts must be made to provide the same kind of education and services that are offered in more technologically advanced nations. It must be recognized, however, that decisions about pregnancy are deeply personal and are influenced by cultural, religious, and social standards. These decisions should be based on free choice.

people who live on Earth. Globally, many experts are concerned that Earth's "carrying capacity" is already surpassed, and experts worry that increasing resource consumption in rapidly developing countries such as India and China will add enormously to the burden of greenhouse gases that threaten to heat the planet (People and the Planet 2006).

Joblessness, environmental devastation, and uncontrolled urban growth are also concerns. In the last decade or two, many countries have attempted to deal with the problem of overpopulation by means of governmental incentives to limit births. However, ethical and moral controversies surround the issue, which is understandably a very delicate and highly personal issue to most individuals.

Regardless of the ethical or moral considerations, however, overpopulation is a serious environmental problem that must be addressed—not only by governmental and private agencies, but by schools as well. Information about family planning and parenthood should be provided to junior high and high school students after a foundation about families and population has been provided at the elementary school level. Children need to understand that our planet will soon be unable to house the growing human population if reproduction continues at the present rate. Although the solutions are not easy and decisions must ultimately be made by each individual, a world perspective should be provided.

▪ Population Control

World population is expanding exponentially. In 1800, about one billon people lived on Earth. The world's population grew to two billion in 1930; to three billion in 1960; to four billion in 1975; to five billion in 1987; and to six billion in 1997. According to the U.S. Census Bureau, the population of the United States is over 300 million people and the global population is more than 6.9 billion people (U.S. Census Bureau 2010).

Pollution of the Ecosphere

Human activity is a major cause of environmental pollution, but humans often experience the results of contamination much less quickly than other organisms in the ecosphere. As a result, although pollution of the environment has been occurring for centuries, only relatively recently has the awareness developed that polluting constitutes self-destructive behavior. The most crucial areas of concern include problems caused by overpopulation, air pollution, water pollution, hazardous chemical pollution, solid waste pollution, radiation pollution, and noise pollution.

■ Air Pollution

Humans—all six-and-a-half billion of us—need air more desperately than any other resource for survival. People can endure drought, famine, and drastic temperature changes, but oxygen deprivation will result in death after only a few minutes. Yet, most of us think very little about the air we breathe, what it is composed of, or how it is replenished and kept clean. Almost no oxygen was present in the atmosphere at the Earth's creation, but an abundance of carbon dioxide was available for sustaining plant life. Photosynthetic microorganisms and green plants were responsible for producing oxygen, a waste product of photosynthesis, such that today's atmosphere is composed of approximately 80 percent nitrogen and 20 percent oxygen. Humans have contributed a variety of harmful gases and other substances to the atmosphere, resulting in air pollution (and thereby some water and soil pollution)—an increasing environmental health problem that affects the ecosphere as a whole, including the plants that provide our oxygen. Exposure to sufficiently high concentrations of air pollutants can cause a variety of health problems ranging from sneezing and coughing to labored breathing and death. The people most sensitive to air pollution are usually older adults and people who have chronic respiratory or cardiovascular conditions.

Major Air Pollutants. Today, the chief air pollutants that impact human health include carbon monoxide and nitrogen oxides, sulfur oxides, hydrocarbons, and particulate matter. Other toxic air pollutants, which are products of technology, include arsenic, mercury, polyvinyl chlorides, and pesticides, all of which can cause cancer and death.

Carbon Monoxide and Nitrogen Oxides. Carbon monoxide, which is a plentiful air pollutant, is a colorless, odorless, and poisonous gas produced by the incomplete burning of carbon in fossil fuels. The chief source of carbon monoxide pollution is internal combustion engines, most of which are gas-powered motor vehicles. Because hemoglobin has a greater affinity for carbon monoxide than for oxygen, carbon monoxide replaces oxygen in the blood. An environment in which heavy traffic is present provides significant levels of carbon monoxide, and diminished physical and mental functioning can result from long-term exposure to carbon monoxide. The effects of carbon monoxide poisoning can range from mild, annoying respiratory symptoms to profound central nervous system dysfunction. Estimates suggest that about one-third of nonfatal cases of carbon monoxide poisoning go undetected and undiagnosed (National Center for Biotechnology Information 2006).

Nitrogen oxides are chemically very similar to carbon monoxide, and poisonous nitrogen oxides, such as nitrogen dioxide and nitric acid, produce comparable physiological disturbances in the circulatory system. Nitrogen oxides cause the formation of ground-level ozone (smog) and combine with water vapor in the air to form nitric acid, a component of acid rain, which is capable of corroding metal and destroying vegetation.

Automobiles and other internal combustion engines produce most human-made carbon monoxide and nitrogen oxides. Most experts agree that shifting away from automobiles as the primary source of transportation is the only way to reduce air pollution significantly. Many cities have encouraged this shift by setting high parking fees, imposing bans on city driving, and establishing high road-use tolls. Local governments have also been implementing plans for electric buses and bicycle lanes to encourage low-impact transportation (Natural Resources Defense Council 2003). Some automobile companies now sell hybrid electric vehicles that use less gas and produce very low emissions.

Sulfur Oxides. Sulfur oxides are a product of combustion of sulfur-containing coal and fuel oil. The major health concerns associated with exposure to high concentrations of sulfur oxides include effects on breathing, respiratory illness, alterations in pulmonary defenses, and aggravation of existing cardiovascular disease. Children, the elderly, and people who have asthma, cardiovascular disease, or chronic lung disease (such as bronchitis or emphysema) are most susceptible to adverse health effects associated with exposure to sulfur oxides (Environmental Protection Agency 2006f).

In the atmosphere, sulfur dioxide is converted to sulfuric acid, which is a major source of acid deposition.

Hydrocarbons. Although no direct ailments or irritations can be directly attributed to the release of hydrocarbons—compounds composed of hydrogen and carbon that result from the incomplete burning of fossil fuels—these substances aid the formation of ground-level ozone. Ground-level ozone can harm health by irritating lung tissue, breathing passages, and mucous membranes. It also aggravates existing respiratory conditions.

Particulate Matter. Particulate matter is any nongaseous pollutant found in the air, whether liquid or solid. These pollutants include substances such as dust, fungi, ash, soot, asbestos, and lead. Prolonged exposure to these pollutants can cause deterioration of the respiratory tract surfaces, particularly the cilia. In particular, lead and asbestos have the following effects:

- **Lead**—Sources of airborne lead are primarily smelters and automobile exhausts. (Unleaded gasoline has somewhat eased the problem of automobile exhaust pollution.) Health hazards from high concentrations of lead include irritability, anemia, convulsions, severe intestinal cramps, loss of consciousness, and kidney and brain damage. Lead enters the body primarily through the respiratory tract and sometimes through the stomach walls. Signs of lead poisoning are behavioral problems, anemia, decreased mental functioning, vomiting, and cramps.

- **Asbestos**—In the past, asbestos was widely used in construction and manufacturing; most exposures occur in occupational settings. Asbestos can cause serious respiratory problems, such as emphysema, and has been implicated in lung cancer.

Damage Resulting from Air Pollution. Air pollution causes serious damage in terms of human well-being, property, and plant and animal life. Air pollution negatively affects such human respiratory illnesses as coughs, colds, asthma, pneumonia, and bronchitis, as well as cancer and even heart disease. Animals and plant life can also be severely harmed by air pollution that interferes with normal physiological functions. Buildings become darkened and discolored and public works of art and monuments are damaged by contaminants. Unfortunately, today's advanced technology produces pollutants faster than the scientific community is able to study their effects. These by-products may pose serious health problems that are currently unknown.

Chemicals. When pesticides are sprayed by crop dusters, typically only one-fourth of the pesticides lands on the crop, less than 1 percent may hit the target insects, and the rest drifts miles away. The pesticides can kill birds, frogs, and beneficial predatory insects. Raptor populations, such as those of falcons and eagles, have been adversely affected by pesticide spraying. Herbicides sprayed on forest lands have caused miscarriages, cancer, and birth defects, and they often wipe out local wildlife as well as pets and livestock. Vegetation may change color or fail to pollinate. Animals grazing on affected land can be contaminated.

Acid Rain. The primary cause of acid rain is the burning of fossil fuels. The sulfur in fuel is converted to sulfur oxides, and sulfur oxides and nitrogen oxides combine with rain, snow, dew, or mist to form sulfuric and nitric acids. Of the two, sulfuric acid is responsible for the most damage. Most sulfur pollution in the United States originates east of the Mississippi River, and much of the pollution that originates in the United States is deposited in Canada. Throughout the eastern parts of Canada and the United States, acid rain changes soil acidity levels and causes lakes and streams to become more acidic. As the water becomes more acidic, life begins to disappear from the water as the lives or reproductive capacities of amphibians and fish are destroyed and the chemical balance of the ecosystem shifts. Mercury levels, for example, tend to rise in acidic waters and thereby also in the organisms living there or that eat food from those sources. In fact, the government has issued warnings against eating fishes from many of these acid-rain-contaminated lakes due to related increased levels of mercury contamination (Environmental Protection Agency 2005).

The impact of acid rain on other aspects of human lives varies widely. Acid rain has accelerated the erosion of limestone buildings and monuments. It corrodes outdoor equipment and mobilizes other toxic elements (such as aluminum and lead) that may then contaminate soil and groundwater supplies. Springtime snowmelt can cause a surge of acid contamination. Forests and other foliage may be damaged by the acid, and even croplands have been affected.

Temperature Inversions. When a warm air mass moves over cooler air that is near the ground, a temperature inversion results. The cooler air cannot be dissipated. Temperature inversions decrease visibility and allow a buildup of pollutants, making the air unsafe for breathing. The pollutants are trapped and subjected to the action of sunlight, which produces other pollutants (known as secondary pollutants) such as ozone. The temperature inversion eventually disperses, but illness and even death have resulted from this situation.

Air Pollution Control. The Environmental Protection Agency (EPA) was established in 1970 by Congress to become the federal environmental enforcement agency. Under the provision of the Clean Air Act of 1970, the EPA set national ambient air quality standards for "criteria" pollutants, or the most common air pollutants. The criteria pollutants are ozone, suspended particulate matter, carbon monoxide, sulfur dioxide, lead, and nitrogen oxides. According to the EPA, at least 74 million people have lived in areas that still exceeded at least one air quality standard, and as many as 140 million people may have lived in areas that had ozone levels or smog in excess of national standards during that year.

Some progress has been made in controlling air pollution through mandating the reduction of pollutants in auto exhaust. This was accomplished by switching to lead-free gasoline and introducing catalytic converters in automobiles. As a result, automobile emissions of carbon monoxide and hydrocarbons have dropped 96 percent and nitric oxide emissions have fallen 88 percent. Emissions from industrial sources are also heavily regulated and have been reduced as new technologies and procedures were implemented.

The EPA also lists "hazardous" air pollutants and establishes safety standards for their emission. For example, asbestos now has been banned in new construction, and materials containing asbestos have been removed from schools and other public buildings (EPA 2006a). Other examples of hazardous pollutants are beryllium, mercury, vinyl chloride, arsenic, benzene, radionucleotides, and coke oven emissions.

▪ Water Pollution

Like air, water is essential to life. The demand for clean water has increased due to population growth, increased irrigation demands, and increased manufacturing. These areas, plus the conversion of land that formerly held water (e.g., wetlands), have caused a significant and dangerous reduction in water tables in many areas of the country.

Most people in the United States have clean water to drink, but there are significant pockets of the country where the water supply is contaminated. About 80 percent of U.S. drinking water has chlorine added to it to prevent outbreaks of waterborne illnesses that were once endemic.

Despite water's importance, we dump everything from fertilizer and detergents to industrial wastes and sewage into our precious water supply. In addition, when pollutants are channeled into nonflowing bodies of water, such as lakes, eutrophication (accelerated growth of algae) occurs. As algae growth skyrockets on a diet of inorganic pollutants, especially nitrogen and phosphorus, a blanket of slime covers the water. Eventual death of the algae results in bacterial decomposition that consumes the oxygen dissolved in water. This oxygen deficit kills fish and other lake inhabitants, many of which are valuable as food resources. Eventually, the body of water becomes contaminated beyond use. Even flowing bodies of water, such as streams and rivers, that undergo natural purification can be badly polluted if sufficient quantities of wastes are dumped into them.

Major Water Pollutants.
There are numerous sources of water pollution. The main ones are industrial wastes, human sewage, and thermal pollution.

Industrial Wastes.
Chemical by-products from the manufacture of paper, steel, oil, pesticides, and the like account for more than half of the water pollution in this country. Despite water pollution laws, an abundance of diverse industrial wastes continues to be deposited in lakes, streams, and rivers throughout the country. Many pollutants, including lead and mercury, are known to be toxic to humans. Of great concern regarding the danger of any industrial waste product is the length of time it takes to be broken down by the environment and the concentration that is tolerable by organisms in the environment, particularly humans.

Human Sewage.
Although contamination of water from human waste is much less pervasive than it once was, it nevertheless can occur in varying degrees if a community's sewage treatment system is antiquated or not inspected regularly. It is recommended that sewage treatment consist of two stages: primary and secondary. The primary stage rids the water, which has been allowed to settle in a holding tank, of large objects through a filtration process of passing the liquid over a series of screens. During the secondary stage of treatment, smaller particles of organic material and microbes are removed through additional filtration techniques, dispersement over beds of stone, and chemical purification. The final step usually involves the addition of chlorine to disinfect the water of any remaining bacteria so it is safe for recycling. There has been rising concern over the presence of antibiotics, prescription medications, and radioactive waste (from medical treatments) in human sewage.

Thermal Pollution.
Numerous industries, including those involved in generating nuclear power, use water as a coolant for their equipment. Water absorbs heat from the equipment and is channeled back to its source, where it raises the temperature of the water source. Although this process seems harmless enough, the warmer the water is, the less oxygen it will absorb; and the less oxygen absorbed, the less quickly the lake or river decomposes its organic material. Because power-generating plants in particular heat large volumes of water, the parent waterway is certainly at risk. In addition, much of the aquatic life is drastically affected by extreme temperature variation from the norm. Many organisms have temperature-controlled behaviors, such as feeding behaviors. When the temperature of their surroundings is changed, the behaviors of the organisms are changed.

Damage Resulting from Water Pollution.
Polluted water can be responsible for transmitting many pathogens. For example, the infectious agents that cause typhoid fever, dysentery, and cholera are just a few of the microorganisms that can be transmitted through polluted water. Viruses from human wastes carried in contaminated water can cause hepatitis. Bacteria found in polluted water can cause intestinal disorders. Parasitic worms and protozoans found in water may cause health problems such as giardiasis, which causes diarrhea. Other materials found in polluted water, such as asbestos fibers, can cause cancer.

Polluted water can be particularly harmful to fishes, birds, and other animals. For example, herbicides, phosphates, fertilizers, sewage, and industrial wastes kill numerous fishes and birds, and some may act as estrogen mimics that disrupt reproductive hormones and even development of reproductive organs. Many of these pollutant products also promote the growth of algae, which changes the ecological balance of an ecosystem and produces odors and foul-tasting drinking water. Aquatic organisms may be affected by rising water temperature, which retards their reproduction, destroys their food supplies, or kills them.

Oil spills are often widely publicized accidents. The devastation to birds and fishes due to oil spills has been apparent. The oil coats the gills of fish, thus killing them. Feathers of birds are coated so that the birds cannot fly, and preening their feathers leads to ingestion of the oil. Oil-covered beaches are also expensive to clean,

| HEALTH HIGHLIGHT | **Analysis of the Effects of Global Climate Change on Human Health in the United States** |

Climate Event	Examples of Possible Impacts	Likelihood of Impact Given Climate Event Occurs	Potential Adaptation Strategies
Extreme temperatures	Heat stress/stroke or hyperthermia	Very likely in Midwest and northeast urban centers	Early watch and warning systems and installation of cooling systems in residential and commercial buildings
Changes in precipitation	Contaminated water and food supplies with associated gastrointestinal illnesses, including *Salmonella* and *Giardia*	Likely in areas with outdated or oversubscribed water treatment plants	Improve infrastructure to guard against combined sewer overflow; public health response to include "boil water" advisories
Hurricane and storm surge	Injuries from flying debris and drowning/exposure to contaminated flood waters and to mold and mildew/exposure to carbon monoxide poisoning from portable generators	Likely in coastal zones of the southeast Atlantic and the Gulf Coast	Increase knowledge and awareness of vulnerability to climate change (e.g., maps showing areas vulnerable to storm surges); public health advisories in immediate aftermath of storm; coordinate storm relief efforts to insure that people receive necessary information for safeguarding their health
Temperature-related effects on ozone	Ozone concentrations more likely to increase than decrease; possible contribution to cardiovascular and pulmonary illnesses, including exacerbation of asthma and chronic obstructive pulmonary disorder (COPD) if current regulatory standards are not attained	Likely in urban centers in the mid-Atlantic and the Northeast	Public warning via air quality action days; encourage public transit, walking, and bicycling to decrease emissions
Wildfires	Degraded air quality, contributing to asthma and COPD aggravation	Likely in California, the intermountain West, the Southwest, and the Southeast	Public health air quality advisories

Source: EPA 2008

and the public loses recreational areas. Floating debris from oil spills and other pollution sources may entangle wildlife or even be mistaken as food and swallowed.

Water Quality Control. Although federal controls regarding water pollution traditionally have not been as extensive as those for air pollution, the enactment of the Federal Water Pollution Control Act in 1973 was conceived as a means of developing a national system that would require any institution, industry, or company that discharges substances into waterways to meet EPA standards. The Safe Drinking Water Act (SDWA) was originally passed by Congress in 1974 to protect public health by regulating the nation's public drinking water supply. The law was amended in 1986 and 1996 and requires the protection of drinking water and its sources—rivers, lakes, reservoirs, springs, and groundwater wells (EPA 2006e). The EPA also provides Internet access to information on water standard violations (National Center for Health Statistics 2000, 123).

▪ Hazardous Chemical Pollution

The hazardous chemicals that pollute our environment are numerous and varied. They include not only the toxins deposited in our air and waterways, but also the pesticides sprayed on crops, the chemicals transported along our railways and highways for use in industry, and those contained in commonly used household products.

▪ Major Hazardous Chemicals

Pesticides. With the 1962 publication of Rachel Carson's *Silent Spring*, people began to become more conscious of the hazards of pesticides, the toxic chemicals that are used to kill insects and other pests that harm or destroy crops. In past decades, the harm caused by the widespread use of chlorinated hydrocarbons such as DDT (dichlorodiphenyl trichloroethane), dieldrin, and chlordane as pesticides was not fully recognized.

Chlorinated hydrocarbons decompose very slowly and remain toxic to a wide variety of animal life for long periods. Organophosphate pesticides such as diazinon, parathion, and malathion exhibit similar properties and are even more poisonous than the chlorinated hydrocarbons are.

Although worldwide food production needs to be increased to meet the demands of a growing population, extensive use of pesticides can cause great harm to environmental health in the process. Questions still need to be answered concerning the implication of long-term exposure to moderate or even minimal levels of pesticides. There is evidence that these chemicals can damage the human reproductive and nervous systems, for example. The use of pesticides must be limited and controlled in order to protect all inhabitants of our ecosphere.

Industrial Chemicals. One of the most dangerous environmental threats is the transportation of industrial chemicals from state to state and from country to country. Although transportation itself is not inherently harmful, leakage or spills of chemical substances most certainly is. For example, accidents involving the transportation of oil and other petroleum products have resulted in several major oil spills that have damaged some of our nation's most beautiful beaches and killed or endangered countless birds and marine life.

In response to this increasingly dangerous threat, many state governments and the federal government have formed special subcommittees to study the problem of transportation of industrial chemicals. Particularly with regard to the movement of radioactive material for industrial and burial purposes, many states have indicated an unwillingness to continue to allow such toxins to cross their borders. More controls and safeguards need to be implemented in transporting hazardous chemicals of any kind, whether by trucks, ships, or trains.

Household Products. Before the ban on spray cans containing propellant chlorofluorocarbons (CFCs) and detergents containing phosphates, numerous household products served as contaminators of the environment by releasing these agents into the air and water, respectively. CFCs destroy the protective ozone layer of the atmosphere that shields us from damaging ultraviolet rays of the sun, while phosphates serve as nutrients for bacteria, protozoa, and algae, promoting eutrophication of lakes, streams, and rivers. These examples serve as an excellent illustration of the dangers involved in releasing seemingly harmless compounds into our surroundings, including household products like cleansers, polishes, waxes, and sprays, without first studying their environmental impact.

Hazardous Chemical Control. Over 20,000 pesticide products are registered for use in the United States. Several federal laws have been passed that have focused on the dangers of pesticides. The Federal Insecticide, Fungicide, and Rodenticide Act (FIFRA), passed originally in 1948 and amended since, provides the overall framework for the federal pesticide regulation program. The Federal Food, Drug, and Cosmetic Act (FFDCA) governs the establishment of pesticide tolerances for food products. These safety standards are measured against the aggregate risk from dietary exposure and other nonoccupational sources of exposure, such as drinking water and residential lawn uses (EPA 1998). As a result, more environmentally sustainable approaches to crop spraying have evolved. Alternative means of pest control are being implemented in the United States and elsewhere, the best known of which is integrated pest management, a combination of controls that include chemical and biological methods. However, the global use of pesticides still poses a danger to environmental health.

In 1976, the U.S. government created the Resource Conservation and Recovery Act (RCRA) to enforce proper management of hazardous wastes. This law has helped to regulate the production, handling, and cleanup of hazardous materials and to reduce illegal disposal of such wastes (Office of Environmental Policy & Guidance 2003).

▪ Solid Waste Pollution

Until recently, the public virtually ignored the problems related to the disposal of solid wastes. The majority of these solid wastes are buried in landfills, many of which have been identified as hazardous waste sites and are associated with unacceptable health risks.

Hazardous waste is defined as waste that has properties that make it dangerous or potentially harmful to human health or the environment. Hazardous wastes can be liquids, solids, contained gases, or sludges, or they can be the by-products of manufacturing processes or discarded commercial products, such as cleaning fluids or pesticides. In regulatory terms, a hazardous waste is a waste that exhibits at least one of four characteristics—ignitability, corrosivity, reactivity, and toxicity. Hazardous waste is regulated under the Resource Conservation and Recovery Act (EPA 2006c).

Today, we use more and more convenience products that are easily disposed of and replaced. Everything from disposable diapers, dishes, and food containers to plastic wraps, sanitary products, and paper napkins are available. The price of this convenience has been the growing problem of solid waste disposal. The unsightly junkyards, dumps, and scattered litter are more than just eyesores. They are a public health hazard as well.

Many solid waste materials are not biodegradable; they remain in the environment for long periods of time because they do not decay or cannot be burned easily. The piles of refuse serve as breeding grounds for microorganisms, rats, insects, and other disease-carrying organisms. In addition, agricultural waste products from orchards, feedlots, and farms add significantly to the total solid waste that must be disposed of each year. How do we rid ourselves of all our refuse?

Solid Waste Control. On December 11, 1980, President Jimmy Carter signed the Comprehensive Environmental Response, Compensation, and Liability Act of 1980 (CERCLA or Superfund), creating the federal government's program to clean up the nation's uncontrolled hazardous waste sites. Through the Superfund program, the EPA and its partners address abandoned, accidentally spilled, or illegally dumped hazardous wastes that pose current or future threats to human health or the environment. There is at least one Superfund site in every state.

Congress passed the Superfund statute, but it is up to the EPA to create and manage the Superfund program. When national media brought attention to such sites as the Valley of the Drums in Kentucky and a chemical explosion in Elizabeth, New Jersey, the EPA took immediate action. Chemical drums were collected and removed, fires were extinguished, and leaks from tanks and waste ponds were stopped. However, responding to emergencies is not the EPA's only challenge. Over the last few decades, the EPA has developed new and innovative ways to conduct cleanups. Research has examined how contamination migrates into groundwater, and new technologies have provided improved methods to treat, store, and dispose of wastes. The EPA has taken steps to ensure that communities near hazardous sites have a strong, meaningful voice in cleanup decisions, including determining how to reuse the land after a cleanup. Finally, the Superfund program has pioneered methods to ensure that the parties responsible for contamination are held responsible for the cleanup. Today, construction work is complete at 62 percent of the Superfund sites, and work is underway at more than 400 additional sites (EPA 2006g).

The United States, like many other nations, is still struggling with the problem of solid waste. Until citizens recognize that many solid waste disposal programs are ineffective or unacceptable, the situation is unlikely to change. Individual efforts toward decreasing the daily use of disposable products that are not easily biodegradable as well as efforts aimed at recycling can assist greatly, but more public awareness and action are needed to draw attention to the problem of solid waste disposal. Current methods of solid waste disposal primarily include dumps, landfills, incineration, and recycling.

Dumps. Most solid waste in this country is deposited in open, minimally managed dumps. Some burning of garbage does take place to condense the material. Besides being unsightly, open dumps can pose a serious threat to a community's health if the subsequent resident insect or rodent population gets out of control. The widespread use of dumps results from the short-term inexpensive nature of this method of solid waste disposal.

Landfills. Unlike the procedures of open disposal in a dump, in a landfill the solid waste is covered by dirt each day after it has been compacted. Once covered with dirt, the landfill is bulldozed to smooth out and compress the area. A properly operated landfill requires predetermined designing and engineering of the site as well as continued daily maintenance from a crew of workers. The benefits of a well-functioning landfill can be numerous. Because refuse is covered daily, risk of a contaminated water supply or of disease due to the breeding of flies, mosquitoes, rats, and the like is diminished considerably. Because burning is not necessary, the technique does not contribute to air pollution. In addition, after the location has been completely filled in, it can serve some other valuable purpose, such as a site for housing, recreation, or industry. (Burial of some types of hazardous wastes in a landfill will preclude its use for some types of construction.)

There are problems, nevertheless, associated with the use of landfills. Land itself is becoming scarcer and more expensive, not all types of terrain are suitable to serve as landfills, and the surrounding water table must be low enough to not be contaminated by chemicals leeching from the landfill. In addition, residents are often opposed to the establishment of a landfill nearby for fear that it will lower property values.

Incineration. Like dumping, incineration is a very old method of waste disposal that adds to environmental pollution because of the release of gases and particulate matter into the atmosphere during burning. Of particular danger is the release of hydrogen chloride from burning plastics, which are mainly composed of polyvinyl chloride. On contact with moisture in the air, hydrogen chloride forms hydrochloric acid, an especially corrosive agent that causes respiratory irritation.

However, the energy and heat produced as by-products of incineration can be used in homes and industry. Incineration of solid wastes has been employed successfully for this purpose in many locations throughout Europe and is now being used in the United States. To accomplish this throughout the entire United States, many incinerators would have to be redesigned and rebuilt. As it stands, incineration is already one of the more costly waste-disposal methods. Nevertheless, incineration as a generator of energy merits more investigation.

Recycling. Many products can be recycled or reused in another mode. For example, paper, glass, and metal products can all be recycled. This method of solid waste control was widespread before World War I and regained some popularity during the environmentally conscious era of the late 1960s and early 1970s. Many communities provide recycling centers to which residents can bring recyclable materials. Some communities merely ask residents to place recyclable materials out for collection in front of their homes. These projects have significantly decreased the amount of solid waste.

Many schools around the country also participate in recycling programs. For example, Madison County in Illinois has implemented the Madison County Solid Waste Recycling Program, which emphasizes recycling,

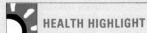

Listed below are facts concerning recycling as presented by the U.S. Environmental Protection Agency (2009).

- Each person creates about 4.34 pounds of waste every single day
- 1.46 pounds of individual daily waste is recycled or composted
- Approximately 9,000 curbside recycling programs exist in the United States
- The amount of recycling in 2009 saved the energy equivalent of 224 million barrels of oil
- Paper was the most commonly recycled nondurable good (those goods that generally last less than three years)

- More than 60 percent of the paper and cardboard generated was recycled
- Eighty-eight percent of newspapers were recycled
- Almost 14 percent of plastic containers and packaging was recycled
- Plastic bottles were the most recycled plastic products
- Recycling one ton of aluminum cans conserves the equivalent of thirty-six barrels of oil, or 1,665 gallons of gasoline
- Lead batteries have one of the highest recycle rates, at 96 percent
- Since 1990, the amount of municipal solid waste going to landfills dropped by more than thirteen million tons

- Through recycling, carbon dioxide equivalent emissions were reduced by 178 million metric tons, equal to removing emissions from almost thirty-three million passenger vehicles
- The number of community composting programs decreased (from 3,227 in 2002 to about 3,000 in 2009)
- Composting recovered twenty-one million tons of waste

Source: U.S. Environmental Protection Agency, *Municipal Solid Waste Generation, Recycling, and Disposal in the United States: Facts and Figures for 2009.* (Full report available at www.epa.gov/epawaste/nonhaz/municipal/pubs/msw2009rpt.pdf.)

---

reduction, and reusing. With regard to recycling, it is suggested that you recycle every item that you can, and be sure to use curbside programs and recycling stations when available. We can reduce the amount of material thrown away by buying items that have less packaging, buying in bulk when possible, avoiding single-use packaging, and packing waste-free lunches by not using paper bags, foil, and/or plastic wraps. Finally, we can use materials and products that can be reused. For example, use lunch containers instead of paper bags, ceramic drinking cups instead of foam, and cloth rags instead of paper towels (Madison County Recycles 2003).

▪ Related Environmental Risks

Radiation Exposure. Individuals are exposed to radiation daily, both from natural sources such as the sun and from human-made sources. The human-made sources of radiation are of most concern. Many radioactive materials release energy in the form of high-energy particles. Alpha and beta radioactive particles do not easily penetrate the human body, but gamma radiation does. Gamma rays are much like X-rays. If an individual is exposed to a sufficiently high dosage of gamma radiation, several adverse effects occur, ranging from nausea, hair loss, and diarrhea to cell mutation, anemia, and death.

Radiation does have some benefits. Radiation is widely used in medicine for diagnosis and treatment of many diseases. Because of the ability of radiation to kill cells, it has also been used in cancer therapy. However, excessive use of radiation in medicine and the development of new techniques that deliver more radiation than may be needed for proper diagnosis remains as a concern for potential increased cancer risk. Researchers are trying to determine if there are health benefits as well as adverse health effects from exposure to low doses of radiation. If such benefits exist, it could change the perception of risk associated with very low doses of radiation.

In the United States, individuals come into contact with radiation mainly through medical testing and X-rays. Although X-rays are generally considered safe, many instances of unnecessary exposure have been reported. Intervals of several months should elapse between exposures to X-rays. Pregnant women, particularly during the first trimester, should avoid being x-rayed if at all possible because radiation can cause cell damage and mutation to the developing fetus. Further, it is well established that exposure of unborn children to radiation during certain stages of fetal development when the major organs are developing results in an increase in birth defects. During the early stages of fetal development radiation exposure results in death of cells that are critical to normal development (CDC 2006).

Because of concerns about radiation exposure, opponents to the use of nuclear power as an energy source are becoming more vocal. They fear both the dangers of mishandling the disposal of nuclear wastes and the potential for a nuclear accident such as those that occurred at

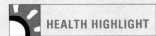

Three Mile Island in Pennsylvania in March 1979 and at the Chernobyl plant in the Soviet Union in April 1986. On the other hand, supporters of nuclear power believe that through the implementation of the Nuclear Regulatory Commission's guidelines nuclear power can be a safe, viable, and much needed energy source for the future.

Radiation Exposure Control. Guidelines exist that indicate allowable ranges of radiation exposure from medical testing, X-rays, and consumer products emitting small amounts of radiation, such as television sets. However, the long-term effects on health of even low or "safe" levels of radiation are still poorly understood. Any radiation at all may in fact be deleterious to health. Certainly as individuals we must become more educated and aware of both the benefits and the dangers of using radiation and nuclear power.

Noise Pollution. With more and more of the U.S. population living in metropolitan areas, the problem of noise as a pollutant is also growing. Noise pollution is a problem for almost every urban dweller and a particular cause of concern among people living near airports, employees working in manufacturing or industry, and commuters who must endure hours of noise each week traveling in cars, trains, buses, and subways. Also, listening to loud music, especially through earphones, is a noise pollutant that can cause hearing loss.

The effect from impulse sound can be instantaneous and can result in an immediate hearing loss that may be permanent. The structures of the inner ear may be severely damaged, and this kind of hearing loss may be accompanied by tinnitus—ringing, buzzing, or roaring in the ears or head—which may subside over time. Hearing loss and tinnitus may occur in one or both ears, and tinnitus may continue intermittently throughout a lifetime.

The damage that occurs slowly over years of continuous exposure to loud noise is accompanied by various changes in the structure of the hair cells that detect sound. This change in structure results in hearing loss and tinnitus. Ear plugs or ear muffs can reduce this damage. Adverse effects of hearing loss include the social consequences of hearing impairment such as:

- the inability to understand speech in daily communication
- disturbance of rest and sleep
- mental health and performance effects
- disruptive effects on residential behavior and annoyance.

People and workers who are continually exposed to noise are at higher risk for developing hypertension and ischemic heart disease. In schools near airports, where children are chronically exposed to noise, children underperform in tasks such as proofreading, persistence in puzzle solving, and some types of reading tests (National Institutes of Health 2006).

Noise Pollution Control. Each individual must exercise personal judgment in deciding how much noise exposure is not only tolerable but safe. Employees in industry are, of course, issued protective ear devices, but the general public is not guaranteed the same protection on noisy highways or in neighborhoods near loud noise sources. Greater awareness of the harmful physical and psychological effects of noise may lead to public action and

> **Creativity in the Classroom**
>
> Split the class into groups. One group has loud conversations, the other group talks in a normal voice or whispers to each other. Can the students follow their conversations, or do they have trouble hearing? Relate this to a discussion of noise pollution in other situations.

Table 25.1 Typical Noise Levels	
Source of Noise	**Decibels**
Whispering	30
Air conditioner at twenty feet	60
Busy traffic	70
Truck noise	90
Airplane overhead	100
Chainsaw	100
Rock band concert, in front of speakers	120
Shotgun blast	140
Rocket pad during launch	180

legislation in the years ahead. Table 25.1 lists some typical noise levels.

Wildlife is also affected by noise pollution. Studies have shown that in response to common human activities that cause large amounts of noise, animals have injured themselves, lost energy due to decreases in food intake, avoided and abandoned their habitat, and suffered reproductive losses. Noise stresses these animals to the point of endangering their population (Noise Pollution Clearinghouse 2003).

Indoor Air Pollution. When people think of pollution, they do not consider their most familiar environment, the indoors, as a factor. Most people do not know that indoor air pollution can also have significant health effects. The EPA has stated that indoor levels of pollutants may be two to five times—and occasionally more than 100 times—higher than outdoor levels. These levels of indoor air pollutants may be of particular concern because most people spend about 90 percent of their time indoors.

In the home, there are many sources of pollution that can have significant effects on health. Tobacco smoke, pet dander, mold, and dust mites are all environmental asthma triggers. Some problems arise from asbestos-containing insulation; household cleaners; gas stoves that emit carbon monoxide; containers of oil, gas, and kerosene; fumes from new carpeting, etc. Any kind of unsanitary conditions, such as excess dirt, old food, and trash, can lead to vermin and insects within the home as well.

Indoor pollution sources that release gases or particles into the air are the primary cause of indoor air quality problems in homes. Inadequate ventilation can increase indoor pollutant levels by not bringing in enough outdoor air to dilute emissions from indoor sources and by not carrying indoor air pollutants out of the home. Radon, a gas that cannot be smelled or tasted, has been a problem in many homes. Breathing air containing radon can lead to lung cancer. High temperature and humidity levels can also increase concentrations of some pollutants. Indoor pollutants are also a concern within schools and classrooms. Chalk dust from boards and erasers, old air-conditioning, old insulation, mildew, and public bathrooms can all contribute to classroom pollution (EPA 2006b).

> **TEACHING TIP**
>
> Environmental health topics offer many opportunities to be developed into exceptional science fair projects.

Preservation of the Ecosphere

Conservation and protection of our natural resources must stem from both individual and public action. Both are needed to stabilize and eventually reverse the harmful cycle of contamination that currently plagues the ecosphere. Legislation and implementation of healthier environmental practices have been instituted. The enactment of additional measures could serve to improve the quality of living for us and for future generations.

Chapter In Review

Summary

- Individuals should act responsibly and diligently with regard to their environment to ensure high-level wellness.
- The environment in which one lives must be free of dangerous levels of pollutants and therefore conducive to quality living, not just mere survival.
- To maintain the natural resources on which all living things depend, we must understand how we interact with and influence our ecosystem, our immediate habitat.
- Many human-made changes have caused havoc in ecological chains or webs within ecosystems.
- Because ecosystems, like the residents within them, are interdependent and thus form one worldwide ecosphere,

the harmful impact of human growth and technology is felt throughout the entire planet.

- Population growth is causing our species to stretch the capacity of land, water, and food supplies to accommodate us.
- Particularly in the highly industrial nations, human lifestyles have resulted in an abundance of pollution problems that cannot be dealt with by the buffering capacities of natural cycles within the ecosphere.
- With our automobiles, we release dangerous pollutants into the air.
- Industry adds still other toxins, and runoff from agriculture and industrial dumping contaminates our water.
- Incidents involving the accidental leakage or spillage of highly lethal substances during transport occur fairly frequently.

- Hazardous waste spills, coupled with problems of solid waste disposal, radiation exposure, noise pollution, and indoor air pollution, have resulted in unprecedented ecological crises.

- Through continued research, education, and responsible action on the part of both governments and individuals, preservation of the ecosphere is possible.

- It is our job as educators to provide instructional and consciousness-raising experiences to the children we teach so that their children and grandchildren will enjoy continued health and well-being in a sound environment.

Discussion Questions

1. Define and differentiate between the terms *environment* and *ecology*.

2. What is the ecosphere, and how do human beings interact with elements of the ecosphere?

3. What impact does overpopulation have on the state of the environment, and what problems directly or indirectly stem from overpopulation?

4. What are the major sources of air pollution? Describe the harmful effects of specific air pollutants on human health.

5. What are the objectives that the U.S. government has set for regulation of contaminants?

6. What individual steps can be taken to more effectively manage and control air pollution?

7. What threats to environmental health does the transportation of hazardous substances pose?

8. What is indoor air pollution? How does it affect environmental health?

9. How can each individual help to preserve the ecosphere? Give specific suggestions.

Critical Thinking Questions

1. After reading this chapter and considering the "Reflections" at the beginning of this chapter, what have you decided are the major environmental hazards that you face personally? What are some steps you have decided to take to protect yourself from these hazards?

2. Are there any environmental hazards to which your behavior may contribute? Consider the Health Highlight box on page 443, "What You Can Do to Protect Our Planet." What are some steps you can incorporate in your lifestyle?

3. The steps to control overpopulation in our world are considered controversial by some. Consider the pros and cons of these steps and your values and beliefs regarding each step.

4. This chapter has challenged you to become proactive in reducing the threat of environmental health problems. Research a piece of environmental health legislation currently being considered by your county or state. Draft a letter to your local or state legislator regarding your stand on this legislation.

Access more material online at www.pearsonhighered.com/anspaugh. At this companion website for *Teaching Today's Health,* you'll find chapter quizzes, web links, flashcards, a glossary, additional Worksheets, and more to help you succeed.

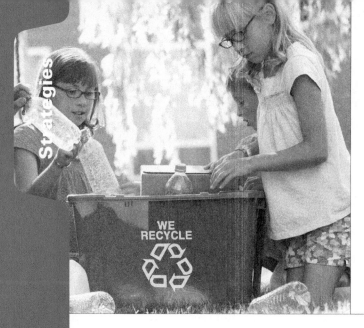

Strategies for Teaching Environmental Health

26

Environmental learning experiences can provide an awareness of who we are and how we relate to the world around us. Studying and exploring the environment teaches our children about the Earth's natural resources while fostering a sense of respect for living things.

NATIONAL HEALTH EDUCATION STANDARDS

1. Students will comprehend concepts related to health promotion and disease prevention to enhance health.

3. Students will demonstrate the ability to access valid information and products and services to enhance health.

4. Students will demonstrate the ability to use interpersonal communication skills to enhance health and avoid or reduce health risks.

5. Students will demonstrate the ability to use decision-making skills to enhance health.

7. Students will demonstrate the ability to practice health-enhancing behaviors and avoid or reduce risks.

8. Students will demonstrate the ability to advocate for personal, family, and community health.

Valued Outcomes

After completion of this chapter, your students should be able to:

- Understand that high levels of wellness can only be sustained if the environment is conducive to well-being.

- Describe how all animals, plants, and natural resources in any habitat form a self-sustaining ecosystem.

- Discuss how all parts of an ecosystem are interdependent.

- Discuss how ecosystems are linked to each other and form a global network called an ecosphere and how a change in one ecosystem has the potential to affect other ecosystems.

- Understand how human activities have the greatest impact on ecosystems.

- Describe the major sources of pollution.

- Discuss how overpopulation has resulted in environmental problems.

- Understand how conservation of natural resources, preservation of ecosystems, and protection of the environment from pollution are essential for preserving the ecosphere.

- Discuss why the preservation of the ecosphere must stem from individual and community action.

Reflections

As you review this chapter, think in terms of where and how the classroom teacher can foster a concern for environmental issues. Where should the emphasis begin and what types of strategies would you use at the lower elementary, upper elementary, and middle school levels?

Fostering Environmental Appreciation

All living species have had to adapt to their environment or face extinction. This adaptation has resulted in an amazing variety of life forms on the planet. Thick-skinned cacti have adapted to the harsh environment of our deserts. Luminescent fish live successfully in the perpetual darkness of the ocean depths. Polar bears carry on their life cycles in the frozen landscape above the Arctic Circle.

Human beings have also had to adapt to the physical environment; but, unlike any other form of life on the planet, human beings can also extensively adapt the environment to suit their needs. We build cities, dam rivers, mine the Earth, and farm the land. To a large extent, we can manipulate and control our environment. This unique ability has sometimes resulted in the misconception that we are the masters of our environment. This has led to abuse of natural resources and consequent pollution, waste, and lowering of environmental quality.

In the last few decades, we have become more aware that human beings are not free to alter the environment—we pay a price. We have recognized that we are part of a worldwide ecosystem, interacting and interrelating with every other part. This increased environmental awareness has not come too soon. We now know all too well that nature's resources are finite and must be conserved and used wisely. We have begun to see that change to any part of the environment can have a wide-ranging impact on many other parts. Failure to understand the consequences could mean disaster not only for ourselves but also for the entire planet.

Students need to learn about the importance of a healthy environment. They must recognize that it is up to each of us to maintain the environment. Doing so will more easily foster high-level wellness. Instruction about environmental health should build a sense of appreciation for all life and natural resources and encourage personal practices that will help to ensure the continued preservation of the ecosphere. The activities suggested in this chapter will help you attain this goal for your students.

Shown to the right of each activity title is the suggested grade level(s) for which the activity might be appropriate. However, many of the suggested activities could be modified for use at various grade levels.

Information Assessment Activities

Ecological Food Chain   Grades 2–6

Valued Outcome: Students will be able to describe an ecological food chain.

National Health Education Standard: 1

Description of Strategy: The following are the major parts of an ecological food chain: predators, scavengers, consumers, and producers. Have the students make a poster illustrating an ecological food chain. Students may add links to make a more elaborate food chain: water, birds, fish, humans.

Materials Needed: paper, markers, and pictures

Processing Questions:

1. What happens when pesticides affect one link in the ecological model?
2. What is an example of an endangered animal that has been affected by pesticides or pollution?
3. What are some ways you can help eliminate environmental pollution?

○ **Integration:** Science

✓ **Assessment:** Students demonstrate their understanding of the workings of the ecological food chain.

Major Environmental Problems   Grades 4–6

Valued Outcome: Students will identify the biggest problem they believe is affecting our environment.

National Health Education Standards: 1, 4, 7

Description of Strategy: Have students research the problems affecting our environment such as overpopulation, pesticides, land pollution, air pollution, water pollution, and noise pollution. Then have a class discussion about each environmental area and the issues associated with each area. After the discussion have the students prepare posters showing the effects of the environmental problems in question. The processing questions are good guidelines for the questions to be answered on the posters. Pictures, graphs, and illustrations should be part of the poster.

Materials Needed: poster board and markers for each student

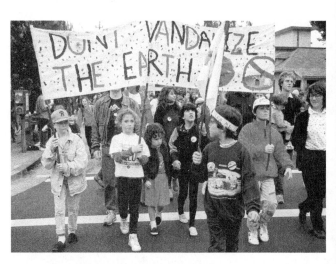

We are the stewards of our land and water.

Our natural resources are important, and there are many things we can do to protect and preserve them. Some things kids can do include the following:

- purchase recycled products
- ask family members to reuse shopping bags
- recycle metals, including all aluminum
- recycle newspapers
- use as few paper products as possible
- recycle cardboard
- recycle plastics
- recycle tin cans
- recycle glass containers

Processing Questions:

1. Why do you believe this is the biggest problem?
2. How is this problem affecting the environment?
3. How does this problem affect you and your family?
4. What can your family do to help relieve this problem?

○ **Integration:** Science, Art

✓ **Assessment:** Students can describe an environmental problem and can both explain how this problem affects them and offer ideas on how they can help relieve the problem.

Using Technology to Teach Environmental Issues
Grades 5–8

Valued Outcomes: Students will utilize technology to develop solutions for dealing with the nation's trash accumulation problems. Students will develop insight into the amount of trash that is accumulated on a yearly basis in the United States.

National Health Education Standards: 5, 7, 8

Description of Strategy: This activity can be used to introduce students to things they can do to address environmental issues. Begin the discussion by asking the students: What are the materials that make up the trash? Continue by developing a list of some possible ways that the trash can be disposed of. Next, ask the students to utilize the Internet to research how material found in the trash can instead be recycled or composted, and to identify products that can be made from recycled materials that people might otherwise throw away. Steer students to trustworthy sites such as www.epa.gov. Help focus student research by providing each student with Worksheet 26.1 (page 505). After completing research each student should submit a short paper summarizing what they have discovered about trash and recycling.

Materials Needed: computer with Internet access and Worksheet 26.1 for each student

Processing Questions:

1. What materials might you find in the trash that could have been recycled?

2. What can some materials often found in trash be use for?
3. How much money can be saved by recycling?
4. Why is it important to recycle certain material? Name some things that it is vital to recycle.

✓ **Assessment:** Students should be able to list methods of disposing of trash and describe products that can be made from recycled materials.

Let's Rank Our Environmental Problems
Grades 6–8

Valued Outcome: Students will be able to identify the most hazardous environmental problems.

National Health Education Standards: 1, 7

Description of Strategy: Have the students rank the environmental problems listed in Worksheet 26.2 on page 506 from most hazardous to least hazardous, with 1 being the most and 3 being the least hazardous. Once the class is finished, write the problems on the board and rank them as a group. Have an open class discussion about the answers.

Materials Needed: Worksheet 26.2 for each student

Processing Questions:

1. Why are some hazards more dangerous than others?
2. What are some ways we can prevent pollution of our environment?

✓ **Assessment:** Students can correctly identify the most hazardous problems on the worksheet.

Decision Stories

Follow the procedure discussed in Chapter 4 (pages 60–62) for presenting decision stories such as the following.

For each of the decision stories, write a list on the board of ideas generated by the class for how each situation should be dealt with. Ask the students to discuss the merits of the methods suggested.

Lesson Title: Recycling Centers

Date: May 14, 2012 **Time:** 10:00 A.M. **Grade:** Three **Teacher:** Wong

I. National Health Education Standards

Health Education Standard 8: Students will demonstrate the ability to advocate for personal, family, and community health.

II. National Health Education Standards Performance Indicator

8.5.2 encourage others to make positive health choices.

III. Valued Outcomes

- Students will discuss their community's recycling plan.
- Students will explain how recycling is helpful to the environment.
- Students will demonstrate recycling habits.

IV. Description of Strategy

1. Discuss with students what they know about recycling. Ask them if any of their families recycle and if so, what types of things they recycle. Ask students to describe how their family recycles.
2. Arrange to have a guest speaker from a local recycling center come in to talk with students. Ask the speaker to describe the activities conducted at the center, what he or she does at the center, and what the students should do to help their community's recycling efforts.
3. As an example of how recycling works, have students bring one recycled item in each day for the rest of the week. Remind students that they should clean the item out and remove labels. Have a box in the classroom where students can place their recyclable items.
4. At the end of the week the students will notice a sizeable pile of recyclables. Tell students to imagine what could happen if recycling were done by everyone every week. Discuss with students some things that they could do to increase the community's recycling efforts.

V. Materials Needed

- recycling box

VI. Formative Evaluation

Benchmarks

- Level 1: Student was able to list some recyclables.
- Level 2: Student was able to list some recyclables and specify some recycling guidelines.
- Level 3: Student was able to list some recyclables and specify some recycling guidelines. Student was able to give examples of recycling programs in the community.
- Level 4: Student was able to list some recyclables and specify some recycling guidelines. Student was able to give examples of recycling programs in the community and describe ways to increase the community's recycling efforts.

VII. Points of Emphasis

1. Explain benefits of everyone doing their part in a recycling program.
2. Explain ways in which recycling is helpful to the environment.
3. Explain the importance of recycling awareness and advocacy.

Teacher Evaluation

1. Keep the lesson as taught? yes _____ no _____

2. What I need to improve _____

3. Next time make sure _____

4. Strengths of lesson _____

TEACHING IN ACTION | **Daily Lesson Plan**

Lesson Title: Water Conservation

Date: May 21, 2012   **Time:** 11:00 A.M.   **Grade:** One   **Teacher:** Nance

I. National Health Education Standards

Health Education Standard 7: Student will demonstrate the ability to practice health-enhancing behaviors and avoid or reduce health risks.

II. National Health Education Standards Performance Indicator

7.2.2 demonstrate behaviors to avoid or reduce health risks.

III. Valued Outcomes

- Students will identify wasteful habits that can easily be changed.
- Students will describe ways to conserve resources to help the environment.
- Students will observe a simple exercise that demonstrates water waste.

IV. Description of Strategy

1. Bring two toothbrushes and a tube of toothpaste to class. Choose two students ahead of time to brush their teeth. Give these students simple instructions so they will be brushing their teeth for approximately the same amount of time. Begin by asking students how many times they should brush their teeth and how many people in their families brush their teeth.
2. Put a bucket under each faucet to catch the water. One student should leave the water running while brushing his or her teeth and the other student should turn the water off.
3. Ask students to compare the amount of water used by each student. Have students predict what would happen to our water supply if everyone wasted water.
4. Have students describe other ways in which we waste water and how we can prevent this from happening. Have them think of ways they use water and ways they could be conserving water.
5. Discuss other limited natural resources. Have students list ways to conserve these resources.

V. Materials Needed

- two toothbrushes/toothpaste
- two buckets

VI. Formative Evaluation

Benchmarks

- Level 1: Student was able to identify a wasteful habit.
- Level 2: Student was able to identify several wasteful habits and give non-wasteful alternatives.
- Level 3: Student was able to identify several wasteful habits and give non-wasteful alternatives. Student was able to describe a way to conserve other resources.
- Level 4: Student was able to identify several wasteful habits and give non-wasteful alternatives. Student was able to describe many ways to conserve other resources.

VII. Points of Emphasis

1. Describe other ways that students can conserve water.
2. Explain that though some waste seems to be very small, waste becomes very large when everyone does it.
3. Describe other limited natural resources.

Teacher Evaluation

1. Keep the lesson as taught?   yes _____   no _____

2. What I need to improve _____

3. Next time make sure _____

4. Strengths of lesson _____

Strategies

✓ **Assessment for Decision Stories:** Students can identify health-enhancing behaviors and exhibit positive decision-making skills.

The Fishing Trip — Grades K–3

Ramon is going fishing with his grandfather and is very excited. They have fixed a picnic lunch because they plan to stay all day. Ramon and his grandfather drive to the river. As they walk along the riverside, Ramon notices some dead fish floating in the water. "Grandfather, what killed those fish?" Ramon asks. "They were killed because people put garbage into the river," Grandfather replies. Then they sit down and start to fish. Ramon and his grandfather catch several fish apiece.

Focus Questions:

1. Should they take the fish home and cook them? Why or why not?
2. What can Ramon and his grandfather do to make the river cleaner?

National Health Education Standards: 5, 7

A Bird's Nest — Grades K–3

Jim and Richard are good friends who live next door to one another. They are now old enough to walk home from school, and today is their first time to do so. On the way home they cut through a small park. Richard discovers a bird's nest with three eggs in it. He wants to take it home. Jim has been taught that it is important not to disturb the natural surroundings, but Richard is such a good friend.

Focus Question: What should Jim do?
National Health Education Standard: 5

Is Recycling Worth the Work? — Grades 3–8

Kathy has heard about a recycling center in her town. People can bring bottles and aluminum cans there. The material is crushed and then sold to industry to be used again. Kathy tells her mother about the recycling center and asks if the family can bring in their bottles and cans. "It sounds like a good idea," Kathy's mother says, "but it's too much work. We would have to clean and sort all our old bottles and cans. Anyway, the recycling center has enough bottles and cans without us."

Focus Question: Should Kathy try to convince her mother that recycling is worth the effort? If so, how could she do this?

National Health Education Standards: 5, 8

Bad Air — Grades 4–6

Esther's mother always comes home from work coughing and wheezing. "What's wrong, Mom?" Esther asks. "It's all that dirty air I have to breathe riding the bus to and from work," her mother replies. "Maybe you could find a job closer to home," Esther says. "It's not that easy to find jobs these days," her mother says. "I guess I'll just have to put up with the bad air on the bus."

Focus Questions:

1. Is there anything Esther can do to help her mother?
2. Who can Esther contact to find out about lowering air pollution?

National Health Education Standards: 5, 8

Dramatizations

Water Pollution: Oil Spills — Grades K–3

Valued Outcome: Students will be able to describe how oil spills hurt the environment.

National Health Education Standards: 1, 7

Description of Strategy: Have five to ten students pretend that they are living plants, fish, animals, and other living things in a body of water. Have three or four other students act as if they are the sun shining on the water and helping the plants and other living things to live. Then have five to ten students come marching in and pretend they are an oil spill in the water. Have each "organism" explain the effect the oil spill will have on its species.

Processing Questions:

1. What exactly happens during an oil spill?
2. What other environmentally dangerous events can oil spills cause?

◯ **Integration:** Science

✓ **Assessment:** Students are able to discuss the environmental impact of oil spills.

Plants and Animals Need Protection, Too — Grades K–3

Valued Outcome: Students will role-play a community of plants and animals in environmental danger.

National Health Education Standard: 1

Description of Strategy: Divide the class into groups and use a story such as "Smokey the Bear," "Bambi," or any other suitable example for the specific grade level to inspire students to role-play a community of plants and animals that is in danger from an environmental threat. Tell students not only to voice their concerns as the animals and plants, but also to try to decide whether they as plants and animals can do anything to either prevent or diminish the environmental threat.

Processing Question: How do environmental health dangers affect animals?

✓ **Assessment:** Students can explain how environmental problems affect plants and animals.

Populations and Resource Use Grades 3–4

Valued Outcome: Students will be able to discuss how to conserve resources.

National Health Education Standards: 7, 8

Description of Strategy: Have three of the students act as if they are horses in the wild. Provide several bottles around the room for water and little snacks such as cereal for food. Tell the horses they must eat and drink to survive. The snacks represent the grass they must have, and the water represents a stream of water. Add three more horses, then three more, and keep going until everyone is a horse. Have them "go to sleep," and tell them that when they wake up there will only be a small amount of water and food left. Ask them to explain to you what they will do. Have several of the horses die. Then ask a variety of questions about what actually happened. Relate the story to human beings and our resources. Explain what happens to other animals and the whole ecological system when resources become limited for a species.

Materials Needed: water bottles, bags of cereal

Processing Questions:

1. What was the problem?
2. What would happen once there was no more food or water?

✓ **Assessment:** Students demonstrate an understanding of the problem of limited resources and can discuss ideas for conservation.

Disaster Preparation Practice Grades 4–6

Valued Outcome: Students will identify an environmental disaster and its effects on communities.

National Health Education Standards: 1, 8

Description of Strategy: Divide the class into groups of five, and assign each group to research an environmental disaster that could affect communities, such as an air pollution crisis, train derailment of hazardous chemicals, or a highly toxic pollutant entering municipal water systems. Ask each group to dramatize a preparation plan that demonstrates the actions that should be taken or contributions that could be made by various community organizations in dealing with the environmental danger, should it ever occur.

Processing Questions:

1. What are examples of environmental danger plans?
2. Does your community have a plan for a radiation disaster or other danger?

○ **Integration:** Social Studies

✓ **Assessment:** Students will be able to discuss steps to be taken in dealing with an environmental danger.

Alien Impressions Grades 4–6

Valued Outcome: Students will be able to discuss how aliens from another planet would react to our environmental conditions.

National Health Education Standard: 1

Description of Strategy: Divide the class into groups of about five students. Tell each group that they are aliens from outer space who have suddenly landed in the heart of the city. Ask the groups to act out their reactions to our earthly surroundings, placing special emphasis on impressions about noise levels, traffic, air pollution, global warming, crowding, and use of natural resources.

Processing Question: How would our environmental conditions appear to someone not familiar with our planet?

✓ **Assessment:** Students demonstrate an understanding of the environmental problems faced by society.

Role-Playing Environmental Hazards Grades 4–6

Valued Outcome: Students will be able to discuss environmental hazards.

National Health Education Standards: 1, 7

Description of Strategy: Divide the class into groups of four to five students. Have the groups pick an environmental hazard, then have one group at a time come up and act out the problem. Examples of hazards that might be used include water pollution and air pollution—pretend to be using hair spray, littering, and so on. The group that can guess what environmental hazard is taking place receives a point. If no one can guess the environmental hazard, then that group receives a point. Have the students draw index cards with the hazards listed on them. Have several cards for each type of hazard. Instruct the students that they may *not* portray the same aspect of that hazard as has already been performed. List hazards on the board. Have students brainstorm to come up with hazards that weren't covered. Keep playing until everyone has had several turns. At the end of the lesson, have the students brainstorm all the hazards and write them down on the board.

Materials Needed: board and marker or overhead projector and pen

Processing Question: Where can environmental hazards be found?

✓ **Assessment:** Students will demonstrate their ability to analyze the effects of various environmental hazards.

Future Lifestyles   Grades 4–8

Valued Outcome: Students will be able to portray what life will be like in the future.

National Health Education Standard: 1

Description of Strategy: Divide the class into small groups; assign each group a different social role—for example, factory workers, business professionals, and small-scale farmers. Ask each group to portray what they think life will be like for their members in fifty years, paying particular attention to possible environmental changes and their influences on the surroundings.

Processing Question: What environmental changes likely will affect people's lives fifty years from now?

○ **Integration:** Social Studies

✓ **Assessment:** Students can discuss the impact of environmental changes on future generations.

City Crisis   Grades 6–8

Valued Outcome: Students will enact a hypothetical dilemma concerning an environmental issue.

National Health Education Standards: 4, 7

Description of Strategy: Provide the class with a hypothetical dilemma involving a voting question about a proposed city ordinance concerning an environmental issue. Give enough detailed information so that the viewpoints of various special interest groups can be developed. Then divide the class into three groups. Assign two groups the task of presenting a scenario and possible solution to the problem at a town meeting; the purpose is to have each group come up with its own solution to the same problem. Let students within each group volunteer to role-play identical characters, such as meeting moderator, mayor, union representatives, and conservation spokespeople. Allow both groups a few days to prepare a fifteen-minute dramatization. Dramatizations are presented as the third group acts as observers. Following the presentations, the third group then objectively critiques the ideas by highlighting strong points of each presentation and suggesting additional alternatives.

Materials Needed: description of hypothetical city and its problems (may be in handout form) for each student

Processing Questions:

1. What environmental concerns are being debated, discussed, and voted on by your city politicians?
2. How will their discussions affect you and your family?

○ **Integration:** Social Studies

✓ **Assessment:** Students demonstrate an understanding of the environmental issues facing metropolitan areas.

Discussion and Report Techniques

Banner   Grades K–5

Valued Outcome: Students will be able to describe the positive and negative environmental aspects of their surroundings.

National Health Education Standards: 1, 7

Description of Strategy: Place a long blank banner on one side of the room and another long banner on the other side of the room. Write Positive on one and Negative on the other. Have the students draw and write positive and negative environmental factors on the correct banners, then have the students volunteer to show what they drew or wrote to the class and discuss each item.

Materials Needed: two long banners, markers or crayons for each student

Processing Questions:

1. What environmental factors in your surroundings should be considered?
2. What are the positive and negative aspects of each of those factors?

✓ **Assessment:** Students can describe the several positive and negative environmental aspects in their lives.

Activities and Their Environmental Effects   Grades 1–3

Valued Outcome: Students will list ten activities and describe how these activities affect the environment.

National Health Education Standards: 1, 7

Description of Strategy: Ask each student to list ten hobbies or activities he or she enjoys doing. After listing the activities, students should examine each activity in terms of its effects, if any, on the environment. As a result of this exercise, students will observe the relationship between their behavior and the environment in which they live.

Materials Needed: pens or pencils and paper for each student

Processing Question: What effects, if any, do your hobbies have on the environment? Are the effects positive or negative?

✓ **Assessment:** Students can name several ways their activities influence the environment.

For the Love of the Earth   Grades 3–6

Valued Outcome: Students will list different things that make up their natural environment and select the ones they think are most important.

National Health Education Standards: 1, 4

Description of Strategy: Conduct a class discussion about the environment: what it is and how it affects our lives. As a group, have students name and list on the board different aspects of our environment (water, air, land, sunshine, petroleum, etc.). After making a comprehensive list, divide the class into groups of three. Have each group name the part of their environment they consider the most important and list three reasons why. Then, have them draw a picture showing this vital resource with the reasons why it is important listed below. Each group will present their completed assignment to the class.

Materials Needed: board and markers or overhead projector and pen; large sheets of butcher paper, markers, crayons, and pencils or pens for each group

Processing Questions:

1. What would our world be like if we did not have the resources we have today?
2. Which resources could we live without? Which ones do we need in order to live?
3. Which resources are most important to you?

○ **Integration:** Art

✓ **Assessment:** Students are able to identify the importance of several natural resources.

Me and My Surroundings   Grades 4–6

Valued Outcome: Students will recognize their perceptions of the environment.

National Health Education Standards: 1, 4, 7

Description of Strategy: Ask each student to keep a daily log for a week about his or her perceptions of environmental influences by writing a short paragraph that describes an event or events of each day in terms of environmental awareness. Students should emphasize not only facts, but also feelings about these influences. For example, "Heavy rain against my window last night sounded nice. The noisy and crowded school bus made me feel irritable." At the end of the week, divide the class into seven discussion groups, each one representing one day of the

week. Have groups compare their logs for that day and summarize major perceptions about surroundings. One group member should then present a five-minute report to the class outlining summary findings for the group.

Materials Needed: pens or pencils and paper for each student

Processing Questions:

1. What environmental influences did you observe?
2. What influences need to be changed in order to protect the environment?

○ **Integration:** Writing

✓ **Assessment:** Students demonstrate an awareness of how the environment impacts their lives.

Can I Recycle?   Grades 4–6

Valued Outcome: Students will become acquainted with a variety of ways to recycle resources on a daily basis.

National Health Education Standards: 7, 8

Description of Strategy: Using the Internet, students will find at least ten different ways to recycle at home and at school. Assign each method to a different group to learn about and describe to the class. Students will discuss how to make each recycling method a part of their daily life.

Materials Needed: computer with Internet access, pens or pencils and paper for each student

Processing Questions:

1. What are some things we can do every day to reduce environmental waste?
2. Why should we consider recycling every day?

✓ **Assessment:** Students can name several ways and places that people can recycle every day.

Energy Savings   Grades 4–6

Valued Outcome: Students will be able to explain how to conserve energy.

National Health Education Standards: 7, 8

Description of Strategy: Have a general class discussion concerning ways to save energy in the United States. Discuss how rising costs of fuel have made Americans more energy conscious in recent years. Individual students may wish to volunteer how their families are doing more to save energy. For older students, ask them to formulate a rationale for why they think their suggestions will save energy.

Processing Questions:

1. What are the types of energy used in your homes?
2. What are ways you and your family can save energy?

○ **Integration:** Social Studies

✓ **Assessment:** Students demonstrate their ability to advocate for instituting energy saving steps in their households.

Solid Waste   Grades 4–6

Valued Outcome: Students will be able to identify the terms associated with handling and disposing of solid waste.

National Health Education Standard: 1

Description of Strategy: Ask the students to identify the terms associated with solid waste. Put the terms on an overhead; discuss each of the terms and provide examples or illustrations of each. After reviewing the terms, pass out a worksheet containing the terms and their definitions (see Worksheet 26.3 on page 507). Have students match the words with the definitions.

Materials Needed: Worksheet 26.3 and pens or pencils for each student

Processing Questions:

1. What three important ideas came out of discussing the solid waste terms?
2. What are ways we can reuse, reduce, or recycle solid waste in our daily lives?
3. Why are biodegradable products important to our environment?

✓ **Assessment:** Students can correctly complete the worksheet.

Environmental Stories   Grades 4–8

Valued Outcome: Students will create a story about the environment.

National Health Education Standard: 4

Description of Strategy: Select a colorful, eye-catching, and appropriate picture depicting an aspect of the

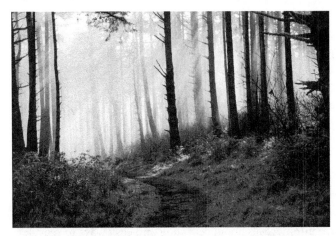

Trees can have a positive influence upon our environment.

environment. Have each student write a story about the picture. Allow about twenty minutes, and encourage both creativity and the exploration of thoughts. Have volunteers read their stories to the class.

Materials Needed: picture of the environment, pens or pencils and paper for each student

Processing Questions:

1. What did you notice about the environment from the picture?
2. Was the environment in the picture a pleasant scene?

○ **Integration:** Writing

✓ **Assessment:** Students can express their experience, feelings, or understanding of the environment in writing.

Population Problems   Grades 4–8

Valued Outcome: Students will be able to discuss overpopulation as an environmental hazard.

National Health Education Standard: 1

Description of Strategy: To stimulate discussion about the concerns of overpopulation for very young students, have them recite the nursery rhyme, "There was an old woman who lived in a shoe./She had so many children she knew not what to do." Have students tell you what this rhyme means to them. Older students can be asked to make a graph of the world's population increases since the beginning of recorded years (see population statistics on page 435). Note especially the trend for the last twenty years. Then provide further information about the problem of overpopulation, and have students discuss suggestions to curb overpopulation.

Materials Needed: pens or pencils and graph paper for each student

Processing Questions:

1. Does your community have an overpopulation problem?
2. What measures can be taken to reduce the overpopulation problem?

○ **Integration:** Social Studies

✓ **Assessment:** Students can articulate the effects of overpopulation.

Hunger Hurts   Grades 4–8

Valued Outcome: Students will be able to discuss world hunger.

National Health Education Standards: 1, 3, 4

Description of Strategy: As a class, have students research information about the impact of hunger on children throughout the world. Ask the librarian to suggest a few sources that each class member can read. Also have students determine the three leading causes of death among infants and children in the United States compared to those of several other countries you select. Be sure to include both European and developing countries. Allow students to discuss their ideas concerning the reason for these differences. You may need to remind students that food, medicine, and access to quality health care are all resources.

Materials Needed: library books

Processing Questions:

1. What is the incidence of hunger in Europe and other countries?
2. Is hunger a problem in our country? In your community?

○ **Integration:** Social Studies, Reading

✓ **Assessment:** Students can cite appropriate and reliable sources to describe the impact of limited resources and overpopulation.

Environmental Newswatch and Commentary
Grades 5–8

Valued Outcome: Students will choose various environmental articles and identify the purpose of the articles.

National Health Education Standards: 3, 7

Description of Strategy: Divide the class into small groups; provide each student with three sheets of colored construction paper. Have them paste an article on an environmental topic onto each sheet. Use of newsletters, supplementary magazines, and books that are written for the students' grade level should be encouraged. Underneath each article, have the students write a caption that describes the purpose of the article. Have each group then compile their articles into a booklet. Similar articles should be grouped within the booklets.

Materials Needed: three sheets of construction paper and pencils or pens for each student, markers, newspapers, magazines, glue

Processing Questions:

1. What were your environmental articles about?
2. Did the stories portray any lessons about conservation?

○ **Integration:** Reading

✓ **Assessment:** Students demonstrate their ability to analyze the purpose of articles about the environment.

Let's Be Creative
Grades 5–8

Valued Outcome: Students will be able to present solutions for various environmental hazards.

National Health Education Standards: 1, 4, 7, 8

Description of Strategy: Have the students draw a cartoon series, write a story, or make up a poem about an environmental problem, then have volunteers share what they did with the class. Discuss what was said, problems, and solutions for the environmental hazard. After completing the activity, have students hang their work around the room. Let them observe each other's displays.

Materials Needed: paper, markers, pens or pencils for each student

Processing Questions:

1. What environmental hazards did you identify?
2. What solutions did you present for each hazard?

○ **Integration:** Art or Writing

✓ **Assessment:** Students' creative projects and discussions demonstrate their ability to seek out and advocate solutions for various environmental problems.

General Pollution Problems
Grades 5–8

Valued Outcome: Students will be able to describe the impact of major environmental problems.

National Health Education Standards: 1, 3, 4

Description of Strategy: Divide the class into several small groups, and assign each group a different major pollution problem. After researching the general aspects of the problem, each group should give a short oral panel presentation. Within the groups, each member is then assigned a specific aspect of the given pollution problem, such as oil spills, effects of sulfides in the air, or the banning of pesticides such as DDT. Have the students prepare individual written reports.

Materials Needed: pens or pencils and paper for each student; references

Processing Question: What are the major environmental problems that directly affect you? That indirectly affect you?

○ **Integration:** Reading, Writing

✓ **Assessment:** Students' reports and presentations demonstrate their understanding of major pollution problems.

Spread the Word
Grades 6–8

Valued Outcome: Students will write and produce their own infomercials about recycling and easy ways to recycle every day.

National Health Education Standards: 7, 8

Description of Strategy: Using the information they have gathered from researching recycling methods on the Internet, students will divide into groups (one for each recycling method) and write their own infomercials about how easy recycling can be, demonstrating their assigned method. The infomercials can be videotaped and played for the class, in other classes, and for special presentations for parents.

Materials Needed: computer with Internet access, pens or pencils and paper for each student, video camera, VCR or DVD player or computer (depending on media type), televisions

Processing Questions:

1. Why do we need to let others know the importance of recycling?
2. What is the best way to get that message across to other people?

○ **Integration:** Social Studies, Writing

✓ **Assessment:** Students' infomercials demonstrate their understanding of the benefits of recycling and their ability to advocate for recycling.

Recycling and You   Grades 6–8

Valued Outcome: Students will design pamphlets that stress the importance of recycling.

National Health Education Standard: 8

Description of Strategy: Divide the class into groups of four or five. Using information they have gathered from the Internet and other sources, have each group design a pamphlet about the importance of recycling. They can include illustrations and suggestions for recycling. When completed, groups present their pamphlets to the class. Additional pamphlets can be made and distributed throughout the school.

Materials Needed: computer with Internet access; research references; colored pens, markers, pencils, tape or glue, and paper for each group

Processing Questions:

1. Why do you think people should recycle?
2. What is the most important aspect of recycling?
3. What can you say that would make others want to recycle?

○ **Integration:** Writing, Art

✓ **Assessment:** Students' pamphlets demonstrate their understanding of the benefits of recycling and their ability to advocate for recycling.

Experiments and Demonstrations

Recyclable Containers   Grades 1–5

Valued Outcome: Students will be able to explain the positive aspects of recycling.

National Health Education Standards: 4, 8

Description of Strategy: Have the students bring a box or paper bag to class to make into a recycle container. Have the students draw, color, or write whatever they want on their containers. Place the containers around the school and in different classes. At the end of the week, collect the recyclable cans and paper. Discuss with the class how they feel about the project and the results from it.

Materials Needed: box or bag, markers, crayons or other writing and drawing tools for each student

Processing Questions:

1. What is the purpose of recycling?
2. How does recycling help our environment?

○ **Integration:** Art

✓ **Assessment:** Students can explain the purpose of recycling and demonstrate the ability to advocate for recycling.

Crowding Problems   Grades 2–6

Valued Outcome: Students will be able to discuss the effects of overcrowding (overpopulation) on the environment.

National Health Education Standards: 7, 8

Description of Strategy: Divide the class into groups, and give each group two milk cartons with the tops cut off and a few holes punched in the bottom for drainage. Ask students to fill each carton about two-thirds full with potting soil, and in one carton plant two or three bean seeds one inch apart just under the surface of the soil. In the other carton, students should plant fifteen seeds about one-half inch apart. Have them water the seeds every four days and record their observations. As an extension of this activity, crowd students into a confined space for a few minutes, and then ask them to describe how it felt.

Materials Needed: two milk cartons for each group, potting soil, bean seeds, water, journals and pen or pencils for each student to record observations

Processing Question: What are the problems of overcrowding as it relates to the use of natural resources?

○ **Integration:** Social Studies

✓ **Assessment:** Students can explain the negative effects of overcrowding and overpopulation.

Product	Frequency	Amount	Ways to Reduce
Paper napkins			
Facial tissues			
Toilet paper			
Notebook paper			

Seasonal Adjustments Grades 3–6

Valued Outcome: Students will be able to explain the environmental influences of trees and plants.

National Health Education Standard: 1

Description of Strategy: Divide the class into small groups, and ask each group to select a favorite tree or shrub in the school yard to observe once a month for the school year. Have groups record their observations in relation to environmental influences on the changes of the tree or shrub.

Materials Needed: journal to record monthly data, and pencils or pens for each group

Processing Questions:

1. What changes take place in trees from season to season?
2. What effects can planting trees have on our environment?

○ **Integration:** Science

✓ **Assessment:** Students can explain the seasonal changes in the environment and the impact of trees on the health of the environment.

Terrariums and Aquariums as Ecosystems Grades 3–6

Valued Outcome: Students will be able to describe the interrelationships involved in ecosystems.

National Health Education Standard: 1

Description of Strategy: As a class project—either in small groups or the entire class—help students make a terrarium or an aquarium. Refer to science textbooks as resources to help you do this. Use the terrarium or aquarium to demonstrate the interrelationships between inhabitants of each ecosystem.

Materials Needed: terrarium(s) or aquarium(s), science textbooks

Processing Question: How do inhabitants in a terrarium or aquarium depend on each other for their existence?

○ **Integration:** Science

✓ **Assessment:** Students can articulate the interrelationships between ecosystem inhabitants.

Resource Reduction Grades 4–6

Valued Outcome: Students will identify common products and compare the usage of different products.

National Health Education Standards: 1, 7, 8

Description of Strategy: Divide the class into small groups, and assign each group a common environmental product or resource, such as paper, plastic, water, electricity, or natural gas. For a few days, ask each group member to keep a daily list of his or her specific uses of the resource or products they use that may impact that resource (such as plastic milk jugs that contain milk to drink, paper towels used to mop up a spill). Have students compare lists. On butcher paper, prepare a master list outlining the most typically used products, the most common uses, the amount students think has been used by the total group, and the ways to reduce the use. Lists might look something like the table on this page.

Materials Needed: daily log for each student, butcher paper and markers

Processing Questions:

1. Did you observe any patterns in your use of the various products?
2. Do you think you can conserve products in order to help the environment?

✓ **Assessment:** Students demonstrate the ability to advocate for conservation of resources and products.

Signs Grades 4–6

Valued Outcome: Students will be able to produce some helpful environmental hints.

National Health Education Standard: 8

Description of Strategy: Have the students make a variety of signs to display around the school—such as, "Turn off the water when you're finished," "Throw away your trash," "Recycle your cans." Ask the students how they might monitor any changes in behavior that might occur in response to their signs, and have them implement their plan. After a week, discuss the results and note any changes in behavior. If there are no changes, ask why. Think of another alternative, and try it. If it works, congratulate them on a job well done.

Materials Needed: paper, markers, pens or pencils for each student

Processing Question: What can we do to help advance the cause of environmental conservation?

✓ **Assessment:** Students demonstrate the ability to model and advocate for environmentally responsible behavior.

Waste Production   Grades 4–8

Valued Outcome: Students will be able to discuss the impact of solid waste (such as household trash) on the environment.

National Health Education Standards: 1, 7

Description of Strategy: Have the students observe in their homes how many bags of trash they fill a day. Have them do this for three days. Every day before class starts, tally up the bags of trash used the day before. After three days, have the students place a recycling container by the trash and ask all family members to put recyclable items in it. Calculate the number of bags of trash for the next three days and keep a class tally as before. Have the students explain what has happened and what they have observed. This will show how much they waste. Tell students how many people were living in the United States at the last population census and point out how much people in our country waste. Discuss what will happen if we keep doing this. Discuss what might happen if we start recycling, or what happens to the recycled products if there is already a recycling program.

Materials Needed: tally sheets, pencils

Processing Questions:

1. What is the impact of solid waste products on our environment?
2. What are some ways you and your family can dispose of or recycle some solid wastes to help protect the environment?

✓ **Assessment:** Students can explain how recycling can reduce the negative impacts of solid waste on the environment.

Noise Levels   Grades 4–8

Valued Outcome: Students will be able to discuss unwanted noise as an environmental hazard.

National Health Education Standard: 7

Description of Strategy: Use a decibel meter to check noise levels in various locations throughout the school.

Record the location, time of day, and meter reading. Noise levels will vary during different times of day. Which locations are noisiest? Are there any sources of particularly loud sounds, such as school bus engines?

Materials Needed: decibel meter, journals, and pencils to record data

Processing Questions:

1. How can some sounds become environmental hazards?
2. What are some ways to diminish noise pollution in the school environment?

○ **Integration:** Science

✓ **Assessment:** Students can list health hazards of high decibel exposure.

Water Impurities   Grades 5–8

Valued Outcome: Students will be able to discuss the environmental implications of impurities in drinking water.

National Health Education Standards: 7, 8

Description of Strategy: Have each student bring in a small glass jar of water from a tap at home. Even though the water may all come from the same municipal supply, there will be differences in the samples because of rust or chemical residues in the water pipes in each home. Examine the water samples using a light microscope.

Materials Needed: glass jars, tap water from each student's home

Processing Questions:

1. What are the implications of impurities in drinking water?
2. How can we ensure that we have safe water to drink?

○ **Integration:** Science

✓ **Assessment:** Students can discuss the importance of maintaining safe drinking water to our quality of life.

Deadly Precipitation   Grades 6–8

Valued Outcome: Students will be able to define acid rain and its potential effects on the environment.

National Health Education Standard: 1

Description of Strategy: Before the class date, assign students to work in groups of five to collect samples of rainwater either at school or at home. Have them also collect and label samples from the school's drinking water, a nearby lake or stream, and other local water sources. (Masking tape labels should include the date and where the sample was collected.) On the activity day, define the term *acid rain* and write the definition on the board. Give each group its own containers for each water source. Have students test the water in each container for acidity by dipping litmus paper into it. Record the results on the label on each container. A pH less than 7.0 is acidic; a pH higher than 7.0 is alkaline (or basic). Water is considered "clean" at 5.4. A pH less than 5.0 is a pollution concern. Have students graph the results for their group and present the data to the class.

Materials Needed: multiple small containers for water samples; water samples; litmus paper, masking tape, graph paper, pencils or pens for each group

Processing Questions:

1. Could acid rain be an environmental hazard in our area?
2. How much of a problem do you think acid rain is in your community?

○ **Integration:** Science

✓ **Assessment:** Students can define acid rain and describe its impact on their community (if any) or its possible impacts in high-risk areas.

Puzzles and Games

Treasure Hunt　　　　　　　　　　Grades 2–8

Valued Outcome: Students will be able to describe the recycling process and how recycling helps protect the environment.

National Health Education Standards: 7, 8

Description of Strategy: Divide the class into groups of five to eight students. On several tables have a variety of items (recyclable, nonrecyclable, hazards, and helpful things for our environment) such as notebook paper, a coin, a leaf, plastic wrap, clean water, rubber stopper, cleansers, oil bottle, and so on. Ask the students various questions about environmental health. Some questions might relate to the items on the table, and some questions may not. Students must write down the answers. An example of a question that might be asked is "Who can show me a recyclable item?" The group with the student who raises a hand first and can give the right answer will get a point. Another example: "Name three types of pollution" (water, air, noise, radiation, chemical, thermal). The game continues until all the questions are answered. The group that answers the most questions correctly is considered the winner.

Materials Needed: a variety of objects that are recyclable, nonrecyclable, harmful, or helpful to the environment; pencils and paper; list of environmental health questions

Processing Questions:

1. What is the purpose of recycling?
2. How does recycling help protect the environment?
3. How can recycling help your health?

○ **Integration:** Science, Social Studies

✓ **Assessment:** Students demonstrate the ability to advocate for recycling by describing why recycling is an important social, economic, and environmental issue.

Health Hazard　　　　　　　　　　Grades 3–8

Valued Outcome: Students will be able to name and suggest solutions to environmental hazards.

National Health Education Standards: 4, 7

Description of Strategy: Ask the students various questions about their environmental health. Examples: How many of you like to drink soda? How many of you recycle your cans when you're done? Why? Why not? How many of you have an electric can opener in your house? Do you think you're wasting electricity by using it instead of a manual one? What are some other hazardous behaviors we have that can threaten our environmental health? (Answers might include not conserving water or electricity; polluting the air, water, environment; not recycling other items; and so on.)

Have a student put on a jersey to represent one of the health hazards in our environment. The student will be "it." He or she will try to tag the other students. Once the students are tagged, they must sit down because they are now health hazards. After two minutes, have all the students who have not been tagged come to you. Ask them to tell you something that we can do to correct the problem. For instance, if the health hazard was "waste," the students may suggest that we recycle. The game starts again with another student as a different health hazard. At the end of the lesson, have three or four health hazards be "it" simultaneously to illustrate that the more health hazards we have, the greater the chance of having a highly unhealthy environment.

Materials Needed: jerseys or bandannas

Processing Question: What are some specific ways that each of us can correct some environmental hazards?

○ **Integration:** Physical Education

✓ **Assessment:** Students can identify environmental hazards and suggest several practical solutions for reducing their impact.

Brainstorm　　　　　　　　　　　Grades 4–6

Valued Outcome: Students will discuss the meaning of several environmental terms.

National Health Education Standard: 1

Description of Strategy: Divide the class into groups of four to six. Write a word on the board, such as *recycle*. Have groups brainstorm everything that comes to their minds when they hear the word *recycle*. Then have each group work as a team and make a list of terms related to the environment—for example, glass, paper, plastic, newspapers, water. After one minute, start with group 1 and have them tell one item on their list. Group 2 will then go, naming a different item. Write all the words on the board for the class.

After each group has been asked, go around the room again. The group that has the most responses gets a point. Then the game starts again with another word. Specific questions can also be asked. For example, what are the effects of water pollution? Answers might include: destroys or injures animals, depletes food supplies, harms reproduction, produces odors, makes foul tasting drinking water, causes diseases, and pollutes beaches.

Materials Needed: paper and pens or pencils for each student; board and markers or overhead projector and pen

Processing Question: What are the effects of various types of pollution on the environment?

✓ **Assessment:** Students' word associations demonstrate their understanding of environmental terminology.

Air Pollution Word Search   Grades 4–6

Valued Outcome: Students will identify words associated with air pollution.

National Health Education Standard: 1

Description of Strategy: After reviewing terms and conditions associated with air pollution, provide the students with a word search and have them find the words. After identifying each word, have them write the definition of the word.

Materials Needed: copy of word search and pencils or pens for each student

Processing Questions:

1. When you found the words, were you able to define them?
2. Of the words on the list, which causes the most air pollution?

✓ **Assessment:** Students can define the words they find in the word search and describe the most egregious influences on air pollution.

Source: Ohio Department of Natural Resources 1990

Other Ideas

Poster Contest   Grades 3–8

Valued Outcome: Students will create a poster with an environmental message.

National Health Education Standard: 8

Description of Strategy: Ask each student to make a poster on a specified environmental topic such as energy, resources, or global warming. Give minimal details about what might be included. Let the students use their creativity. Number each poster anonymously and hang each around the room. Have another class view the posters and select the five best, which are then hung in the hallway or school library.

Materials Needed: poster board, markers, crayons for each student

Processing Question: What are some environmental messages we can portray through posters?

○ **Integration:** Art

✓ **Assessment:** Students demonstrate their ability to advocate for environmentally responsible behavior.

Illustrating Environmental Aspects   Grades 4–6

Valued Outcome: Students will illustrate ideas concerning various environmental resources.

National Health Education Standards: 4, 8

Description of Strategy: Create a handout from the list below and give one to each student. Then ask the class to draw or illustrate their ideas about the items on the list. Have students share their pictures with each other to compare ideas.

- most important environmental resource
- most abundant environmental resource
- most depleted environmental resource
- most dangerous environmental threat to the world
- most environmentally helpful family measure practiced
- least environmentally helpful family measure practiced
- most environmentally helpful personal measure practiced
- least environmentally helpful personal measure practiced

Materials Needed: pencils or pens, paper, handout for each student

Processing Questions:

1. What did you learn from this activity that will help protect our environment?
2. What can you personally do to protect the environment?

○ **Integration:** Art

✔ **Assessment:** Students demonstrate an awareness of how their efforts to make good choices affect the environment.

Survival Lists   Grades 4–6

Valued Outcome: Students will be able to compile a list of supplies needed in the time of an environmental disaster.

National Health Education Standards: 3, 7

Description of Strategy: Divide the class into small groups. Ask each group to prepare two lists. One list should include necessary supplies for a family of four to survive on the Earth for the next year in the event of a disaster. The other list should include the twenty most important items to take on a trip to outer space. Let groups compare lists and discuss ideas. If enough agreement can be reached, make a class master list.

Materials Needed: paper and pens or pencils foreach student

Processing Questions:

1. What are some environmental disasters that might necessitate the prior accumulation of supplies?
2. What supplies would be the most important to gather prior to such a disaster?

Integration: Social Studies

✔ **Assessment:** Students can list the most important supplies needed in the event of an environmental disaster.

Epilogue

A coordinated approach to addressing students' health can become one of the means to meet a shared outcome: productive and capable students. Similarly, a primary objective of health care reform is cost savings; health education and prevention play central roles in accomplishing that goal.[*]

It is the intention of the authors that this textbook portrays the necessity for providing a sound framework for health education complemented by opportunities for weighing and formulating a value system. This weighing and formulating of a value system is imperative because the authors view attitudes and values as predispositions to action or behavior. In other words, we act on or do those things that we view as important to us, whether those things are positive or negative in nature. By enabling students to assess the importance and ramifications of information and potential actions, we enable them to begin to make more intelligent decisions pertaining to their health. The message is that all teaching efforts are aimed at the development of a value system resulting in a positive and healthy lifestyle.

Attitudinal formation is essential since our attitudes provide the predisposition for us to act or carry out a behavior. If we value positive health habits and view those habits as life enhancing, there is a high probability that we will follow a positive behavior.

Ultimately, the decisions about lifestyle rest with each individual. Although the ability of children to fully control their health patterns may be limited, the seeds of critical thinking, wise decision making, and positive health choices must be planted and nourished. It is the teacher's professional, societal, and personal responsibility to facilitate the understanding of a wellness lifestyle that will result in the highest possible quality of life for every student.

We believe that health education should be viewed as a planned series of experiences that promote disease prevention behaviors and reinforce positive health experiences in each student. The ultimate goal of health education is to have students accept responsibility for their lives, take charge of their health, and seek to promote the well-being of themselves, their families, and their communities. To accomplish this goal, our nation must strive for the development of a coordinated school health education program with a comprehensive health education curriculum as part of this model. A comprehensive health education program begins in kindergarten and continues through grade 12. Each step in the educational ladder should be predicated on what has previously occurred in the learning situation. Health is the most fundamental of topics. Health education must be allotted time in the same manner as mathematics, reading, and science.

The content areas of health education are many and varied. Health is not just physical education, although this is an important component. Truly healthy individuals are more able to accept themselves and others, are more physically fit, and are more capable of making informed decisions concerning the many components of living a healthier, wellness type of lifestyle. Without the best possible health, people become less productive, less satisfied in their personal lives, and less capable of contributing to other people's lives and the society of which they are a part.

As health educators, we should seek to enhance the life of each person we touch. It is our desire to help people feel better about themselves, to enhance their personal esteem, to help them select positive health habits, and to become better critical thinkers. We now have the blueprint to accomplish these goals, through adoption of the the National Health Standards, which provide the framework for formulating and accomplishing quality health education. Each state, many school systems, and individual teachers have plans and strategies that can serve as springboards to better provide responsible health education.

Each year new crises evolve requiring health educators' efforts. New needs and new knowledge are continually evolving. Childhood obesity and diabetes should be primary concerns among parents and educators. Nationwide crime statistics indicate that American children are still at danger for violence while at school, en route to and from school, and at school-related events. Also school administrators and teachers need to address the possibility of terrorist threats at school. Challenges in the areas of HIV education, nutrition

[*]Marx, E., and S. F. Wooley, eds. with D. Northrop. 1998. *Health is academic: A guide to coordinated school health programs.* New York: Teachers College Press.

education, substance abuse education, sexuality education, and environmental education continually arise.

The one constant in all of this upheaval is the classroom teacher. His or her professional dedication and love for the student must remain if health education is to be successful. Other than parents, no one person has a greater impact on a child than a teacher. What children learn about themselves, others, and their society begins with the classroom teacher.

We hope this book helps point out the necessity for health education and provides part of the blueprint for becoming successful in the teaching of health education. After all, each teacher deals with our most precious of resources—our children.

—*David J. Anspaugh and Gene Ezell*

If our values are straight and we value human health above all else, then health education becomes one of the master areas in all of American education, along with language. It deals, or should deal, with all those phenomena indigenous to being human, that develop or retard, create or kill. Nothing is more important. Time must be found for it.

—*Delbert Oberteuffer, April 24, 1982*

Appendix A: Index of Teaching Strategies

Method	Method Description
Information Assessment Activities	Information assessment activities are designed to help children develop their critical thinking skills. This often involves individual research or coursework, or small group discussions.
Decision Stories	Decision stories are open-ended vignettes that describe a values-related dilemma and ask students to suggest a course of action.
Dramatizations	Dramatizations are action-oriented strategies that can be used to enliven health instruction. Plays, skits, and puppet shows are all examples of dramatization techniques.
Discussion and Report Techniques	Discussion and report strategies help students to generate ideas about a topic or issue, and to enhance their writing and verbal/presentation skills.
Experiments and Demonstrations	Experiments and Demonstrations can help make verbal explanations more meaningful by allowing students to view, examine, and touch health-related materials.
Puzzles and Games	Puzzles are useful seatwork devices for building vocabulary and reinforcing concepts. Games can stimulate interest in a topic while providing a review of concepts learned through other strategies. Worksheets for some of these activities are now available through the Companion Website to this book, www.pearsonhighered.com/anspaugh.
Other Ideas	There are some activities that don't neatly fit into other categories; either they combine multiple strategies, or they involve primarily individual work on the part of the student (such as art collage projects). These can often be useful to assign as take-home activities for students to complete with their families.

Chapter 7   Strategies for Teaching Mental Health and Stress Reduction

Method	Sample Strategies Provided
Information Assessment Activities	Special Me Happy or Sad Helping Others Looking at Me Voting Questions Name Tag Descriptors Using Technology to Understand Mental Health and Stress Friends Should Be… Relationship Collage The Time of My Life
Decision Stories	Handling Stress Where Did I Put Them? I Dare You New Girl in School A Nasty Note
Dramatizations	Appropriate Personality Traits Guess My Trait Truth and Consequences Body Language Emotional Reactions Hidden Messages The Decision Giving and Gaining Refusal Skills

Method	Sample Strategies Provided
Discussion and Report Techniques	Ups and Downs Emotions and Me Caring Getting to Know You Who Can I Turn To? We Are Different People Picture the Emotion Living By the Rules Cartoon Personalities Who Am I? Stories Who Am I? Worksheets State of Mind "Me" Poster Question Box Steps to the Top Coping with Stress How to Handle Peer Pressure Musical Compliments Understanding Bullying I Understanding Bullying II Coping with and Controlling Stress Stress Feelings
Experiments and Demonstrations	Unique! That's Me! Costume Party Mental Health in Music Human Scavenger Hunt Hearing Is Not Always Listening
Puzzles and Games	Emotional Musical Chairs Silent Steps
Other Ideas	Facial Forecasts How Do I See Myself? Stress Facial Forecasts Emotions Bag

Chapter 10 Strategies for Teaching Body Systems and Personal Health

Method	Sample Strategies Provided	
Information Assessment Activities	**Body Systems:** Values Voting Sun Safety Art Project Being Good to Me Rank-Ordering Health Practices Body Image Sentence Completion	**Personal Health:** Smiley/Sad Face Good Health/Bad Health Personal Health Voting Exercise and Sleep Attitude Scale Dental Health/Good Self-Confidence Relaxation Ranking What Sleep Means to Me Self-Portrait Personal Health Sentence Completion
Decision Stories	**Body Systems:** Mary's Father Rita's Dilemma	**Personal Health:** Vision Problems Teeth and Truth Fitness Decision Story The Christmas Party

Continued

Chapter 10   Strategies for Teaching Body Systems and Personal Health, *continued*

Method	Sample Strategies Provided	
Dramatizations	**Body Systems:** Circulatory System Digestive System Dramatizing the Circulatory System Senses Activity Excretory System The Nervous System Inside-Out	**Personal Health:** Immunization Tanning Booths Wearing Braces
Discussion and Report Techniques	**Body Systems:** The Five Senses How Does the Heart Work? Sense of Touch Learning about the Five Senses Identifying Leaves (Sight) Review of the Senses My Five Senses Tracing Body Systems Effects of Smoking on the Lungs Which Organ Am I? Tracing the Blood Flow Muscular System Debate Voluntary Health Organization Panel Virtual Body	**Personal Health:** Presentation by Health Professionals Sleeping and Relaxing Fitness for Life Screening Procedures
Experiments and Demonstrations	**Body Systems:** Properties of Skin Seeing Is Important Follow Your Nose Body Drawings Bone Transformation Brain Viewing Nerve Messages Joint Experiment Ears Help Us Hear	**Personal Health:** Covering Sneezes and Coughs Germs Four Kinds of Teeth Fingerprints Daily Water Intake Dental Hygiene Pupil Dilation and Constriction Sound Localization Shadow Play Health Habits Aerobic and Anaerobic Activities Demonstration of Correct Brushing Teeth Problems Teeth and Digestion Sleep Needs
Puzzles and Games	**Body Systems:** The Sound Matching Game I See Blood Jeopardy Body Parts Puzzle Body Organs Game Memory Game Bean Bag Toss	**Personal Health:** Take Time for Personal Health
Other Ideas	**Body Systems:** Body Builders	**Personal Health:** Dressing for the Weather

Chapter 12   Strategies for Teaching Sexuality Education

Method	Sample Strategies Provided
Information Assessment Activities	Finding Answers Through Technology Rights and Responsibilities Attitude Inventory—How Do I Feel? Getting to Know Me How My Decisions Affect Others That's My Opinion Me and My Self-Confidence Legal Rights
Decision Stories	Am I Stuck with Me? The Crush John's World Stories or Facts Being Friendly Fooling Around The Party
Dramatizations	The Answer Is No Superkid How Would You Handle It? Understanding Others
Discussion and Report Techniques	Being My Own Perfect Friend Solving Problems Opportunities for All Dictionary with a Difference Growing Up Individual Reports
Experiments and Demonstrations	Guppies
Puzzles and Games	Word Search for the Reproductive System Reproductive System Crossword Puzzle Scrambled Sentences Matching Parts and Functions True or False
Other Ideas	Family Activities Collage Growing Up Families Are Different Inherited Traits My Family Tree Caught in the Act Responsibility Helping Others The Menstrual Cycle Why Are They Like That? Why Not? Family Rules Advice Column

Chapter 14   Strategies for Teaching about Substance Use and Abuse

Method	Sample Strategies Provided
Information Assessment Activities	Where Do You Stand? Sentence Completion Smoking and the Law Smoking and You Drug Abuse Prevention Newspaper Living without Drugs Living with Drugs Drug Rating Scale
Decision Stories	Drugs in the Neighborhood Mom Drinks Too Much Want a Smoke? Sleepover Problems at Home
Dramatizations	I'm No Dummy Drug Abuse Prevention Decision Story Presentation Peers Helping Other Peers Drug Court What Would Happen If...? Dangers of Huffing Past, Present, and Future Drug Users and Abusers Public Service Messages
Discussion and Report Techniques	Presentation by Health Professionals Dealing with Problems Who Influences Your Decisions? The Question Box Smoking Resiliency Skills Blog Saying No to Drugs Effects of Drug Use Smoking Marijuana Preventing Drinking and Driving Dangers of Smoking The Space Colony Individual Reports Defending Yourself from Pressure Just Saying No Is Our Final Answer! Researching Drug Abuse Debating Drug Abuse
Experiments and Demonstrations	Smoking Machine Goldfish Demonstration Breathalyzer Demonstration Saying No! Impaired Sobriety Testing Stations Smoking Aerobics How to Say No to Smoking
Puzzles and Games	Drugs Spell Trouble Smoking Crossword Puzzle Let's Play Tic-Tac-Toe Safe Use of Medicines
Other Ideas	My Choice, Your Choice...Consequences! Dealing with Peer Pressure Affirmations Informational Interviews and Presentations Slogans Drug Collage

Chapter 16 Strategies for Teaching about Infectious and Noninfectious Conditions

Method	Sample Strategies Provided
Information Assessment Activities	Facts and Myths How Did I Get It? Values Statements The Help I Get
Decision Stories	Play Ball Moles Can Change Your Heart's Eating Habits
Dramatizations	Betty Bacteria "Catching" Cold
Discussion and Report Techniques	Name That Disease Disease Search What Should Be Done?
Experiments and Demonstrations	Draw a Bug Things I Know, Things I'd Like to Know The Anatomy of the Heart Using Technology to Understand Infectious Diseases Analyzing Cigarette Smoke Mini-Documentary for Infectious and Noninfectious Diseases
Puzzles and Games	Heart Word Search Cancer Crossword Puzzle Hidden Message to Help Prevent Heart Disease

Chapter 18 Strategies for Teaching Nutrition

Method	Sample Strategies Provided
Information Assessment Activities	Nutrition Self-Portraits Healthy Food Voting Rank-Ordering Favorite Foods What's for Lunch? A Healthy Breakfast Nutrition Sentence Completion Nutrition Podcasts Values Continuum
Decision Stories	What to Drink? Fast Food
Dramatizations	Foods That Keep the Body Healthy Role-Playing Nutrients Garden Puppet Show Dieting Puppets and Eating Disorders Star Search Caffeine and Sleeping Cafeteria Selection Choosing from a Menu Eating for Special Needs Selling a Product Nutrients on Trial Stranger in a Strange Land

Continued

Chapter 18   Strategies for Teaching Nutrition, *continued*

Method	Sample Strategies Provided
Discussion and Report Techniques	Classifying Nutritious and Nonnutritious Snacks
	Grocery Shopping
	Healthy Breakfasts
	Nutrition
	Breakfast Book
	Eating for Healthy Teeth
	Food Preference
	Food Labels in the Classroom
	Assess Your Food Intake
	Snack Machines in the Schools Debate
	Food Basket Turnover
	Food Journal
	Nutrition IQ
	Being Healthy!
	Foods From Around the World
	Diet Goals
	School Cafeteria Menus
	Diet Modification
	Diet and Athletic Performance
	Food Label Activity
	Weight Management Programs
Experiments and Demonstrations	Food and the Five Senses
	Say Cheese
	Is It Healthy or Not?
	Sugar and Salt Detectives
	Differences in Milk
	Fats and the Heart
	Foods Eaten in the Cafeteria
	Food Waste
	Our Bodies Need Water
	Complete Proteins
Puzzles and Games	Food Alphabet
	MyPlate Bingo
	Online Nutrition Games
	Wheel of Food
	Alphabet Game
	Learning MyPlate
	What Kind of Food Am I?
	Label Scavenger Hunt
	Cultural Foods Game
	Balanced Meals
Other Ideas	Field Trips
	Poster Contest

Chapter 20   Strategies for Teaching about Injuries: Accident and Violence Prevention

Method	Sample Strategies Provided
Information Assessment Activities	Stranger Safety Safety Habits Beliefs Safety Values Escaping a Home Fire Learning about Personal Safety and Strangers How to Stay Safe Online Field Trip Documentaries School Safety Newspaper Pool Safety
Decision Stories	Show and Tell Around the Neighborhood Fire! The Hill Cyberbullying Safety Belts The Stranger Emergency Care Violence Prevention Presentation
Dramatizations	Safety Puppet Show School Bus Behavior Looking for Hazards Phoning for Help Disaster Drama Safety Attitudes
Discussion and Report Techniques	Home-Alone Safety Accidents around the Home Bike Safety Laws Resiliency Skills Blog Disaster Demonstration Holiday Safety Diary School Safety Books Don't Touch That! Emergency! Safety Belt Discussion
Experiments and Demonstrations	Natural Disasters Fire Safety Pedestrian Safety Lesson Plan Safe Crossing Demonstration Fire Safety at Home Cuts, Scratches, and Abrasions Strains and Sprains Backpack Safety Resuscitation Annie Fire Extinguishers The Hug of Life
Puzzles and Games	Safe Route Home
Other Ideas	Traffic Safety Obstacle Course Field Trips

Chapter 22　Strategies for Teaching Consumer Health

Method	Sample Strategies Provided
Information Assessment Activities	Why Do I Buy? Assessing Attitudes I'm a Wise Consumer Because… Health Fact or Fiction Use Technology to Make Wise Consumer Decisions Where Is the Help? What Is Best? Budget Diary What Is Really Happening? Techniques That Sell What Is in There?
Decision Stories	Broken Promises Vitamins for Vera? Munch or Lunch Shampoo of the Stars Spots and Shaun
Dramatizations	Finding a Doctor Medicine Safety Rules Now for This Commercial Message Complaints
Discussion and Report Techniques	Health Myths Do Only Ducks Quack? Advertising: Don't Buy It Hook, Line, and Sinker Health News The Laws of Advertising Labels Are Important How Are Your Health Habits? Health Promotion Agencies Health Options Where Can I Go for Help?
Experiments and Demonstrations	Is There Any Difference? Comparison Shopping Listen Carefully Which Is Better?
Puzzles and Games	Consumer Health Tic-Tac-Toe Consumer Riddles Scrambled-Up Health Shopping Game
Other Ideas	Packaging The Pharmacist and You Slogans—Do They Sell?

Chapter 24	Strategies for Teaching about Aging, Dying, and Death

Method	Sample Strategies Provided	
Information Assessment Activities	**Aging:** How Does It Feel to Be Old? Aging Voting Rank-Ordering Sentence Completion Aging Collage Value Voting	**Dying and Death:** Values Statements Personal Views on Suicide On Living and Dying
Decision Stories	**Aging:** Going for a Visit	**Dying and Death:** A Gift of Life Sally's Grief
Dramatizations	**Aging:** Elderly Puppet Show Grandparents and Grandchildren Now I Am Old	**Dying and Death:** Suicide Talk Can Help Only One Week to Live
Discussion and Report Techniques	**Aging:** Age, Dying, and Death Life Collage Quality Time with Elderly Friends or Relatives Challenges Facing the Elderly Services for the Elderly Fountain of Youth The Elderly in the Media The Science of Aging Caloric Comparison	**Dying and Death:** Ding: True/False My Pet Died How It Felt to Go to a Funeral The Five Stages of Grief Mourning and Funerals Why Should I Have a Will? Organ and Tissue Donation Why People Die
Experiments and Demonstrations	**Aging:** Last Year's Clothing Aging in Humans Life Cycle of a Frog	
Puzzles and Games	**Aging:** Aging Word Search	
Other Ideas	**Aging:** Adopt a Grandparent Elderly Health Fair What Was It Like Then?	**Dying and Death:** Poetry Field Trip to a Nursing Home What Does a Funeral Director Do? Obituary

Chapter 26 Strategies for Teaching Environmental Health

Method	Sample Strategies Provided
Information Assessment Activities	Ecological Food Chain Major Environmental Problems Using Technology to Teach Environmental Issues Let's Rank Our Environmental Problems
Decision Stories	The Fishing Trip A Bird's Next Is Recycling Worth the Work? Bad Air
Dramatizations	Water Pollution: Oil Spills Plants and Animals Need Protection, Too Populations and Resource Use Disaster Preparation Practice Alien Impressions Role-Playing Environmental Hazards Future Lifestyles City Crisis
Discussion and Report Techniques	Banner Activities and Their Environmental Effects For the Love of the Earth Me and My Surroundings Can I Recycle? Energy Savings Solid Waste Environmental Stories Population Problems Hunger Hurts Environmental News Watch and Commentary Let's Be Creative General Pollution Problems Spread the Word Recycling and You
Experiments and Demonstrations	Recyclable Containers Crowding Problems Seasonal Adjustments Terrariums and Aquariums as Ecosystems Resource Reduction Signs Waste Production Noise Levels Water Impurities Deadly Precipitation
Puzzles and Games	Treasure Hunt Health Hazard Brainstorm Air Pollution Word Search
Other Ideas	Poster Contest Illustrating Environmental Aspects Survival Lists

Worksheets

Shield Activity for Identifying and Assessing Values

Name:

Date:

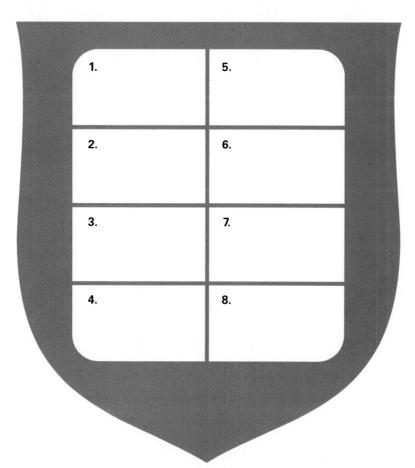

1. Name or draw something that you do well.

2. Name or draw something that you are trying to get better at.

3. Write down a feeling that would be very hard for you to change.

4. Write the thing that you are most proud of having done.

5. Tell about a happy thing that happened to you.

6. Tell about a sad thing that happened to you.

7. Tell what you want to do with your life.

8. Write three words that best tell about who you are.

Emotions and Me

Name:

Date:

Under each face, write the word for how the person in the picture is feeling.

happy   **sad**   **angry**   **excited**   **contented**   **scared**

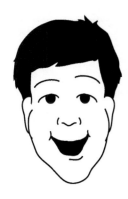

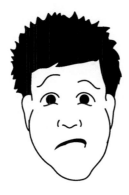

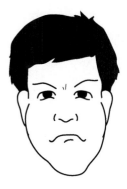

_____

_____

_____

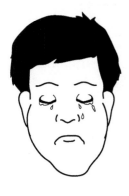

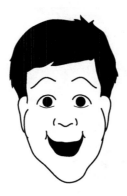

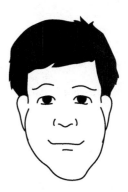

_____

_____

_____

Who Am I?

Name:	
Date:	

Answer the questions below. After you are done, the teacher will share your answers with the class to see if other students can guess who wrote the answers.

1. My two favorite things to do are _____

_____

2. My favorite food is _____

_____

3. My favorite TV program is _____

_____

4. My best subject in school is _____

_____

5. What I like best about myself is _____

_____

6. Friends should _____

_____

7. If I could change one thing about me, it would be _____

_____

8. I am special because _____

_____

9. I have brothers/sisters who _____

_____

10. My favorite activity is _____

_____

11. Three words I would use to describe myself are _____

_____

Stress Feelings

Name:

Date:

Use this worksheet to write about a stressful event that happened to you.

Stressful event: _____

Time of day: _____

What occurred: _____

_____

_____

_____

_____

_____

_____

How I handled the event: _____

_____

_____

_____

_____

_____

_____

Tracing the Blood Flow

Name:

Date:

Identify each part of the blood flow through the heart as labeled on the diagram. Use words from the bank below. Each word will be used once.

1. _____

2. _____

3. _____

4. _____

5. _____

6. _____

7. _____

8. _____

9. _____

10. _____

11. _____

12. _____

13. _____

14. _____

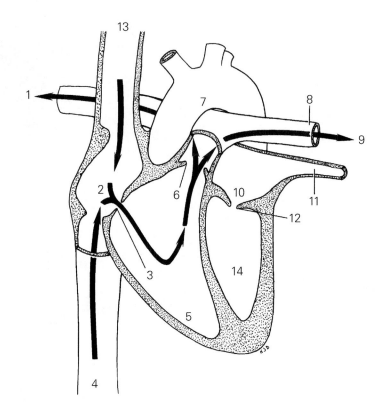

Word Bank

to left lung
right ventricle
right atrium
tricuspid valve
to right lung
pulmonary artery
pulmonary valve

pulmonary vein
mitral valve
left atrium
inferior vena cava
aorta
left ventricle
superior vena cava

My Family Tree

Name:

Date:

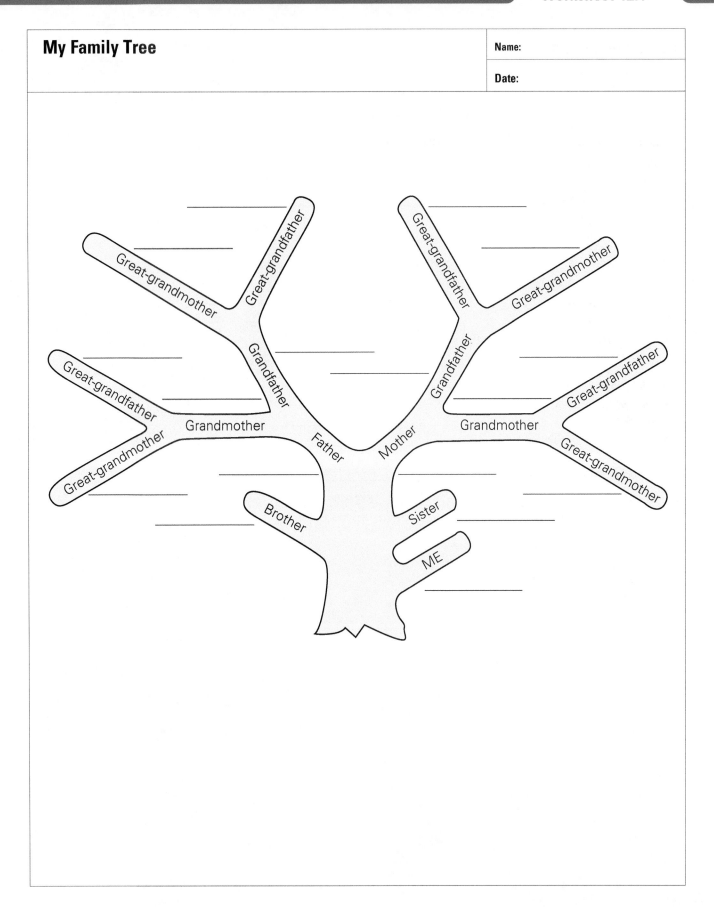

Caught in the Act

Name:

Date:

Write in the names of the people you see using the behaviors listed below.

Being Responsible

- *Returned something that was borrowed*
- *Admitted making a mistake*
- *Finished all schoolwork and turned it in on time*

Who Did It?

_____

_____

_____

Being Cooperative

- *Followed the line leader*
- *Worked well with someone to get a job done*
- *Tried hard in a game or in physical education*

Who Did It?

_____

_____

_____

Being Courteous

- *Helped someone who had a problem*
- *Waited for his or her turn in line*
- *Gave someone else a compliment for doing something well*

Who Did It?

_____

_____

_____

Responsibility

Write your name and the names of your family members in the top row. Put an "X" in each column that includes the responsibility each person has in your home. If you need to, add other responsibilities in the blank lines or other columns to include more family members.

Family Member				
Cooking				
Washing Clothes				
Doing Dishes				
Paying Bills				
Taking Out Trash				
Cleaning Bathroom				
Other				

Helping Others

Name:

Date:

What can you do to make life easier or better for the people around you?

Who I Can Help	How I Can Help	How Many Times I've Helped
Parents	_____	_____
Grandparents	_____	_____
Brother or sister	_____	_____
My teacher	_____	_____
My best friend	_____	_____
A neighbor	_____	_____

The Menstrual Cycle

Name:

Date:

The figure below shows a 28-day menstrual cycle. Put the letter of each phase listed below on the corresponding segment of the diagram.

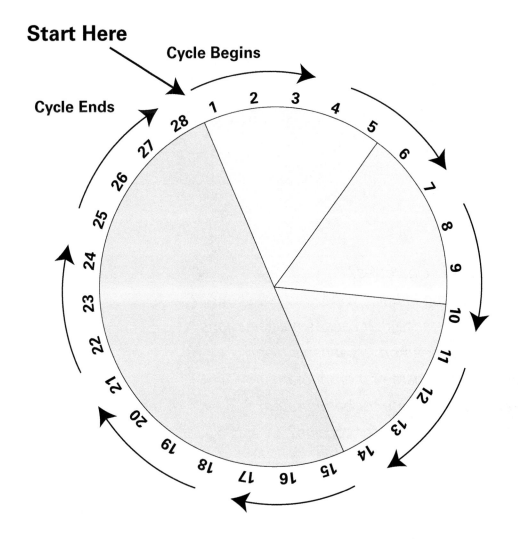

A. *Uterine lining is very thin.*

B. *Menstruation takes place.*

C. *Lining becomes thicker as egg travels.*

D. *Uterine lining begins thickening and ovulation takes place.*

Source: The Menstrual Cycle Worksheet, © 1989 Tambrands, Inc. Used by permission of Procter & Gamble.

Drugs Spell Trouble Puzzle

Name:

Date:

Fill in the blanks to find out what drugs really spell.

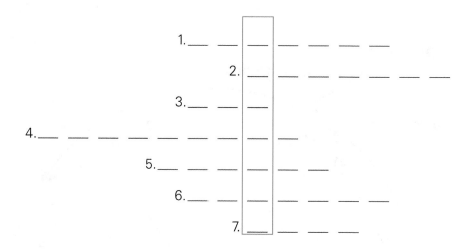

1. What drug is in cigarettes?
2. What is the drug in beer, wine, and whiskey?
3. What is a substance that causes hallucinations?
4. What drug comes from a cannabis plant?
5. What is a street name for amphetamines?
6. What is a street name for barbiturates?
7. What is a street name for cocaine?

Let's Play Tic-Tac-Toe

Name:

Date:

Write a T in the square for each statement that is true. Write an F in the square for each statement that is false.

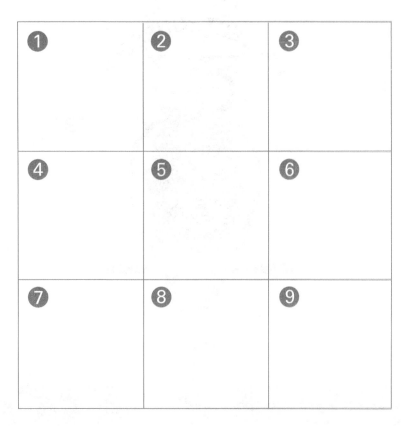

1. A person's family does not cause a drug-dependent person to take drugs.
2. Drug dependency does not occur in good families.
3. Talking to someone you trust about a drug problem is helpful.
4. Family members of drug-dependent people never need help.
5. Drug-dependent people may be unable to stop taking drugs unless they get special help.
6. Family members can make drug-dependent people stop taking drugs by being good and by doing nice things.
7. A drug-dependent person has an illness.
8. Bad children cause their parents to drink.
9. Drug-dependent people do not love their families.

The "Bert Bird Knows" Mobile	Name:
	Date:

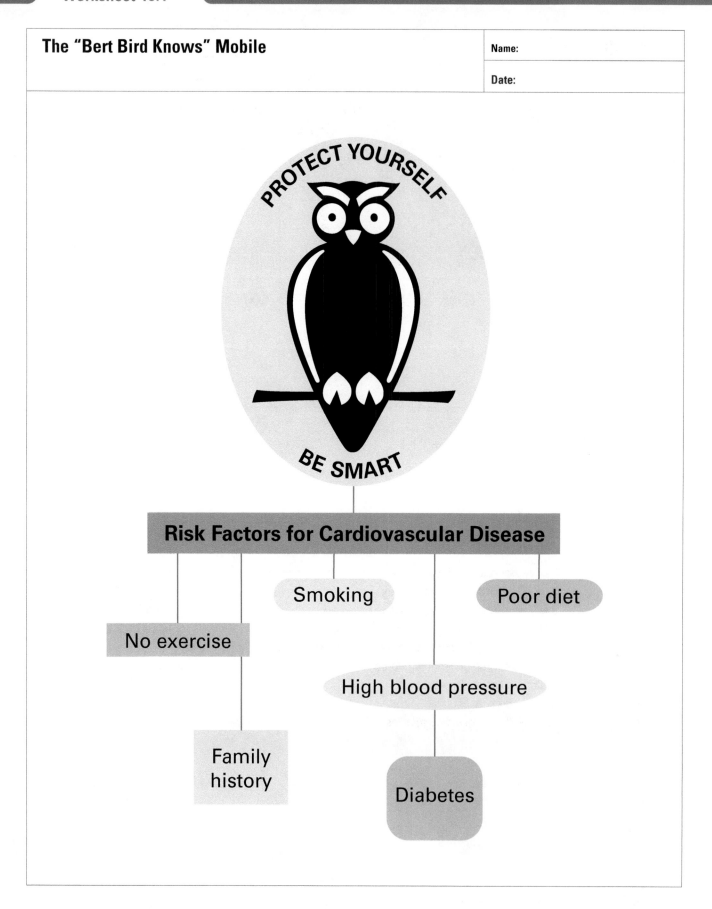

Values Statements

Name:

Date:

Finish the statements in your own words. These will then be discussed in class.

My heart is _____.

Smoking is _____.

Having someone sneeze on me will _____.

I go to the doctor when _____.

A good diet will _____.

People with diabetes should _____.

Cancer is _____.

If a friend had cancer, I would _____.

Preventing heart disease is _____.

AIDS is _____.

If I had a friend with AIDS, I would _____.

Someone who is not feeling well should _____.

The Help I Get

Name:

Date:

A. pain _____

_____

B. tears _____

_____

C. sweat _____

_____

D. saliva _____

_____

E. skin _____

_____

F. stomach acid _____

_____

G. urine _____

_____

H. bleeding _____

_____

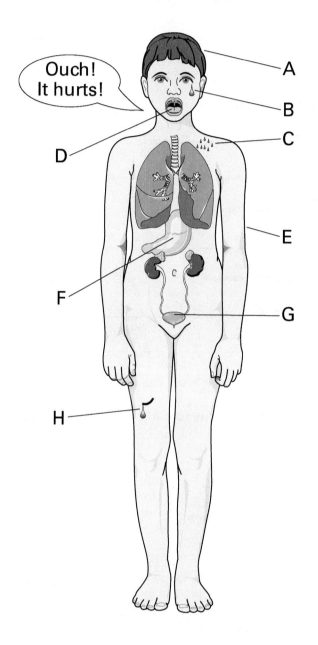

Ouch! It hurts!

A

B

C

D

E

F

G

H

Things I Know, Things I'd Like to Know

Name:

Date:

What five things do you think you know about this disease? What five things would you like to find out about the disease? After doing research and filling in your answers, did you find you knew a great deal or very little of the information?

Disease or Condition:

Things I know	**True**	**False**
1. _____	T	F
2. _____	T	F
3. _____	T	F
4. _____	T	F
5. _____	T	F

Things I'd like to know

1. _____

2. _____

3. _____

4. _____

5. _____

Answers

_____

_____

_____

_____

_____

_____

_____

_____

_____

_____

_____

Using Technology to Understand Infectious Diseases

Name:

Date:

Epidemiological Triangle

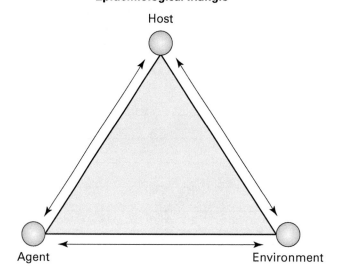

Host

Agent

Environment

Disease to investigate: _____

What factors could have influenced the development of this disease?

Host factors identified:

_____

_____

Agent factors identified:

_____

_____

Environmental factors identified:

_____

_____

Research sources:

_____

_____

Nutrition

Match the items on the left with one of the six essential nutrients on the right. Nutrients may be used more than once, and food items may match more than one nutrient.

_____   *1. peanuts*

_____   *2. watermelon*

_____   *3. calcium*

_____   *4. whole wheat pasta*

_____   *5. corn oil*

_____   *6. folic acid*

_____   *7. sodium*

_____   *8. brown rice*

_____   *9. butter*

_____   *10. vitamin D*

_____   *11. chicken*

_____   *12. potatoes*

_____   *13. potassium*

_____   *14. eggs*

_____   *15. vitamin C*

A. carbohydrates

B. proteins

C. fats (lipids)

D. water

E. vitamins

F. minerals

Food Labels in the Classroom

Name:

Date:

Answer the following questions using the food label shown.

Nutrition Facts
Serving Size: 1 cup (228g)
Servings Per Container: 2

Amount Per Serving

Calories 260   Calories from Fat 120

	% Daily Value*
Total Fat 12g	20%
Saturated Fat 5g	25%
Trans Fat 3g	
Cholesterol 30g	10%
Sodium 660mg	28%
Total Carbohydrate 31g	10%
Dietary Fiber 0g	0%
Sugars 5g	
Protein 5g	

Vitamin A	4%
Vitamin C	2%
Calcium	15%
Iron	4%

* Percent Daily Values are based on a 2,000 calorie diet. Your Daily Values may be higher or lower depending on your calorie needs:

	Calories:	2,000	2,500
Total Fat	Less than	65g	80g
Sat Fat	Less than	20g	25g
Cholesterol	Less than	300mg	300mg
Sodium	Less than	2,400mg	2,400mg
Total Carbohydrate		300g	375g
Dietary Fiber		25g	30g

1. How many grams of fat are in one serving of this food?

_____

2. What percentage of the Daily Value for carbohydrates is in this food?

_____

3. How many grams of sugar are in one serving?

_____

4. What are two vitamins found in this food?

_____

5. What are three minerals found in this food?

_____

6. How many total cups of food are in this container?

_____

7. What percentage of the Daily Value for saturated fat is in this food?

_____

8. How many total calories are in each serving of this food?

_____

9. How much is one serving size?

_____

10. How many grams of dietary fiber are in one serving of this food?

_____

Nutrition IQ

Name:

Date:

What do you really know about nutrition? Mark each statement true or false. These will then be discussed in class.

True or False

T/F   1. You can get proper nourishment if you just eat a variety of foods.

T/F   2. People who don't eat meat, poultry, or fish can still stay healthy.

T/F   3. Food eaten between meals can be just as good for your health as food eaten at regular meals.

T/F   4. Fresh vegetables are always more nutritious than canned or frozen vegetables.

T/F   5. A high-protein, low-carbohydrate diet is ideal for losing weight.

T/F   6. When dieting, avoid starchy foods, such as bread and potatoes.

T/F   7. If you weigh what you should (according to accepted weight standards), you're getting proper nourishment.

T/F   8. Milk contains all the essential elements of a good diet.

T/F   9. Give a child all the foods he or she wants, and the child will never suffer from malnutrition.

T/F   10. Dark bread has the same caloric value as white bread.

T/F   11. Once a person stops exercising, muscle fibers change to fat.

T/F   12. Women in their childbearing years need more iron than men do.

Stranger Safety

Name:

Date:

Color or mark the box under Yes for something that is OK to do. Color or mark the box under No if it is not OK to do.

	Yes	No
1. *I would take candy or gifts from someone I did not know.*		
2. *I would take a ride from someone I did not know.*		
3. *I would talk to my mother's friend.*		
4. *I would let someone I did not know into my house.*		
5. *I would help someone find his or her puppy, even if I did not know that person.*		
6. *I would talk to my school counselor.*		
7. *I would tell someone I have met on the Internet where I go to school.*		
8. *I would tell my mom or dad if I thought someone was following me home from school.*		
9. *I would talk to someone my own age whom I didn't know.*		
10. *I would walk away from someone who made me uncomfortable, even if I had met him or her before.*		

Safety Habits Beliefs

Name:

Date:

How do you feel about safety? Complete the following statements. You may be asked to volunteer your answers to discuss them in class.

1. *I wear a helmet when I ride a bicycle because* _____.

2. *I can avoid falling by* _____.

3. *I think the most dangerous type of safety violation is* _____.

4. *The safest place to walk is* _____.

5. *I always swim with an adult present because* _____.

6. *The most important thing I can do when mowing the lawn is* _____.

7. *The best thing I can know when there is a fire is* _____.

8. *The best place for poisons to be kept is* _____.

9. *In case of an emergency, I need to know how to call the local emergency numbers because* _____

    _____.

10. *I always fasten my safety belt in the car because* _____.

11. *I think the most important thing that I can do to try to remain safe is* _____

    _____.

12. *All students should be required to participate in disaster drills (for fire, tornado, hurricane, etc.) because* _____

    _____.

13. *To me, safety education means* _____.

14. *Accidents are the result of* _____.

15. *As a pedestrian, I should know* _____.

Assessing Attitudes

Name:

Date:

	Agree	Disagree	Not Sure
1. Most television commercials give accurate information about the product advertised.	____	____	____
2. If my friends have a certain product, I usually want to buy that product, too.	____	____	____
3. I only buy products that I need.	____	____	____
4. Advertisers must tell the truth.	____	____	____
5. Only products and services that are useful are sold.	____	____	____
6. I sometimes buy things that I don't need.	____	____	____
7. There is not much point to saving money.	____	____	____
8. Sometimes I buy things without knowing very much about how good they are.	____	____	____
9. Health care products are always safe to use.	____	____	____
10. The products I buy for myself can affect my health.	____	____	____

Health Promotion Agencies

Name:

Date:

Write the letter of the health promotion agency next to the description of its functions. Not all terms in the lettered list will be used.

_____ 1. enforces laws for labeling and safety of cosmetics, medicines, and food

_____ 2. responsible for inspecting and grading meat and poultry

_____ 3. prevents false advertising from being sent through the mail

_____ 4. has offices all over the country to handle consumer complaints and keep track of businesses engaged in fraudulent practices

_____ 5. involved in examining and testing electrical devices to ensure safety in operation

_____ 6. in charge of coordinating federal efforts in the field of health care

_____ 7. promotes cancer research and educational programs dealing with all aspects of cancer

_____ 8. under the guidance of the United Nations, oversees programs dealing with disease, nutrition, and sanitation in all member countries

_____ 9. establishes regulations on the manufacture and sale of biological products, researches health problems and provides information to the public, and assists local and state health departments

_____ 10. within a specific political division, maintains clinics, laboratories, and staffs of nurses and other personnel to aid in the prevention and control of disease

a. Better Business Bureau

b. Department of Health, Education, and Welfare

c. U.S. Postal Service

d. National Association for the Prevention of Blindness

e. Underwriters Laboratory

f. American Heart Association

g. American Cancer Society

h. Public Health Service

i. Food and Drug Administration

j. World Health Organization

k. U.S. Department of Agriculture

l. state and local health departments

Shopping

Name:

Date:

START			
Buy mouthwash. Spend $2.	**END** ←	Spend allowance on video games. Spend $10. ←	Go to HMO. Save money and get $50 back.
Buy unneeded vitamin pills. Spend $8.	Buy defective product. Waste $50. →	Have everything you need. No buying.	Buy most expensive shampoo. Spend $7.
Waste money on junk food. Spend $4.	Buy a new shirt that shrinks so it no longer fits. Waste $15.	Find cheaper and better brand of toothpaste. Save $2. (Get $2 back.)	Buy a worthless acne cure. Waste $6.
Do comparison shopping. Save $12.	Resist silly commercial for cold remedy. No money spent.	Buy a new coat that you like on sale. Receive $25.	Buy a present for a family member. Spend $15.
Go fishing. No cost.	Buy a toy that breaks. Waste $11.	Visit the dentist for a check-up. Spend $30. Receive $50 if dental problem avoided.	Buy a book that you want. Spend $7.
Develop dental problem you could have prevented. Spend $100. →	Buy a new brand of soap. Save $1. (Get $1 back.)	Buy a new bicycle. Spend $120 but get $20 back because of sale. →	Consult a quack. Spend $100.

Values Statements about Death and Dying

Name:

Date:

1. When I think about death, I _____
   _____
   _____
   _____.

2. To me, death means _____
   _____
   _____
   _____.

3. If I could choose how I will die, I would _____
   _____
   _____
   _____.

4. My greatest fear about dying is _____
   _____
   _____
   _____.

5. When I think about relatives who have died, I _____
   _____
   _____
   _____.

Challenges Facing the Elderly

Name:

Date:

Fill in the following blanks based on the clues below.

1. ____ ____ ____ ____ C ____ ____ ____

2. H ____ ____ ____ ____ ____ ____

3. ____ ____ A ____ ____ ____

4. ____ ____ ____ ____ L ____ ____ ____ ____ ____

5. ____ ____ ____ ____ L ____ ____ ____ ____

6. E ____ ____ ____ ____ ____ ____ ____

7. ____ ____ N ____ ____ ____ ____

8. ____ ____ G ____ ____ ____ ____

9. ____ ____ E ____

Clues

1. Financial assistance for medical care provided by the U.S. government

2. Examples are owned homes, apartments, nursing homes, and assisted living facilities

3. These types of problems are due largely to the aging process and affect relationships, income-producing ability, and leisure pursuits

4. This has increased among seniors as the need for their financial resources has increased

5. Can enhance a person's health; examples are vitamins, minerals, and antioxidants

6. Regular _____ increases strength, endurance, and flexibility

7. Lack of this pushes the elderly to seek employment well into their retirement years

8. The term for discriminating against someone based on his or her age

9. One's _____ and eating the right foods can prevent premature aging

Municipal Solid Waste in the United States

Name:

Date:

How can the disposal of municipal solid waste in the U.S. be improved?

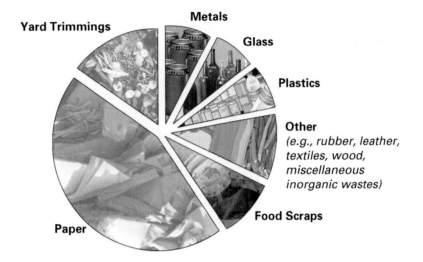

Yard Trimmings

Metals

Glass

Plastics

Other
(e.g., rubber, leather, textiles, wood, miscellaneous inorganic wastes)

Food Scraps

Paper

Table of Trash Types and Percentages*

Trash Type	Percentage	Tonnage
paper	40.4%	71.6 million tons
yard trimmings	17.6%	31.6 million tons
metals	8.5%	15.3 million tons
plastics	8.0%	14.4 million tons
food scraps	7.4%	13.2 million tons
glass	7.0%	12.5 million tons
other	11.6%	20.8 million tons (e.g., rubber, leather, textiles, wood, miscellaneous inorganic wastes)

*Numbers are based on 2011 data from the United States Environmental Protection Agency

Let's Rank Our Environmental Problems

Name:

Date:

For each group below, rank the environmental problems in order, from most hazardous to least hazardous.

Air Pollution

_____ carbon monoxide and nitrogen

_____ sulfur oxides

_____ lead

Water Pollution

_____ animal fertilizers

_____ human sewage

_____ industrial wastes

Solid Waste Pollution

_____ dump

_____ landfills

_____ recycling

Hazardous Chemical Pollution

_____ pesticides

_____ industrial chemicals

_____ household products

Solid Waste

Name:

Date:

Place the correct letter in the blank to the left.

_____ 1. biodegradable

_____ 2. compost

_____ 3. conservation

_____ 4. decompose

_____ 5. ecosystem

_____ 6. garbage

_____ 7. incinerator

_____ 8. landfill

_____ 9. leachate

_____ 10. microorganisms

_____ 11. recycle

_____ 12. reduce

_____ 13. reuse

_____ 14. solid waste

_____ 15. wasteland

a. ravaged land that is unable to support life

b. a material that can be broken down by microorganisms into simpler forms

c. the things that we throw away such as trash, yard and kitchen waste, and old machinery

d. a mixture of degraded organic materials such as grass, leaves, and garden and kitchen wastes; the mixture is usually used as fertilizer

e. to extend the life of an item by repairing it or creating a new use for it

f. the preservation and wise use of natural resources to minimize loss and waste

g. to decrease the amount of trash or waste produced by buying only what is needed and contained in packages that are not excessively wrapped

h. to rot or break down into the simplest form possible

i. to make materials such as plastic, glass, and paper into new products

j. a unit of the environment that consists of living and nonliving things that interact with each other

k. minute living organisms that can be seen only through a microscope

l. solid waste or trash; things that we throw away

m. a solution of water that streams through a dump or landfill and picks up pollutants and other soluble molecules along the way

n. a furnace used for burning waste

o. a place where solid waste or trash is dumped and covered with dirt

Worksheet Answer Key

Worksheet 4.1: Shield Activity for Indentifying and Assessing Values

Answers will vary. Accept all reasonable answers.

Worksheet 7.1: Emotions and Me

1. happy
2. scared
3. angry
4. sad
5. excited
6. contented

Worksheet 7.2: Who Am I?

Answers will vary. Accept all reasonable answers.

Worksheet 7.3: Stress Feelings

Answers will vary. Accept all reasonable answers.

Worksheet 10.1: Tracing the Blood Flow

1. to right lung
2. right atrium
3. tricuspid valve
4. inferior vena cava
5. right ventricle
6. pulmonary valve
7. aorta
8. pulmonary artery
9. to left lung
10. left atrium
11. pulmonary vein
12. mitral valve
13. superior vena cava
14. left ventricle

Worksheet 12.1: My Family Tree

Answers will vary. Accept all reasonable answers.

Worksheet 12.2: Caught in the Act

Answers will vary. Accept all reasonable answers.

Worksheet 12.3: Responsibility

Answers will vary. Accept all reasonable answers.

Worksheet 12.4: Helping Others

Answers will vary. Accept all reasonable answers.

Worksheet 12.5: The Menstrual Cycle

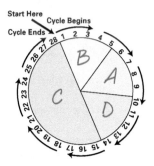

Worksheet 14.1: Drugs Spell Trouble Puzzle

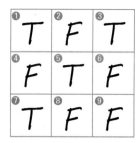

Worksheet 14.2: Let's Play Tic-Tac-Toe

① T	② F	③ T
④ F	⑤ T	⑥ F
⑦ T	⑧ F	⑨ F

Worksheet 16.1: The "Bert Bird Knows" Mobile

This worksheet does not have answers.

Worksheet 16.2: Values Statements

Answers will vary. Accept all reasonable answers.

Worksheet 16.3: The Help I Get

Answers will vary. Accept all reasonable answers.

Worksheet 16.4: Things I Know, Things I'd Like to Know

Answers will vary. Accept all reasonable answers.

Worksheet 16.5: Using Technology to Understand Infectious Diseases

Answers will vary. Accept all reasonable answers.

Worksheet 18.1: Nutrition

1. B, C
2. D, E
3. F
4. A, E
5. C, E
6. E
7. F
8. A, E, F
9. C
10. E
11. B, F
12. A, E, F
13. F
14. B, C, E, F
15. E

Worksheet 18.2: Food Labels in the Classroom

1. 12 g
2. 10%
3. 5 g
4. vitamin A, vitamin C
5. sodium, calcium, iron
6. 2 cups
7. 25%
8. 260 Calories
9. 1 cup
10. 0 g

Worksheet 18.3: Nutrition IQ

1. T
2. T
3. T
4. F
5. F
6. F
7. F
8. F
9. F
10. F
11. F
12. T

Worksheet 20.1: Stranger Safety

1. no
2. no
3. no
4. no
5. no
6. yes
7. no
8. yes
9. yes
10. yes

Worksheet 20.2: Safety Habits Beliefs

Answers will vary. Accept all reasonable answers.

Worksheet 22.1: Assessing Attitudes

Answers will vary. Accept all reasonable answers.

Worksheet 22.2: Health Promotion Agencies

1. I
2. K
3. C
4. A
5. E
6. H
7. G
8. J
9. H
10. L

Worksheet 22.3: Shopping

This worksheet does not have answers.

Worksheet 24.1: Values Statements about Death and Dying

Answers will vary. Accept all reasonable answers.

Worksheet 24.2: Challenges Facing the Elderly

1. M E D I C A R E
2. H O U S I N G
3. H E A L T H
4. E M P L O Y M E N T
5. S U P P L E M E N T S
6. E X E R C I S E
7. I N C O M E
8. A G E I S M
9. D I E T

Worksheet 26.1: Municipal Solid Waste in the United States

Answers will vary. Accept all reasonable answers.

Worksheet 26.2: Let's Rank Our Environmental Problems

Answers will vary. Accept all reasonable answers.

Worksheet 26.3: Solid Waste

1. B
2. D
3. F
4. H
5. J
6. L
7. N
8. O
9. M
10. K
11. I
12. G
13. E
14. C
15. A

Glossary

A

Acne A skin disease caused by inflammation of the oil glands in the skin and at the base of hair. The skin pores become clogged with oil, and bacteria grow in the blocked pores and cause swollen blemishes to appear.

Ageism Discrimination against a person based on his or her age.

Air pollution Chemicals present in the atmosphere in higher than usual concentration, due to human activities, that can cause irritation and diseases such as asthma or cancer when breathed. It can also cause environmental damage, such as acid rain or temperature inversions. Examples of air pollutants include sulfur oxides, hydrocarbons, lead, asbestos, and nitrogen oxides.

Allergy A hypersensitivity or exaggerated response to an antibody-forming substance. Hay fever is one example of a relatively harmless allergy to plant pollen.

Alzheimer's disease A progressive and irreversible disease involving the death of nerve cells and deposition of plaques of amyloid (a protein) in the brain.

Angina pectoris Chest pain. It is not a heart attack or a disease unto itself, but often is a symptom of existing heart disease.

Angioplasty A procedure where a flexible tube (catheter) with a balloon at the tip is inserted into a blocked artery. When the balloon is inflated it compresses the blockage against the artery wall and restores blood flow.

Anorexia nervosa The eating disorder is characterized by self-starvation, food preoccupation and rituals, compulsive exercising, and often an absence of menstrual cycles in women.

Antibody A substance made by specialized cells in the body that defends against infections due to viruses, bacteria, and other foreign substances.

Antigen A foreign substance that invades and causes the body to react to it.

Antigen An antibody-forming substance.

Antioxidants Compounds in the body that act as scavengers, binding up free radicals and thereby preventing damage to cells. Vitamins C, E, and beta-carotene, a precursor of vitamin A, are all examples.

Anvil (incus) The ossicle (bone of the middle ear) that is connected to both the hammer and stirrup bones.

Arteriosclerosis A generic term for diseases impacting the body's arteries. These diseases are also known as "hardening of the arteries."

Artificial immunity Immunity developed through vaccination to a disease.

Assessment Evaluations of the learning process in the classroom that include the use of standards, benchmarks, and performance indicators to gauge each student's progress in learning and mastering tasks in specific content.

Asthma A disease characterized by spastic contractions of the air passageways to foreign substances found in the air. For 70 percent of people under age thirty, the main cause of this is pollen allergy.

Astigmatism A condition of the eye where an irregularly shaped cornea causes blurry focusing. It can be treated with corrective lenses (glasses) or, sometimes, with surgery.

Atherosclerosis The buildup of fat and other deposits (plaques) in the body's arteries. Over time this causes the arteries to thicken and harden, which diminishes their ability to dilate and constrict. It can lead to blood clots, heart attacks, and strokes.

Attention Deficit Hyperactivity Disorder (ADHD) A common psychiatric disorder appearing in children. Children with ADHD cannot stay focused on a task or activity, demonstrate impulsive behavior, and experience difficulty with finishing a task. It is most often diagnosed between ages six and twelve.

Attitude scale A testing instrument that requires the student to choose between alternatives on a continuum. Two polar choices, such as yes/no, may be provided and are known as a forced-choice scale. A Likert scale provides a range of choices.

Auditory learner Person who may learn best by listening to instructors lecture and students discuss materials. Auditory learners should be encouraged to record lessons when possible for later review and to speak out loud while studying on their own time.

B

B cells A type of white blood cell that makes antibodies to destroy antigens.

Basal metabolism The minimum amount of energy required by the body to maintain essential body functions (e.g., to maintain a normal body temperature, muscle tone, respiration) when at rest.

Benign Noncancerous.

Bereavement A state of experiencing grief.

Biopsy A procedure where a tissue specimen is taken from the body for microscopic examination.

Bodily-kinesthetic intelligence One of the nine multiple intelligences. A child whose strength is in this area enjoys games, movement, and hands-on tasks such as building something. They may be labeled overly active in the traditional classroom, in which they are told to sit and be still.

Body odor The odor from excreting sweat through the aprocrine glands that are located under the arms and around the groin.

Bulbourethral glands (Cowper's glands) A male gland that produces an alkaline substance that lubricates and neutralizes the acidity of urine as part of semen.

Bulimia nervosa Eating disorder characterized by recurring periods of binge eating, during which large amounts of food are consumed in a short period of time, followed by purging through self-induced vomiting, abuse of laxatives and/or diuretics, or periods of fasting.

Bullying Intimidation and domination of one person by another (or a group) through repeated hostile or disrespectful acts. Abuse can be verbal, physical, or emotional in nature and can happen in person or through other means (such as through technology).

Bundle of His (AV bundle) The area of the heart that receives the electrical impulse from the pacemaker (sinoatrial node) and then causes the ventricles to contract.

C

Cancer A group of diseases characterized by uncontrolled growth and spread of abnormal cells or neoplasms that often form a mass of tissue called a tumor.

Carcinoma The most common type of cancer, which includes cancers of the skin, breast, uterus, prostate, lungs, stomach, colon, and rectum.

Cartilaginous joints The places where bones come together are called joints. Cartilaginous joints have articulating surfaces that are covered with cartilage and permit a moderate amount of flexibility. Examples are the junctions between the ribs and vertebrae.

Cellular immunity Protection provided by T cells that attack microbes such as viruses or abnormal cells such as tumors.

Chemotherapy The use of drugs, often in combination, to treat cancer.

Choroid plexus A thin network of blood vessels that provide the retina with a steady supply of oxygen and sugar.

Clitoris A small structure at the top of the *labia minora* that facilitates sexual stimulation. Part of the female reproductive system.

Cochlea A tube that is part of the inner ear that is shaped like a shell and is concerned with hearing.

Collagen A strong protein found in abundance in the dermis layer of the skin.

Combined type ADHD In this version of Attention Deficit Hyperactivity Disorder, children exhibit both inattentive and hyperactive and/or impulsive problems.

Complementary protein ingestion A dietary strategy that ensures each food supplies some amino acids that others lack. For example, corn is deficient in the amino acids isoleucine and lysine, so it is often eaten with beans, which contain those amino acids but lack tryptophan and methionine found in corn.

Conception Occurs when a single sperm fertilizes an egg to produce a zygote.

Concurrent validity (of tests) The degree to which the scores on a given test are related to the scores on another test.

Congenital heart defects A form of heart disease resulting when a fetus's heart does not develop normally, resulting in septum or valve malformations.

Conjunctiva The flexible membrane that seals the eyeball from the outside world. It attaches to the skin at the corners of the eye.

Consumer health The intelligent purchase and use of products and services that will directly affect one's health.

Content standards The knowledge and skills expected of students at certain stages in their education.

Cornea The front, circular, transparent part of the eyeball that refracts (bends) light back toward the retina.

Coronary atherectomy A procedure where a flexible tube (catheter) with a high-speed rotary cutting blade attached to the end is inserted into a blocked artery. The tool cuts or shaves off plaque in the blockage, thereby restoring blood flow.

Coronary bypass A surgical procedure whereby heart blood flow is restored by transplanting a vein taken from a patient's leg into the heart, bypassing an existing, blocked artery.

Coronary heart disease The leading cause of death in the U.S., coronary heart disease refers to buildup of plaques and hardening of the coronary vessels, rather than the heart itself.

Coronary stent A flexible, metallic tube implanted into a diseased artery that restores healthy blood flow.

Cyber bullying Use of the Internet, phone texting, and other technologies to intimidate, isolate, or dominate another person.

D

Decision-commitment The cognitive component or decision a person makes about being in love and committing to a relationship.

Defense mechanism A behavior a person uses to avoid confronting a situation or problem.

Dementia The general term for loss of cognitive and intellectual functions that is caused by a variety of factors, the most common of which is structural brain disease.

Depression Loss of interest in things that generally bring enjoyment to life and feelings of extreme or overwhelming sadness.

Dermis The inner layer of skin directly under the epidermis.

Dietary fiber A generic term for nondigestible carbohydrates (including cellulose, lignin, and pectin) found in plants. It has important health benefits in childhood, especially in promoting normal bowel movements.

Distress A forms of stress generated by negative events.

Drug Any substance that has mind-altering properties or in other ways interacts with and modifies the structure and function of the body.

Drug abuse If a person uses an illegal drug for any reason. Also, chronic, excessive use of a drug; may also refer to a person's intent when using a drug (such as excessive alcohol consumption for the purpose of getting drunk).

Drug misuse The unintentional or inappropriate use of prescribed or nonprescribed medicine that results in the impaired physical, mental, emotional, or social well-being of the user.

Drug use Implies that a drug is being used legally, the user is following the directions on the label or directions from the health care provider, and the drug is being used for a legitimate, medical reason.

E

Eardrum A thin, fibrous, circular membrane covered with a thin layer of skin in the ear. It vibrates in response to changes in air pressure that constitute sound.

Embolus A free-moving clot within an artery, usually composed of an air or gas bubble, a clump of bacteria, tissue, tumor, or thrombus. If they get stuck in an artery they can block blood flow and result in a heart attack or stroke.

Emotional abuse Any attitude or behavior that interferes with a child's mental health or development. This includes yelling, screaming, name calling, shaming, negative comparisons to others, and telling a child that he or she is "bad," "no good," "worthless," or a "mistake."

Emotional health A component of mental health that relates to the ability of a person to deal constructively with reality, regardless of whether the situation is good or bad.

Emotional neglect Failure to provide affection and support necessary for the development of emotional, social, physical, and intellectual well-being.

Emotional wellness The ability to control stress, recognize and accept feelings appropriately, and not be immediately defeated by setbacks or failures.

Environmental wellness Having safe water, food, and air in which one can live and carry out daily activities.

Epidermis The outermost layer of the skin.

Epididymis A structure attached to the top of each testis. These tightly coiled tubes allow mature sperm to pass to vas deferens, which serves as a storage area and allows the sperm to then pass on to the urethra.

Epilepsy A seizure disorder of the central nervous system.

Essay test A test requiring students to organize and write information about a given subject in a systematic fashion.

Eustress A form of stress generated by positive events.

Euthanasia The act of ending a life or permitting a death ("death with dignity").

Evaluation The use of measurements to make a decision.

Existential intelligence One of the nine multiple intelligences. A child whose strength is in this area enjoys tackling the deep questions of human existence, such as what is the meaning of life, why do we die, and how did we get here. These children learn in the context of where humankind stands in the "big picture" of existence.

External locus of control The sense that one is primarily not in control of the factors impacting the quality of his or her own life.

F

Fats Triglycerides that remain solid at room temperature. They are a ground of chemical compounds that contain fatty acids. Some fatty acids are needed for body processes, and the body stores fat deposits throughout the body, including a layer just below the skin, so it has energy set aside for use.

Fibrous joints The places where bones come together are called joints. Fibrous joints provide the least flexibility because they are joined together with fibrous tissue, such as what is found between teeth and their bony sockets. Sutures of the skull are fibrous joints.

Fitness The ability to perform daily tasks vigorously and alertly, with energy left over for enjoying leisure-time activities and meeting energy demands.

Forced-choice scale An attitude scale that provides only two answer options per question, such as agree/disagree, true/false, or yes/no. This is an appropriate scale for use with young children, who may not have the developmental ability to handle more complicated attitude scales.

Formative evaluation Formative evaluation is gathering data for the purpose of improving specific aspects of the teaching/learning process.

Free radical An atom or group of atoms with an unpaired electron. Electrons usually function in pairs, so these free radicals are very prone to binding to other substrates. When this happens in the human body, cellular damage occurs.

Funeral An organized, group-centered response to a death that usually involves a ceremony during which the body of the deceased is present.

G

General adaptation syndrome (GAS) A three-stage process by which the body responds to a stressor. The first stage is alarm, when the body first detects and prepares to deal with an event. The second stage is resistance, when the stressor is dealt with through increased strength and sensory capacity. The third stage, exhaustion, occurs when stress is chronic or traumatic enough to require the body to need to restore itself in order to avoid serious health impacts such as high blood pressure, heart and stomach problems, or achy muscles and joints.

Gestational diabetes This type of diabetes occurs in pregnant women. It is usually controlled through careful diet and exercise. It resolves on its own after childbirth, but puts a woman at greater risk of developing diabetes later in life.

Grading A method physicians use to determine the severity of a cancer.

Grief The sorrow, mental distress, and related feelings that are caused by a death.

H

Hammer (malleus) This ossicle (bone of the middle ear) connects the eardrum to the anvil with a broad joint.

Hazardous chemical pollution Toxic substances deposited in our air and waterways through various human activities that cause damage to the ecosystem, impacting the health of humans, animals, and plants. They include pesticides intended for crops that end up in water, industrial chemicals, and household products such as cleaning sprays or detergents.

HDL cholesterol High-density lipoproteins are often referred to as the "good" cholesterol because having large amounts of it in your bloodstream seems to protect against heart disease.

Health An integrated method of functioning that is oriented toward maximizing an individual's potential across the spiritual, social, physical, environmental, and intellectual aspects of life.

Health education Learning that enables people to make informed decisions, and modify and change social conditions in ways that are health enhancing.

Health literacy The ability of an individual to obtain, interpret, and understand basic health information and services and to act on that knowledge by making health-enhancing decisions.

Health promotion Educational, economic, political, or organizational interventions designed to bring about behavioral and environmental changes conducive to health.

Heart attack Also known as a myocardial infarction. An event often caused by blocked blood flow that causes some portion of heart tissue to die. Since heart tissue is thought not to regenerate, scar tissue that forms in strategic areas may prevent full recovery.

Heart murmurs Abnormal heart sounds that result from abnormal heart valves or an incomplete closure of a congenital hole in the heart's septum. Most heart murmurs are benign in nature, but some indicate problems that may require surgical repair.

HECAT The Health Education Curriculum Analysis Tool (HECAT) is a diagnostic tool that helps officials compare and rate health education curricula. It is used at the state, regional, or local level.

Homeostasis A state of physiological balance the body strives to maintain.

Hormone therapy A type of cancer treatment where drugs are taken to interfere with hormone production and action as a way to stop the growth of certain cancers. This modality is sometimes classified as a type of chemotherapy.

Humoral immunity Protection provided by antibodies derived from B cells.

Hunger A physiological and psychological state that occurs when food needs are not met satisfactorily.

Hyperglycemia High blood sugar levels. This is a hallmark sign of the disease diabetes.

Hyperopia (farsightedness) Light focuses in the eye behind the retina. Symptoms include clear distance vision, blurred near vision, frontal headaches, and eyestrain with near work. Glasses or surgery can treat it.

Hypersensitivity An allergy, or exaggerated response, to an antibody-forming substance. Hay fever is one example of a relatively harmless type of allergy.

Hypertension The condition of having blood pressure within the arteries that is too high. It can lead to congestive heart failure and put a person at high risk for other heart problems if not treated.

I

Immunity The state of being protected against diseases through activities of the immune system.

Immunotherapy The use of a variety of substances to trigger an individual's own immune system to fight the cancer.

Impetigo A common bacterial infection in children characterized by a red, oozing rash that often appears as small blisters. It is commonly found on the face and can be itchy. It is treated with antibiotics.

Indoor air pollution Chemicals or substances present in the home or office (the indoor environment) that can cause health problems or disease in people. Examples of indoor air pollutants include tobacco smoke, carbon monoxide, radon, mold, mildew, or excessive amounts of dust.

Insulin shock A condition that diabetics can develop when too much insulin is present in the bloodstream. Disorientation, convulsions, and loss of consciousness may result.

Integumentary system This protective outer body system includes the skin and, for humans, also the nails and hair. It is designed to be a barrier from the outside world to germs and a cushioning layer for the inner organs, as well as a method of temperature control and excretion of wastes.

Intellectual wellness The ability to learn and use information effectively for personal, family, and career development. It involves striving for continued growth and learning to deal with new challenges.

Internal locus of control The sense that one is primarily in control of the factors impacting the quality of his or her own life.

Interpersonal intelligence One of the nine multiple intelligences. A child whose strength is in this area enjoys learning cooperatively in groups or with a partner. He or she may be labeled as talkative or too concerned with being social in a traditional classroom.

Intimacy The emotional feeling of closeness to others.

Intrapersonal intelligence One of the nine multiple intelligences. A child whose strength is in this area can be self aware and tune into his or her inner feelings, beliefs, and thinking processes. These children may appear reserved but are quite intuitive about what they learn and how it relates to themselves.

Iris The colored part of the eyeball.

Ischemia The narrowing of an artery, usually due to plaque buildup (atherosclerosis). This leads to diminished blood flow and increased risk of blood clot (thrombus).

K

Ketone body When fat is metabolized without sugar, a residue called a ketone body develops, increasing acid in the bloodstream. This is a problem that people with diabetes suffer. High enough amounts of ketone bodies in the bloodstream can cause diabetic coma and death.

Kilocalories (calorie) The amount of heat energy required to raise the temperature of a kilogram of water one degree Celsius. All foods have specific caloric values, and a given amount of food will produce a certain number of kilocalories when broken down by the body. Also referred to as a calorie.

Kinesthetic learner People who learn best by replicating an action or repeating something that an instructor demonstrates. They may struggle to learn by reading or listening, but tend to perform well at experiments, physical activities, art, and acting.

L

Labyrinth The inner ear, composed of a delicate series of structures deep within the bones of the skull.

Latchkey child A child who is regularly left without direct adult supervision before or after school.

LDL cholesterol Low-density lipoproteins are often referred to as the "bad" cholesterol because having a large amount of it in your bloodstream increases risk of fat deposits in the arteries and related heart disease.

Learning disability (LD) A learning disability (LD) is a neurological disorder that impacts a child's ability to receive, process, store, and respond to information. It is not a single disease but a group of disorders.

Learning strategies An activity or experience that teachers use to interpret, illustrate, or facilitate learning. They make content and objectives come alive.

Lens The part of the eye behind the iris that contracts to alter its shape and permit fine focusing of an image on the retina.

Leukemia Cancers that affect blood cells.

Likert scale An attitude scale that provides a range of choices about each issue. For example, a question may request students either strongly agree, agree, disagree, or strongly disagree with a statement.

Lipids Organic compounds that do not easily dissolve in water. Based on their solubility, they are classified as triglycerides (fats), phospholipids, or sterols.

Lipocytes These fat-storing cells form a layer under the dermis that cushions muscles, bones, and inner organs against shocks and acts as an insulator and source of energy during lean times.

Lipoproteins This is the method by which cholesterol is transported through the bloodstream—via large fat and protein molecules.

Lymphocytes White blood cells responsible for much of the human immune response.

Lymphomas Cancers that affect the lymph nodes.

M

Major minerals Inorganic compounds needed by the body for proper nutrition. The major ones needed are calcium, phosphorus, potassium, sulfur, sodium, chloride, and magnesium.

Malignant Cancerous.

Malnutrition An imbalance of proper nutrients.

Matching test A test that calls for the answers given in one column to be paired with a corresponding term or item in another column.

Mathematical-logical intelligence One of the nine multiple intelligences. A child whose strength is in this area enjoys numbers, reasoning, and problem solving. These children do well in the traditional classroom when teaching is logically sequenced and students are asked to conform.

Measurement The collection of information upon which a decision is based. Aptitude tests, rating scales, checklists, and observation techniques are all methods of measurement used in schools.

Medicaid Funded by state and federal taxes, this program is run by states and provides limited health insurance to people with certain disabilities, as well as people who are eligible for assistance from the Aid to Families with Dependent Children and Supplementary Security Income programs.

Medicare A form of socialized health care that is financed by Social Security taxes in the United States. It is designed to provide health insurance for retired people, as well as the blind and severely disabled.

Mental health The ability to perceive the world as it is, respond to its challenges, and develop rational strategies for living.

Metastasis The spread of cancer cells throughout the body from the original location of the abnormal cells.

Michigan Model for Health Based on several behavior-change models and the Adapted Health Belief Model, the Michigan Model is designed as a component of a school's core curriculum. It includes age-appropriate lessons for grades K–12, as well as family resource sheets. This model has been adopted by most Michigan public schools, as well as other public and private schools throughout the United States. Over one million students have taken part in the program.

Monounsaturated fatty acid A type of fatty acid where a double bond exists between two of the carbon atoms and therefore is lacking a pair of the hydrogen atoms found in saturated fatty acids.

Mourning Culturally defined acts, such as a funeral or memorial service, performed when a death occurs.

Multiple-choice test A test consisting of questions that require the student to pick the correct answer options from a series of suggested responses.

Myocardial infarction Also known as a heart attack. An event often caused by blocked blood flow that causes some portion of heart tissue to die. Since heart tissue is thought not to regenerate, scar tissue that forms in strategic areas may prevent full recovery.

Myopia (nearsightedness) Light focuses in the eye before it reaches the retina. Symptoms include blurred distance vision, clear near vision, squinting, and poor night vision. Glasses and, at times, surgery can be used to treat it.

N

Narrative grading A student-generated dialog between student and teacher about the quality of the work. This grading method is thought to aid in the student taking ownership once a concept is verbalized.

Natural immunity Immunity to a future infection developed through contracting and fighting off the disease previously.

Naturalist intelligence One of the nine multiple intelligences. A child whose strength is in this area enjoys the outdoors, nature, animals, and field trips. They also like to pick up on subtle differences in meanings.

Neoplasms Abnormal cells.

Noise pollution Too much sound in the human environment, often from traffic, manufacturing, industry, construction, or airport activities. People who are continually exposed to high levels of noise are at higher risk for developing hearing loss, hypertension, and ischemic heart disease.

Nutrients Substances in food that are needed to support life functions.

O

Obsessive compulsive disorder (OCD) A person with recurrent thoughts or fears (obsessions) or a need to perform a specific action (compulsions). Examples include a person who develops rituals, such as repeatedly checking the door to see if it is locked or constant hand washing.

Oils Triglycerides that remain liquid at room temperature. The body requires some fat for body processes, and it stores it in deposits, including a layer just below the skin.

Oncogenes Genes responsible for specialization, replication, repair, and suppression that have been shown to also carry increased risk of cancer development.

Ossicles The smallest bones in the human body, ossicles are tiny, linked, moveable bones of the middle ear.

Ovaries Produce ova and secrete hormones that bring about the development of the female secondary sex characteristics, such as the rounding of the female figure, breast development, and pubic hair. Part of the female reproductive system.

Oxidation reactions A type of chemical reaction where an oxygen atom adds an electron to a group of atoms or a molecule (a substrate). Additionally, it is a chemical reaction where a hydrogen atom removes an electron from a substrate. The result is a substrate with a charge.

P

Panic disorder A mental health disorder characterized by unexpected and repeated periods of intense fear and discomfort, accompanied by racing heartbeat and shortness of breath.

Passion Feelings of romantic or sexual attraction to another individual.

Patient's Bill of Rights Patients have a right to information disclosure, a choice of providers and plans, access to emergency services, participation in treatment decisions, respect/nondiscrimination, confidentiality of information, and a right to complain and appeal an issue with their health plan, doctors, hospitals, or other medical personnel.

Pediculosis (lice infestation) Lice infestation happens when very small parasitic insects attach themselves to human hair shafts. They feed by biting the scalp, causing itching. Lice spread through direct contact or the sharing of hats or other clothing.

Penis The male organ for sexual intercourse and consists of spongy vascular material called erectile tissue, which swells when blood fills the vascular spaces in response to psychological and/or physical stimulation. The head of the penis is called the *glans penis*.

Performance indicators A list of criteria that students should be able to demonstrate or perform to show that the intended instruction and learning took place.

Performance tasks Hands-on demonstrations, written projects, and portfolios a school system uses to determine whether a student has met the content standards.

Performance-based evaluation This evaluation method is contingent on how students show they have learned something, as opposed to the students' recall of information. Examples include portfolios, exhibitions, and critical-thinking essays.

Phagocytosis The destruction of pathogens by white blood cells.

Physical abuse Any intentional injury done to a child. This includes hitting, slapping, kicking, shaking, burning, pinching, hair pulling, biting, choking, throwing, shoving, whipping, and paddling.

Physical bullying Repeated physical attacks, including pushing, shoving, and hitting, with the intent to intimidate and dominate.

Physical neglect Failure to provide for a child's needs in the form of supervision, housing, food, clothing, medical care, and hygiene.

Physical wellness The ability to carry out daily tasks, develop cardiovascular fitness and muscular fitness, maintain adequate nutrition and weight, and avoid the abuse of alcohol, drugs, and tobacco.

Polyunsaturated fatty acid A type of fatty acid where a double bond exists between two of the carbon atoms and therefore is lacking a pair of the hydrogen atoms found in saturated fatty acids.

Posture The graceful, efficient movement of the body, including standing up straight and walking correctly to maintain good balance.

Predictive validity (of tests) The degree to which a test can predict how well a student will do in a particular situation.

Predominately hyperactive-impulsive type ADHD In this version of Attention Deficit Hyperactivity Disorder, children do not show significant inattention, but are hyperactive.

Predominately inattentive type ADHD In this version of Attention Deficit Hyperactivity Disorder, children do not show significant hyperactive or impulse problems, but are inattentive.

Prostate gland Provides a highly alkaline milky fluid that helps neutralize the highly acidic vagina and facilitates the movement of sperm. Part of the male reproductive system.

Protein A molecule composed of amino acids, eight of which are considered essential to the biological processes of cells in adults.

Pupil The hole at the center of the eye's iris that changes diameter in response to light intensity in order to control how much light enters the eye.

R

Radiation A cancer treatment that utilizes high-energy X-rays or gamma rays to destroy or damage cancerous tissue so it cannot replicate.

Radiation exposure and control Exposure to gamma radiation (such as X-rays) via medical tests or use of computers/cell phones. Too much sort-term radiation exposure can lead to nausea, anemia, cell mutation, hair loss, and even death. Prolonged radiation exposure also increases the chance of cell mutation and cancer.

Regulatory genes The part of the genetic code of cells that controls orderly replacement of cells in the body. If one of these genes fails to regulate the specialization and replication process correctly, cancers can result.

Retina A nerve-tissue structure at the back of the eye on which images are focused by the cornea and the lens.

Retrovirus A variety of RNA virus that invades a host cell and reverse transcribes its RNA into DNA. Some varieties are known to alter certain human genes in a way that can lead to cancer.

Rheumatic heart disease The common childhood disease called strep throat can result in rheumatic fever if left untreated. Rheumatic fever, in turn, can lead to damage to one or more heart valves—a condition called Rheumatic heart disease.

Rhythmic intelligence One of the nine multiple intelligences. A child whose strength is in this area enjoys rhythm, pitch, and timber. These children learn well through songs, patterns, rhythms, instruments, and other musical expression.

Ringworm (*tinea*) A fungal infection of the skin, hair (scalp), or nails characterized by a ring-shaped rash. Athlete's foot and jock itch are commonly occurring varieties of the disease.

Rubrics The criteria used to assess and evaluate how a student performs in the health education and instructional process. Rubrics describe a set of fixed measurements and criteria, which are accompanied by examples of products that represent different levels of accomplishment or skill acquisition. It is a useful tool for assessing complex and subjective criteria.

S

Sarcomas Cancers of the connective tissues, including bones, muscles, and cartilage. These cancers occur less frequently than carcinomas but, when they do arise, tend to spread to surrounding tissues more quickly.

Saturated fatty acid This molecule has the maximum possible number of hydrogen atoms attached to every carbon atom, so it is said to be saturated with hydrogen atoms. These contain only single bonds between the carbon atoms.

Sclera The tough outer coating of the eyeball.

Scope The breadth and arrangement of essential health topics and concepts across grade levels.

Scrotum The saclike structure that contains the testicles.

Self-esteem A combination of self confidence and self respect that allows a person to feel they are capable of coping with life's challenges and are worthy of happiness.

Semen An ejaculatory fluid containing sperm and other substances from the prostate gland, Cowper's glands, and seminal vesicles.

Semicircular canals The rear part of the inner ear that is concerned with balance.

Seminal vesicles These produce a simple sugar, fructose, which adds volume to the ejaculatory fluid (semen), and activates the movement of the sperm. Part of the male reproductive system.

Sequence The logical progression of health knowledge, skills, and behaviors to address at each grade level from grades K through high school.

Sexual abuse Any sexual act between an adult and child. This includes fondling, penetration, intercourse, prostitution, group sex, oral sex, or forced observation of sexual acts.

Sexuality education A lifelong process of acquiring information and forming attitudes, beliefs, and values. It encompasses sexual development, sexual and reproductive health, interpersonal relationships, affection, intimacy, body image, and gender roles.

Short-answer test A test consisting of a number of statements that have certain key words or phrases omitted that the student must provide. Also known as completion tests.

Sinoatrial node Also known as the pacemaker, this area of the heart is responsible for controlling the rhythm of beats.

Social bullying Repeated spreading of rumors, leaving people out of group conversations or activities on purpose, and attempts to break up friendships.

Social wellness The ability to interact successfully with people and one's personal environment. Intimacy, respect, and tolerance for those with different opinions or beliefs are all aspects of social wellness.

Solid waste pollution Items or substances discarded by humans that are reactive, corrosive, toxic, or ignitable, and therefore can cause damage to the environment or illness and disease in humans, plants, or animals. Current methods for dealing with solid waste disposal include dumps, landfills, incineration, and recycling.

Sperm Male reproductive cells produced in the testes.

Spiritual wellness Includes such aspects as meaning and purpose in life, self awareness, and connectedness with self, others, and a larger reality.

Staging A numerical method indicating the extent to which a cancer has spread; helps determine the prognosis and best form of treatment.

Sterol Lipid compounds, some of which play important roles in the body. One example is cholesterol.

Stirrup (stapes) The ossicle (bone of the middle ear) closest to the inner ear.

Strabismus (crossed eyes) A muscular misalignment of the eyes that causes them to not point at the same place at the same time. It is most commonly seen in children.

Stress The body's physical or emotional response to a demand, a change, or other unanticipated or stimulating event.

Stroke A shortage of blood to the brain usually caused by a blood clot (either an embolus or thrombus). Resulting damage can impact any organ system, including cognition and the ability to move or speak normally.

Summative evaluation Summative evaluation is the collecting of data at the end of a unit of instruction.

Synovial joints The places where bones come together are called joints. Synovial joints have a fluid-filled cavity and are very flexible. Examples are the hip and shoulder, which have a wide range of rotation.

T

T cells A type of white blood cell that circulates through the lymphatic system and bloodstream to neutralize antigens.

T helpers These white blood cells increase the response of other lymphocytes.

T suppressor cells These white blood cells decrease the response of other lymphocytes.

Teaching unit An organized method for developing lesson plans for a particular group of students. It is a specific plan for student learning developed by the classroom teacher, as opposed to a curriculum committee.

Test administration and scoring The ease of giving and evaluating the test results. Note that a test that is easy to administer may not automatically be easy to score. For instance, an essay test is difficult to score, but may be a better assessment of some concepts than the easier-to-score multiple-choice test on the same concepts.

Test comprehensiveness The degree to which a test adequately covers the material in question.

Test construct validity The degree to which a test actually measures a hypothetical construct, such as intelligence.

Test content validity The degree to which a test actually measures an intended content area.

Test discrimination Evaluating test items based on answers from high, middle, or low performing students to determine if a test item is appropriate (too easy, too difficult, or acceptable for the mid range of students).

Test objectivity The degree of fairness to students that a test has. For instance, a test with correct reading level and that is written clearly, so there is no debate about correct answers, is considered objective.

Test reliability The degree to which test results are consistent, or can be duplicated. For instance, if the results for a test are the same when it is given to the same person on two different occasions, then the test is considered reliable.

Test validity The idea that a test actually measures what it is designed to measure.

Testes/testicles The main sexual male endocrine glands. They produce sperm.

Thrombus A stationary blood clot in an artery. These can lead to heart attacks or stroke.

Trace minerals Inorganic compounds needed by the body. The body needs less of these compounds than the major minerals, but they are still important for health. They include iron, zinc, selenium, magnesium, copper, iodine, fluorine, chromium, molybdenum, and manganese.

Trans **fatty acid** A type of fatty acid not found in nature but created via food processing, where missing hydrogen atoms are put back into polyunsaturated fats. As a result, vegetable oils can be made to be solid at room temperature.

True-false test A test consisting of declaratory statements that are either true or false. Students must decide whether each test item is true or false, and answer accordingly.

Tumor A mass of abnormal cells (neoplasms) that may be malignant (cancerous) or benign (noncancerous).

Type 1 diabetes This type of diabetes develops when the pancreas does not secrete insulin. People with this variety of diabetes usually develop it before age thirty-five and must carefully monitor blood sugar levels and regularly inject insulin.

Type 2 diabetes This type of diabetes often occurs in obese people. The pancreas provides some, but not adequate, insulin production. This version of the disease is usually controlled via diet and exercise. Often when adequate weight loss is achieved, the person no longer has diabetes.

U

Undernutrition The lack of sufficient nutrients for a body to carry out its necessary daily processes.

Urethra A tube that runs the length of the penis and is used to transport both urine and semen.

Uterus (womb) A pear-shaped organ where the fetus develops. The uterus has three layers: the *perimetrium* (outer layer), the *myometrium* (muscular middle layer), and *endometrium* (inner layer). Part of the female reproductive system.

V

Vagina An elastic canal extending from just behind the cervix to the opening of the external genitalia. It serves as the organ for sexual intercourse and as the birth canal. Part of the female reproductive system.

Verbal bullying Repeated name calling or teasing done to intimidate and dominate a victim.

Verbal-linguistic intelligence One of the nine multiple intelligences. A child whose strength is in this area enjoys language arts, speaking, writing, reading, and listening. This child does well in the traditional classroom.

Visual learner People who may think in pictures and may learn best from PowerPoint presentations, diagrams, illustrations, and handouts. They often prefer to take detailed notes when learning and do better on written tests than oral ones.

Visual-spatial intelligence One of the nine multiple intelligences. A child whose strength is in this area enjoys seeing what you are talking about in order to understand. They like puzzles, graphs, charts, maps, and tables.

Vitamins Organic compounds required by the body to maintain health and prevent disease. They include A, C, D, E, K, niacin, riboflavin, cobalamin, pyridoxine, folic acid, and biotin.

W

Water pollution Chemicals and other by-products from human activities that concentrate in water (lakes, rivers, aquifers, or the ocean) and can cause disease and damage to the ecosystem, humans, plants, or animals. Examples include human sewage, industrial wastes, and thermal pollution.

Wellness Another term for health. Components of wellness are spiritual, social, physical, environmental, emotional, and intellectual.

References

Chapter 1: The Need for Health Education

Centers for Disease Control and Prevention (CDC). 2011. SHPPS: School health policies and practices study, 2006. Atlanta, GA: CDC.

Centers for Disease Control and Prevention (CDC). 2011. *Coordinated School health–key strategies.* Atlanta, GA: CDC.

———. 2002a, August 30. Healthy youth: An investment in our nation's future.

———. 2002b. *Comprehensive health education curriculum.*

———. 2006a. *Healthy youth: Coordinated school health program.* Atlanta, GA: CDC.

———. 2006b. *Surveillance 2011—Trends in reportable sexually transmitted diseases, 2011.* Atlanta, GA: CDC.

———. 2006c. *YRBSS: Trends in the prevalence of marijuana, cocaine, and other illegal drug use.* Atlanta, GA: CDC.

———. 2009d. *YRBSS: Trends in the prevalence of sexual behaviors.* Atlanta, GA: CDC.

———. 2009. *YRBSS: Trends in the prevalence of behaviors that contribute to unintentional injury.* Atlanta, GA: CDC.

Kann, L., Brener N., and H. Wechsler. 2007. Overview and summary: School health policies and programs study 2006. *Journal of School Health.* October 2007, vol.77:8. American School Health Association.

Federal Interagency Forum on Child and Family Statistics. 2006. *America's children in brief: Key national indicators of well-being, 2006: Summary list of recent indicator changes.* www.childstats.gov/americaschildren/index.asp. (May 2009).

Gold, Robert. 2002, January. Report of the 2000 joint committee on health education and promotion terminology (Special Report). *Journal of school health* (January 2002).

Joint Committee on Health Education Standards. 1995. *The national health education standards: Achieving health literacy.* Atlanta, GA: American Cancer Society.

Joint Committee on Health Education Terminology. 1991. Report of the 1990 joint committee on health education terminology. *Journal of health education* 22: 97–108.

National Center for Health Fitness. 2006. *Definition of health promotion.* Washington, DC: American University.

National Education Goals Panel. 2002, March. Goals. www.negp.gov/page3.htm (23 January 2003).

Northern California Society for Public Health Education. 2006. *Health education is . . .* San Francisco, CA: NCSOPHE.

Office of Disease Prevention and Health Promotion. 2010. *Healthy people 2020. National health promotion and disease prevention objectives.* U.S. Department of Health and Human Services. www.cdc.gov/nchs/healthy_people.htm

U. S. Department of Education, Office of Planning, Evaluation and Policy Development. 2010. ESEA Blueprint for Reform. Washington, D.C: DHHS.

U.S. Department of Health and Human Services. 2011. Let's move: America's move to raise a healthier generation of kids. Washington, DC: U.S. Department of Health and Human Services.

Chapter 2: The Role of the Teacher in Coordinated School Health Programs

Brener ND, McManus T, Foti K, Shanklin SL, Hawkins J, Kann L, Speicher N. School Health Profiles 2008: Characteristics of Health Programs Among Secondary Schools. Atlanta: Centers for Disease Control and Prevention. www.cdc.gov/healthyyouth/profiles/2008/profiles_report.pdf (November 2011).

California Commission on Teacher Credentialing. Revised 2010. Health Science Teacher Preparation in California: Standards of Quality and Effectiveness for Subject Matter Programs: A Handbook for Teacher Educators and Program Reviewers. California Commission on Teacher Credentialing: Sacramento, CA. www.ctc.ca.gov/educator-prep/standards/SSMP-Handbook-Health.pdf (October 2011).

Institute for Educational Leadership. 2011. "Issues Facing People of Color in Education." Institute for Educational Leadership, University of Northern Iowa: Cedar Falls, Iowa. www.uni.edu/coe/iel/monographs/col.html (October 2011).

National Commission for Health Education Credentialing, Inc. 2010. Responsibilities and Competencies of Health Educators. National Commission for Health Education Credentialing, Inc.: Whitehall, PA. www.nchec.org/credentialing/responsibilities/ (October 2011).

Minnesota Office of the Revisor of Statutes. 2011. Minnesota Administrative Rules. Part 8700.7500 Code of Ethics for Minnesota Teachers. State of Minnesota: Minneapolis, MN. www.revisor.mn.gov/rules/?id=8700.7500 (October 2011).

National Task Force on the Preparation and Practice of Health Educators. 1988. *A framework for the development of competency-based curricula for entry-level health educators.* New York, NY: National Task Force on the Preparation and Practice of Health Educators.

National Transition Task Force on Accreditation in Health Education. 2004. *Transition task force charge.* Reston, VA: American Association for Health Education.

The National Commission for Health Education Credentialing, Inc. 2002. *Credentialing & benefits of certification.* Whitehall, PA: The National Commission for Health Education Credentialing, Inc.

United States Department of Labor, Bureau of Labor Statistics. 2011. "Occupational Outlook Handbook, 2010-11 Edition." U. S. Bureau of Labor Statistics: Washington, DC. www.bls.gov/oco/ocos063.htm (October 2011).

Wechsler, Howell, McKenna, Mary L., Lee, Sarah M., and Diet, William H. December 2004, pages 4-12. The Role of Schools in Preventing Childhood Obesity. The State Education Standard. National Association of State Boards of Education: Arlington, Virginia. www.cdc.gov/healthyyouth/physicalactivity/pdf/roleofschools_obesity.pdf (October 2011).

Chapter 3: Planning for Health Instruction

American Association for Health Education (AAHE). 2006. *National health education standards.* Reston, VA: AAHE.

American Cancer Society. 2008. *National health education standards.* Atlanta, GA: American Cancer Society.

Anderson, L.W. and D. R. Krathwohl (Eds). 2001. A taxonomy for learning, teaching, and Assessing: A revision of Bloom's Taxonomy of educational objectives. New York: Longman.

Association for the Advancement of Health Education (AAHE). 1995. *National health education standards—achieving health literacy.* Reston, VA: AAHE.

Bloom, B. S. 1956. *Taxonomy of educational objectives, handbook I: Cognitive domain.* New York, NY: McKay.

Centers for Disease Control and Prevention (CDC). 2009. *Health curriculum analysis tool (HECAT).*

Center for Disease Control and Prevention (CDC). 2011. Characteristics of an effective health education curriculum. Atlanta, GA: CDC.

———. 2010. *Health curriculum analysis tool (HECAT).* Atlanta, GA: CDC.

Dave, R. H., in R. J. Armstrong et al. 1970. Developing and writing behavioral objectives. Tucson, AX: Educational Innovators Press.

Division of Adolescent and School Health (DASH) 2005. *Healthy youth: An investment in our nation's future 2005.* February 2006. www.cde.gov/HealthyYouth/about/healthyyouth.htm.

Educational Materials Center (EMC). 2011. The Michigan model for health. Mount Pleasant, MI: Central Michigan University.

Ferrara, S., and J. McTighe. 1992. Assessment: A thoughtful process. In *If minds matter: A forward to the future,* H. Sasta, J. Bellanca, and R. Togarty, eds., 337–48. Palatine, IL: Skylight.

Harrow, A. J. 1972. A taxonomy of the psychomotor domain. New York: David McKay Co.

Iowa State University Extension. 2006. *Child development.* www.extension.iastate.edu (20 March 2006).

Joint Committee on National Health Standards. 1995. *Achieving health literacy: An investment in the future.* Atlanta, GA: American Cancer Society.

Lochner, J. 1981. Growth and development characteristics. In *A pocket guide to health and weight problems in school physical activities.* Kent, OH: American School Health Association.

Lohrmann, D. 2006. Personal interview conducted by authors on February 10, 2006.

Chapter 4: Strategies for Implementing Health Instruction

Barth, R. P. 2004. *Reducing the risk—Building skills to prevent pregnancy, STD and HIV.* Santa Cruz, CA: ETR Associates.

Carr, R. 1992. *Peer helper handbook to accompany just for me.* Bloomington, IN: AIT.

Concept to classroom: Tapping into multiple intelligence—Implementation. 2002, June 15. www.thirteen.org/edonline/concept2class/mi/index.html (October 2011).

Curtis, J., and R. Papenfuss. 1980. *Health instruction: A task approach.* Minneapolis, MN: Burgess.

Evertson, C. M., E. T. Emmer, B. S. Clements, and M. E. Worsham. 2008. *Classroom management for elementary teachers.* 8th ed. Boston, MA: Allyn & Bacon.

Foder, G. T., and G. T. Dalis. 1989. *Health instruction: Theory and application.* 4th ed. Philadelphia, PA: Lea & Febiger.

Gardner, H. 2011. *Frames of mind: The theory of multiple intelligence.* New York, NY: Basic Books.

Gold, R. S. 1991. *Microcomputer applications in health education.* Dubuque, IA: Brown.

Greenberg, J. S. 1989. *Health education—Learner-centered instructional strategies.* Dubuque, IA: Brown.

Hamrick, M., D. Anspaugh, and D. Smith. 1980. Decision making and the behavioral gap. *Journal of school health* 50: 455–58.

Hochbaum, G. M., S. M. Rosenstock, and S. S. Kegeles. 1960. *Determinants of health behavior.* Washington, DC: White House Conference on Children and Youth, 1960.

Komoski, P. K., and E. Plotnik. 1995. *Seven steps to responsible software selection.* ERIC Digest. ERIC Clearinghouse on Information and Technology, Syracuse, NY. www.ericdigests.org/1996-1/seven.htm (October 2011).

McKenzie, W. 1999. *It's not how smart you are—It's how you are smart!.* http://surfaquarium.com/MI/nine_intelligences.pdf (October 2011).

National School Boards Association, American Association of School Administrators, American Cancer Society, and National School Health Education Coalition. 1995. *Be a leader in academic achievement.* Alexandria, VA: National School Boards Association, American Association of School Administrators, American Cancer Society, and National School Health Education Coalition.

Price, G. E., and R. Dunn. 1997. *Learning style inventory (LSI): An inventory for the identification of how individuals in grades 3 through 12 prefer to learn.* Lawrence, KS: Price Systems.

Rivard, J. D. 1998. *Allyn & Bacon quick guide to the Internet for educators.* Boston, MA: Allyn & Bacon.

Smith, D., M. Hamrick, and D. Anspaugh. 1981. Decision story strategy: Practical approach for teaching decision making. *Journal of school health* 51(10): 637–43.

Stone, D., L. O'Reilley, and J. Brown. 1980. *Elementary school health education.* Dubuque, IA: Brown.

Strowage, J. 2002. *Qualities of effective teachers.* Alexandria, VA: Association for Supervision and Curriculum Development.

Timmreck, T. 1978. Creative health education through puppetry. *Health education* 9(1): 40–41.

Wagner, B., S. Gregory, M. Daniel, and J. Sapers. 1997. Where computers do work. *U.S. News & World Report* 121(22): 82–93.

Whitaker, T. 2004. *What great teachers do differently—14 things that matter most.* Larchmont, NY: Eye on Education.

Chapter 5: Measurement and Evaluation of Health Education

Arter, J., and J. McTighe. 2001. *Scoring rubrics in the classroom: Using performance criteria for assessing and improving student performance.* Thousand Oaks, CA: Corwin Press, Inc.

Barrett, Helen. 2004. *Electronic portfolios as digital stories of deep learning.* http://electronicportfolios.org/digistory/epstory.html (October 2011).

Centers for Disease Control and Prevention. 2011. *Characteristics of an effective health education curriculum.* Atlanta, GA: Centers for Disease Control and Prevention. www.cdc.gov/healthyyouth/SHER/characteristics/index.htm (October 2011).

Coffey, Heather. 2011. *Benchmark assessments.* Chapel Hill, NC: LEARN NC, University of North Carolina at Chapel Hill. www.learnnc.org/lp/pages/5317 (October 2011).

Council of Chief State School Officers. 2011. Health education assessment project. www.ccsso.org/Resources/Programs/Health_Education_Assessment_Project_(HEAP).htm (October 2011).

Council of Chief State School Officers. 2002. *The health education assessment project.* www.ccsso.org/scass/p_heap (October 2011).

Council of Chief State School Officers. 2006. *Health education assessment project (HEAP).* scassheap.org (October 2011).

Indiana Department of Education. 2010. *Licensing rules 2011.* www.doe.in.gov/educatorlicensing/ (October 2011).

Indiana Department of Education. 2011. Supporting student success. www.doe.in.gov/educatorlicensing/jstandards.html (October 2011).

Linn, R., and N. Gronlund. 2004. *Measurement and assessment in teaching.* 9th ed. Upper Saddle River, NJ: Prentice Hall.

Marzano, R., and J. Kendall. 1996. *A comprehensive guide to designing standards-based districts, schools, and classrooms.* Aurora, CO: McREL.

McCown, R., M. Driscoll, and P. G. Roop. 1996. *Educational psychology—A learning-centered approach to classroom practice.* 2d ed. Boston, MA: Allyn & Bacon.

McTighe, J. 2010. An introduction to understanding by design. www.mtace.org/pirday_sept2010/Intro%20to%20UBD%20Handout.pdf (October 2011).

McTighe, J., and S. Ferrara, 2011. Performance-based assessment in the classroom. http://jaymctighe.com/wordpress/wp-content/uploads/2011/04/Performance-Based-Assessment-in-the-Classroom.pdf (October 2011).

Milwaukee Country Nutrition and Physical Activity Coalition. 2009. Role modeling action guide: Promoting healthy eating and physical activity. Milwaukee, WI.

Morrow, J. R., A. W. Jackson, J. G. Disch, and D. P. Mood. 2005. *Measurement and evaluation in human performance.* Champaign, IL: Human Kinetics.

National Council on Measurement in Education. 2002, October. www.ncme.org.

Peer Evaluation: National Board for Professional Teaching Standards. 2008. www.nbpts.org/become_a_candidate/assessment_process (October 2011).

Rhode Island Department of Elementary and Secondary Education. 2008. K-12 literacy, restructuring of the learning environment at the middle and high school levels, and proficiency based graduation requirements (PBGR) at high schools. www.ride.ri.gov/Regents/Docs/RegentsRegulations/HS%20 Regulations%20September,%202008.pdf (October 2011).

Rocky Mountain Center for Health Promotion and Education. Content standards: Purposes and intended audiences. *RMC health educator* 1(2, Winter 2001).

Rocky Mountain Center for Health Promotion and Education (RMC Health). 2007 RMC analytic rubrics for national health education standards. Reprinted with permission. For information call 303-239-6494 or email info@rmc.org.

Sanchez, W., et al. 1995. *Working with diverse learners and school staff in a multicultural society.* Greensboro, NC: ERIC Clearinghouse on Counseling and Student Services. www.ericdigests.org/1996–3/working.htm (October 2011).

Shor, I. 1992. *Empowering education: Critical teaching for social change.* Chicago, IL: University of Chicago Press.

Social Solidarity. 2008. *Bogardus' Social Distance Scale.* www.csudh.edu/dearhabermas/bogardus02.htm (October 2011).

Tappe, Marlene K. 2010. The importance of standards-based health education. RMC Health Educator. http://blog.rmc.org/?p=183 (October 2011).

Tennessee.gov. *Tennessee's K–8 healthful living curriculum standards.* www.tennessee.gov/sbe/2008Aprilpdfs/IIIHHealthEducationPreK-8CurriculumStds.pdf (October 2011).

University of California Santa Cruz. 2011. *The narrative evaluation system: Evaluation of academic performance.* Santa Cruz, CA: University of California Santa Cruz. http://planning.ucsc.edu/irps/Stratpln/WASC94/a/sec2.htm (October 2011).

Utah State Office of Education. 2011. *Performance assessment for science teachers.* Salt Lake City, UT: Utah State Office of Education. www.schools.utah.gov/CURR/science/Elementary/Kindergarten/K-2ScienceCoreCurriculum.aspx (October 2011).

Chapter 6: Mental Health and Stress Reduction & Chapter 7: Strategies for Teaching Mental Health and Stress Reduction

American Academy of Child and Adolescent Psychiatry. 2004. *Panic disorder in children and adolescents.* www.aacap.org/cs/root/facts_for_families/panic_disorder_in_children_and_adolescents (October 2011).

———. 2008a, December 15. *Children's major psychiatric disorders.* www.aacap.org/cs/resource.centers (October 2011).

———. 2011. *Children's major psychiatric disorders.* www.aacap.org/cs/root/facts_for_families/children_and_divorce (October 2011).

———. 2008c. *Children's major psychiatric disorders.* www.aacap.org/cs/root/facts_for_families/teen_suicide (October 2011).

American Psychiatric Association (APA). 1987. *Diagnostic and statistical manual of mental disorders.* 3d ed., rev. Washington, DC: APA.

———. 1999, December 20. *Depression.* www.psych.org.

Bean, R. 1992. *The four conditions of self-esteem in the classroom: A handbook for teachers and parents.* Santa Cruz, CA: ETR Associates.

Bender, W. 1997. *Understanding ADHD: A practical guide for teachers and parents.* Upper Saddle River, NJ: Merrill/Prentice Hall.

Chandler, C., and C. Kolander. 1989. Depression. *Mayo Clinic health letter—Medical essay.*

Deming, W. E. 1994. *The new economics for industry, government, education.* Cambridge, MA: W. Edwards Deming Institute.

Department of Health and Human Resources. 2011. Stop bullying. Stopbullyingnow.gov (October 2011).

DeSpelder, L., and A. Strickland. 1987. *The last dance.* 2nd ed. Mountain View, CA: Mayfield.

Fredlund, B. S. 1984. Children and death from the school setting viewpoint. In *Death and dying in the classroom: Reading for reference,* J. L. Thomas, ed. Phoenix, AZ: Oryx Press.

Goodwin, L., W. Goodwin, and J. Cantrill. 1988. The mental health needs of elementary school children. *Journal of school health* 58(7): 282–87.

Hales, D. 2011. *An invitation to health.* Redwood City, CA: Benjamin Cummings.

Hamrick, M., D. Anspaugh, and G. Ezell. 1986. *Health.* Columbus, OH: Merrill.

Jones, J. 1985. *Promoting mental health of children and youth through the schools.* Paper presented at the American School Health Association Convention, October, Little Rock, AR.

Katz, L. G. 2002. *How can we strengthen children's self-esteem?* www.kidsource.com/kidsource/content2/strengthen_children_self.html (October 2011).

Kuersten, J. 1999. Healthy young minds: Rx for children's emotional and mental health. *Our children magazine.* Taken from www.selectivemutism.org/resources/library/Parenting%20 Issues/RX%20for%20Emotional%20Health.pdf (October 2011).

Magg, J. W., and S. R. Forness. 1991, September. Depression in children and adolescents: Assessment and treatment. *Focus on exceptional children* 24:14–19.

Maslow, A. 1983. *The farther reaches of human nature.* New York: Penguin Books.

National Center for Learning Disabilities, 2008. www.ncld.org.

National Institute of Mental Health, 2011. *Attention deficit hyperactivity disorder.* www.nimh.nih.gov/publicat/adhd.cfm (October 2011). Washington, DC: National Institute of Mental Health.

Nelson, R. E., and B. Crawford. 1991. Suicide among elementary school-age children. *Elementary school guidance and counseling* 25:123–28.

Olsen, L., K. Redican, and C. Baffi. 1986. *Health today.* 2d ed. New York, NY: Macmillan.

Page, R. M., and T. S. Page. 2006. *Fostering emotional well-being in the classroom.* Boston, MA: Jones & Bartlett.

Patros, P. G., and T. K. Shamoo. 1989. *Depression and suicide in children and adolescents: Prevention, intervention, and postvention.* Boston, MA: Allyn & Bacon.

Payne, W. A., and Hahn, D. B. 2010. *Understanding your health.* 10th ed. Boston, MA: McGraw-Hill.

Psychological Trauma Center. 2002, June 26. *Terrorism. What does one say to children?* http://ptcweb.org/terror-whattosay.html (October 2011).

Ricci, I. 1982. *Mom's house, Dad's house.* New York, NY: Macmillan.

Rinholm, J. 1999. *Classroom behavior strategies—Self-esteem building.*

Selye, H. 1975. *Stress without distress.* New York, NY: New American Library.

Stepfamily Foundation. 2003. *Ten steps for steps.* www.stepfamily.org.

Stroher, D. B. 1986. Latchkey children: The fastest-growing special interest group in the schools. *Journal of school health* 56(1): 16.

U.S. Department of Health and Human Services. 2002. *Child health USA 93.* Washington, DC: U.S. Government Printing Office.

U.S. Department of Education. 2011. *Teaching children with attention deficit hyperactivity disorder: Instructional strategies and practices.* Washington, DC: U.S. Government Printing Office.

Wallerstein, J., and J. Kelly. 1981. *Surviving the break-up.* New York, NY: Basic Books.

Chapter 8: Body Systems

Hootman, J. M. 2007, September. These old bones-A growing public health problem. *Journal of Athletic Training.* 2007, Jul-Sep; 42(3): 325–326. Dallas, TX: National Athletic Trainers' Association, Inc.

Jennings, W., and G. Phillips. 2008. *Indelible learning.* braincompatiblelearning.org/wp-content/uploads/2008/08/indelible-learning.pdf (October 2011).

Lutz, B. 2008. *Your unique body story.* www.bodytalkcentral.com/articles/Your%20Unique%20Body%20Story.pdf (October 2011).

National Heart Lung and Blood Institute. 2008, June. *Are you at risk for heart disease?* Bethesda, MD: National Heart Lung and Blood Institute. www.nhlbi.nih.gov/health/public/heart/other/latino/chd/action.htm (October 2011).

U.S. National Institutes of Health. 2011, January 4. Inside the human brain. Bethesda, MD: National Institutes of Health. www.nia.nih.gov/Alzheimers/Publications/Unraveling/Part1/inside.htm (October 2011).

U.S. National Institutes of Health. 2010, July 27. Skin care and aging. Bethesda, MD: U.S. National Institutes of Health. www.nia.nih.gov/HealthInformation/Publications/skin.htm (October 2011).

U.S. National Institutes of Health. 2011, March 28. Chest X-ray. Bethesda, MD: National Institutes of Health. www.nlm.nih.gov/medlineplus/ency/article/003804.htm (October 2011).

U.S. National Institutes of Health. 2011, March 28. Chest X-ray. Bethesda, MD: National Institutes of Health. www.nlm.nih.gov/medlineplus/ency/article/003804.htm (October 2011).

U.S. National Institutes of Health. 2011, March 28. Diabetes. Bethesda, MD: National Institutes of Health. www.nlm.nih.gov/medlineplus/ency/article/001214.htm (October 2011).

U.S. National Institutes of Health. 2011, May. Teacher's guide: Information about the musculoskeletal and skin systems. Bethesda, MD: National Institutes of Health. http://science-education.nih.gov/supplements/nih6/bone/guide/info_musculo_skin-a.htm (October 2011).

Chapter 9: Personal Health

American Academy of Dermatology. 2011. Nails. Schaumburg, IL: American Academy of Dermatology. www.aad.org/media-resources/stats-and-facts/prevention-and-care/nails/nails (October 2011).

American Alliance for Health, Physical Education, Recreation and Dance (AAHPERD). 2011, April. Improving Health and Academic Performance. www.aahperd.org/letsmoveinschool/ (October 2011).

AAHPERD. 2011, April. Overview of a comprehensive school physical activity program. www.aahperd.org/letsmoveinschool/about/overview.cfm (October 2011).

AAHPERD. 2011, April. Physical activity during school. www.aahperd.org/letsmoveinschool/about/paclassroom.cfm (October 2011).

Centers for Disease Control and Prevention (CDC). 2011. *School Health Guidelines to Promote Healthy Eating and Physical Activity.* www.cdc.gov/healthyyouth/npao/strategies.htm (October 2011).

Centers for Disease Control and Prevention. 2010. Your eyes are the windows to your health: Schedule an eye exam today Atlanta, GA: Centers for Disease Control and Prevention. www.cdc.gov/Features/HealthyVision/ (October 2011).

Centers for Disease Control and Prevention. 2011. How much sleep do I need? www.cdc.gov/sleep/about_sleep/how_much_sleep.htm (October 2011).

Centers for Disease Control and Prevention. 2011. Obesity. www.cdc.gov/chronicdisease/resources/publications/aag/obesity.htm (October 2011).

———. 2008. Perspectives in disease prevention and health promotion status of the 1990 Physical Fitness and Exercise Objectives.

www.cdc.gov/MMWR/preview/mmwrhtml/00000600.htm (October 2011).

MedicineNet.com. 2011, April 27. Definition of nail care. www.medterms.com/script/main/art.asp?articlekey=7745 (October 2011).

President's Council on Physical Fitness and Sports, U.S. Department of Health and Human Services, Office of Public Health and Science, Washington, DC. www.fitness.gov (October 2011).

U.S. Department of Health and Human Services. 2008, October 17. Physical activity guidelines for Americans: At-a-glance: A fact sheet for professionals. Washington, DC: U.S. Department of Health and Human Services. www.health.gov/paguidelines/factsheetprof.aspx (October 2011).

U.S. Department of Health and Human Services. 2011. *Healthy people 2020 objectives.* Washington, DC: Office of Public Health and Science.

U.S. Department of Health and Human Services. 2011, May. Healthy people 2020: Physical activity. Washington, DC: U.S. Department of Health and Human Services. http://healthypeople.gov/2020/topicsobjectives2020/pdfs/PhysicalActivity.pdf (October 2011).

Chapter 10: Strategies for Teaching Body Systems and Personal Health

A to Z Teacher Stuff, LLC. 2002a, November. *Glitter germs.* www.atozteacherstuff.com/lessons/GlitterGerms.shtml.

———. 2002b, November. *Stay away tooth decay.* www.atozteacherstuff.com/lessons/ToothDecay.shtml.

American Heart Association (AHA). 1996. *Heart power, kindergarten through second grade level.* Dallas, TX: AHA.

Bajah, S., and IICBA Organization. 2011. *School Health Guidelines to Promote Healthy Eating and Physical Activity.* www.cdc.gov/healthyyouth/npao/strategies.htm (October 2011).

Berenstain, S., and J. Berenstain. 1981a. *The Berenstain bears go to the doctor.* New York, NY: Random House.

———. 1981b. *The Berenstain bears visit the dentist.* New York, NY: Random House.

Calvert County Public Schools (Prince Frederick, MD). 2002, November. www.calvertnet.k12.md.us.

Health Strategies, Inc. 2002a, February 2. Home page. www.healthteacher.com/

———. 2002b, February 9. Home page. www.healthteacher.com.

———. 2002c, March 2. www.healthteacher.com

Mace-Matluck, B. J., and N. G. Hernandez. 1993. Five senses in *Integrating mathematics, science, and language (Paso Partners): An instructional volume I (Grades K–1).* Austin, TX: Southwest Education Development Laboratory. www.sedl.org/scimath/pasopartners/senses/ (October 2011).

MEDtropolis. 2011. *Virtual body.* www.medtropolis.com/Vbody.asp. (October 2011).

Merritt, K. 2002, October. *Dental health.* Information Institute of Syracuse, ERIC Clearinghouse on Information & Technology, Syracuse University, Syracuse, NY.

Sevaly, K. 1997. *February idea book.* Riverside, CA: Teacher's Friend.

Smoak, D. W. 2002, October. *Brushing and flossing to a healthy smile.* Information Institute of Syracuse, ERIC Clearinghouse on Information & Technology, Syracuse University, Syracuse, NY.

South Carolina State University. 2002, May 10. *Body systems.* http://askeric.org (2002).

Chapter 11: Sexuality Education

Administration for Children & Families. 2011. www.childwelfare.gov/can/statistics/ (October 2011). Washington, DC: U.S. Department of Health and Human Services.

Allen, L. S., and R. A. Gorski. 2002. Sexual orientation and the size of the anterior human brain. *Proceedings of the National Academy of Sciences USA* (15):7199–202.

American Academy of Child and Adolescent Psychiatry. 2006. *Gay and lesbian adolescents*. www.aacap.org/cs/root/facts_for_families/gay_lesbian_and_bisexual_adolescents (October 2011).

Byer, C. O., and L. W. Shainberg. 2001. *Dimensions of human sexuality*. Madison, WI: Brown and Benchmark.

Childhelp USA. 2011. *Child abuse*. www.childhelpusa.org/ (June 2011).

Eshleman, J. 2003. *The family: An introduction*. 8th ed. Boston, MA: Allyn & Bacon.

Fromm, E. 1989. *The art of loving*. New York, NY: Harper & Row.

Gevinger-Woititz, J. 1993. *The intimacy struggle*. Dearfield Beach, FL: Health Communications.

Guttimacher Institute. 2011. State policies in brief: Sex and HIV education. New York, NY: Guttimacher Institute.

Haas, K., and A. Haas. 2003. *Understanding sexuality*. St. Louis, MO: Mosby.

Henry J. Kaiser Foundation, The. 2002. *Talking with kids about tough issues: A national survey of parents and kids*. New York, NY: The Henry J. Kaiser Foundation.

Kelly, G. F. 2006. *Sexuality today: The human perspective*. 8th ed. New York, NY: McGraw-Hill.

Kilander, F. H. 1968. *Sex education in the schools*. Toronto, Canada: Macmillan.

Nelson, K. L. 1996. The conflict over sexuality education: Interviews with both sides of the debate. *Sexuality Information and Education Council of the United States (SIECUS) Report*, 24(6): 12–16. New York, NY: SIECUS.

Office of the Attorney General. 1985. *Child abuse prevention handbook*. Sacramento, CA: Office of the Attorney General.

Prevent Child Abuse America. 2011. *Fact sheet: Sexual abuse of children*. www.preventchildabuse.org (1 June, 2011).

Scales, P. 1984. *The front line of sexuality education*. Santa Cruz, CA: Network Publications.

Sexuality Information and Education Council of the United States (SIECUS). 2011. *Guidelines for comprehensive sexuality education: Grades K–12*. New York, NY: SIECUS.

———. 2006. *SIECUS special report: A revamped federal abstinence-only-until marriage program goes into existence*. www.siecus.org (20 July, 2006).

———. 2002. *State mandates: Sex education and HIV/AIDS/STD education*. www.siecus.org/ (December, 2002.)

———. 2004b. *Updated guidelines for comprehensive sexuality education: Grades K–12*. New York, NY: SIECUS.

Single Parent Central. *Did you know?* www.singleparentcentral.com (16 December, 2002).

Spalt, S. W. 1996. Coping with controversy: The professional epidemic of the nineties. *Journal of school health* 66(9): 339–340.

Strong, B., C. DeVault, and B. Sayad. 2004. *Human sexuality: Diversity in contemporary America*. Mountain View, CA: Mayfield.

U.S. Bureau of the Census. 2011. *Statistical abstract of the United States*. Washington, DC: U.S. Government Printing Office. www.census.gov/compendia/statab/ (October 2011).

U.S. Department of Health and Human Services. 2008. *Child maltreatment 2006*. U.S. Department of Health and Human Services, Administration on Children, Youth and Families. Washington, DC: Government Printing Office.

U.S. Census Bureau. 2005. *Examining American Household Composition: 1990 and 2000*. www.census.gov/prod/2005pubs/censr-24.pdf (October 2011).

Chapter 12: Strategies for Teaching Sexuality Education

Heesacker, M. 1994. *Portraits of adjustment*. Boston, MA: Allyn & Bacon.

Sexuality Information and Education Council of the United States (SIECUS). 2004. *Guidelines for comprehensive sexuality education: Grades K–12*. New York, NY: SIECUS.

Chapter 13: Substance Use and Abuse

Abadinsky, H. 2001. *Drugs: An introduction*. 4th ed. Belmont, CA: Wadsworth.

American Cancer Society. 2010. Smokeless tobacco and how to quit. Atlanta, GA: American Cancer Society. www.cancer.org/acs/groups/cid/documents/webcontent/002979-pdf.pdf (October 2011).

American Lung Association. 2008. New CDC report demonstrates urgency for all states and cities to become smokefree. Washington, DC: American Lung Association. www.lungusa.org/press-room/press-releases/new-cdc-report-demonstrates.html (October 2011).

Barry, J. D. 2002. Barbiturate abuse. *eMedicine consumer journal* 3(3) (March 2002).

Bliss, Donna Leigh. 2009. Beyond the disease model: Reframing the etiology of alcoholism from a spiritual perspective. *Journal of Teaching in the Addictions*: (8) 1&2: 10–26. www.informaworld.com/smpp/content~db=all?content=10.1080/15332270903396556 (October 2011).

California State University Northridge, Department of Education. 2011. Why do women smoke? www.csun.edu/~ams36455/whysmoke.htm (October 2011).

CDC. 2010. Tobacco use by young people: Tobacco use and the health of young people. Atlanta, GA: CDC. www.cdc.gov/HealthyYouth/tobacco/facts.htm (October 2011).

CDC. 2011. Tobacco use: Targeting the nation's leading killer at a glance, 2011. Atlanta, GA: CDC. www.cdc.gov/chronicdisease/resources/publications/aag/osh.htm (October 2011).

CDC. 2010. Vital and health statistics. Summary health statistics for U.S. adults: National health interview survey, 2009. Atlanta, GA: CDC. www.cdc.gov/nchs/data/series/sr_10/sr10_249.pdf (October 2011).

CDC. 2010. World no tobacco day. Atlanta, GA: CDC. www.cdc.gov/Features/WorldNoTobaccoDay/ (October 2011).

CDC. 2011. Youth and tobacco use. Atlanta, GA: CDC. www.cdc.gov/tobacco/data_statistics/fact_sheets/youth_data/tobacco_use/index.htm (October 2011).

Centers for Disease Control and Prevention (CDC). 2011. Adolescent and school health. Atlanta, GA: CDC. www.cdc.gov/HealthyYouth/ (October 2011).

Education Development Center, Inc. 2011. What is a coordinated school health program? Newton, MA: Education Development Center, Inc. www2.edc.org/makinghealthacademic/cshp.asp (October 2011).

GovTrack.us. 2006. *S. 3546 [109th]: Dietary supplement and nonprescription drug consumer protection act*. www.fda.gov/RegulatoryInformation/Legislation/FederalFoodDrugandCosmeticActFDCAct/SignificantAmendmentstotheFDCAct/ucm148035.htm (October 2011).

National Cancer Institute. U.S. National Institutes of Health. 2011. Smoking and tobacco control monograph no. 14: The role of tobacco advertising and promotion in smoking initiation. cancercontrol.cancer.gov/tcrb/monographs/14/m14_13.pdf (October 2011).

National Institute on Drug Abuse (NIDA). 1980. *Research monograph series 31*. www.drugabuse.gov/pdf/monographs/31.pdf. (October 2011).

National Institute on Drug Abuse. 2007. Marijuana: Facts parents need to know. Bethesda, MD: National Institute on Drug Abuse. www.nida.nih.gov/marijbroch/marijparentstxt.html (October 2011).

National Institute on Drug Abuse. 2009. Research report series: Tobacco addiction. Bethesda, MD: National Institute on Drug Abuse. www.nida.nih.gov/PDF/TobaccoRRS_v16.pdf (October 2011).

National Institute on Drug Abuse. 2010. NIDA InfoFacts: Cocaine. Bethesda, MD: National Institute on Drug Abuse. www.nida.nih.gov/infofacts/cocaine.html (October 2011).

National Institute on Drug Abuse. 2010. NIDA InfoFacts: Methamphetamine. Bethesda, MD: National Institute on Drug Abuse. www.drugabuse.gov/infofacts/methamphetamine.html (October 2011).

National Institute on Drug Abuse. 2010. Research report series: Marijuana abuse. Bethesda, MD: National Institute on Drug Abuse. www.drugabuse.gov/ResearchReports/Marijuana/marijuana2.html#scope (October 2011).

National Institute on Drug Abuse. 2010. Research report series: Marijuana abuse. Bethesda, MD: National Institute on Drug Abuse. www.nida.nih.gov/researchreports/marijuana/marijuana4.html (October 2011).

National Institute on Drug Abuse. 2011. Commonly abused drugs. Bethesda, MD: National Institute on Drug Abuse. www.nida.nih.gov/drugpages/drugsofabuse.html (October 2011).

National Institute on Drug Abuse. 2011. Preventing drug abuse among children: Examples of research-based drug abuse prevention programs. drugabuse.gov/prevention/examples.html (October 2011).

National Institute on Drug Abuse. 2011. Public service announcements: Keep your body healthy. Bethesda, MD: National Institute on Drug Abuse. www.nida.nih.gov/drugpages/psahome.html (October 2011).

National Institute on Drug Abuse. 2011. Real teens ask: What are designer drugs? Bethesda, MD: National Institute on Drug Abuse. http://teens.drugabuse.gov/blog/real-teens-ask-designer-drugs/ (October 2011).

National Institutes of Health (NIH). National Institute on Alcohol Abuse and Alcoholism. 2011. FAQs for the general public: Is alcoholism inherited? Bethesda, MD: NIH. www.niaaa.nih.gov/FAQs/General-English/Pages/default.aspx (October 2011).

National Reye's Syndrome Foundation. 2008, December 12. What is the role of aspirin? National Reye's Syndrome Foundation, United States. www.reyessyndrome.org/aspirin.html (October 2011).

———. 2008a, February. *NIDA Infofacts: Inhalants.* http://www.nida.nih.gov/Infofacts/Inhalants.html. (October 2011).

National Library of Medicine. 2005. *Self-healing, patents, and placebos.* www.nlm.nih.gov/hmd/emotions/self.html. (October 2011).

Office of National Drug Control Policy. 2011. Prevention. Rockville, MD: Office of National Drug Control Policy. www.whitehousedrugpolicy.gov/prevent/index.html (October 2011).

Office of the Surgeon General. 2006. The health consequences of involuntary exposure to tobacco smoke: A report of the surgeon general, Chapter 5: Reproductive and developmental effects from exposure to secondhand smoke. Atlanta, GA: Office of the Surgeon General. www.surgeongeneral.gov/library/secondhandsmoke/report/chapter5.pdf (October 2011).

Ray, O., and C. Ksir. 2002. *Drugs, society, and human behavior.* 9th ed. Boston, MA: WCB McGraw-Hill.

Substance Abuse and Mental Health Services Administration. 2010. Results from the 2009 National Survey on Drug Use and Health, volume I. Summary of national findings (Office of Applied Studies, NSDUH Series H-38A, HHS Publication No. SMA 10-4586Findings). Rockville, MD. www.oas.samhsa.gov/NSDUH/2k9NSDUH/2k9ResultsP.pdf (October 2011).

U.S. Department of Health and Human Services, Substance Abuse and Mental Health Services Administration, Center for Substance Abuse Prevention. 2011. Underage drinking: The basic facts. Washington, DC: U.S. Department of Health and Human Services. www.toosmarttostart.samhsa.gov/teens/facts/myths.aspx (October 2011).

U.S. Department of Justice. 2011. *Drugs of abuse.* www.justice.gov/dea/pubs/drugs_of_abuse.pdf (October 2011).

U.S. Food and Drug Administration (FDA) 2011. *Consumer education: Over-the-counter medicine.* www.fda.gov/Drugs/ResourcesForYou/Consumers/default.htm (October 2011).

U.S. Food and Drug Administration. 2010, April 5. FDA approves new formulation for OxyContin. Silver Spring, MD: U.S. Food and Drug Administration. www.fda.gov/NewsEvents/Newsroom/PressAnnouncements/2010/ucm207480.htm (October 2011).

U.S. Drug Enforcement Agency. 2011. "Medical" marijuana — The facts. U.S. Washington, DC: Drug Enforcement Agency. www.justice.gov/dea/ongoing/marinol.html (October 2011).

United States Food and Drug Administration. 2010. Medication guide: Vyvanse. Silver Spring, MD: United States Food and Drug Administration. www.fda.gov/downloads/Drugs/DrugSafety/ucm089823.pdf (October 2011).

———. *OxyContin information.* www.fda.gov/Drugs/DrugSafety/PostmarketDrugSafetyInformationforPatientsandProviders/ucm207196.htm (October 2011).

White House Initiative on Educational Excellence for Hispanic Americans. 2011. Helping your child be drug free. Washington, DC: White House Initiative on Educational Excellence for Hispanic Americans. www.yesican.gov/ (October 2011).

Chapter 14: Strategies for Teaching about Substance Use and Abuse

American Lung Association. 2002. *Teens against tobacco use (TATU).* www.lungusa.org/smokefreeclass/index.html.

———. 2003, January. *State of the air—2002.* www.lungusa.org/tobacco/teenager_factsheet99.html.

———. 1995–2003b. *Smoking stinks.* www.kidshealth.org/kid/watch/house/smoking.html (October 2002).

PE Central. 2000. *Smoking aerobics.* www.pecentral.org/lessonideas/ViewLesson.asp?ID=930.

U.S. Department of Education. 2001. *The gateway to educational material.* www.thegateway.org.

Wolfanger, S. 2001, August 24. *Impaired.* www.pecentral.org/LessonIdeas/ViewLesson.asp?ID=931.

Chapter 15: Infectious and Noninfectious Conditions

American Cancer Society. 2011. *Cancer prevention and early detection facts and figures 2011.* Atlanta, GA: American Cancer Association.

American Cancer Society. 2011. *What is staging?* www.cancer.org (October 2011).

American Diabetes Association. 2011. *Fact sheet.* www.diabetes.org (October 2011).

American Heart Association. 2006. *Cholesterol and atherosclerosis in children.* www.heart.org/HEARTORG/ (October 2011).

Anderson, K. N., L. E. Anderson, and W. D. Glanze, eds. 1998. *Mosby's medical, nursing, & allied health dictionary.* 5th ed. Boston, MA: Mosby.

Brooks, G. F., J. S. Butel, and S. A. Morse. 2001. *Jawetz, Melnick, & Adelberg's medical microbiology.* 22d ed. New York, NY: McGraw-Hill.

Centers for Disease Control and Prevention (CDC). 2011. America Responds to AIDS. *AIDS prevention guide—Deciding what to say to younger children.* Atlanta, GA: CDC.

Center for Disease Control and Prevention (CDC). 2011. Preventable diseases and the vaccines that prevent them. www.cdc.gov/vaccines/spec-grps/hcp/conv-materials.htm (October 2011).

CDC. 2011. Recommended immunization schedule for 2011. www.cdc.gov/vaccines/recs/schedules/child-schedule.htm (September 2011).

———. 2006. *Twenty-five years of HIV-AIDS, United States 1981–2006.* 55(21): 585–589.

———. 2008. *HIV and AIDS in the United States: A picture of today's epidemic* www.cdc.gov/hiv/topics/surveillance/pdf/us_media.pdf (October 2011).

———. 2011. *Viral hepatitis.* www.cdc.gov/hepatitis/ (October 2011).

Cray, D., and A. Park. 1996. The exorcists. *Time,* Special Issue 148(14): 64–68.

Crocker, A. C., A. T. Lavin, J. S. Polfrey, S. M. Porter, D. M. Shaw, and K. S. Weill. 1994. Support for children with HIV infection in school: Best practices guidelines. *Journal of school health* 64(1): 33–34.

Crowley, L. 2010. *An introduction to human disease: Pathology and Pathophysiology Correlations.* 8th ed. Boston, MA: Jones and Bartlett.

Elster, A. B., and N. J. Kuznets. 1994. *AMA guidelines for adolescent prevention services (GAPS).* Baltimore, MD: Williams & Wilkins.

Guyton, A. C., and J. E. Hall. 2005. *Textbook of medical physiology of disease.* 10th ed. Philadelphia, PA: W. B. Saunders.

Lichtenstein, P., N. V. Holm, P. K. Verasalo, A. Iliadou, J. Kaprio, M. Koskenvuo, Z. Pokkala, A. Skythe, and K. Hemmink. 2000. Environmental and heritable factors in the causation of cancer—Analysis of cohorts of twins from Sweden, Denmark, and Finland. *New England journal of medicine* 343(2):78–85.

Mange, E. J., and A. P. Mange. 1990. *Basic human genetics.* Sunderland, MA: Sinauer Associates.

Margolis, S., and C. D. Saudek. 2009. *The John Hopkins white papers: Diabetes mellitus-2009.* Baltimore, MD: John Hopkins Medical Institutions.

National Institute of Allergy and Infectious Diseases. 2011. HIV/AIDS treatment. www.naid.nih.gov (July 2011).

National Institute of Allergy and Infectious Diseases. 2011. *Understanding HIV/AIDS.* www.niaid.nih.gov/topics/HIVAIDS/Understanding/Pages/Default.aspx (October 2011).

Peterman, T. A. 1986. Sexual transmission of human immunode-ficiency virus infection in the United States. *Journal of the American medical association* 256: 2222–26.

Scott, R., and A. D. Kessler. 1988. *A child with sickle cell anemia in your class.* Washington, DC: Center for Sickle Cell Disease, Howard University College of Medicine.

Seeley, R. R., T. D. Stephens, and P. Tate. 2007. *Anatomy and physiology.* 8th ed. Boston, MA: WCB McGraw-Hill.

Spence, A. P., and E. B. Mason. 1992. *Human anatomy and physiology.* 4th ed. New York, NY: West Publishing Company.

Thibodeau, G. A., and K. T. Patton. 2009. *Anatomy and physiology.* St. Louis, MO: Mosby.

U.S. Department of Health and Human Services. 2011. *Recommended HIV treatment regimens.* www.aidsinfo.nih.gov/ContentFiles/RecommendedHIVTreatmentRegimens_FS_en.pdf (October 2011).

Chapter 16: Strategies for Teaching about Infectious and Noninfectious Conditions

White, D. M., and L. Rudisill. 1987. Analyzing cigarette smoke. *Health education* (August–September): 50–51.

Chapter 17: Nutrition

Acaloriecounter.com. 2011. Fast food restaurants & nutrition facts compared. www.acaloriecounter.com/fast-food.php (October 2011).

American Dietetic Association. 2009. Health implications of dietary fiber. *Journal of the American Dietetic Association.* February 2009: 109(2): 350.

American Heart Association. 2010. Eating fast food. www.heart.org/HEARTORG/GettingHealthy/NutritionCenter/DiningOut/Eating-Fast-Food_UCM_301473_Article.jsp (October 2011).

American Heart Association. 2011. *What do my cholesterol levels mean?* www.heart.org/idc/groups/heart-public/@wcm/@hcm/documents/downloadable/ucm_300301.pdf (October 2011).

California Department of Health Care Services. 2006. California food guide: Health and dietary issues affecting Latinos. www.dhcs.ca.gov/dataandstats/reports/Documents/CaliforniaFoodGuide/16HealthandDietaryIssuesAffectingLatinos.pdf (October 2011).

CDC. 2009, August. U.S. schools show decreasing availability of junk food and promoting physical activity.

Centers for Disease Control and Prevention (CDC). 2011, February. Iron and iron deficiency. www.cdc.gov/nutrition/everyone/basics/vitamins/iron.html (October 2011).

Glickman, D. 2002, January 31. *Healthy eating helps you make the grade!* U.S. Department of Agriculture.

MedlinePlus. 2011. Bulimia. Bethesda, MD: National Library of Medicine and National Institutes of Health. www.nlm.nih.gov/medlineplus/ency/article/000341.htm (October 2011).

National Institute of Health. National Library of Medicine. 2011. Vitamin supplementation and megadoses.

National Institutes of Health, Office of Dietary Supplements. 2007, August. Dietary supplement fact sheet: Iron. ods.od.nih.gov/factsheets/iron/ (October 2011).

National Institutes of Health. National Cancer Institute. 2004. Antioxidants and cancer prevention: Fact sheet. www.cancer.gov/cancertopics/factsheet/prevention/antioxidants (October 2011).

National Institutes of Health. National Cancer Institute. 2011, March. Dietary antioxidants, redox tone and health promotion: An orthomolecular study of interactions. http://clinicaltrials.gov/ct2/show/NCT01315977 (October 2011).

National Institutes of Health. National Library of Medicine. 2011. Anorexia nervosa. www.nlm.nih.gov/medlineplus/ency/article/000362.htm (October 2011).

Rahman, K. 2007. Studies on free radicals, antioxidants, and co-factors. *Clinical Interventions in Aging.* June 2007; 2(2): 219–236. Dove Medical Press. www.ncbi.nlm.nih.gov/pmc/articles/PMC2684512/ (October 2011).

Satcher, D. Department of Health and Human Services. 1998, February 13. *Progress review: Nutrition.*

Stewart, S., Noel Blissard, and Dean Jolliffe. 2006, October. Let's eat out. Economic information bulletin no. (EIB-19) 16 pp, October 2006. U. S. Department of Agriculture, Economic Research Service. www.ers.usda.gov/publications/eib19/eib19_reportsummary.pdf (October 2011).

———. U.S. Department of Agriculture (USDA). 2006. *USDA celebrates school breakfast week.* www.usda.gov/wps/portal/usda/usdahome?contentidonly=true&contentid=2006/03/0065.xml (October 2011).

———. 2008. *Food and nutrition: Research briefs.* www.ars.usda.gov

U. S. Department of Agriculture. 2011. MyPlate background. www.cnpp.usda.gov/Publications/MyPlate/Backgrounder.pdf (October 2011).

U. S. Department of Agriculture. Food and Nutrition Service. 2010, June. Children's diets in the mid-1990s: Dietary intake and Its relationship with school meal participation. www.fns.usda.gov/ora/menu/published/CNP/FILES/ChilDietsum.htm (October 2011).

U.S. Department of Agriculture. 2011, June. A brief history of USDA food guides. www.choosemyplate.gov/downloads/MyPlate/ABriefHistoryOfUSDAFoodGuides.pdf (October 2011).

U. S. Department of Health & Human Services. Office of the Surgeon General. 2007, January. Overweight in children and adolescents. www.surgeongeneral.gov/topics/obesity/calltoaction/fact_adolescents.htm (October 2011).

U. S. Department of Health and Human Services, National Center for Chronic Disease Prevention and Health Promotion. 2010, June. Healthy youth! Health topics: Childhood obesity. www.cdc.gov/healthyyouth/obesity/facts.htm (October 2011).

U. S. Department of Health and Human Services, National Institutes of Health. 2011, March. Food for thought: Good nutrition begins. www.hhs.gov/news/nutrition_month11_508.pdf (October 2011).

U. S. Department of Health and Human Services, Office on Women's Health. 2011. Anorexia nervosa. www.womenshealth.gov/faq/anorexia-nervosa.cfm (October 2011).

U. S. Department of Health and Human Services. 2011. Healthy People 2020 Summary of Objectives: Nutrition and weight status. www.healthypeople.gov/2020/topicsobjectives2020/pdfs/NutritionandWeight.pdf (October 2011).

U.S. Food and Drug Administration (FDA). 2005. *Revealing trans fats.* www.fda.gov/downloads/Food/ScienceResearch/ResearchAreas/ConsumerResearch/UCM080413.pdf (October 2011).

U. S. Food and Drug Administration. 2011, June. Lowering salt in your diet. www.fda.gov/ForConsumers/ConsumerUpdates/ucm181577.htm (October 2011).

U. S. Food and Drug Administration. 2011, May (update). Food labeling and nutrition: Guidance for Industry. www.fda.gov/Food/GuidanceComplianceRegulatoryInformation/GuidanceDocuments/FoodLabelingNutrition/default.htm (October 2011).

United States Department of Agriculture. 2011. Expanding school breakfast: Talking points. www.fns.usda.gov/cnd/breakfast/expansion/breakfast_talkingpoints.pdf (October 2011).

United States Department of Agriculture, Food and Nutrition Service. 2011. *National school lunch monthly data.* www.fns.usda.gov/pd/36slmonthly.htm.

United States Department of Agriculture, Food and Nutrition Service. April 19, 2011. Healthier U.S. School Challenge. http://teamnutrition.usda.gov/healthierus/vision.html (October 2011).

United States Department of Agriculture. Food and Nutrition Service. 2011, January. National School Lunch Program. www.fns.usda.gov/cnd/lunch/ (October 2011).

United States Department of Agriculture, Food and Nutrition Service. 2011, January. School Superintendents Are Important to School Breakfast! www.fns.usda.gov/cnd/breakfast/expansion/stakeholderfactsheets.pdf (October 2011).

United States Department of Agriculture. 2011, January. The School Breakfast Program. www.fns.usda.gov/cnd/breakfast/AboutBFast/SBPFactSheet.pdf (October 2011).

United States Department of Agriculture. 2011, May. Dietary Guidelines for Americans, 2010. www.cnpp.usda.gov/DGAs2010-PolicyDocument.htm (October 2011).

United States Food and Drug Administration. 2011, March. How to understand and use the nutrition facts label. www.fda.gov/food/labelingnutrition/consumerinformation/ucm078889.htm#twoparts (October 2011).

University of Pittsburgh. Schools of the Health Sciences. 2011, March. Grapefruit diet (Hollywood Diet). www.upmc.com/healthatoz/pages/healthlibrary.aspx?chunkiid=201796 (October 2011).

White House.gov. December 2010. Child nutrition reauthorization healthy, hunger-free kids act of 2010. www.whitehouse.gov/sites/default/files/Child_Nutrition_Fact_Sheet_12_10_10.pdf (October 2011).

Chapter 18: Strategies for Teaching Nutrition

Dairy Council of California. 2011. Kids games. www.dairycouncilofca.org/Tools/KidsLearningTools.aspx (October 2011).

Health Strategies, Inc. 2002. *Nutrition.* www.healthteacher.com.

MeYou Health. 2011. Munch 5-a-DAY. http://munch5aday.com/ (October 2011).

Medical University of South Carolina. 2011. MUSC health audio podcasts: Overweight: Nutritional guidance for overweight children. Charleston, SC. Medical University of South Carolina: www.muschealth.com/multimedia/Podcasts/displayPod.aspx?podid=582&autostart=false (October 2011).

National Dairy Council. 2011. Explore the world of nutrition with nutrition explorations. www.nutritionexplorations.org/kids/activities-main.asp (October 2011).

PodcastDirectory.com. 2011. Kids, sports and nutrition episode. www.podcastdirectory.com/podshows/1419765 (October 2011).

Roger, K. 1994. *Food labels in the classroom.* ERIC Clearinghouse on Reading and Communication Skills. http://askeric.org/cgi-bin/printlessons.cgi/Virtual/Lessons/Health/Consumer_Health/COH0001.html.

Teacher Store. 1999. *A to Z Teacher Stuff Network.* www.lessonplanz.com.

United States Department of Agriculture, Center for Nutrition Policy and Promotion. 2011. Dietary guidance. Washington, DC. United States Department of Agriculture: http://fnic.nal.usda.gov/nal_display/index.php?info_center=4&tax_level=1&tax_subject=256 (October 2011).

Utah Education Network. 1996. *Breakfast.* www.uen.org/Lessonplan/preview.cgi?LPid=4482 (October 2011).

Chapter 19: Injuries: Accident and Violence Prevention

Centers for Disease Control and Prevention. 2011. Injuries among children and adolescents. www.cdc.gov/ncipc/factsheets/children.htm (October 2011).

Centers for Disease Control and Prevention. 2011, March. *Injuries and violence are leading causes of death: Key data & statistics.* www.cdc.gov/injury/overview/data.html (October 2011).

Centers for Disease Control and Prevention, National Institute for Occupational Safety and Health. 2011. *NIOSH workplace safety and health topics: Asbestos.* www.cdc.gov/niosh/topics/asbestos/ (October 2011).

Los Angeles County Department of Children and Family Services. 2011. Frequently asked questions. http://dcfs.lacounty.gov/faq.html#5 (October 2011).

Michigan Department of Labor and Economic Growth. 2006. *Accident proneness.* Lansing, MI: Michigan Occupational Safety and Health Administration, Consultation Education & Training Division.

National Center for Education Statistics, Bureau of Justice Statistics. 2010. *Indicators of school crime and safety: 2010.* http://nces.ed.gov/pubs2011/2011002.pdf (October 2011).

National Safety Council. 2011, June. Skateboarding Safety Tips. http://downloads.nsc.org/pdf/factsheets/Skateboarding_Safety_Tips.pdf (October 2011).

U.S. Department of Education. National Center for Education Statistics. 2011. *Crime, violence, discipline, and safety in U. S. public schools: Findings from the school survey on crime and safety: 2009-10.* http://nces.ed.gov/pubs2011/2011320.pdf (October 2011).

U.S. Department of Education. National Center for Education Statistics. 2011. *Indicators of school crime and safety: 2010. Indicator 11: Bullying at school and cyber-bullying anywhere.* http://nces.ed.gov/programs/crimeindicators/crimeindicators2010/ind_11.asp (October 2011).

U.S. Department of Education. National Center for Education Statistics. 2011. *Indicators of school crime and safety: 2010.* http://nces.ed.gov/programs/crimeindicators/crimeindicators2010/index.asp (October 2011).

U.S. Department of Health and Human Services Administration for Children and Families. 2007. *Leaving your child home alone.* www.childwelfare.gov/pubs/factsheets/homealone.cfm (October 2011).

U.S. Department of Health and Human Services. 2011. *Healthy people 2020 topics and objectives: Injury and violence prevention.* www.healthypeople.gov/2020/topicsobjectives2020/overview.aspx?topicid=24 (October 2011).

U. S. Department of Justice, National Criminal Justice Reference Service. 2011. *Motor vehicle accidents and self-control.* www.ncjrs.gov/App/Publications/abstract.aspx?ID=126761 (October 2011).

Chapter 20: Strategies for Teaching Injuries: Accident and Violence Prevention

Arizona Rural Metro Fire Department. 2011. Lesson Plans. www.rmfire.com/lesson_plans/2nd.pdf (October 2011).

Governale, F. 2002, July 25. *Number bingo.* http://askeric.org/cgi-bin/printlessons.cig/Virtual/Lessons/Foreign–Language/French/FRN0202.html.

Help Keep Kids Safe. 2011. Lesson plans. www.helpkeepkidssafe.org (October 2011).

SafeKids.org. 2011. Lesson plans. www.safekids.org (October 2011).

University of Northern Iowa. 2003. *National program for playground safety.* www.uni.edu/playground/home.html.

Virginia Department of Education. 2011. Lessons: Life skills. http://learninglab.org (October 2011).

Chapter 21: Consumer Health

Anspaugh, D. J., M. Hamrick, and F. D. Rosato. 2011. *Wellness: Concepts and Applications.* 8th ed. Boston, MA: McGraw-Hill.

Barrett, S., W. London, R. Baratz, and M. Kroger. 2006. *Consumer health: A guide to intelligent decisions.* 8th ed. New York, NY: McGraw-Hill.

Butler, J. T. 2012. *Consumer health: Making informed decisions.* Sudbury, MA: Jones and Bartlett.

Devita, E. 1995. The decline of the doctor–patient relationship. *American health* 13(7): 63–65, 105.

FirstGov for Consumers. 2006. *Patients bill of rights.*

Howard, T. 2009. Push is on to end prescription drugs ads targeting consumers. *USA Today* (10 August, 2009). Gannett Co., Inc.

Payne, W. A., and D. B. Hahn. 2006. *Understanding your health.* 8th ed. Boston, MA: McGraw-Hill.

Propecia. 1998. Propecia and Rogaine: Extra strength for alopecia. *The medical letter* 40 (February 27): 25–27.

Rubin, A. 2005. *Research and marketing of drugs.* www.cato.org/pubs/regulation/regv28n2/v28n2-5.pdf (October 2011).

Woolley, John T, and Gerhard Peters. 1999–2011. *The American presidency project* [online]. Santa Barbara, CA. www.presidency.ucsb.edu/ws/?pid=9108 (July 2011).

Chapter 23: Aging, Dying, and Death

American Association of Retired Persons. 2010, October. Take charge of your future: Legal documents you need now! Washington, DC: American Association of Retired Persons. www.aarp.org/relationships/caregiving/info-09-2010/legal_documents_women_long_term_care.html (July 2011).

American Association of Suicidology. 2011. Know the warning signs. Washington, DC: American Association of Suicidology. www.suicidology.org/web/guest/stats-and-tools/warning-signs (July 2011).

Center for American Progress. 2008, July 30. Elderly poverty: The challenge before us. Washington, DC: Center for American Progress. www.americanprogress.org/issues/2008/07/elderly_poverty.html (July 2011).

Centers for Disease Control and Prevention. 2008, August 7. Suicide prevention: Youth suicide. Atlanta, GA: Centers for Disease Control and Prevention. http://www.cdc.gov/ncipc/dvp/suicide/youthsuicide.htm (July 2011).

Centers for Disease Control and Prevention. 2011, March 16. National vital statistics reports: Volume 59, number 4. Atlanta, GA: Centers for Disease Control and Prevention. www.cdc.gov/nchs/data/nvsr/nvsr59/nvsr59_04.pdf (July 2011).

Centers for Disease Control and Prevention. 2011. Healthy aging: Helping people to live long and productive lives and enjoy a good quality of life. Atlanta, GA: Centers for Disease Control and Prevention. www.cdc.gov/chronicdisease/resources/publications/AAG/aging.htm (July 2011).

Encyclopaedia Britannica, Merriam-Webster, Inc. 2011. Euthanasia. Chicago, IL: Encyclopaedia Britannica. www.merriam-webster.com/dictionary/euthanasia (July 2011).

Encyclopedia of Death and Dying. 2011. Anxiety and fear. Encyclopedia of death and dying: deathreference.com. www.deathreference.com/A-Bi/Anxiety-and-Fear.html (July 2011).

Iowa Department on Aging. 2011. End-of-life care conversations. Des Moines, IA: Iowa Department on Aging. www.aging.iowa.gov/Documents/Publications/EndOfLifeCareConversations.pdf (July 2011).

National Center for Biotechnology Information, U.S. National Library of Medicine. 2010, August. Reflecting on God: Religious primes can reduce neurophysiological response to errors. www.ncbi.nlm.nih.gov/pubmed/20558751 (July 2011).

National Cancer Institute. 2005. *Model of life-threatening illness.* www.cancer.gov.

National Institutes of Health, National Library of Medicine. 2010, August 15. Aging changes in the bones, muscles and joints. Rockville, MD: National Institutes of Health. www.nlm.nih.gov/medlineplus/ency/article/004015.htm (July 2011).

National Institutes of Health, National Library of Medicine. 2010, December 13. Aging changes in body shape. Rockville, MD: National Institutes of Health. www.nlm.nih.gov/medlineplus/ency/article/003998.htm (July 2011).

National Institutes of Health. National Institute of Neurological Disorders and Stroke. 2011 NINDS dementia information page: Dementias. Bethesda, MD: National Institutes of Health. www.ninds.nih.gov/disorders/dementias/dementia.htm (July 2011).

National Institutes of Health. National Institute of Neurological Disorders and Stroke. 2011. NINDS Alzheimer's disease. Bethesda, MD: National Institutes of Health. www.ninds.nih.gov/disorders/alzheimersdisease/alzheimersdisease.htm (July 2011).

Project America. 2008. Seniors: Living arrangements. Florence, MS: Project America. www.project.org/info.php?recordID=128 (July 2011).

Pruitt, B., and J. Stein. 1999. *Health styles: Decisions for living well.* 2d ed. Boston, MA: Allyn & Bacon.

The National Women's Health Information Center, U.S. Department of Health and Human Services: Office on Women's Health. 2010, February 17. Organ donation and transplantation. Washington, DC: U.S. Department of Health and Human Services. www.womenshealth.gov/faq/organ-donation.cfm (July 2011).

U.S. Census Bureau. 2011. 2010 census: The elderly population. Washington, DC: U.S. Census Bureau. www.census.gov/population/www/pop-profile/elderpop.html (July 2011).

U.S. Census Bureau. 2011. Population profile of the United States. Washington, DC: U.S. Censure Bureau. www.census.gov/population/www/pop-profile/elderpop.html

U.S. Congressional Budget Office. 2008. April 17, Growing disparities in life expectancy. Washington, DC: U.S. Congressional Budget Office. www.cbo.gov/ftpdocs/91xx/doc9104/04-17-LifeExpectancy_Brief.pdf (July 2011).

U.S. Department of Health and Human Services. 2003. *Organ donation.* www.organdonor.gov.

U. S. Department of Health and Human Services. 2011. The need is real: Data. Washington, DC: U.S. Department of Health and Human Services. www.organdonor.gov/aboutStatsFacts.asp (July 2011).

U.S. Department of Health and Human Services, Administration on Aging. 2003a. *An overview of programs and initiatives sponsored by DHHS to promote healthy aging: A background paper for the blueprint on aging for the 21st century Technical Advisory Group (TAG) meeting.* www.aoa.gov

U.S. Department of Health and Human Services: Administration on Aging. 2011. A profile of older Americans: 2010. Washington, DC: U. S. Department of Health and Human Services.

U.S. Department of Health and Human Services, Administration on Aging. 2011, February 25. Washington, DC: U.S. Department of Health and Human Services. www.aoa.gov/aoaroot/aging_statistics/Profile/2010/6.aspx (July 2011).

U.S. Department of Health and Human Services: Administration on Aging. 2011 January 14 (updated). Older Americans 2010: Key indicators of well-being. Washington, DC: U.S. Department of Health and Human Services. www.aoa.gov/agingstatsdotnet/Main_Site/Data/2010_Documents/Health_Status.aspx (July 2011).

U.S. Department of Health and Human Services, Substance Abuse and Mental Health Services Administration. 2006. *Substance abuse by older adults: Estimates of future impact on the treatment system.* www.oas.samhsa.gov/aging/chap1.htm. (October 2011).

U.S. Department of State. 2007, July. Caring for elderly parents. Washington, DC: U.S. Department of State. www.state.gov/m/dghr/flo/c23141.htm (July 2011).

U.S. Food and Drug Administration. 2010, March 9. Medicines and you: A guide for older adults. Silver Spring, MD: U.S. Food and Drug Administration. www.fda.gov/Drugs/ResourcesForYou/ucm163959.htm (July 2011).

Youth Suicide Prevention. 2001. *Youth.*

Chapter 24: Strategies for Teaching about Aging, Dying, and Death

Science NetLinks. 2002, January. *Aging2: How scientists study aging.* www.sciencelinks.com

Wacona Elementary School. 2003. Ideas for Integrating with KidPix. Wacona Elementary School: Waycross, GA. www.wacona.com/kidpix/kidpix.html (July 2011).

Chapter 25: Environmental Health

Madison County Recycles. *Madison county recycling.* www.madison-countyrecycles.com (27 March 2003).

National Academy of Sciences. 2008. *Global warming and climate.* www.nas.edu.

National Center for Biotechnology Information. 2006. *CO poisoning.* www.ncbi.nlm.nih.gov/entrez/query.fcgi?cmd=Retrieve&db=PubMed&list_uids=12126326&dopt=Abstract.

National Center for Health Statistics. 2000. *Healthy people 2000 review, 1998–99.* Washington, D.C.: National Center for Health Statistics.

National Institutes of Health. 2006. *Noise-induced hearing loss.* http://healthlink.mcw.edu/article/965928293.html.

Natural Resources Defense Council. *Clean air and energy: Transportation.* www.nrdc.org/air/transportation/brief.asp (27 March 2003).

Noise Pollution Clearinghouse. *NPC online library.* www.nonoise.org/library.htm (27 March 2003).

Office of Environmental Policy & Guidance. *Federal Environmental Laws.* www.tis.eh.doe.gov/oepa (27 March 2003).

PeopleandPlanet.net. 2006. *Population and human development: The key connections.* www.peopleandplanet.net/doc.php?id=199&section=2.

U.S. Census Bureau. 2006. *U.S. and world population clocks: POPClocks.* www.census.gov/main/www/popclock.html.

U.S. Environmental Protection Agency. 1998. *Laws affecting EPA's pesticide programs.* www.epa.gov/pesticides/factsheets/legisfac.htm.

———. 2002. *Global warming.* http://yosemite.epa.gov/oar/globalwarming.nsf/content/index.html.

———. 2005. *Mercury poisoning in fish.* http://yosemite.epa.gov/opa/admpress.nsf/d9bf8d9315e942578525701c005e573c/0e9aa92b45c2501a8525707d0066551e!OpenDocument.

———. 2006a. *Asbestos in schools.* www.epa.gov/asbestos/pubs/asbestos_in_schools.html#1.

———. 2006b. *Global warming: Kid's site.* www.epa.gov/globalwarming/kids/difference.html.

———. 2006c. *Hazardous waste.* www.epa.gov/epaoswer/osw/hazwaste.htm#hazwaste.

———. 2006d. *Safe Drinking Water Act.* www.epa.gov/safewater/sdwa/basicinformation.html.

———. 2006e. *Sulfur dioxide.* www.epa.gov/air/aqtrnd95/so2.html.

———. 2006f. *Superfund's 25th anniversary: Capturing the past, charting the future.* www.epa.gov/superfund/25anniversary/.

Chapter 26: Strategies for Teaching Environmental Health

Ohio Department of Natural Resources. 2008. Project learning tree. www.ohiodnr.com.

Index

Page numbers followed by *fig* indicate figures
Page numbers followed by *t* indicate tables

Photo Credits

p. 1, Randy Faris/Corbis; p. 8, Comstock Images/Thinkstock; p. 17, Chris Schmidt/istockphoto; p. 22, Stephen McBrady/PhotoEdit, Inc.; p. 24, zhang bo/istockphoto.com; p. 26, michaeljung/Shutterstock; p. 46, Stockbyte/Getty Images; p. 49, amana images inc./Alamy; p. 74, Jacek Chabraszewski/Fotolia; p. 90, Stockbroker/Digital Vision/Getty Images; p. 101, Anne Vega/Pearson Education; p. 104, Comstock/Jupiter Images; p. 110, Monkey Business Images/Shutterstock; p. 119, Charles Gupton/Corbis; p. 129, Randy Faris/Corbis; p. 144, Frans Rombout/istockphoto.com; p. 147, Peter Glass/Alamy; p. 171, GWImages/Shutterstock; p. 181, szeyuen/Fotolia; p. 182, Paula Connelly/istockphoto.com; p. 192 (top), Dmitriy Shironosov/Shutterstock; p. 192 (bottom), George Doyle/Stockbyte/Getty Images; p. 202, Monkey Business Images/Fotolia; p. 212, Digital Vision/Getty Images; p. 219, Efrem Lukatsky/AP Wide World; p. 238, AP Photo/The Hawk Eye, John Lovretta; p. 257, Elena Rostunova/Shutterstock; p. 258, Image Source/Getty Images; p. 264, michaeljung/Shutterstock; p. 269, Yuri Arcurs/Shutterstock; p. 281, LWA/Dann Tardi/Jupiter Images; p. 288, Thinkstock/Jupiterimages; p. 293, Blend Images/Alamy; p. 314, Image 100/Jupiter Images; p. 321, Manuel Balce Ceneta/AP Wide World Photos; p. 335, CandyBox Images/Shutterstock; p. 336, Bob Daemmrich/PhotoEdit, Inc.; p. 341 (top), Gary Buss/Jupiter Images; p. 341 (bottom), Richard Susanto/Shutterstock; p. 347, Joshua Hultuqist/Stockbyte/Getty images; p. 349, Christina Kennedy/PhotoEdit Inc.; p. 357, Berc/Dreamstime.com; p. 363, Syracuse Newspapers/Michaelle Gabel/The Image Works; p. 367, West Coast Surfer/AGE Fotostock; p. 369, Felicia Martinez/Photoedit, Inc.; p. 375, Patrick Olear/PhotoEdit; p. 381, Myrleen Pearson/PhotoEdit; p. 391, Ryan McVay/Getty Images; p. 398, Noam/Fotolia; p. 403, Lisa S./Shutterstock; p. 406, Thinkstock; p. 408, Les Stone/The Image Works; p. 415, Tom Grill/Corbis; p. 416, auremar/Shutterstock; p. 422, David Anspaugh; p. 432, Bob Daemmrich/PhotoEdit, Inc.; p. 435, Jan kranendonk/Shutterstock.com; p. 446, Morgan Lane Photography/Shutterstock; p. 447, Lisa Law/The Image Works; p. 455, Kristin Piljay